BEVERAGES IN NUTRITION AND HEALTH

NUTRITION ◊ AND ◊ HEALTH
Adrianne Bendich, Series Editor

Beverages in Nutrition and Health

Edited by

Ted Wilson, PhD

Department of Biology,
Winona State University, Winona, MN

and

Norman J. Temple, PhD

Centre for Science, Athabasca University, Athabasca,
Alberta, Canada

Foreword by

David R. Jacobs, Jr., PhD

School of Public Health, University of Minnesota,
Minneapolis, MN

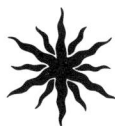

Humana Press
Totowa, New Jersey

Cover design by Patricia F. Cleary.
Production Editor: Jessica Jannicelli.

For additional copies, pricing for bulk purchases, and/or information about other Humana titles, contact Humana at the above address or at any of the following numbers: Tel.: 973-256-1699; Fax: 973-256-8341; E-mail: humana@humanapr.com or visit our website at http://humanapress.com

This publication is printed on acid-free paper. ∞
ANSI Z39.48-1984 (American National Standards Institute) Permanence of Paper for Printed Library Materials.

Printed in the United States of America. 10 9 8 7 6 5 4 3 2 1

E-ISBN: 1-59259-415-8

Library of Congress Cataloging-in-Publication Data

Beverages in nutrition and health / edited by Ted Wilson and
    Norman J. Temple ; foreword by David R. Jacobs, Jr.
      p. ; cm. -- (Nutrition and health)
    Includes bibliographical references and index.
    ISBN 1-58829-173-1 (alk. paper)
    1. Beverages--Health aspects.   I. Wilson, Ted. II. Temple,
Norman J. III. Series: Nutrition and health (Totowa, N.J.)
    [DNLM: 1. Beverages. 2. Dietary Supplements. 3. Consu-
mer Product Safety. 4. Food Labeling--standards. 5. Health
Promotion. 6. Nutritive Value.   WB 433 B571 2004]
QP144.B48B48 2004
613.2--dc21

                                                            2003012468

DEDICATION

In a stream we fish for trout, but in nutrition we fish for the truth. These chapters
are the flies we use to fish for healthier lives. Let our wisdom guide our
understanding of how to use this information appropriately. Special thanks to my
father for indirectly helping me understand this on the Big Horn River in
Montana and my mom.

—Ted

To Alf and Esther, thanks for the genes and the dreams.

—Norman

Series Introduction

The *Nutrition and Health* series of books has an overriding mission to provide health professionals with texts that are considered essential because each includes: (1) a synthesis of the state of the science; (2) timely, in-depth reviews by the leading researchers in their respective fields; (3) extensive, up-to-date, fully annotated reference lists; (4) a detailed index; (5) relevant tables and figures; (6) identification of paradigm shifts and the consequences; (7) virtually no overlap of information between chapters, but targeted, interchapter referrals; (8) suggestions of areas for future research; and (9) balanced, data-driven answers to patient/health professionals' questions that are based on the totality of evidence rather than the findings of any single study.

The series volumes are not the outcome of a symposium. Rather, each editor has been asked to examine a chosen area with a broad perspective, both in subject matter as well as in the choice of chapter authors. The international perspective, especially with regard to public health initiatives, is emphasized where appropriate. The editors, whose trainings are both research and practice oriented, have the opportunity to develop a primary objective for their book, define the scope and focus, and then invite the leading authorities from around the world to be part of their initiative. The authors are encouraged to provide an overview of the field, discuss their own research, and relate the research findings to potential human health consequences. Because each book is developed *de novo*, the chapters are coordinated so that the resulting volume imparts greater knowledge than the sum of the information contained in the individual chapters.

Beverages in Nutrition and Health, edited by Ted Wilson and Norman J. Temple clearly exemplifies the goals of the *Nutrition and Health* series. In fact, this is the most unique topic currently in the *Nutrition and Health* series. Containing 28 comprehensive chapters that examine beverages such as water, both tap and bottled; alcoholic beverages; teas, such as green, black, and herbal; juices, including orange, grapefruit, tomato, and cranberry; milks, both animal and plant-based, with and without probiotics; chocolate drinks; sodas; oral rehydration and nutritional support drinks, this volume is clearly the most comprehensive treatise available concerning the role of beverages in human health. As the editors and chapter authors remind the reader, beverage consumption is essential for life, and the care that is given to assure the safety of the water supply is extensively reviewed. Regulation of beverages on a global perspective is also included, with a most informative chapter on the beverage categories in Japan. This important text provides practical, data-driven resources in well-organized tables and figures that assist the reader in evaluating the nutritive value of the beverages discussed as well as the up-to-date science on the potential for beverages, especially in at-risk populations, to optimize health and prevent disease. The overarching goal of the editors is to provide fully referenced information to health professionals so they may have a balanced perspective on the value, or lack thereof, of many beverages that are routinely consumed.

Wilson and Temple, who have edited many important volumes in the past, have organized the volume into 10 areas of focus that reflect the beverages that are reviewed in this text. Unique areas of focus include regulatory and ethical aspects of beverage labeling and distribution. Certain of these chapters are controversial in their position; however, these are supported by extensive references to the published literature and national epidemiological surveys. Other chapters present the scientific arguments for or against the use of beverages such as probiotic-containing milks, herbal teas, bottled water, and soda. Each chapter includes a discussion of the chemical composition of the actives contained in the beverage, the physiology of the response to the beverage, the effects in populations that could benefit and/or be at risk with consumption, pertinent drug–beverage interactions, especially with grapefruit juice, coffee, alcohol, and other relevant drinks. At the end of each chapter there is a summary entitled Main Points for Primary and Clinical Review, which readers will find exceptionally helpful.

Beverages in Nutrition and Health sets the benchmark for providing the most critical data on the health role of the myriad of beverages available for human consumption. This important information is provided in extensive, well-organized tables and figures that are captured in the extensive index. The editors have taken special care to use the same terms and abbreviations between chapters, and provide clear reference to relevant material between chapters.

Understanding the complexities of the beverage industry, water treatment standards, and the regulations that are in place to assure the safety of the public certainly is not simple and the standards used can often seem daunting. However, the editors and authors have focused on assisting those who are unfamiliar with this field in understanding the critical issues and important new research findings that can impact their fields of interest. Drs. Wilson and Temple have carefully chosen the very best researchers from around the world who can communicate the relevance of specific beverages to nutrition's role in health. The authors have worked hard to make their information accessible to health professionals interested in public health, geriatrics, nursing, pharmacy, psychology, as well as nutrition-related health professionals. The well-referenced tables and figures, as well as the detailed references, add great value to this text. Many of the tables provide health professionals with guides to assessment of the nutritional content of the beverages, and also are helpful in assessing the potential for problems when regulations are not followed carefully. Several chapters include unique tables of information that were not available previously, such as the three-page table on the medical claims that have been made for chocolate. Discussions of the metabolic fate of the active constituents of several juices are included, and the epidemiological as well as clinical study literature is reviewed in each chapter.

In conclusion, *Beverages in Nutrition and Health* provides health professionals in many areas of research and practice with the most up-to-date, well-referenced, and easy-to-understand volume on the importance of beverages for optimal health. This volume will serve the reader as the most authoritative resource in the field to date and is a very welcome addition to the *Nutrition and Health* series.

Adrianne Bendich, PhD, FACN, *Series Editor*

FOREWORD

Most people, certainly including myself, do not read technical books from cover to cover. Thanks to a welcome invitation from the editors to write this foreword, however, I have done exactly that: read *Beverages in Nutrition and Health* from cover to cover. I have found it to be a rewarding, informative, and enriching experience. What makes a body of information of real value is when it reaches a wider audience. This is perhaps the real value of edited books such as this one. The authors have read, digested, and analyzed a vast number of studies and have synthesized the findings into a collection of reviews that are accessible to a broader audience of such people as health professionals, academics, and food scientists, the very people who are in most need of this information. Reading groups of related chapters for specific information will also be useful for readers with narrower interests, for example, those writing articles about topics covered in this book, or as part of a class, or in product development and marketing. The reference lists alone are a treasure trove.

Why a comprehensive book about the nutrition of beverages? There are, after all, plenty of academic nutrition books and plenty of books about the nutrition of foods generally. But there is a difference between eating and drinking, hunger and thirst. The need for water is distinct from the need for energy- and nutrient-bearing foods. Hydration and consumption of nutrients can be thought of as distinct aspects of nutrition. I can be hungry, but not thirsty, or I can be thirsty, but not hungry. Liquid vs solid form of the consumable is nearly, but not exactly, the key here: drinking a milkshake (liquid form) will satisfy hunger, while eating an apple (solid form) will reduce thirst at least somewhat. The same amount of sugar appears to have different effects on satiation in a soft drink vs a sweet solid dessert. Therefore, the question of beverages and health is not entirely subsumed under the question of food and health. This book is unique in that it constitutes a comprehensive review of an underappreciated nutritional subfield, namely the nutrition of beverages.

I list several categories of beverages, with different implications for interpretation. First are beverages that are extracts of whole foods. These extracts might contain less nutritional value than the whole food, but they also might extract just what is nutritionally important. Second are foods that arise only as beverages, including most importantly water itself. Also included here are extracts such as coffee, wherein the whole bean is rarely eaten, and a fermentation product: alcohol. Third are designer beverages, in which I include beverages for rehydration of the elderly or ill and those for rehydration and enhanced performance in sport and other activities demanding high-energy expenditure. In this category falls also soft drinks or liquid sugar. Besides comments on these three categories of beverages, the book offers one chapter on the sociology of drinking beverages and pieces of several chapters that comment on issues surrounding labeling and marketing of various beverages.

The book covers a wide variety of topics. It demonstrates the role that beverages have played historically in the evolution of modern day society. It goes on to highlight positive and negative effects of alcohol generally and of wine consumption more particularly. The health effects of cranberry, orange, and tomato juices are characterized. Cautionary notes are presented concerning the shelf life of orange juice. Interesting interactions are noted of grapefruit juice with some medications, either facilitating uptake or allowing lower dose for the same medical effect. Tea, coffee, cocoa, and herbal drinks are widely consumed and therefore have great potential to affect health. This potential is extensively reviewed with an emphasis on their phytochemical content and potential health benefits.

Especially enlightening is the examination of milk from cow, human, and soy sources, with a further consideration of probiotic organisms that are often added to cow's milk. The point is made by Friel that human milk has many characteristics associated with a "tissue," in that it is responsive to the biological needs of the infant. An interesting aspect of cow's milk is therefore that it must contain myriad substances aimed at the health of the calf. Vegetable milk substitute formulations, particularly soy milk, are interesting in that they avoid some of the potentially deleterious aspects of animal products (e.g., saturated fat and cholesterol), but with a possible tradeoff of more limited biological versatility.

Consideration of beverage impact on weight control, nutritional support, optimal physical performance, and rehydration is important in light of the explosion of products marketed for these purposes. A comprehensive review of potential effects of tap and mineral waters is included, wherein bottled water has also been the subject of much recent marketing effort. The discussion of the important role of marketing is carried forward in chapters by Jacobson and by Balay-Karperien, Temple, and Nestle. Marketing has played a major role in the explosion of soft drink consumption. Finally, the interaction of marketing, health claims, and health is decisively reviewed in chapters on the legalities of presentation of beverage content and labeling claims in the United States and Japan. In the light of nutritional and financial forces on beverage consumption, a final summary chapter asks whether it is possible to have a society in which beverages promote both a healthy economy and a healthy population.

A strength of this book is that most sections contain several chapters that provide complementary views on each topic. In several cases, there are chapters with different perspectives from a group or author in academia and another in industry. Although some chapters might be interpreted to paint an overly rosy picture, and some an overly glum picture, this strategy provides balance, providing competing views and interpretations, and therefore pushes scientific discourse forward. Despite extreme efforts by all authors for scientific objectivity, in the end scientific inference is an art; there are always unknown facts. This art proceeds by discourse. In my view, the essence of scientific discourse is putting facts, interpretations and opinions on the table; then discussing them. *Beverages in Nutrition and Health* is a step forward in scientific discourse.

David R. Jacobs, Jr., PhD
School of Public Health, University of Minnesota,
Minneapolis, MN

PREFACE

In this high-tech era of molecular biology and designer drug therapies, it remains a basic fact that good nutrition is the single most cost-effective way to improve the health and well-being of the greatest number of individuals on our planet *(1,2)*. *Beverages in Nutrition and Health* is the first book dedicated to helping us discover how different beverages impact our basic nutrition and the risk of disease. This book also helps explain the potential value of these beverages for the promotion of optimal human health and well-being. In addition, it discusses developments in the formulation of beverages and the likely implications on human health.

During the last century, we have vastly improved the palatability and variety of beverage choices available to a population that is expanding in size, demands, and affluence. We have also seen many changes in the state of our health, sometimes for the better and sometimes for the worse. It has only been in the last 100 years that the Western diseases have become prominent in the cultures that have embraced the new diet of affluence *(3)*, and beverages are very much a part of that diet of affluence.

Beverages have been an integral part of life since animals left the sea and moved onto dry land. The first period of human life occurs bathed in a sea of fluids; indeed as a fetus we begin to drink even before birth has occurred. Beverage consumption starts for most of us immediately after we are born with breast milk. For the rest of our lives, we will continue to require approx 1.2 mL of water per dietary calorie spent per day.

Until modern times, our choices of beverages were fairly limited and included water, alcoholic drinks, milk, and a few fermented milk products. The history of the human use of these drinks is discussed in Chapter 1 by Grivetti and Wilson. However, in recent years, there has been an explosion in the number of beverage choices available for acquiring our daily fluid requirements. This has been made possible by using such industrial processes as carbonation, processing to add ingredients, such as high-fructose corn syrup, vitamins, and minerals, and the development of new processing and preservation methods. But what has the impact of these changes been on our ability to obtain proper nutrition and maintain health? These impacts are the focus of *Beverages in Nutrition and Health*.

Alcohol has been a part of our diet for thousands of years. In recent years, we have come to a new understanding of how alcohol affects our health, and how the amounts and types of alcoholic beverages that increase or decrease mortality rates. This is discussed in Chapter 2 by Rimm and Temple. Research has revealed mechanisms by which substances in wine may have specific health benefits, a topic reviewed in Chapter 3 by Walzem and German.

Recent advances in ideas and methods for investigation available to researchers in the food sciences and medicine have provided new insights into how fruit and vegetable juices affect disease outcomes in both beneficial and potentially deleterious ways. Wilson, in Chapter 4, discusses how cranberry juice has been clinically determined to prevent urinary tract infections and possibly other diseases. McGill, Wilson, and Papanikolaou, in Chapter 5, review how citrus juice consumption affords protection against various diseases, whereas Johnston, in Chapter 6, discusses how processing methods and storage may actually limit the availability of vitamin C and flavonoids from these same juices. The observation that some citrus juices may actually create harmful interactions with prescription drugs is another possibly important ancillary issue and is discussed in Chapter 7 by Kane. In addition, the intriguing associative link between tomato juice consumption and reduced risks of prostate and other cancers is explored by Hadley, Schwartz, and Clinton in Chapter 8.

How do coffee and tea and the caffeine and other substances they contain affect our health? The health effects of green and black teas are discussed in Chapter 10 by Afaq, Adhami, Ahmad, and Mukhtar. In Chapter 9, Tavani and La Vecchia discuss the general lack of associations between coffee intake and cancer. They also discuss the complex relation between coffee and heart disease. Chocolate was originally consumed in the form of a drink and its consumption in a liquid form remains popular. In Chapter 11, Schmitz, Kelm, and Hammerstone investigate this topic from a historical and health-related point of view. In Chapter 12, Weinberg and Bealer discuss the health effects of the caffeine that is a ubiquitous component of these and numerous other beverages. Finally, in Chapter 13, Craig discusses the health risks and some of the benefits that may be obtained from the increasing number of herbal teas that are available.

A variety of milks and milk products have been in the diet of many human cultures for millenia. Chapter 14 by McBean, Miller, and Heaney provides an optimistic view of how cow's milk can provide some degree of protection against osteoporosis, obesity, and heart disease, and discuss some of the claims and counterclaims that have emerged in regard to milk consumption. The potential of probiotic organisms in dairy and fermented dairy products to impact the health qualities of beverages is discussed by Heller in Chapter 17. Finally, because many persons avoid dairy products for health or religious reasons, substitutes are needed and Woodside and Morton, in Chapter 15, discuss the health qualities of the most commonly consumed substitute, soy milk.

Different beverages become more important as we pass from neonate to adult to elderly adult. Friel reviews the current state of affairs in the heated and continuing breast milk vs neonate/infant formula debate, fueled on one side by our traditional habits and on the other by commercial forces. As we enter middle age, weight management becomes a problem for many of us and Chapter 18 by Stubbs and Whybrow discusses how particular beverages can contribute to weight problems, whereas others may become part of the solution. Finally, Johnson and Glassman, in Chapter 19, look at what happens when an elderly person's diet is unable to meet his or her nutrient needs. They describe the often overrated value of nutritional support beverages for helping us achieve our required intake of vitamins and minerals.

Beverages have also evolved to meet specific physiological functions and needs for simple hydration. The topic of sports beverage content and effectiveness is reviewed in Chapter 20 by Maughan. Ramakrishna considers the factors that have helped oral electrolyte-carbohydrate rehydration therapies save more lives on our planet every year than any other medical treatment. In Chapter 21, our transition to living in an urbanized, and sometimes affluent, culture has created new opportunities for safe water and at the same time created potential exposure to new water-borne pathogens, a topic discussed in Chapter 23 by Chauret. Our affluence and concern about water safety has led many to consume bottled water. In Chapter 20, Jamal and Eisenberg discuss some surprising facts regarding the quality and content of these products.

The consumption of soft drinks has recently been linked to a wide range of health problems, especially for children and young adults. This problem is discussed in Chapter 24 by Jacobson from the watchdog organization the Center for Science in the Public Interest. In that chapter, as well as in Chapter 25 by Balay-Karperien, Temple, and Nestle, the authors discuss marketing practices used to promote the consumption of these products.

Regulation of beverage content and marketing practice has been a part of American life for nearly a century since the establishment of the US Food and Drug Administration and the original "Snake Oil Laws" of the 1920s. These laws sought to limit the use of bogus health claims that manufacturers used to market their products. The fast growing popularity of "functional foods" (including beverages) has created a resurgence of concern and interest in the area of regulation. Chapter 27 by Krasny provides a current update of the status of these laws and regulations with regards to how beverages can be marketed in the United States. Other nations have similar laws, and in Chapter 26, Ohki, Nakamura, and Takano provide a review of the status of the recreational and tonic beverage industry in Japan and how the laws of Japan regulate beverage-health claims on products sold there.

In recent decades, researchers have made considerable progress in our understanding of possible associations between beverages and the Western diseases. This book provides an overview of the field. In that respect it continues from our previous books *(2,3)*. Every one of us will undoubtedly (unless we want to die) continue to consume beverages and experience potentially beneficial or possibly detrimental effects related to our choices. Readers of this book will have a better understanding of how to optimize their beverage consumption for optimizing health. *Beverages in Nutrition and Health* is also intended to help the reader understand how current and probable future innovations in the beverage industry have the potential to affect our health in both positive and negative ways. At the risk of stating the obvious, beverage nutrition research is very much an ongoing activity. As a result, there are many contrasting views on aspects of the field, and the significance of some of these contrasts is discussed in the final chapter (28) by Jacobs, Temple, and Wilson. An important means of resolving these contentious areas is by debate. To some extent this debate can be found on the pages of this book. Accordingly, the editors make no apology if the reader finds that statements in one chapter may contradict those in another.

Ted Wilson, PhD
Norman J. Temple, PhD

REFERENCES

1. Wilson T. What types of nutrition research give the best results? Nutrition 2002;18:352.
2. Wilson T, Temple NJ, eds. Nutritional health: Strategies for Disease Prevention. Humana Press, Totowa, NJ, 2002.
3. Temple NJ, Burkitt DP, eds. Western Diseases: Their Dietary Prevention and Reversibility. Humana Press, Totowa, NJ, 1994.

CONTENTS

CONTRIBUTORS

VAQAR M. ADHAMI, PhD • *Department of Dermatology, University of Wisconsin, Madison, WI*

FARRUKH AFAQ, PhD • *Department of Dermatology, University of Wisconsin, Madison, WI*

NIHAL AHMAD, PhD • *Department of Dermatology ,University of Wisconsin, Madison, WI*

AUDREY BALAY-KARPERIEN, BS • *Edwards, CA*

BONNIE K. BEALER, BA • *Philadelphia, PA*

CHRISTIAN CHAURET, PhD • *Department of Natural, Mathematical, and Information Sciences, Indiana University Kokomo, Kokomo, IN*

STEVEN K. CLINTON, MD, PhD • *Division of Hematology and Oncology, The James Cancer Hospital and Solove Research Institute, The Ohio State University, Columbus, OH*

WINSTON J. CRAIG, PhD, RD • *Nutrition Department, Andrews University, Berrien Springs, MI*

MARK J. EISENBERG, MD, MPH • *Division of Clinical Epidemiology, Jewish General Hospital, McGill University, Montreal, Canada*

JAMES K. FRIEL, PhD • *Department of Human Nutritional Sciences, University of Manitoba, Winnipeg, Manitoba, Canada*

J. BRUCE GERMAN, PhD • *Department of Food Science and Technology, University California, Davis, CA; and Nestle Research Centre, Lausanne, Switzerland*

PETER GLASSMAN, MBBS, MSc • *Department of Medicine, University of California Los Angeles, Los Angeles, CA*

LOUIS E. GRIVETTI, PhD • *Department of Nutrition, University of California, Davis, CA*

CRAIG W. HADLEY, PhD(C) • *Department of Food Science and Technology, The Ohio State University, Columbus, OH*

JOHN F. HAMMERSTONE, BS • *Analytical and Applied Chemistry, Mars Incorporated, Hackettstown, NJ*

ROBERT P. HEANEY, MD • *Osteoporosis Research Center, Creighton University Medical Center, Omaha, NE*

KNUT J. HELLER, PhD • *Institute for Microbiology, Federal Dairy Research Centre, Kiel, Germany*

MICHAEL F. JACOBSON, PhD • *Executive Director, Center for Science in the Public Interest, Washington, DC*

DAVID R. JACOBS, JR., PhD • *Division of Epidemiology, School of Public Health, University of Minnesota, Minneapolis, MN*

SHELINA M. JAMAL, BSc • *McGill University, Montreal, Canada*

CARRIE JOHNSEN, MPH, RD • *Nutrition and Food Service, Veterans Administration Greater Los Angeles Healthcare System, Los Angeles, CA*

CAROL S. JOHNSTON, PhD • *Department of Nutrition, Arizona State University, Mesa, AZ*

GARVAN C. KANE, MB, BCh, BAO • *Departments of Medicine and Molecular Pharmacology and Experimental Therapeutics, Mayo Clinic, Rochester, MN*

MARK A. KELM, PhD • *Analytical and Applied Chemistry, Mars Incorporated, Hackettstown, NJ*

LESLIE T. KRASNY, MA, JD • *Keller and Heckman LLP, San Francisco, CA*

CARLO LA VECCHIA, MD • *Istituto di Ricerche Farmacologiche Mario Negri, Milan, Italy*

RON J. MAUGHAN, PhD • *School of Sport and Exercise Sciences, Loughborough University, Loughborough, UK*

LOIS D. MCBEAN, MS, RD • *Nutrition Consultant, Ann Arbor, MI*

CARLA R. MCGILL, PhD, RD • *Principal Nutrition Scientist, Tropicana Products, Bradenton, FL*

GREGORY D. MILLER, PhD • *Senior Vice President, National Dairy Council, Rosemont, IL*

MICHAEL S. MORTON, PhD • *Department of Medical Biochemistry, University of Wales College of Medicine, Cardiff, Wales*

HASAN MUKHTAR, PhD • *Department of Dermatology, University of Wisconsin, Madison, WI*

YASUNORI NAKAMURA, PhD • *Research and Development Center, Calpis Co. Ltd., Sagamihara, Japan*

MARION NESTLE, PhD, MPH • *Department of Nutrition and Food Studies, New York University, New York, NY*

KOHJI OHKI, PhD • *Research and Development Center, Calpis Co. Ltd., Sagamihara, Japan*

YANNI PAPANIKOLAOU, MHSc, PhD • *Director, Nutritional Strategies, Toronto, Canada*

B. S. RAMAKRISHNA, MD, DM, PhD • *Department of Gastrointestinal Sciences, Christian Medical College, Vellore, India*

ERIC RIMM, PhD • *Department of Nutrition, Harvard School of Public Health, Boston, MA*

HAROLD H. SCHMITZ, PhD • *Analytical and Applied Chemistry, Mars Incorporated, Hackettstown, NJ*

STEVEN J. SCHWARTZ, PhD • *Department of Food Science and Technology, The Ohio State University, Columbus, OH*

JAMES STUBBS, PhD • *Energy Balance and Obesity Division, The Rowett Research Institute, Aberdeen, Scotland*

TOSHIAKI TAKANO, BA • *Research and Development Center, Calpis Co. Ltd., Sagamihara, Japan*

ALESSANDRA TAVANI, Biol Sci D • *Istituto di Ricerche Farmacologiche "Mario Negri," Milan, Italy*

NORMAN J. TEMPLE, PhD • *Centre for Science, Athabasca University, Athabasca, Canada*

ROSEMARY L. WALZEM, RD, PhD • *Center for Nutrition, Health and Food Genomics, Texas A&M University, College Station, TX*

BENNETT ALAN WEINBERG, JD • *Philadelphia, PA*

STEPHEN WHYBROW, PhD • *Energy Balance and Obesity Division, The Rowett Research Institute, Aberdeen, Scotland*

ALISSA M. R. WILSON, PhD, RD • *Nutrition Scientist, Tropicana Products, Bradenton, FL*

TED WILSON, PhD • *Department of Biology, Winona State University, Winona, MN*

JAYNE V. WOODSIDE, PhD • *Department of Medicine, Queens University Belfast, Belfast, Northern Ireland*

I INTRODUCTION TO BEVERAGES

1 A Brief History of Human Beverage Consumption

Prehistory to the Present

Louis E. Grivetti and Ted Wilson

The humans arise after periods of fitful sleep. They climb down from tree-top lairs and amble toward nearby water holes. Alert to the potential presence of predators, they kneel, brush algal scum from the pond surfaces, fill their cupped hands, and take their first drinks of the day ...

Two million years later ...

The humans arise after periods of fitful sleep. They dress and walk across the dirt floors of their huts. They grasp crude pottery cups, walk outside, and meet others at the village cisterns. They fill their cups with polluted water, and take their first drinks of the day ...

Six thousand years later ...

The humans arise after periods of restful sleep. They dress and walk across their spotless upscale kitchens. They prepare their favorite morning beverages. They sit on breakfast-nook stools with mugs filled with steaming goodness, and take their first drinks of the day ...

1. INTRODUCTION

How did humans learn to drink? Are drinking preferences instinctive? How did humans learn which beverages were safe to drink? Did the earliest humans watch and imitate the drinking behavior of animals? How did early humans know whether a pond of standing water was suitable to drink? At the dawn of human history, life spans were short and illness from drinking polluted water was not associated with bacteria or toxins. Then, as now, aesthetics and a well-developed sense of smell and taste determine our beverage selection.

How does one drink? The earliest humans had no cups or ways to store water, so, by necessity, they frequented water holes or other sources of standing or running water. It

From: *Beverages in Nutrition and Health*
Edited by: T. Wilson and N. J. Temple © Humana Press Inc., Totowa, NJ

is presumed that the earliest humans channeled run-off rain, drank melted snow, and consumed rainfall collected from tree crotches or natural depressions. Simple observations on the timing and quality of rainfall and the probability of water at any specific geographical location would have served ancient humans well. Eventually through observation and trial and error, early humans learned to predict sources of water even in subsurface deposits beneath the sands of dry stream beds and also learned which fruits and succulents/cacti in arid lands offered refreshing lifesaving fluids to drink.

Since remote antiquity, there has existed a world of different beverages: fresh water, fresh plant juices, fresh animal fluids (whether blood, milk, sometimes urine), fermented plant and animal products, and various mixtures. Some beverages are primarily water, but others were prepared from myriad fresh or dried barks, flowers, pods, resins/saps, and roots and resins. Some are drunk to satisfy thirst or provide simple pleasures, and some are drunk for cultural and religious significance, whereas still others for their medicinal value. For reviews on specific fruit and vegetable juice effects on health and nutrition, *see* the chapters by Wilson (Chapter 4), McGill et al. (Chapter 5), Johnston (Chapter 6), and Hadley et al. (Chapter 8).

The purpose of this introductory chapter is not to review all of the effects that beverages have had on human health and nutrition, but to discuss how widespread these effects have been and to make the reader consider how beverages influence various aspects of our lives.

2. WATER

Water is one of the oldest known beverages and one of the first to be medicinally characterized with respect to effect on health. For reviews on the topic of water, *see* the chapters by Jamal and Eisenberg (Chapter 22) and Chauret (Chapter 23). The Chakara-Samhita document *(1)* is the oldest known Asian medical text (c. 1500 BCE). The text presents a classification of common beverages for physicians and addresses their presumed medical properties and attributes:

> *"Water (jala), by nature has six qualities: cold, pure, wholesome, palatability, clean, light. When water falls to earth it depends for its properties on the containing soil. Water in white soil is astringent. Water in pale soil is bitter. Water in brown soil is alkaline. Water in hilly areas is pungent. Water in black soil is sweet. Water derived from rain, hailstone, and snow has unmanifested rasa (taste); Fresh rainwater of the rainy season is heavy, blocks body channels, and is sweet; ... Rivers with water polluted with soil, feces, insects, snakes, and rats, and carrying rain water aggravate all dosas."* (1).

For a modern review of rehydration therapy for these dosas, *see* Chapter 21 by Ramakrishna.

The *Nei-Ching* dates to Han dynasty times (207 BCE–220 CE) in ancient China and demonstrates the wide range in beverage choices that had rapidly become available and how they were closely associated with medicine and the healing process *(2)*. The ancient Chinese medical system defined five organs (heart, liver, lung, kidney, and spleen) and integrated factors of hot-cold, wet-dry, male-female, set within a complex integration of Yang, Neutrality, and Yin. Alcoholic beverages (except beer) and coffee are classified as Yang or hot/heating, whereas fruit juices, milk, tea, and unboiled water are classified as Yin or cold/cooling *(3)*. Furthermore, Chinese Buddhist monks followed strict dietary codes that limited their eating time to morning hours, and the foods/beverages forbidden to them included: fermented items, milk, cream, fish, and meat *(4)*.

3. THE ORIGINS OF MILKING

For millions of years, breast milk has been the first beverage (*see* Chapter 16 by Friel). Replacement with animal milk carried tremendous implications and potential nutritional advantages. The first irrefutable evidence for milking domesticated livestock and, by implication, human use of milk and the manufacture of dairy products, dates to approx 4000 BCE and is based on Stone Age rock art produced in the central Sahara region of Africa *(5)*. By 1500 BCE, milk use was widely distributed, and in India, many of milk's qualities had already been described in the Charaka-Samhita *(1)*.

> *"Cow milk has ten properties: sweet, cold, soft, fatty, viscous, smooth, slimy, heavy, dull, and clear. Buffalo milk is heavier and colder than that from cow; useful to cure sleeplessness and excessive digestive power. Camel milk is rough, hot, slightly saline, light, and prescribed for hardness in the bowels, works against worms ... Milk from one-hooved animals [donkey; horse] is hot, slightly sour, saline, rough, light, promotes strength, stability, alleviates* vata *in extremities. Goat milk is astringent ..."*

Anthropologists, geographers, and physicians have written on the physiologic and dietary implications of humans using animal milks and use or nonuse of favored particular societies. With our ability to feed grass to livestock and the use the milk in its raw form or as fermented cheese, humans expanded into new areas of habitation and increased population density. The majority of other human populations—following the standard mammalian pattern—lose the ability to maintain lactase production and, therefore, cannot digest fresh animal milks easily, a pattern evidenced by most Asians, West Africans, Southern European Mediterraneans, and most Central and South Americans *(6–8)*. However, some human populations now maintain lactase production throughout their lives, a physiologic characteristic that links peoples and cultures as diverse as east African cattle pastoralists (e.g., the Masai, Suk, and Turkana) with northern European Scandinavians (e.g., Danes, Norwegians, and Swedes).

Different cultures have widely diverging views regarding the suitability of animal milks as human foods or beverages. For some, it is a question of identification: because animal milks are for the young of specific animals, it is wrong to mix these foods because the consumer may take on characteristics of the animal. For others, it is an issue of ethics: taking milk from cows, ewes, or mares deprives the young of those species and, therefore does harm to the young thus breaking the tenet of ahimsa (i.e., nonviolence toward animals). For still others, milk is rejected for two linked, but opposing, viewpoints: disgust and purity. Regarding the element of disgust, milk is rejected because it is perceived akin to other disgusting body excretions, such as feces, mucus, and urine. Regarding purity, milk is rejected because it is pure, something to be offered to deities, and a product not for humans. Some also reject processed milk because they believe that pasteurization "devitalizes" the milk. However, this practice is not without danger, given the difficulties of maintaining cleanliness within the environmental setting of traditional, even modern, dairies *(9)*. Heaney et al., in Chapter 14, review some of the modern health implications of cows milk consumption. More recently, vegetable origin milk substitutes have become popular. Chapter 15 by Woodside and Morton reviews soy milk.

4. FERMENTED BEVERAGES

4.1. General

Fermentation can be used to produce both plant-based and animal-based beverages. As with most issues, there are two sides, especially with the fermentation product alcohol. The moral and ethical considerations of overindulgence with alcohol have been touted since antiquity, whereby ancient Egyptian sages admonished young men not to overindulge and to be respectful of their elders who became intoxicated. The health-related properties of alcoholic beverages, however, extend well beyond current 21st-century reports related to the so-called French Paradox. The chapters by Rimm and Temple (Chapter 2) and Walzem and German (Chapter 3) review modern interpretations of alcohol and wine effects.

4.2. Wine and the Start of Trade and Commerce

The earliest evidence for the preparation/manufacture of fermented beverages predates writing (i.e., c. 3200 BCE). During recent decades, excavations in northwestern Iran at Godin Tepe provided the first unequivocal evidence for the presence of wine. Analysis of residues at the bottom of large jars retrieved there reveal the presence of tartaric acid, a characteristic chemical signature confirming that the vases once contained juice from *Vitis vinifera (10,11)*. Based on the ancient Iranian data, trade in fermented beverages developed during the late Stone Age or early Copper Age (Chalcolithic), perhaps 4000 BCE. Increased demand and production created a prosperous wine trade, promulgating the establishment of many Roman trade routes. Wrecks from the Roman era on the southern coast of France provided partially intact amphorae that still contained traces of red pigment presumed to have been wine *(11)*. Similiar deposits in amphorae were found in Upper Egyptian tombs *(12)*.

Fermentation of barley and wheat for beer and distillation remains the primary source of fermented beverages in much of the modern world. However, fermented beverages are also prepared from other materials. The ancient people of Meso-America, among them the Maya, Mexica (Aztecs), Mixtecs, Toltecs, and Zapotecs, as well as the Inca of the Peruvian highlands, prepared fermented beverages from corn/maize. African cultures from the Sahel south through the equatorial regions into Southern Africa prepared their fermented beverages from local grains, among them millet (*Pennisetum glaucum*) and sorghum (*Sorghum bicolor, S. vulgare*), whereas the Amhara people of highland Ethiopia fermented honey to make their traditional beverage called *tej*.

4.3. Social Implications of Fermented Beverages

Throughout the ages, social attitudes toward fermented beverages—especially wine—have taken two distinctly divergent forms. The first view holds that moderate use of alcoholic beverages enlivens the human spirit, arouses creativity, and enhances social and personal behaviors. Alternatively, fermented beverages have also been seen as something evil, where overindulgence and repeated intoxication lead to illness, social disgrace, and early death. Expectedly, wine has been called the food with two faces *(13,14)*. Attempts to address these divergent views in the United States led to the Temperance Movement, the Volstead Act of 1919, and a temporary ban on alcohol sales.

Athenaeus, the third-century CE Greek social commentator born in the Egyptian delta city of Naucratis, provided numerous positive examples whereby moderate use of fermented beverages improved the human condition. Athenaeus wrote that wine possessed the power to forge friendships and that drinking wine warmed and fused the human soul *(15)*. He also noted that wine drinking improved creativity, whereby poets received their muse, and if writers wished to produce anything of quality, they—by definition—should drink wine and should, likewise, avoid drinking water *(15)*.

The dark side of wine use, drinking to intoxication and resulting alcoholism, can also be traced to remote antiquity. Egyptian tomb art depicts elegantly dressed, bejeweled beautiful women turning their heads to vomit because of excessive drinking, whereas tombs also depict other guests who have passed out because of intoxication and show the drunkards being carried out of the banquet halls, borne on the shoulders of their comrades *(16)*. The ancient Egyptian scribe Ani condemned intoxication: "Boast not that you can drink a jug of beer. You speak, and an unintelligible utterance issues from your mouth … you are found lying on the ground and you are like a child" *(17)*.

5. HISTORIC NONALCOHOLIC BEVERAGES

5.1. General

Several beverages, specifically cocoa, coffee, cola, and tea, have been lauded through the centuries for their flavor, effects, and medicinal, recreational, and social roles. These beverages have also affected the current status of trade and culture in the world today. For reviews on coffee, cocoa, and tea, *see* the chapters by Tavani and La Vecchia (Chapter 9), Muhktar et al. (Chapter 10), and Schmitz et al. (Chapter 11), respectively.

5.2. Cocoa

All chocolate was prepared in liquid form as beverages until the mid-1830s when it became technically possible to remove cocoa fat and collect the solids. The original introduction of chocolate to Europe during the 16th century, therefore, was only in beverage form. Chocolate appeared for the first time in Europe in 1544 when introduced to the Spanish court by Mayan nobles who greeted Prince Philip *(18)*. The Mayan word *cacao* entered scientific nomenclature in 1753 when Linnaeus published his taxonomic system and coined the genus and species, *Theobroma cacao*, terms translated as "food of the gods" *(19)*.

The Florentine Codex provides recipes on how to prepare cocoa and reports: "When ordinary quantities are drunk, [cacao] gladdens, refreshes, consoles, and invigorates" *(20)*. During the past 450 yr, chocolate beverages have been used to treat four consistent medical-related conditions: (1) to restore flesh to emaciated patients, especially those suffering from tuberculosis; (2) to stimulate the nervous systems of patients identified as feeble, exhausted, or apathetic; (3) to calm patients identified as overstimulated; and (4) to improve digestion and elimination *(19)*.

5.3. Coffee

From earliest times, coffee has been a medicinal drug and social beverage. The origins of coffee are lost to legend, as some tales identify an Ethiopian goat shepherd as the first person to notice the effects that natural coffee beans had on his goats, whereas other stories advance the claim of Arab traders or Christian monks as the first people to make coffee. Still other legends relate that the angel Gabrielle presented coffee to the prophet, Mohammed, to replace drinking wine. Whatever the origin, Muslim traders ultimately were responsible for the geographic spread of coffee throughout the Islamic world, whereas others beyond the realm of Islam spread the beverage globally *(21)*.

Historically, coffee has been used as a medicine to cure eye disorders, gout, and even scurvy *(21)*. By the early 1900s, scientific investigations on coffee had identified caffeine as being responsible for its stimulant effects. During the 1970s, the use of coffee/caffeine as an ergogenic aid became popular after a large body of literature indicated that caffeine improved endurance performance *(22)*. The effect of caffeine on sports performance is so pronounced that the International Olympic Committee has set maximum caffeine blood levels for its athletes *(23,24)*. For a review of how caffeine is used in sports beverages, *see* the chapters by Maughan (Chapter 20) and Weinberg and Bealer (Chapter 12); for a review of the effects of coffee on health, *see* Chapter 9 by Tavani and Le Vecchia.

5.4. Cola

Cola nitida and *C. acuminata* trees of Africa produce cola nuts that are both chewed and prepared as beverages for their stimulant properties. Muslim physicians of the 12th century reported that cola powder prepared as a beverage-treated colic and stomachache. Subsequent writers stated that cola reduced thirst pangs and, when mixed with milk cured headache, relieved fatigue and increased the appetite *(25)*. In recent decades, medical reports have extolled the use of cola beverages to treat indigestion, infection, migraine and nervous headache, and ulcers. In Western Africa, decoctions of cola bark are drunk to reduce labor pains during childbirth *(25)*.

The use of cola as a flavoring for beverages dates to the 1870s when mixtures of cola, sugar, and vanilla were served as tonics for people who were invalid. In 1886, John S. Pemberton invented the beverage Coca-Cola, which initially was prepared using a combination of coca (i.e., cocaine, *Erythroxylum coca*) and cola, and was initially dispensed as a drugstore remedy to cure headache and hangover *(25)*. Coca-Cola has since become one of the most widely distributed soft-drink products in the world, and the Coca-Cola company has become one of the world's largest corporate entities. One may even ponder how much our culture has to thank the Coca-Cola company for its portrayal of Santa Claus in a red robe with a bottle of Coca-Cola. For a review of how these soft drinks affect our health, *see* Chapter 24 by Jacobson and Chapter 25 by Nestle et al.

5.5. Tea

The eighth-century CE Chinese author Yu Lu produced one of the important texts on the properties of tea and how to serve this beverage *(26)*. His *Cha Ching* [classic of tea] considers a range of issues on how to make the best tea:

> *"On the question of what water to use I would suggest that tea made from mountain streams is best, river water is all right, but well-water tea is quite inferior ... Water from the slow-flowing streams, the stone-lined pools or milk-pure springs is the best of mountain water"* (26).

Tea has long been touted for its healthful properties and, according to some scholars, may be the most commonly drunk beverage in the world after water *(27)*. Tea is clearly healthful, because the water used to prepare it is boiled. The medicinal roles of tea in the 21st century include use to alleviate the common cold and various infections, and tea may have a role in preventing or fighting cancers of the esophagus, lung, and stomach *(28–30).* Up-to-date reviews of the effects of various types of tea can be found in Chapter 10 by Muhktar et al. and Chapter 13 by Craig.

6. EFFECT OF BEVERAGES ON THE DEVELOPMENT OF CULTURE

6.1. General

Why are certain beverages associated with certain cultural events, festivals, or seasons? How are beverages used in these events? How do these traditions continue to affect us today?

6.2. Art, Dance, Literature, Song, and Theater

Depiction of beverages in art are legion, from the tomb art of Ancient Egypt to depictions of drinking in Aztec and Mayan Codices, painted before the conquest of Mexico. Most art galleries throughout the world present lithographs, mosaics, paintings, and prints that depict people dining, eating, and drinking. From Da Vinci's masterpiece *The Last Supper* to Edgar Degas's *L'Absinthe* to Salvador Dali's *The Wines of Gaea*, beverages are depicted as an integral part of human life and culture.

The identification of beverages in poetry and song are too extensive to document completely. From the *Rhyme of the Ancient Mariner* ("Water, water everywhere but not a drop to drink"), to sage expressions ("Never drink good water when whisky abounds") to the clever turn of phrase ("Candy is dandy, but liquor is quicker"), beverages have been ever-present. Songs that have beverages as their central content are also numerous; several that come to mind are: "Beer Barrel Polka," "Cool Water, Drink to Me Only With Thine Eyes," "Mountain Dew," "99 Bottles of Beer on the Wall," "Scotch and Soda," and "Tea for Two."

Beverages have been an integral and often fatal part of the creative spirit in the arts and literature. Jack London, Ernest Hemingway, and F. Scott Fitzgerald are all examples of great authors who consumed large amounts of alcohol, had alcohol as a theme in many of their greatest works, and had problems with alcoholism. In the late 1800s, the art world was also modified by another addictive and mind-altering beverage produced from Algerian wormwood root: the greenish drink absinthe. The problems associated with this beverage influenced Edgar Degas to use it as the subject of his *L'Absinthe* (1876), a controversial social commentary on the deleterious effect of this beverage on the culture of the time. Ultimately, social pressures led to the abolition of absinthe in most Western countries by 1915 *(31).*

6.3. Beverages and the Rites of Passage and Other Rituals

Beverages form part of the life cycle of humans and are integrated into birth, rites of passage, coming of age, marriage, and death. The birth of children worldwide is celebrated by offering beverages to guests who come to visit and inspect the newborn and to offer pleasantries and good wishes to the new parents: fresh water in some cultures, freshly brewed coffee or tea in others, sometimes fermented beverages, whether beer or wines (e.g., champagne), in other societies.

Coming of age, that mysterious and dangerous time of life, is also marked by beverages in different societies. At 21, the question of maturity arises in many American youth, some of whom, with the incautious abandon of youth, coupled with the lack of awareness of physiology, celebrate their 21st birthday by downing 21 shots of liquor, the infamous 21/21, that has led to many alcohol-related deaths.

Other beverage-related initiations worthy of note include the smashing of a bottle of champagne during the launching of ships; the three-martini "power lunch" that once served as the central point for business discussions and sealing deals; blessings of Holy Water sprayed over assembled worshipers; the preparation of eggnog and wassail bowls by Christians; the use of green food coloring to "spruce-up" beer on St. Patrick's day; and even the rituals associated with bathing in asses' milk.

6.4. Beverages and Hospitality

Social activities require hospitality, and beverages play important roles in cementing bonds of hospitality between individuals and nations. This can be summed up in the words: "Let's drink to it." Individuals invited into homes are served a multitude of beverages, depending on the country, geographic region, and period in history. In Egypt, the host and hostess serve guests a range of beverages, sometimes specially brewed coffee (accompanied with a glass of water), and other times, juices from fresh fruits or sugar cane. In Mongolia, the tradition is an offering of hot tea to visitors (Wilson, unpublished observations). Beverages are also important on a larger diplomatic scale, where toasts of rice wine were the social highlights of President Nixon's initial visit to the Peoples Republic of China and, of course, vodka toasts are central to diplomatic missions to Russia. Although innocent to some, the guise of hospitality, alcohol, and sensitivity to alcoholism was often used to procure favorable treaties, often resulting in a complete loss of land rights for indigenous peoples. The disputes over treaties signed in the guise of hospitality remain in the courts of Australia, Canada, and the United States to this day.

7. BEVERAGE IMPACT ON RELIGIONS

7.1. General

In Christianity, red wine used in religious celebrations is symbolic of the blood of Jesus. In Judaism, almond milk (*mizo*) drunk to break the fast of Yom Kippur is symbolic of purity, whereas wine remains central to Jewish religious ritual. Muslims reject wine (and by extension, other alcoholic beverages), but were responsible for the spread of coffee during the seventh century to other societies of the Middle East, North Africa, and southern and eastern Europe. Much of the debate within different religious communities followed two themes. For Christians, the debate was whether sacramental wines identified in the Scripture texts were fermented. For Muslims, Christians, and some other religions, the debate focused on "being ready, or being in a state of grace," to receive *The Word*, or to be in the proper frame of mind to act as a witness for the faith.

7.2. Judaism

Wine is central to Jewish religious traditions. Examination of the Torah (Books of Moses) and other Old Testament books reveals more than 230 references to wine *(32)*. Wine is respected throughout Judaism for its religious, medical, and social uses, yet it is a beverage surrounded by specific ethical and moral behavior codes, with specific admonitions regarding intoxication that date to the earliest Jewish texts *(33)*. References to wine are also found in other Talmud literature of the sixth-century CE, and Medieval commentaries that include a range of views *(34)*:

> *"People who are suffering from a strong mid-line headache or the like, secondary to thick blood, or coldness of the face, will be overtly benefited by drinking undiluted wine, either after a meal or during the meal. Their pain will be alleviated by the warming effect of the wine and its thinning [effect on the blood]"* (35).

Of special interest to Maimonides was the role of wine in matters of human reproduction and cohabitation:

> *"Of greater benefit than any food or medicine for [male erection] is wine. There is no substitute for it in this respect, because the blood that is produced [by wine] is warm and moist and rejoices the soul, and strongly incites to sexual intercourse because of its special characteristic ... This is especially so if one takes some [wine] after the meal, and when one leaves the bath, for its effect in this regard is far greater than anything else"* (36).

7.3. Christianity

Within Christianity, wine and bread are symbolic of the blood and body of Christ *(37,38)*. Sacramental wine is viewed by many faithful Mediterraneans as having curative properties; it may be poured over the body of Catholic believers thought to be possessed. Among faithful Greek Orthodox, wine is used to cleanse and wash the body of the deceased and to make an offering linking the deceased with Christ's resurrection *(39)*. Vines, grapes, and wine have served as symbolic icons throughout the centuries of Christian art.

Despite the dual attitude toward wine expressed historically throughout Christian literature, early Christian physicians recommended wine for therapeutic properties. Perhaps the most important influential early Christian doctor was Ibn Ishaq. Known in the west as Hunayn Ibn Ishaq (809–873 CE) he was a member of the Nestorian (Diophysite) Christian sect. His primary medical text, *Questions on Medicine for Scholars*, defined types of beverages prescribed by physicians, presented an unusually clear view of physiology, debated the medical properties of wine and how it warmed the body, and then described the effects of intoxication:

> *"How many kinds of beverages [are there]? Three: some like water, serve only as drinks; some, like fermented beverages and wine, serve as nutrients; and others ... serve in the same way as the preceding two and, in addition, as medicines"* (40).

Other early Christians (nonphysicians) took ethical-moral viewpoints regarding wine. One of these, Gregory of Nyssa (later St. Gregory), a religious scholar of the fourth century CE, wrote that wine, taken to excess, was the drug of madness, it poisoned the soul, led to the destruction of the mind and the ruin of nature, and was "the danger of youth, the disgrace of old age, and the shame of women" *(41)*.

Tradition holds that Mary, the mother of Jesus, gave birth inside a cave located within the precinct of Bethlehem in ancient Palestine. The story is commonly related that when Mary initiated breastfeeding, some of her milk spilled onto the floor of the cave and turned the stones white. For at least a millennium, this site has been called the *Milk Grotto* and receives tens of thousands of visitors yearly. It has remained customary through the centuries for Christian and Muslim women visitors who are nursing to collect the white stones that form the floor of the cave, take them home, grind them to dust, mix them with water, and drink as a medical beverage in the belief that the volume of their breast milk will be increased (Grivetti L, unpublished observations, 1995).

7.4. Islam

Despite Koran and Hadith injunctions against wine, Muslim physicians of the Middle Ages extolled the merits and healthful properties of this beverage. Specifically prohibited to believers is wine: "O believers, wine and arrow-shuffling, idols and diving-arrows are an abomination, some of Satan's work" *(42)*. Although the specific Arabic term used in the Koran is *khmr*, the prohibition has been generally extended to include alcoholic beverages. However, some Muslims argue just the opposite, and because the term is so specifically defined, it is not uncommon to encounter devout Muslims who drink wine and consume a range of potentially intoxicating beverages *(43)*. Positive therapeutic uses of wine abound in texts attributed to devout Medieval Muslim physicians. Despite the Koran's ban on wine, the great Muslim physicians of the Middle Ages prescribed wine and wrote on its positive and negative attributes.

Ibn Sina of Afshena (937–1037 CE) is perhaps the preeminent Muslim physician of the Middle Ages. He wrote extensively on beverages, partically the medical-dietary role of wine. In regard to wine's positive and negative attributes, Ibn Sina said: "The advantage of wine is that it excites the secretion of urine, thus removing the bilious humor with it, and that it moistens the joints" *(44)*. However, he did point to some negative effects: "To take wine after a meal is very unsatisfactory, for it is rapidly digested and enters the blood quickly and carries food on into the blood before it is properly digested" *(44)*. He added: "To give wine to youths is like adding fire to a fire already prepared with matchwood. Young adults should take it in moderation. But elderly persons may take as much as they can tolerate. Wine is borne better in a cold country than in a hot one" *(44)*.

Finally, young students attending traditional Islamic schools throughout the Middle East and elsewhere transcribe Koran passages on to slate tablets using chalk, alternative locally prepared vegetable inks are used to write the sacred texts onto smoothed boards. When the daily lessons are concluded and the passages memorized, the words are erased, and the fine chalk dust is commonly eaten as a form of religious pica. Across the Sahel states of western Africa, the students' wooden boards are washed clean at the conclusion of the lesson, the holy words removed by damp cloths, and then the cloths containing the vegetable inks are soaked, rinsed, and the fluid is caught in a small bowl and subsequently drunk (Smith G, personal communication).

8. BEVERAGES, SOCIAL CONFLICT, AND WAR

Access to water has always been critical in warfare. Since antiquity, generals have sent detachments in advance of the main body of troops to secure and protect water holes and lakes. The pattern has also been to deny advancing armies access to water; when an army is in retreat, the common practice has been to defile local wells by tossing bodies of animals or soldiers into the water to make it putrid. Expectedly, technological inventions of water-purification tablets (e.g., halazone during World War II), became an advantage, thereby making once putrid, unsafe waters safe. One might also remember the so-called "Jerry Can" invented by the Germans to carry water during their World War II campaigns.

There are numerous military references to the importance of water. For example, Sun Tzu wrote his classic on tactics and deception, *The Art of War*, c. 500 BCE. He noted: "When soldiers stand leaning on their spears, they are faint from want of food. If those who are sent to draw water begin by drinking themselves, the army is suffering from thirst" *(45)*.

A classic of Eastern Roman military tactics and logistics was written by Publius Flavius Vegetius Renatus during the fifth-century CE. His critical observations included the following: "Neither should the army use bad or marsh water, for bad drinking water, like poison, causes disease in the drinkers" *(46)*. He added: "Shortages of grain, wine-vinegar, wine and salt should be prevented at all times" *(46)*.

Marshal Maurice de Saxe commanded his troops during the early decades of the 18th century when more than one-third of his soldiers perished—not in battle—but because of dysentery, and he believed that he knew the cause:

> "In the year 1718 we entered the camp at Belgrade with 55,000 men. On the day of the battle, August 18th, there were only 22,000 men under arms; all the rest were dead or unable to fight. It is the change of climate that causes it. There were no such examples among the Romans as long as they had vinegar [for their water]. But just as soon as it was lacking they were subject to the same misfortunes that our troops are at present. This is a fact to which few persons have given any attention ... The Romans distributed several days' supply [of vinegar] among their men by order, and each man poured a few drops in his drinking water. I leave to the doctors the discovery of the causes of such beneficial effects" (47).

Indeed, deprivation of access to beverage luxuries has also brought nations to war. America's War of Independence was, in part, precipitated by British Stamp Taxes on the colonial luxury of tea. This ultimately led to the Boston Tea Party of 1765 and the events that brought independence to what became the United States of America.

Every summer, armies of tourists consume beverages of unknown origin and composition, purchased from street vendors in many nations of the world, especially in the tropics. What may be advertised as fruit juice, sugar-cane juice, and even potable water, may be adulterated with water contaminated with a host of potential disease organisms. Furthermore, when ice vendors sell chunks of ice, they hack off chips from the block—chips that fall onto the filthy street—and then wipe the chips clean with their unwashed hands, and sell the chips to beverage vendors to cool the product they are selling to the occupying army (Grivetti L, unpublished observations, 1964–1967; 1969; 1979; 1993). Of course, the best advice is for tourists and visitors in the tropics to rehydrate with bottled beverages (without ice) and to never consume fresh fruit juices prepared by street vendors when on vacation *(48)*. For an updated review on rehydration therapy, *see* Chapter 21 by Ramakrishna.

9. ATHLETICS, SPORTS, AND HYDRATION

Although descriptions of training regimens of ancient athletes have been documented for centuries, accounts of foods and beverages used by ancient elite athletes are rare.

One of the most complete passages to describe the diets of ancient athletes was by Philostratos Flavius: "An excess of wine in the athletes' bodies requires moderate exercise to bring on sweating. We should not make people in this condition take hard exercise, but we should not excuse them from their workout entirely" *(49)*.

Epictetus, a philosopher of the first- and second-century CE, provided a challenge to athletes who strived to win at the Olympic games: "If you do, you will have to obey instructions, eat according to regulations, keep away from desserts, exercise on a fixed schedule at definite hours, in both heat and cold; you must not drink cold water nor can you have a drink of wine whenever you want" *(50)*.

Turning to elite athletes of the modern era, more reasonable information on food and beverage use can be obtained. At the Berlin Olympic Games held in 1936, data are available on 42 of the 49 nations that competed. Strong coffee was part of the training tables of only 7 countries: Argentina, Australia/New Zealand, Brazil, Estonia, Greece, India, and Italy. Ironically, coffee was not a significant component of the diet of athletes from so-called "coffee-drinking" cultures, specifically Austria, Mexico, Peru, Switzerland, Turkey, or the United States. Milk in quantities greater than 2 L/d was consumed by athletes who represented Afghanistan, Bermuda, Brazil, Finland, Holland, Iceland, India, Norway, South Africa, and the United States. Whiskey in undefined quantities was a dietary component of Canadian athletes, whereas wine in undefined quantities appeared on the training tables of French and Italian athletes. Chinese athletes drank limited quantities of milk and drank iced tea and orange juice, whereas Japanese athletes did not drink tea at all *(51,52)*. More recently, the Atlanta Olympic Games of 1996 were managed by ARAMARK Corporation of Philadelphia, who provided milk (70,000 lbs) and bottled water (550,000 gal) to American and visiting athletes *(53)*.

Fluid replacement beverages were developed in the 1960s, beginning with Gatorade. Currently, numerous sports beverages are marketed in the United States, among them AllSport, POWERade, and Sport Toddy *(53–55)*. The United States has also seen a growth in beverages marketed to maintain specific weights or to aid in losing weight. These topics are reviewed in Chapter 18 by Stubbs and Whybrow and Chapter 20 by Maughan.

It is perhaps appropriate to also note how beverages are used at the conclusion of certain sporting events, where the traditional beverage of victors in the Indianapolis 500 is milk, and winners of the Tour de France drink champagne, then shake the bottle and spray their fans with a champagne mist. Who does not delight in (or is repelled by) the relatively recent US pattern accorded National Football League coaches who win the Super Bowl of being drenched in a cascade of ice-chilled Gatorade.

10. BEVERAGES AND SPACE FLIGHT

Several key problems must be overcome before embarking on periods of extended space flight, e.g., the mission to Mars. In addition to the well-known problems of calcium metabolism and bone loss, potential radiation, and food-energy balance, water balance is perhaps the most critical: one may survive for several months on limited food supplies, but only days without water.

Early estimates and calculations for water needs of astronauts were conducted in the 1960s when decisions were made to produce closed systems that recycled waste water from human urine and exhaled air for drinking, cooking, and washing needs. The estimated daily water requirement for drinking and cooking needs was 5000 mL/d/astronaut *(56)*.

Beverages developed and served to the early Mercury Program astronauts were Spartan and not particularly fine tasting, whereas Gemini Program astronauts (1965–1966) fared substantially better. Food product developers realized it was impractical to associate specific consumables with earthbound concepts of breakfast, lunch, and dinner. Accordingly, astronauts were presented with 3-d menu cycles for each 24-h period. This included a range of beverages: cocoa, grapefruit drink, orange drink, orange-grapefruit drink, and tea *(57,58)*. Indeed, the need to create a flavorful drink in space from recycled water led to the development of the orange-drink beverage Tang, now popular with more earthbound consumers.

Astronauts associated with the Sky Lab Program experienced substantial improvements in both variety and presentation. Sky Lab astronauts could select from cocoa, cocoa-flavored liquid instant breakfast, coffee (black), grape drink, grapefruit (soluble crystal form), lemonade, orange (soluble crystal form) *(59)*. The value for daily water needs by Skylab and some shuttle crew astronauts has been established at 2000–2500 mL/d, with intakes increased depending on activity level *(60)*. Still, there remains a basic question: In the centuries to come, what will the traditional beverages become once colonies are established on the Moon and Mars?

11. CODA

Beverages, whether from animal, plant, or natural sources, have served humans well through the millennia. Historically, water was identified as one of the four great elements: air, earth, fire, and water. Water and related companion beverages have been the focus of development and scientific scrutiny for centuries, dating well before the invention of writing. Water—such a simple compound, just three atoms—two hydrogens and an oxygen—but without water, humans could not exist.

Three hundred years from today …

Humans arise after periods of restful sleep, dress, and walk across their spotless living quarters. In their ergogenic-fitted workspace, they grind coffee beans grown hydroponically from recycled waste water. They nestle into their ergogenic chairs, molded to accommodate their bodies, and gaze outward through thick, meteoroid-resistant tempered windows and view the ongoing construction taking place on the red dusty landscape of the Martian surface, and take their first drink of the day...

12. MAIN POINTS FOR PRIMARY AND CLINICAL REVIEW

1. Water is the primordial drink after breast milk, and it remains the most ubiquitous, despite the many new beverage choices created in the last millennium.
2. Beverages have developed though human history: our primordial drinks lead to the use of animal milk, fermented drinks, teas, coffee, and, today, an ever-expanding set of choices, tastes, and drinks with diverse nutritional qualities.
3. In addition to its obvious impact on nutrition, beverage usage and choice has been central to the development of culture, commerce, science, the arts, and religion.
4. From the ancient Greeks and Romans to the armies and athletes of the Modern World, an understanding of the importance of safe and healthy beverages has been central to clarifying the military and athletic success that has determined the identity of the world today.

5. Recent diversification of choices ensures that beverages will continue to dominate what we as people, nations, and a planet have become, both on earth and in space.

REFERENCES

1. Caraka-Samhita. Agnivesa's treatise refined and annotated by Caraka and redacted by Drdhabala. Vol. 1. Sutrasthana to Indriyasthana. Edited by P Sharma. Chaukambha Orientalia, Delhi, India, 1981.
2. Nei-Ching. The Yellow Emporers classic of internal medicine. Translated by I. Veith. University of California Press, Berkley, CA, 1996.
3. Grivetti LE. Nutrition past—nutrition today. Prescientific origins of nutrition and dietetics. Part 3. Legacy of China. Nutr Today 1991;26:6–17.
4. Beal S. A catena of Buddhist scriptures from the Chinese. Translated by S Beal. Cheng wen Publishing Company, Taipei, Republic of China, 1970.
5. Simoons FJ. The antiquity of dairying in Asia and Africa. Geographical Rev 1971;61:431–439.
6. Simoons FJ. Primary adult lactose intolerance and the milking habit: a problem in biological and cultural interrelations. Part I. Review of the medical research. Am J Dig Dis 1969;14:819–836.
7. Simoons FJ. Primary adult lactose intolerance and the milking habit: a problem in biological and cultural interrelations. Part II. A culture historical hypothesis. Am J Dig Dis 1970;15:695–710.
8. Johnson JD, Kretchmer N, Simoons FJ. Lactose malabsorption: its biology and history. In: Advances in Pediatrics. Schulman I (ed.). 21st Ed. Year Book Medical Publishers, Chicago, IL, 1974, pp. 197–237.
9. Reed BA, Grivetti LE. Controlling on-farm inventories of bulk-tank raw milk. An opportunity to protect public health. J Dairy Sci 2001;83:1–4.
10. Badler V. The archaeological evidence for winemaking, distribution, and consumption at Proto-Historic Godin Tepe, Iran. In: The Origins and Ancient History of Wine. McGovern PE, Fleming SJ, and Katz SH (eds.). Gordon and Breach Publishers, Newark, NJ, 1995, pp. 45–56.
11. Formenti F, Duthel JM. The analysis of wine and other organics inside amphoras of the Roman Period. In: The Origins and Ancient History of Wine. McGovern PE, Fleming SJ, Katz SH (eds.). Gordon and Breach Publishers, Newark, NJ, 1995, pp. 79–85.
12. McGovern PE, Michel, RH. The analytical and archeological challenge of detecting ancient wine: two case studies from the ancient Near East. In: The Origins and Ancient History of Wine. McGovern PE, Fleming SJ, Katz SH (eds.) Gordon and Breach Publishers, Newark, NJ, 1995, pp. 57–65.
13. Grivetti LE. Wine: the food with two faces. In: The Origins and Ancient History of Wine. McGovern PE, Fleming SJ, Katz SH (eds.). Gordon and Breach Publishers, Newark, NJ, 1995, pp. 9–22.
14. Grivetti LE. Wine in health and social commentary. From Hippocrates to Athenaeus. Laetaberis, in press.
15. Athenaeus. The Deipnosophists. Translated by CB Gulick. 7 vols. G. P. Putnam & Sons, New York, NY, 1927–1941.
16. Darby WJ, Ghalioungui P, Grivetti LE. Food. The Gift of Osiris. Academic Press, London, 1977.
17. Erman A. The literature of the ancient Egyptians. Translated by AM Blackmn. Methuen, London, 1927.
18. Coe SD, Coe MD. The true history of chocolate. Thames and Hudson, London, 1996.
19. Dillinger TL, Barriga P, Escarcega S, Jimenez M, Lowe DS, Grivetti LE. Food of the gods: cure for humanity? A cultural history of the medicinal and ritual use of chocolate. J Nutr 2000;130(Suppl): 2057S–2072S.
20. Sahagen B. General history of the things of New Spain. Santa Fe, NM. The School of American Research, the University of Utah, and the Museum of New Mexico; 1590/1981.
21. Topik SC. Coffee. In: The Cambridge World History of Food. Kiple KF, Ornelas KC (eds.). Cambridge University Press, Cambridge, England, 2000, pp. 641–653.
22. Costill DL, Dalsky G, Find W. Effects of caffeine ingestion on metabolism and exercise performance. Med Sci Sports Exer 1978;10:155–158.
23. Williams MH. The use of nutritional ergogenic aids in sports. Is it an ethical issue? Int J Sport Nutr 1994;4:120–131.
24. Applegate EA, Grivetti LE. Search for the competitive edge. A history of dietary fads and supplements. J Nutr 1997;127(Suppl):869S–873S.
25. Abaka E. Kola nut. In: The Cambridge World History of Food. Kiple KF, Ornelas KC (eds.). Cambridge University Press, Cambridge, England, 2000, pp. 684–692.

26. Yu L. Classic of Tea. Translated by FR Carpenter. Little, Brown, and Company, Boston, MA, 8th century CE/1974.
27. Weisburger JH, Comer J. Tea. In: The Cambridge World History of Food. Kiple KF, Ornelas KC (eds.). Cambridge University Press, Cambridge, England, 2000, pp. 712–720.
28. Katiyar SK, Mukhtar H. Tea consumption and cancer. World Rev Nutr Dietetics 1996;79:154–184.
29. Weisburger JH. Tea and health. A historical perspective. Cancer Let 1997;114:315–317.
30. Yang CS, Lee MJ, Chen I, Yang GY. Polyphenols as inhibitors of carcinogenesis. Env Health Persp 1997;4:971–976.
31. Bell MA. Art. JAMA 1984;252:1838.
32. Goodrick EW, Kohlenberger JR, III. The New Complete Concordance. The Complete English Concordance to the New International Version. Zonderuan, Grand Rapids, MI, 1981.
33. Malka M, Monnier J, Moron P, Jarrige A. Les Juifs et l'alcool. Annales Societe Medico-Psychologique 1979;5:496–502.
34. Kottek SS. Talmudic aphorisms on diet III: What should we drink? Israel J Med Sci 1994;30:732–733.
35. Maimonides. The Medical Aphorisms of Moses Maimonides. Translated and Edited by F Rosner and S Muntner. Bloch, New York, 1970–1971.
36. Maimonides. Treatise on cohabitation. In: F Rosner, trans. Treatises on Poisons, Hemorrhoids, Cohabitation. Maimonides' medical writings. The Maimonides Research Institute, Haifa, Israel, 1984.
37. Child H, Colles D. Cing and milk use in southern Asia. Anthropos 1970;65:547–593.
38. Murray R. Symbols of Church and Kingdom. A Study in Early Syriac Tradition. University Press, Cambridge, England, 1975.
39. Danforth LM. The Death Rituals of Rural Greece. Princeton University Press, Princeton, NJ, 1982.
40. Ibn Ishaq H. Al Masa'il fi al-Tibb lil Muta'allimin [Questions on medicine for scholars]. Translated by P Ghalioungui. Al-Ahram Center for Scientific Translations, Cairo, Egypt, 1980.
41. Keenan ME. St. Gregory of Nyssa and the medical profession. Bull History Med 1944;15:150–161.
42. Koran. The Koran Interpreted. Translated by AJ Arberry. The Macmillan Company, New York, 1955.
43. Grivetti LE. Flavor and culture. The importance of flavors in the Middle East. Food Tech 1975;29:38–40.
44. Ibn Sina. Avicenna's Poem on Medicine. Translated by HC Krueger. Charles C. Thomas, Springfield, IL, 1963.
45. de Saxe M. My reveries upon the art of war. In: Phillips TR (ed.). Roots of Strategy. The 5 Greatest Military Classics of All Time. Stackpole Books, Harrisburg, PA, 1985, pp. 177–300.
46. Sun Tzu. The art of war. In: Roots of Strategy. The 5 Greatest Military Classics of All Time. Phillips TR (ed.). Stackpole Books, Harrisburg, PA, 1985, pp. 130–163.
47. Vegetius Renatus PF. Epitoma Rei Militaris [Epitome of Military Science]. Translated by NP Milner. Vol. 16. Translated Texts for Historians. Liverpool University Press, Liverpool, England, 5th century CE/1993.
48. Simopoulos AP, Bhat RV. Street foods. World Rev Nutr Dietetics 2000;86:1–175.
49. Philostratus F. Concerning Gymnastics. Translated by T Woody. American Physical Education Association, Ann Arbor, MI, 1936.
50. Epictetus. The Discourses of Epictetus, With the Enchiridion and Fragments. Translated by G Long. AL Burt, New York, 1888.
51. Schenk P. Die Verpflegung von 4700 Wettkämpfern aus 42 Nationen im Olympischen Dorf wärend der XI. Olympischen Spiele 1936 zu Berlin. Meunch Med Wochenschr 1936;83:1535–1539.
52. Schenk P. Bericht über die Verpflegung der im óOlympischen Dorfó untergebrachten Teilnehmer an den XI. Olympischen Spielen 1936 zu Berlin. Die Ernaehrung, 1937;2:1–24.
53. Grivetti LE, Applegate EA. From Olympia to Atlanta. A cultural-historical perspective on diet and athletic training. J Nutr 1997;127(Suppl):860S–868S.
54. Grandjean AC. Diets of elite athletes. Has the discipline of sports nutrition made an impact? J Nutr 1997;127(Suppl):874S–877S.
55. Cade R, Spooner G, Schlein E, Pickering M, Dean R. Effect of fluid, electrolyte, and glucose replacement during exercise on performance, body temperature, rate of sweat loss, and compositional changes of extracellular fluid. J Sports Med Phys Fit 1972;12:150–156.
56. Taylor AA, Finkelstein F, Hayes RE. Food for space travel. Examination of current capabilities and future needs. Air Research and Development Command, Washington, DC, 1960.

57. Klicka MV, Hollender HA, Lachance PA. Development of space foods. 4th International Congress of Dietetics, Stockhom, Sweden, 15 July, 1965. Ekonomiforestandarinnors Tidskrift 1966;1:3–12.
58. Klicka MV, Hollender HA, Lachance PA. Foods for astronauts. J Am Dietet Assoc 1967;51:238–245.
59. Heidelbaugh ND, Smith MC Jr., Rambaut PC, et al. Clinical nutrition applications of space food technology. J Am Dietet Assoc 1973;62:383–389.
60. Lane HW, Leach C., Smith SM. Fluid and electrolyte homeostasis. In: Lane HW, Schoeller DA (ed.). Nutrition in Spaceflight and Weightlessness Models. CRC Press, Boca Raton, FL, 2000, pp. 119–139.

II HEALTH EFFECTS OF ALCOHOLIC BEVERAGES

2

What Are the Health Implications of Alcohol Consumption?

Eric Rimm and Norman J. Temple

The harmful effects of alcohol are far better known that its beneficial effects. This is scarcely surprising: it requires no training in epidemiology to recognize the devastating harm that often comes with both drunkenness and chronic alcohol abuse. However, findings that have emerged in recent years have uncovered several surprising associations between moderate alcohol intake and enhanced health and well being.

In this chapter, the American definition of a drink, namely 12.5–13.0 g of alcohol, is used. This quantity of alcohol is approximately the amount contained in 12 oz (356 g) of regular beer, 4–5 oz (118–148 g) of wine, or 1.5 oz (42 g) of spirits. We also use the US Department of Agriculture (USDA) dietary guidelines' definition of moderate alcohol consumption as up to two drinks a day for men and one drink a day for women.

1. HARMFUL EFFECTS OF ALCOHOL

1.1. Accidents, Violence, and Suicide

It is well established that abuse of alcohol is associated with accidents, violence, and suicide. The most dramatic evidence of this has come from Russia. Between 1984 and 1994, there was serious economic decline and great political turmoil. During this period, life expectancy fell by 4 yr in men and by 2 yr in women. A major factor contributing to this decline was widespread alcohol abuse, particularly binge drinking, which led to large increases in deaths from accidents, homicide, and suicide, as well as cardiovascular disease [1,2].

In 1999 in the United States, there were approx 15,800 alcohol-related traffic accidents, approx 38% of all traffic fatalities. This is a decrease of 30% when compared with 1989 [3]. Stricter enforcement of existing legal codes and the passage of new laws have been suggested as promoting these beneficial changes.

1.2. Chronic Alcohol Abuse

For many people, years of alcohol abuse eventually lead to chronic health and nutritional problems. Alcohol is rich in calories and typically devoid in nutrients, especially alcohol-rich and sugar-rich hard liquors. The body often compensates for the high caloric intake by decreasing the stimulus to eat regular nutrient-rich foods. As a result, there is

From: *Beverages in Nutrition and Health*
Edited by: T. Wilson and N. J. Temple © Humana Press Inc., Totowa, NJ

a high probability of malnutrition, especially of folate and thiamin. The thiamin deficiency associated with alcohol abuse is known as Wernicke-Korsakoff syndrome. Liver disease is also a likely result, with a downward spiral from fatty liver to alcoholic hepatitis and, eventually, to cirrhosis.

1.3. Fetal Alcohol Syndrome

Pregnancy is another situation in which alcohol misuse can have tragic consequences. This induces fetal alcohol syndrome (FAS). FAS encompasses several symptoms, including prenatal and postnatal growth retardation, abnormal facial features, and an increased frequency of major birth defects. Children born with FAS never recover.

A subclinical form of FAS is known as fetal alcohol effects (FAE). Children with FAE may be short or have only minor facial abnormalities or develop learning disabilities, behavioral problems, or motor impairments.

FAS occurs at a level of alcohol intake that in a nonpregnant woman would not be considered alcohol abuse. Approximately four drinks per day pose a real threat of FAS, whereas one or two drinks per day may still retard growth, although the epidemiological data are weaker and somewhat inconsistent at these lower consumption levels. Although women who have an occasional drink during pregnancy should not fear they are doing irreparable harm to their fetuses, it is now generally accepted that any woman who is or may become pregnant should abstain from alcohol.

1.4. Cancer

Alcohol increases the risk of cancer of the mouth, throat, and esophagus *(4,5)*. It also acts as a cocarcinogen with cigarette smoke *(6)*. It is likely that among heavy alcohol consumers, the alcohol or one of its metabolites, acetaldehyde, is toxic to mucosal epithelial cells. Alcohol also increases the risk of cancer of the liver, ovary, and breast *(4,5)*. The risk ratio (RR) with an alcohol intake of four drinks per day is estimated to be 2.3 for cancer of the mouth, throat, and esophagus; 1.7 for breast cancer; and 1.15–1.35 for cancer of the stomach, colon-rectum, liver, and ovary *(5)*. For all cancer combined, a significant risk is seen starting at an alcohol intake of two drinks per day, with a RR of 1.22 at four drinks per day *(5)*. For breast cancer, it is less likely that ethanol is toxic, because the increase has been seen at relatively low levels. It is more likely that alcohol influences circulating estrogen levels, which may affect disease occurrence *(7,8)*.

Emerging evidence also indicates that alcohol, even in moderation, may suppress circulating folate levels, which could affect DNA synthesis and gene expression. Several recent large prospective studies of breast cancer *(9,10)* show that an adequate folate intake ameliorated the carcinogenic action of alcohol *(see Fig. 1)*. As with breast cancer, the effect of alcohol on colon cancer may be muted or eliminated completely if the diet has sufficient folate or methionine (both methyl donors) *(11)*.

1.5. Obesity

Alcohol, of course, is a source of calories (7 kcal/g). It is important to remember that alcoholic beverages also contain carbohydrates that add additional calories. A half liter of wine contains approx 350 kcal, whereas three cans of beer supply approx 250–450 kcal, clearly enough to tip the energy balance well into positive territory. These numbers explain the popularity of low-calorie "light beers." It is predictable, therefore, that alcohol con-

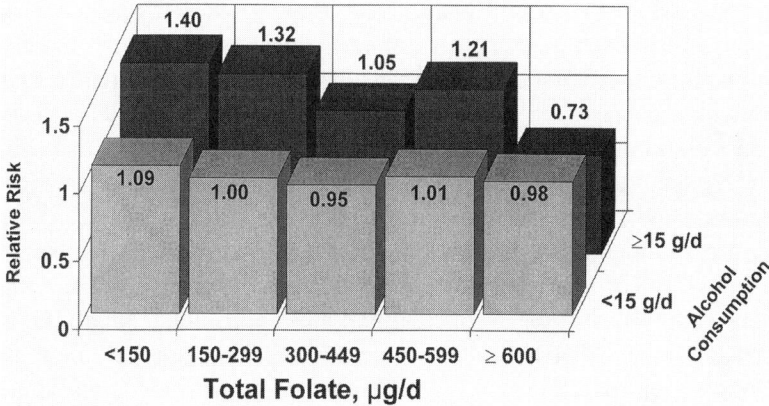

Fig. 1. Multivariate relative risk of breast cancer by total folate intake and alcohol consumption. The reference group for all comparisons was women who consumed 150–299 µg/d of total folate and fewer than 15 g/d alcohol.

sumption should be associated with excess weight gain. But, as so often happens in nutrition, predictions collapse in the face of reality. A solid body of evidence from mostly cross-sectional studies has demonstrated that alcohol intake actually has an inverse association with body mass index (an index of weight relative to height) *(12–14)*. However, when diet, physical activity, and other lifestyle factors are not examined prospectively, it can be difficult to interpret whether the association is causal. Thus, more longitudinal studies of alcohol and weight gain are needed. Intervention studies are inconclusive, although Cordain et al. *(15)* reported that supplementation with 35 g of alcohol per day (a little less than three glasses of wine) to the daily energy requirements for a period of 6 wk did not affect body weight and/or energy metabolism. It is feasible that the increase in basal metabolic rate caused by moderate alcohol consumption may offset the additional calories from consuming alcohol-containing beverages *(16)*.

2. PROTECTIVE EFFECTS OF ALCOHOL

2.1. Coronary Heart Disease

A convincing body of evidence suggests that the risk of coronary heart disease (CHD) is reduced by 10–40% in persons who consume alcohol in moderation *(17)*. In some populations, this association can be skewed if individuals at higher risk for CHD reduce or eliminate alcohol consumption due to a diagnosis of a related chronic disease (e.g., hypertension or diabetes). This is frequently described as the "sick quitter" syndrome and can create a spurious artificial inverse association between alcohol and CHD *(18)*. Because conditions like hypertension and diabetes increase the risk of CHD by twofold to threefold, a study that does not consider these conditions may find that moderate drinkers have as much as 50–70% less heart disease. However, even in large cohort studies where sick quitters are removed or moderate drinkers are compared to lifelong abstainers, alcohol has had strong cardiovascular benefits *(19)*.

There has been much speculation that wine may be more potent than beer or spirits in preventing CHD. This is largely based on findings from ecological studies (i.e., countries like France that have a high intake of wine have relatively low CHD rates) *(17)*. It has been repeatedly shown that such associations can easily be spurious. This is indicated by the findings from case-control and cohort studies: these show no clear trend for one type of alcohol to be more consistently associated with protection from CHD *(17)*. Where one type of alcohol does manifest a stronger association than other types, this is likely due to confounding by such factors as smoking and drinking pattern or to differences in other lifestyle factors, such as eating patterns or physical activity.

Short-term experimental studies have helped to explain the mechanisms by which alcohol prevents CHD *(20)*. First and foremost, alcohol causes an increased level of high-density lipoprotein (HDL) cholesterol. This explains approximately half of the association between alcohol and CHD. Another protective mechanism is that alcohol exerts an antithrombotic action by reducing hepatic production of fibrinogen and other clotting proteins. There is also some evidence indicating that alcohol may lower low-density lipoprotein (LDL) cholesterol levels *(21)*, but findings are not consistent.

Alcohol has been reported to elevate the blood homocysteine level, a relatively new CHD predictor. This was seen with 6 wk of consumption of a moderate level of alcohol (30 g/d) *(22)*. Red wine and beer had a greater effect than spirits. This action of alcohol is predicted to partly counter its protective benefit on CHD.

As with cancer, there is a suggestion of an alcohol-folate interaction: the beneficial effects of alcohol on CHD may be strongest among those with folate-sufficient diets *(23,24)*. Because alcohol may suppress folate levels leading to a subsequent increase in homocysteine, individuals with high folate intakes may benefit the most from a moderate alcohol intake because they will have low levels of homocysteine from the extra folate yet still reap the beneficial effects of alcohol on lipids, coagulation factors, and insulin sensitivity.

Recent findings from the Physicians' Health Study reveal a genetic component to the relationship between alcohol intake and risk of CHD *(25)*. The enzyme alcohol dehydrogenase is crucial to the metabolism of alcohol. Approximately 15% of the population is homozygous (or has two copies of the gene) for the form of the gene that induces a slow rate of alcohol metabolism. Slow metabolizers have higher plasma HDL cholesterol levels than fast metabolizers, and, among those in the Physicians' Health Study who drink moderately there is a dramatically low risk of CHD. This is one of the first diet-gene interactions to be reported in the literature and provides strong evidence that the ethanol component of alcohol-containing beverages is responsible for the benefit rather than other components in wine, beer, or spirits.

2.2. Blood Pressure and Stroke

A relatively high alcohol intake (>4 drinks/d) is associated with elevated blood pressure *(26,27)* and an increased risk of stroke. Recent evidence from cohort studies suggest that the association between alcohol and hypertension may be J-shaped, such that light and moderate drinkers have a modestly reduced risk of developing hypertension, although the exact mechanism for this effect is unknown *(28)*. Studies on the association between moderate alcohol consumption and stroke have been mixed. Several case-control and cohort studies have seen a reduced risk of stroke among moderate drinkers. Yet others find little benefit in the moderate range. In studies that find benefit, the reduction is usually limited to ischemic rather than hemorrhagic stroke *(4,29–31)*.

Clearly, the data support no increase in ischemic risk at moderate levels, but more work is needed to determine if drinking patterns influence risk of stroke (i.e., frequent consumption of small amounts of alcohol vs binge drinking).

2.3. Impotence

The relationship between excessive alcohol intake and poor erectile function is well known. As Shakespeare wrote: "It provokes the desire, but takes away from the performance" (Macbeth). However, as in the case of alcohol and blood pressure, recent findings have revealed an apparently beneficial effect, or at least no ill effects, of moderate alcohol consumption. Preliminary data from the Health Professionals' Follow-up Study, a prospective cohort study of more than 50,000 US male health professionals, show a modest U-shaped relationship between alcohol intake and erectile dysfunction. Like CHD, the strongest risk reduction was among those who consumed one to two drinks per day *(32)*. Although erectile dysfunction was originally believed to be purely pyschogenic in nature, 80–90% of the dysfunction is likely the result of biological factors that may share a similar profile to atherosclerosis.

2.4. Gallstones

Most studies that have examined this question have reported a protective association between alcohol and risk of gallstones. For instance, Leitzmann et al. *(33)* observed that men who consume alcohol frequently (5–7 d/wk) have a reduced risk of gallstones but not those who consume alcohol less frequently (1–2 d/wk). These findings indicate that frequency of alcohol consumption rather than quantity is the critical factor.

2.5. Bone Health

Although findings are not consistent, several studies have reported an inverse association between moderate alcohol intake and bone mineral density, especially in women who are postmenopausal *(34,35)*. This suggests that alcohol may help prevent osteoporosis. However, as osteoporosis is so dependent on lifetime diet, physical activity, obesity, and other factors, it is probable that alcohol does not play an important role in osteoporosis. In contrast to the situation with osteoporosis, high levels of drinking cause loss of balance and falls, leading to an increased risk of hip or wrist fracture.

2.6. Hearing Loss

A cross-sectional study of subjects aged 50–91 years reported that moderate alcohol intake was associated with better hearing *(36)*. Again, like bone health, many other environmental and genetic effects play a more important role in the etiology of hearing loss.

2.7. Cognitive Function

Findings from the Framingham study, conducted among older adults, suggested that alcohol is associated with enhanced cognitive ability, especially in women *(37)*. This was seen at an intake of two to four drinks per day in women and four to eight drinks per day in men, an intake above what is usually considered moderate. An earlier study observed that this benefit was seen only in women *(38)*. It is well known that higher intakes have a damaging effect on brain function. Once again, therefore, alcohol manifests a U-shaped or J-shaped relationship. An even more revealing study that had detailed measures of cognitive function and dementia also reported benefits of alcohol consumption. In a 6-yr follow-up of 8000 middle-aged and older men and women in the Netherlands, Ruitenberg et al. *(39)* found that men and women consuming 1–3 drinks per day had a 42% lower risk than abstainers of developing dementia (mainly Alzheimer's disease).

2.8. Benign Prostatic Hyperplasia

A cohort study reported that moderate alcohol intake (2.5–4 drinks/d) was associated with a reduced risk of benign prostatic hyperplasia (RR of 0.59) *(40)*. The mechanisms for this action are speculative but may include the effects of alcohol on steroid hormone levels.

2.9. Diabetes

Cohort studies have suggested that alcohol may be protective against type 2 diabetes. A British *(41)* and an American *(42)* cohort study indicated that moderate alcohol consumption reduces risk of the condition by approx 40% in men but less so among American women *(43)*. Interestingly, there have been several recent studies suggesting that moderate alcohol consumption among men and women with type 2 diabetes is also associated with a much reduced risk of subsequent CHD, the leading killer of people with diabetes *(44–47)*.

2.10. Lung Disease

Alcohol may also be protective against chronic obstructive pulmonary disease (COPD). A cohort study of middle-aged men in Finland, the Netherlands, and Italy revealed a protective association between alcohol intake and risk of death from COPD *(48)*. The lowest risk was seen at an intake of up to approximately three drinks per day. Alcohol intake has also been observed to manifest a protective association with emphysema in smokers *(49)*.

3. EFFECT OF ALCOHOL ON TOTAL MORTALITY

When alcohol intake is moderate, the beneficial health effects on the cardiovascular system outweigh most detrimental effects. As a result, the net effect of alcohol on total mortality is a J-shaped curve, with minimum mortality associated with a moderate alcohol intake but with a rising curve as consumption increases. A major study by the American Cancer Society reported that in each gender, persons consuming one drink daily had a risk of death from all causes approx 20% below those of nondrinkers *(4)*. To put this in perspective, among American men and women aged 35–69 yr, a moderate consumption of alcohol prevents approximately one death for every six deaths caused by smoking *(4)*.

The alcohol intake corresponding to the nadir for mortality is still unclear but in people aged 50–80 is approx 0.7–1.2 drinks per day in men and 0.3 drinks per day in women *(50)*. However, because this is based on self-reported intake, which represents a substantial underestimation, the true nadir is almost certainly higher *(50)*.

The benefits of alcohol are most apparent in the middle-aged and elderly. This is because alcohol reduces risk of CHD and stroke, the first and third leading causes of death, respectively, in that age group. By contrast, the leading cause of death in Americans under age 40 yr is accidents, with homicide and suicide also being major causes, especially in men. These are all associated with alcohol. This age effect is illustrated by a report from the Nurses' Health Study. A moderate alcohol intake has a protective relationship with total mortality in women aged over 50 yr (RR is 0.80–0.88) but is associated with a doubling of the risk of death in those aged 34–39 yr (51). Similar findings were reported from England and Wales. A net favorable mortality outcome was seen only in men over age 55 and women over 65 yr (52).

4. DRINKING PATTERNS

More recently, research has focused on the importance of drinking pattern on risk of health outcomes. Not surprisingly, alcohol is most protective when consumed in small regular amounts rather than binge or episodic drinking. This was demonstrated in a cohort study in the United States (53). People who engaged in occasional heavy drinking had a higher risk of death than persons with the same alcohol intake but who did not engage in binge drinking. Similar observations were made on cardiovascular disease in Canada. The data from that study revealed that although alcohol consumption has a protective association with both CHD and hypertension, binge drinking increases the risk of both, especially in men (54). In a recent study of US male health professionals, frequency of consumption (d/wk) was more important than quantity consumed. Men who consumed alcohol at least 4 d/wk had the lowest risk of type 2 diabetes, regardless of the total amount consumed (55). These findings are hardly surprising: many dietary components cause no harm in small frequent doses but are toxic when a large dose is taken.

5. CONCLUSIONS

Clearly, alcohol can do much good but also much harm. It is important to remember that the harmful effects of alcohol frequently occur at a much younger age than the benefits. Consequently, if the effects of alcohol are measured in terms of quality years of life (lost or gained), then the harm done to one (usually younger) person by alcohol may be far greater than the benefit gained by another (usually older) person.

The majority of the harmful effects of alcohol can be avoided by sensible drinking, by not smoking, by drinking in moderation, and by avoiding alcohol when driving. For the person who can drink sensibly and can avoid alcohol's negative side effects, alcohol can be of considerable benefit. Like so much else in life, it's a matter of balance. Although alcohol should perhaps not be prescribed (56), neither should it be proscribed.

Australian researchers estimated that for people aged over 60 yr, the cost per life year gained by moderate consumption of alcohol was A$5700 (US $2900) in men and A$19,000 (US $9600) in women (57). On this basis, alcohol can be considered a cost-effective medication. For instance, it is many times more cost-effective than medication with statins for treatment of hypercholesterolemia (58).

The findings discussed in this chapter have implications for public health policy. But what are these implications? One possible policy is the following: all adults aged over 40 yr should be encouraged to consume moderate amounts of alcohol daily, unless there is a specific reason to the contrary, such as religion, medication use, or a history of alcohol abuse. The problem with such a policy is the risk of causing a rise in the prevalence of alcohol abuse. Typically, approx 5–10% of people in any society where alcohol is available become abusers of the beverage. The actual proportion is related to the mean alcohol intake: the higher the mean alcohol intake, the higher the proportion of alcohol abusers *(59)*. Thus, a policy that encourages greater alcohol use will likely also lead to more problems associated with abuse.

Arguably, the most prudent policy is one that explains that alcohol in moderation will likely have several health benefits for people who are middle age and older, while also stressing the hazards of abuse.

6. MAIN POINTS FOR PRIMARY AND CLINICAL REVIEW

1. An alcoholic drink is generally considered to contain 12.5–13 g of alcohol (ethanol); this amount is found in a 12-oz (356 g) beer, 4–5-oz (118–148 g) wine, or 1.5-oz (42 g) of distilled spirits.
2. The US Department of Agriculture defines moderate alcohol consumption as 2 drinks/day for men or 1 drink/day for women.
3. Alcohol creates many social problems, such as violence and accidents, as well as negative health effects, most notably those related to cancer and fetal alcohol syndrome.
4. Although persons with alcoholism should perhaps never drink, moderate alcohol consumption is associated with significant protective effects with respect to cardiovascular disease, several other diseases, and overall mortality.
5. The alcohol intake associated with the lowest overall mortality is 0.7–1.3 drinks/day in men and approx 0.3 drinks/day in women, but this is probably an underestimate.

REFERENCES

1. Leon DA, Chenet L, Shkolnikov VM, et al. Huge variation in Russian mortality rates 1984-94: artefact, alcohol, or what? Lancet 1997;350:383–388.
2. Walberg P, McKee M, Shkolnikov V, Chenet L, Leon DA. Economic change, crime, and mortality crisis in Russia: regional analysis. BMJ 1998;317:312–318.
3. Available at website: http://www.nhtsa.dot.gov/people/ncsa/factprev.html. Accessed June 6, 2002.
4. Thun MJ, Peto R, Lopez AD, et al. Alcohol consumption and mortality among middle-aged and elderly U.S. adults. N Engl J Med 1997;337:1705–1714.
5. Bagnardi V, Blangiardo M, Vecchia CL, Corrao G. A meta-analysis of alcohol drinking and cancer risk. Br J Cancer 2001;85:1700–1705.
6. World Cancer Research Fund/American Institute for Cancer Research. Food, Nutrition and the Prevention of Cancer: A Global Perspective. American Institute for Cancer Research, Washington, DC, 1997.
7. Hankinson SE, Willett WC, Manson JE, et al. Alcohol, height, and adiposity in relation to estrogen and prolactin levels in postmenopausal women. J Natl Cancer Inst 1995;87:1297–1302.
8. Dorgan JF, Baer DJ, Albert PS, et al. Serum hormones and the alcohol-breast cancer association in postmenopausal women. J Natl Cancer Inst 2001;93:710–715.
9. Zhang S, Hunter DJ, Hankinson SE, et al. A prospective study of folate intake and the risk of breast cancer. JAMA 1999;281:1632–1637.
10. Sellers TA, Kushi LH, Cerhan JR, et al. Dietary folate intake, alcohol, and risk of breast cancer in a prospective study of postmenopausal women. Epidemiology 2001;12:420–428.
11. Giovannucci E, Rimm EB, Ascherio A, Stampfer MJ, Colditz GA, Willett WC. Alcohol, low-methionine—low-folate diets, and risk of colon cancer in men. J Natl Cancer Inst 1995;87:265–273.
12. Colditz GA, Giovannucci E, Rimm EB, et al. Alcohol intake in relation to diet and obesity in women and men. Am J Clin Nutr 1991;54:49–55.
13. Williamson DF, Forman MR, Binkin NJ, Gentry EM, Remington PL, Trowbridge FL. Alcohol and body weight in United States adults. Am J Public Health 1987;7:1324–1330.
14. Hellerstedt WL, Jeffery RW, Murray DM. The association between alcohol intake and adiposity in the general population. Am J Epidemiol 1990;132:594–611.

15. Cordain L, Bryan ED, Melby CL, Smith MJ. Influence of moderate daily wine consumption on body weight regulation and metabolism in healthy free-living males. J Am Coll Nutr 1997;16:134–139.
16. Klesges R, Maaler CZ, Klesges LM. Effect of alcohol intake on resting energy expenditure in young women social drinkers. Am J Clin Nutr 1994;59:805–809.
17. Rimm EB, Klatsky A, Grobbee D, Stampfer MJ. Review of moderate alcohol consumption and reduced risk of coronary heart disease: is the effect due to beer, wine, or spirits? BMJ 1996;312:731–736.
18. Shaper AG, Wannamethee G, Walker M. Alcohol and mortality in British men: explaining the U-shaped curve. Lancet 1988;2:1267–1273.
19. Rimm E. Alcohol and cardiovascular disease. Curr Atheroscler Rep 2000;2:529–535.
20. Rimm EB, Williams P, Fosher K, Criqui M, Stampfer MJ. Moderate alcohol intake and lower risk of coronary heart disease: meta-analysis of effects on lipids and haemostatic factors. BMJ 1999;319:1523–1528.
21. Castelli WP, Doyle JT, Gordon T, et al. Alcohol and blood lipids: the cooperative lipoprotein phenotyping study. Lancet 1977;2:153–157.
22. Bleich S, Bleich K, Kropp S, et al. Moderate alcohol consumption in social drinkers raises plasma homocysteine levels: a contradiction to the "French Paradox"? Alcohol Alcohol 2001;36:189–192.
23. Rimm EB, Willett WC, Hu FB, et al. Folate and vitamin B6 from diet and supplements in relation to risk of coronary heart disease among women. JAMA 1998;279:359–364.
24. Koehler KM, Baumgartner RN, Garry PJ, Allen RH, Stabler SP, Rimm EB. Association of folate intake and serum homocysteine in elderly persons according to vitamin supplementation and alcohol use. Am J Clin Nutr 2001;73:628–637.
25. Hines LM, Stampfer MJ, Ma J, et al. Genetic variation in alcohol dehydrogenase and the beneficial effect of moderate alcohol consumption on myocardial infarction. N Engl J Med 2001;344:549–555.
26. Ascherio A, Rimm EB, Giovannucci EL, et al. A prospective study of nutritional factors and hypertension among US men. Circulation 1992;86:1475–1484.
27. Puddey IB, Beilin LJ, Vandongen R, Rouse IL, Rogers P. Evidence for a direct effect of alcohol consumption on blood pressure in normotensive men. A randomized controlled trial. Hypertension 1985;7:707–713.
28. Thadhani R, Camargo CA Jr, Stampfer MJ, Curhan GC, Willett WC, Rimm EB. Prospective study of moderate alcohol consumption and risk of hypertension in young women. Arch Intern Med 2002;162:569–574.
29. Berger K, Ajani UA, Kase CS, et al. Light-to-moderate alcohol consumption and the risk of stroke among U.S. male physicians. N Engl J Med 1999;341:1557–1564.
30. Sacco RL, Elkind M, Boden-Albala B, et al. The protective effect of moderate alcohol consumption on ischemic stroke. JAMA 1999;281:53–60.
31. Camargo CA. Case-control and cohort studies of moderate alcohol consumption and stroke. Clin Chim Acta 1996;246:107–119.
32. Rimm EB, Bacon C, Giovannucci E, Kawachi I. Waist circumference, physical activity, and alcohol consumption in relation to erectile dysfunction among US male health professionals. Annual Meeting of the American Urological Association, May 2, 2000, Atlanta, GA.
33. Leitzmann MF, Giovannucci EL, Stampfer MJ, et al. Prospective study of alcohol consumption patterns in relation to symptomatic gallstone disease in men. Alcohol Clin Exp Res 1999;23:835–841.
34. Rapuri PB, Gallagher JC, Balhorn KE, Ryschon KL. Alcohol intake and bone metabolism in elderly women. Am J Clin Nutr 2000;72:1206–1213.
35. Feskanich D, Korrick SA, Greenspan SL, Rosen HN, Colditz GA. Moderate alcohol consumption and bone density among postmenopausal women. J Women Health 1999;8:65–73.
36. Popelka MM, Cruikshanks KJ, Wiley TL, et al. Moderate alcohol consumption and hearing loss: a protective effect. J Am Geriatr Soc 2000;48:1273–1278.
37. Elias PK, Elias MF, D'Agostino RB, Silbershatz H, Wolf PA. Alcohol consumption and cognitive performance in the Framingham Heart Study. Am J Epidemiol 1999;150:580–590.
38. Dufouil C, Ducimetiere P, Alperovitch A. Sex differences in the association between alcohol consumption and cognitive performance. EVA Study Group. Epidemiology of vascular aging. Am J Epidemiol 1997;146:405–412.

39. Ruitenberg A, van Swieten JC, Witteman JC, et al. Alcohol consumption and risk of dementia: the Rotterdam Study. Lancet 2002;359:281–286.
40. Platz EA, Rimm EB, Kawachi I, et al. Alcohol consumption, cigarette smoking, and risk of benign prostatic hyperplasia. Am J Epidemiol 1999;149:106–115.
41. Wannamethee SG, Shaper AG, Perry IJ, Alberti KGMM. Alcohol consumption and the incidence of type II diabetes. J Epidemiol Community Health. 2002;56:542–548.
42. Conigrave KM, Hu BF, Camargo CA Jr, Stampfer MJ, Willett WC, Rimm EB. A prospective study of drinking patterns in relation to risk of type 2 diabetes among men. Diabetes 2001;50:2390–2395.
43. Stampfer MJ, Colditz GA, Willett WC, et al. A prospective study of moderate alcohol drinking and risk of diabetes in women. Am J Epidemiol 1988;128:549–558.
44. Tanasescu M, Hu FB, Willett WC, Stampfer MJ, Rimm EB. Alcohol consumption and risk of coronary heart disease among men with type 2 diabetes mellitus. J Am Coll Cardiol 2001;38:1836–1842.
45. Ajani UA, Gaziano JM, Lotufo PA, et al. Alcohol consumption and risk of coronary heart disease by diabetes status. Circulation 2000;102:500–505.
46. Solomon CG, Hu FB, Stampfer MJ, et al. Moderate alcohol consumption and risk of coronary heart disease among women with type 2 diabetes mellitus. Circulation 2000;102:494–499.
47. Valmadrid CT, Klein R, Moss SE, Klein BE, Cruickshanks KJ. Alcohol intake and the risk of coronary heart disease mortality in persons with older-onset diabetes mellitus. JAMA 1999;282:239–246.
48. Tabak C, Smit HA, Rasanen L, et al. Alcohol consumption in relation to 20-year COPD mortality and pulmonary function in middle-aged men from three European countries. Epidemiology 2001;12:239–245.
49. Pratt PC, Vollmer RT. The beneficial effect of alcohol consumption on the prevalence and extent of centrilobular emphysema. Chest 1984;85:372–377.
50. White IR. The level of alcohol consumption at which all-cause mortality is least. J Clin Epidemiol 1999;52:967–975.
51. Fuchs CS, Stampfer MJ, Colditz GA, et al. Alcohol consumption and mortality among women. N Engl J Med 1995;332:1245–1250.
52. Britton A, McPherson K. Mortality in England and Wales attributable to current alcohol consumption. J Epidemiol Community Health 2001;55:383–388.
53. Rehm J, Greenfield TK, Rogers JD. Average volume of alcohol consumption, patterns of drinking, and all-cause mortality: results from the US National Alcohol Survey. Am J Epidemiol 2001;153:64–71.
54. Murray RP, Connett JE, Tyas SL, et al. Alcohol volume, drinking pattern, and cardiovascular disease morbidity and mortality: is there a U-shaped function? Am J Epidemiol 2002;155:242–248.
55. Conigrave KM, Hu BF, Camargo CA Jr, Stampfer MJ, Willett WC, Rimm EB. A prospective study of drinking patterns in relation to risk of type 2 diabetes among men. Diabetes 2001;50:2390–2395.
56. Wannamethee SG, Shaper AG. Taking up regular drinking in middle age: effect on major coronary heart disease events and mortality. Heart 2002;87:32–36.
57. Simons LA, McCallum J, Friedlander Y, Ortiz M, Simons J. Moderate alcohol intake is associated with survival in the elderly: the Dubbo Study. Med J Aust 2000;173:121–124.
58. Thompson A, Temple NJ. Ethics, Medical Research, and Medicine: Commercialization Versus Social Justice and Environmentalism. Kluwer Academic Publishers, Dordrecht, the Netherlands, 2001, pp. 95–116.
59. Colhoun H, Ben-Shlomo Y, Dong W, Bost L, Marmot M. Ecological analysis of collectivity of alcohol consumption in England: importance of average drinker. BMJ 1997;314:1164–1168.

3 The French Paradox

Mechanisms of Action of Nonalcoholic Wine Components on Cardiovascular Disease

Rosemary L. Walzem and J. Bruce German

1. THE FRENCH PARADOX

Epidemiologic studies of populations in most developed countries show that dietary intakes of high amounts of cholesterol, saturated fat, total fat, and calories are associated positively with mortality from cardiovascular disease (CVD) *(1)*. In France, a paradoxical epidemiological situation was identified because despite high intakes of saturated fat and high serum cholesterol concentrations, mortality from heart attacks was only one third of the average in other Western countries. This low incidence of CVD mortality, despite consumption of dietary fats and possession of blood lipid profiles that would predict otherwise, has become known popularly as the "French Paradox" *(2)*.

The French Paradox was identified during a period of rapid progress in CVD research. Scientists soon speculated that nonalcoholic compounds (NAC) of wine were actively protective against CVD *(3–5)*. The alcoholic component of wine has several health effects and is discussed in specific detail in Chapter 2 by Rimm and Temple.

Several physiological processes were initially identified as beneficially responsive to wine NAC, including various antioxidant, and antiaggregatory or vasorelaxing mechanisms *(3–6)*. This scientific grounding for health claims was largely responsible for the 44% increase in red wine sales in the United States after the original broadcast report of the French Paradox in 1991 *(7,8)*. By 1997, United States consumers drank 7.3 gal of all types of wine per capita per year and ranked 36th worldwide in per capita consumption *(9)*. France ranked number two in per capita wine consumption, averaging 15.9 gal/yr *(9)* or one and a half 750-mL bottles of wine per week. Studies involving wine NAC continue to expand as more is learned about CVD mechanisms, and indeed, in 1998, certain mechanisms of action were proposed that are distinct from those originally identified during the 1980s and early 1990s *(10)*.

From: *Beverages in Nutrition and Health*
Edited by: T. Wilson and N. J. Temple © Humana Press Inc., Totowa, NJ

This chapter provides limited compositional information for different types of wine. More exhaustive reviews on the effects of cultivation and processing techniques on wine NAC are available *(11–13)* and should be consulted to completely appreciate these aspects of wine quality development. The research portfolio on wine and CVD protection assembled to date includes chemical, in vitro, ex vivo, and in vivo animal and clinical studies. Each type of data has its strengths and weaknesses, and no one test is adequate to describe the biological effects of wine on human health. Therefore, we present key or recent studies that provide evidence for protective effects of several wine NAC against CVD, as well as describe the limitations in data and methodology that prevent our complete understanding of the relationships between wine and CVD pathogenesis. Moreover, efforts by growers, producers, or marketing agents to make "extra healthy" wine must critically consider the role of the spectrum of phytochemicals on the color and organoleptic properties of wine. These aspects may be connected to a singular feature of the epidemiology of wine, namely that benefits observed epidemiologically are associated with consumers freely choosing to drink wine in an open food and beverage marketplace. Thus, any change in composition must be considered for the broad impact that it might have on the value that each consumer finds in a truly beautiful and delicious glass of wine with regard to their decisions on how and why to continue to consume it.

2. ACTIVE COMPONENTS OF WINE AND MECHANISMS OF ACTION

2.1. Active Components

General chemical compositions of red and white wines were recently tabulated in detail *(1)*. *See* Table 1 for an abbreviated summary. Wine NAC, currently believed to possess CVD protective effects, include phenolic compounds *(5,12,14)*, and nonphenolic components (e.g., betaine) *(15)*. Phenolics are organic compounds containing one or more hydroxyl groups attached to an aromatic or a carbon ring and are classified into two groups: the flavonoids and the nonflavonoids (Fig. 1). Nonflavonoid phenolic compound classes include hydroxybenzoic acids, hydroxycinnamic acids, and stilbenes. Flavonoid compound classes include flavonols, flavanols, and anthocyanins. Plants metabolize the amino acid phenylalanine via the phenylpropanoid pathway to synthesize disparate phenolic compounds (Fig. 2).

The concentration of compounds in source grapes is influenced by environmental and horticultural practices *(11)* as well as by plant genetics. The betaine and glycerol content of wine relate to vintification techniques more than to grape constituents *(16)*. After vintification, polymeric aggregation gives rise to the viniferins (potent antifungal agents) and procyanidins (strong, in vitro antioxidants that also inhibit platelet aggregation) (Fig. 1). The environmental factors with the greatest influence on grape phytochemical content and composition are the availability of sunlight and water. Sunlight stimulates phytochemical synthesis as many of these compounds are protective for the berry. Other environmental factors can also alter berry phytochemical content. The stilbene resveratrol is a phytoalexin, so its synthesis increases as part of the plant's defense against fungal attack. Water application can also alter total phytochemical content. For example, vines watered after the onset of ripening show decreased total phenolic content, probably through dilution. Overproduction *per se*, leaving too many berries on the vine, also results in lower total phenolics and an inferior spectrum of phenolics for color and flavor.

Table 1
Nonalcoholic Wine Components

Component	Red wine (mg/L)	Nonphytochemical (g/L)	White wine (mg/L)
Total phenols and phenolic acids	1200 (900–2500)[a]		200 (190–290)
Nonflavonoid[b]	240–500		160–260
Flavonoids, total[b]	750–1060		25–30
Flavonoids, anthocyanin[b,c]	281 (20–500)		0
Water		800–900	
Carbohydrate[d]		<1–200	
Glycerol[e]		3–14	
Betaine: single value from ref. *12*		0.010–0.011	
Organic acids:		3–11	
tartaric, lactic, succinic, acetic,			
p-hydroxyglutaric, galacturonic,			
amino, malic, citric, fumaric, oxalic,			
α-ketoglutaric, aconic, citra-malic,			
malonic, pyrorocemic, pantothenic.			
Nitrogenous compounds		0.1–0.9	
Minerals[f]		1.5–4.0	

[a] Tabular values summarized from ref. *1*. Mean values were calculated from literature reports; the range of values contributing to the mean is in parentheses.

[b] *See* Fig. 1 for structural variants.

[c] Anthocyanins impart a red color to wine. Includes 3-monoglucosides of aglycone forms.

[d] Concentration varies with style of wine—dry (low carbohydrate) or sweet (high carbohydrate). Dessert wines are the sweetest and contain 140–240 g sugar/L; in contrast, a dry red might contain 2.5 g sugar/L. Residual sugar may appear on the label.

[e] Glycerol imparts mouthfeel to a wine. A dry white wine contains approx 5 g glycerol/L.

[f] Varies with location of vineyard and equipment used in winemaking.

Red and white wines are prepared using different methods. There is epidemiologic evidence that red wine offers greater protection than white wine, beer, or spirits *(17,18)*. White wine is not fermented on the skin as is red wine; as a result, red wine has a total phenolic content 6- to 12-fold greater than that of white wine and is more efficient at protecting low-density lipoprotein (LDL) from oxidation in vitro *(19)*. The fractional composition of red and white wine NAC differ *(20)*; red wine contains some NAC that are not in white wine and those compounds contribute to its antioxidant properties *(21)*. However, when corrections for concentration differences are made, white wines— *tested on a phenol-equivalent molar basis*—have an antioxidant capability similar to red wines *(22)*. For these reasons it is unlikely that white wine—*consumed on an equal-volume basis*—would ever have an equivalent effect to red wine in concentration-dependent wine NAC bioactivities, although nontraditional white wine preparations might allow for equivalence *(23)*. White wine provides similar amounts of alcohol as red wine, and if consumed in regular moderate amounts in conjunction with an otherwise phytochemical-rich diet, its actions may be indistinguishable from those of regular moderate red wine consumption in epidemiologic studies *(24)*.

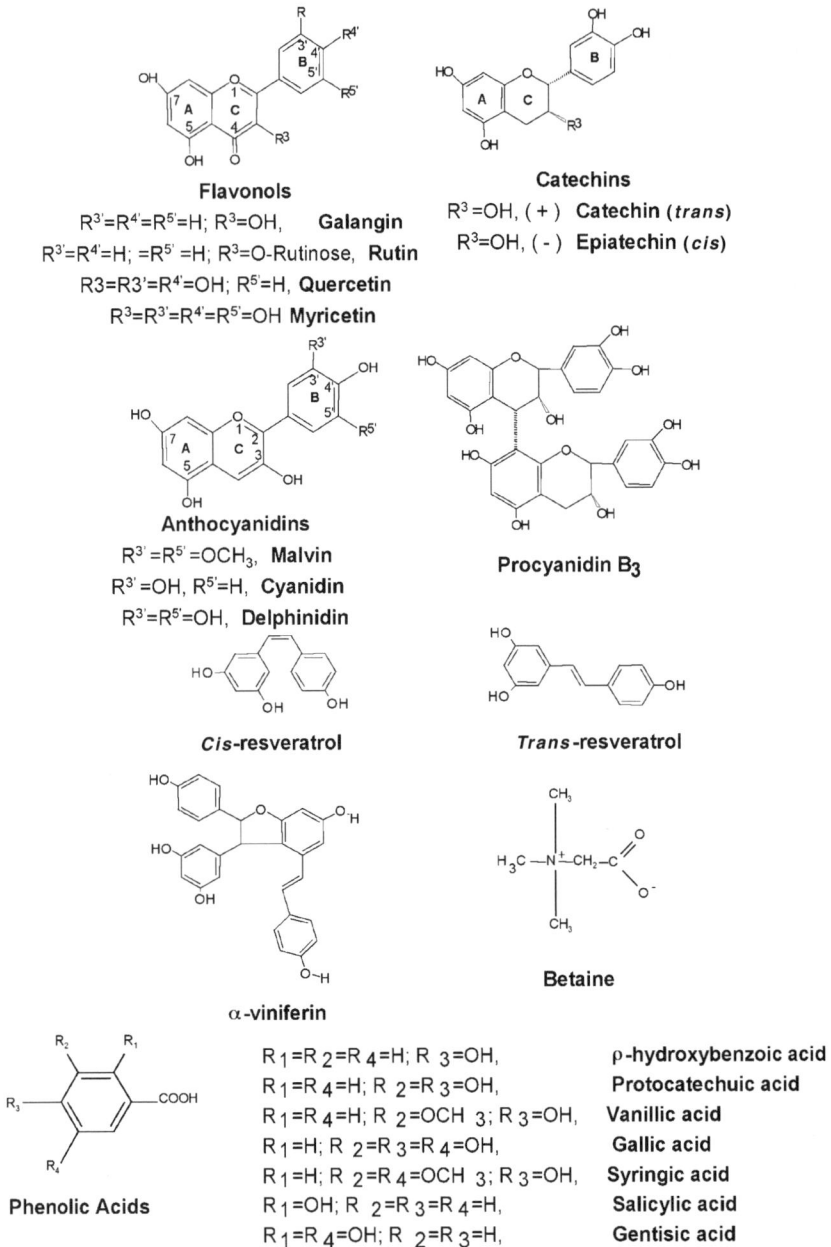

Fig. 1. Generalized structures for flavonoid and nonflavonoid phytochemicals found in wine.

At present, there is a vastly superior body of knowledge on the effects of plant genetics, cultivation, harvesting, and vintification on wine NAC and the relationship of those compounds to wine quality and stability than there is on the relationships to various biological activities. The compositional measurements needed to improve wine quality and stability differ somewhat from those that seek to determine bioactivities and mechanism of action. As a result, more detailed compositional information is needed for all types of wine.

Shikimic acid Pathway

↓

L-Phenylalanine
                                      Psoralin

↓ *PAL**   *furanoncoumarins*

trans-Cinnamic acid

Ferulic acid   ↓   ↑ + mevalonate

↑

Caffeic acid ← p-Coumaric acid → Coumarin

↓   + 3 malonates

↓

Dihydroflavonol ← Chalcone

↓   ⇅

Flavonol   *Flavanone* → *Flavone*

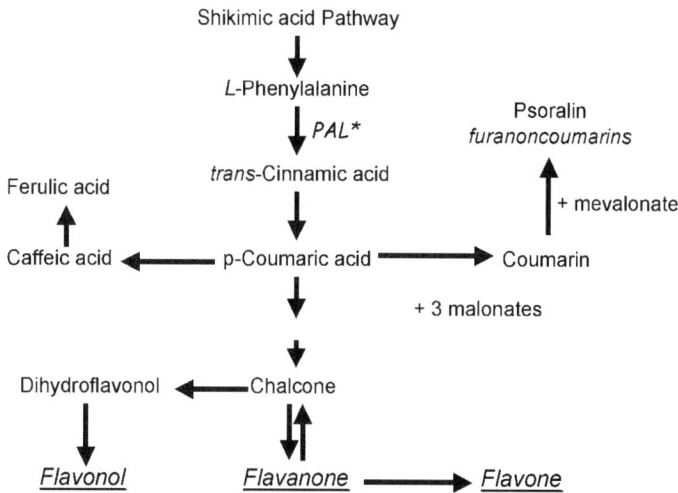

*Phenylalanine: ammonia lyase.

Fig. 2. Polyprenoid pathway of phenolic acid and flavonoid synthesis.

2.2. Antioxidant Capacity of Wine

Early epidemiological studies suggested a protective role for antioxidant vitamins (ascorbate and tocopherol) and fiber, in addition to the "classical" deleterious role of dietary cholesterol and saturated fat, in CVD development *(25)*. Antioxidants hold the potential to limit CVD development because many of the steps involved in the formation and progression of arterial lesions result from dysfunction in oxygen use in the body *(1,26)* (Fig. 3). It is now believed that CVD develops as part of the vascular wall's response to injury in the form of damage caused by oxidative compounds that form through the metabolic activities of the body itself *(1,27)*. How and when injury occurs remains highly debatable, but multiple mechanisms are most likely. It is for this reason that the disparate array of wine NAC may be particularly effective: each molecule may influence an individual mechanism to a greater or lesser extent, but a complex spectrum of compounds may net a "best effect" on several mechanisms simultaneously. It is also important to recognize that the damage from these various mechanisms must occur nearly constantly for lesions to progress in size and complexity as normal defense and repair mechanisms act continuously to maintain vascular wall health.

Among otherwise healthy individuals, a primary mechanism leading to vascular wall damage is believed to be delayed clearance of lipoproteins, such as LDL, and the metabolic responses that occur as a consequence *(27–29)*. Delays in LDL-type lipoprotein clearance are believed to underlie lipoprotein retention in the subendothelial space, a region of the vascular wall where many oxidizing metabolites accumulate and can damage susceptible lipoproteins. Damaged or "oxidized" LDLs provoke defense and repair responses that remove them from the vascular wall, thereby promoting cholesterol accumulation in the arterial wall *(30)*. As part of this response, monocytes migrate into the subendothelial space and become macrophages that engulf oxidized LDL. Possibly, this process can occur at some tolerable level at or below which no vascular lesions form.

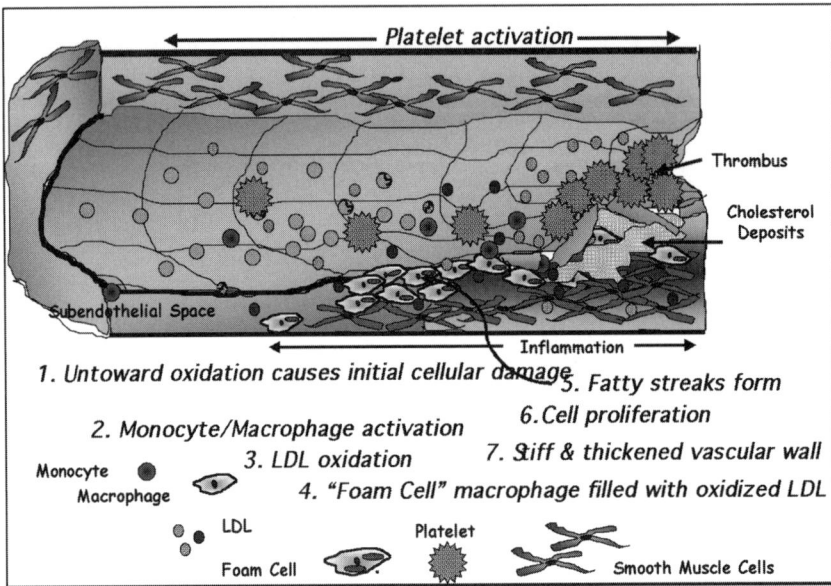

Fig. 3. Key steps in atherosclerotic damage of an artery.

However, above that putative threshold, the system becomes overwhelmed and macrophages become engorged with oxidized LDL-type lipoproteins to become what is termed "foam cells." If progression is not halted, the body finds itself unable to remove the foam cells through reverse cholesterol transport process in high-density lipoprotein (HDL) particles, and a fatty streak forms *(30)*. Again, if the insults continue and fat (primarily cholesteryl esters) continues to accumulate as foam cells under the endothelial lining of the artery, an elevated lesion (plaque) forms that narrows the lumen of the artery. At this point, metabolism of the cells in the lesion produces many new oxidizing compounds and the cells may die by necrosis; as a result, those compounds may be widely disseminated, causing further damage to the vascular wall *(31)*. This unrelenting attack causes numerous changes in the functioning of all cell types present in the vascular wall, and, as a result, it becomes progressively thicker, less compliant, and develops a narrower lumen. Ultimately, the fibrous cap of material covering the plaque can rupture and release cholesterol and oxidized lipids into the bloodstream, which in turn causes blood clotting (thrombus formation) that can occlude the vessel, causing ischemia and death in the surrounding tissue *(32)*.

Some of the factors influencing CVD processes are believed to occur immediately after eating *(33)*. Therefore, antioxidant food components that are available when an individual eats hold the potential to provide highly effective protection. The polyphenolic compounds naturally present in vegetables, fruits, and beverages, such as wine and tea, can act as antioxidants in various in vitro systems. Diets rich in phytochemicals can increase circulating concentrations of phytochemicals *(34,35)*. It was suggested that when regularly consumed, the general antioxidant actions of dietary polyphenols from several sources partially account for the varying risk of death from CVD in elderly men *(14)*. Wine, particularly red wine, represents a concentrated and storage-stable source of dietary phenolic acids and polyphenols.

Dietary antioxidants, including wine NAC, act at nearly every step of CVD development and participate in the body's antioxidant defense system. Wine NAC inhibit LDL oxidation caused by macrophages and other cell types *(36)* and inhibit foam cell formation in vitro *(37)*. Other in vitro studies have shown that the flavonoid (+)-catechin (Fig. 1) and red wines rich in (+)-catechin effectively prevent oxidation of vitamin E in plasma. Carbonneau et al. *(38)* reported that the antioxidant capacity of plasma and the vitamin E content of LDL increases with ingestion of red wine polyphenolics by human subjects consuming low but adequate amounts of vitamins C and E. Such results support the concept that wine NAC can contribute to the antioxidant status of human plasma *(39)*.

Considerable efforts have been expended to identify and characterize a single phenolic constituent of grapes and/or red wine as the active component responsible for any and all CVD-protective benefits. Results suggest that the logic of this pursuit is flawed. CVD has a multifactorial etiology, and effective dietary prevention is likely to be best accomplished by the summed effects of multiple beneficial components that act through multiple and various mechanisms *(1)*. Numerous natural antioxidants are present in grapes and the wines made from them, and it is likely that this disparate spectrum of compounds is a particular strength of wine. The ability of different wine varieties to act as free-radical scavenging antioxidants in vitro varies as a function of total phenolic acid and polyphenol content *(20)* and cannot be attributed to a single constituent. Flavonols (e.g., quercetin) were suggested as major contributors to the antioxidant potential of red wines *(40)* but are probably present in insufficient quantities to be major contributors to their total antioxidant capacity *(41,42)*. The same is true for resveratrol *(20, 43–46)*. It was also argued *(47)* that the antioxidant effect of alcoholic beverages in general is connected to the contents of proanthocyanidins, epicatechin, and ferulic acid. However, recent analysis of 16 red wines *(48,49)* reconfirmed that the widely differing antioxidant capacities of individual wines parallel total phenolic content *(20)*.

There is often a failure to marry information on food composition and molecule bioavailability in the area of phytochemical research. This lack of knowledge can lead to unreal expectations of benefit and, in some cases, potentially unsafe situations. This lack of safety is particularly true when compound concentrations employed in vitro are greater than what are possible through consumption of foods and beverages in the amounts suggested in epidemiologic studies associated with health benefit. Use of physiologically irrelevant concentrations within in vitro assays is common in studies with resveratrol (3,4',5-trihydroxystilbene; Fig. 1) *(50)*. Resveratrol exhibits many of the activities through which other polyphenols are believed to confer cardiovascular benefit *(51)*. However, the concentrations and chemical forms used in these tests to demonstrate activity were not always physiologically relevant *(4,52–57)*. Resveratrol was also suggested to limit CVD by inhibiting endogenous cholesterol biosynthesis *(58)*. However, a sufficient resveratrol concentration is unlikely to be achievable through diet alone. In fact, if a sufficiently high concentration were achieved, it would inhibit a key drug-metabolizing enzyme, CYP3A4, based on observations using a different model system *(59)*. Inhibition of CYP3A4, a member of the P450 superfamily, by grapefruit phytochemicals is known to provoke adverse drug effects *(60)*, and so limit other health benefits that resveratrol might provide. These observations are not unexpected as many of the anticarcinogenic effects of phytochemicals are thought to be mediated through altered P450 carcinogen activation

(60). However, the observations remind us that humans and animals employ several complex and highly integrated chemical and enzymatic systems to sustain life. As such, ingested phytochemicals cannot be assumed to interact exclusively with the system indicated by in vitro studies. Therefore, individual phytochemicals might have different effects in the whole animal than would be predicted by in vitro data. Resveratrol again provides a case in point because atherosclerosis was accelerated in hypercholesterolemic rabbits supplemented with the compound *(61)*.

Observations such as these emphasize how critical it is to: (1) conduct in vitro tests at physiologically relevant concentrations of chemical forms present in foods before claiming effects relevant to human health, and (2) appreciate that individual effects studied in model systems may not adequately describe the total effect of a phytochemical on a whole animal. We are still at an early stage of understanding how individual phytochemicals—let alone the complex phytochemical mixtures presented through diets rich in plant materials—interact with overall diet composition, environment, and physiological state to produce biological effects. It is also appropriate to recall that many phytochemicals currently being investigated for potential health benefit have also been studied in connection with their toxic potential *(62)*.

If in vitro antioxidant actions relate to protective activities in vivo, then wine NAC could reduce the risk of CVD. Disease indices in animal models of CVD improve when wine NAC are included in the diet at physiological concentrations *(63–72)*. However, human trials on the antioxidant effects of polyphenolic-rich beverages, such as red wine, fruit juice, or tea, have provided inconclusive or contradictory results *(73)*. Lack of consensus whether phenolics exert biological effects by altering oxidation is due in part to the limited availability of validated measures of biologically relevant oxidative targets. As a result, measurements such as one termed "total antioxidant capacity" are often used in human studies. This nonspecific assay strategy measures the chemical potential of plasma to decrease oxidation of an indicator molecule. No information is obtained about individual wine NAC molecules *per se*, so this measure cannot be used alone to determine the mechanisms of wine NAC action. The test does serve as a crude indicator of whether ingested materials influence plasma redox chemistry *(74)*. Importantly, total antioxidant capacity fails to show proportionality to the amounts of polyphenols ingested, and the measure is generally unable to describe the complex interplay of biological redox systems that operate in vivo *(75,76)*. Several technical and methodological limitations are known *(38,77–80)*. An integrated review is available *(1)*.

Design of unequivocal experiments is, in many cases, limited by incomplete knowledge regarding the variables affected by wine consumption *(81,82)*. Changes in concentrations of specific redox-active chemicals may correlate better with transient oxidative events occurring during the postprandial period. Acute meal-related events may have a complex relationship to long-term processes such as vasorelaxation or vascular inflammation that could also be influenced by wine. Wine NAC may produce chronic or systematic effects on cells or tissues that reduce oxidant production or alter lipoprotein metabolism to enhance clearance rates, stabilize HDL-linked antioxidant enzymes, or alter tissue-lipid exchange rates. Although not acting directly during the postprandial period, such systemic actions could lead to lower average meal-related oxidant formation or limit other atherosclerosis-promoting processes. Indeed, wine NAC are likely to operate as both general chemical reductants/antioxidants and systemic modifiers of metabolism. A similar dichotomy in biological effects is well known for essential nutrients, such as ascorbic acid, which has nonspecific reducing actions in several systems and specific actions in enzymatic hydroxylation *(83)*. Only time and additional research will reveal the relative importance of each mechanism of wine polyphenol action and its overall physiological effect. As these actions and relationships are discovered, it will become possible to model disease processes under various dietary patterns *(27)*.

2.3. Effect of Wine on Blood Clotting/Platelet Aggregation

Maintaining blood in a liquid state while also retaining the ability to rapidly transform it into a solid clot is a remarkable physiological ability. This ability leads to platelet aggregation and clot formation only when a clot is needed; inappropriate clot formation can lead to thrombus formation, including myocardial infarction or stroke. Studies in humans *(84)* and animal models *(68,85)* show that grapes and wine contain compounds that limit platelet aggregation and blood clotting in several ways, including modulation of platelet cAMP levels *(86)*, phospholipase C-signaling *(87)*, and cytokine production *(88)*. NAC may also reduce clotting by increasing the local production of nitric oxide that inhibits platelet aggregation *(84)*.

Intermittent heavy alcohol consumption causes decreased platelet-derived nitric oxide release and as a result platelet hyperaggregability. This inappropriate clotting phenomenon is termed "platelet rebound" and is associated with risk of sudden death and acute nonfatal cardiac events *(6)*. Platelet rebound in humans was prevented when red wine was the alcohol abused *(65)*. The biologic activity of wine NAC in this protective effect was confirmed in animals by addition of grape phenolics to alcohol *(89)*. However, red wine NAC did not protect against binge-associated impairments in fibrinolytic (clot destroying) activity *(90)*, reemphasizing the importance of avoiding binge drinking. It is often assumed that other aspects of a typical Western diet promote clotting *(91)*. Therefore, the anticlotting activity of wine NAC is believed to be of net benefit in populations consuming Western-type diets. Clearly, this may not be the case for all individuals.

Ex vivo studies have not produced a unified explanation for the antiplatelet aggregation actions of wine. To do so, study designs must control for whether alcohol or nonalcoholic components are responsible for the antiaggregatory effects and assign fractional activities or synergies as they occur. Moreover, synergism among wine NAC and other dietary components has been poorly studied but could influence CVD protective effects of wine. Special care must therefore be taken to account for variation and confounding effects of prior diet in humans.

A recent study with 20 patients with type 2 diabetes used liquid formula feeding to control prior diet *(92)*. In that study, 300 mL of red wine minimized the effect of meal-induced oxidative stress and reduced associated increases in plasma thrombotic indices (levels of prothrombin fragments 1 + 2 and activated factor VII) and susceptibility of LDL to in vitro oxidation. Separate studies showed that drinking one to two cups of purple grape juice daily for a week decreased ex vivo platelet aggregation by an average of 77% *(93)*. Orange juice and grapefruit juice were also tested but had only one third the total polyphenolic content of purple grape juice and did not affect platelet aggregation.

Despite the lack of explicit knowledge of the mechanisms responsible or doses required for the effects, polyphenols consistently exhibit antiaggregative actions. The significant inhibition of platelet aggregation by wine and wine NAC in particular can partially explain the protective effect of red wine against CVD. Clearly, physiological activity dose–response effects relative to different types of polyphenols needs further study.

2.4. Effect of Grape Juice and Wine on Vasodilation

Flow-mediated vasodilation indicates the ability of the vascular wall to relax after external constriction. Stiff and incompliant vessels cannot relax effectively, and this incapacity indicates the presence of CVD. Compounds that enhance vasorelaxation often act by enhancing nitric oxide production or its effects, because that molecule is largely responsible for vasorelaxation of smooth muscle in the vascular wall. Wine NAC or similar compounds found in purple grape products possess an alcohol-independent ability to cause vasorelaxation in animal models *(69,70,94)* and humans *(95,96)*. These actions are associated with reduced blood pressure in normotensive rats *(94)*. However, vasorelaxation was not observed in coronary microvessels that control blood flow to the heart in a rabbit model *(97)*.

Stanley and Mazier *(98)* extensively reviewed the evidence suggesting that some wines, grape juices, and grape-skin extracts contain vasorelaxant components. Both crude mixtures of wine phenolics and various purified flavonoids consistently modulate the properties of isolated vessels and endothelial cells in culture *(69,99)*. Wine NAC promoted nitric oxide-dependent vasorelaxation in an isolated artery *(69)*.

The relationships between antioxidant activity, vasodilation activity, and phenolic content were compared in 16 red wines *(48)*. The total phenol content, measured by both high-performance liquid chromatography (HPLC) and colorimetry, correlated with the antioxidant *(48,100)* and vasodilation activities *(48)*. The antioxidant activity was best associated with total phenols and flavonoid subclasses. The rank order was not wholly uniform in the two laboratories, and the reasons for this are not apparent. Interestingly, only total phenolic content and total anthocyanin content were correlated with vasodilation activity (Table 2). Thus, it is not possible to say what constitutes a "best" spectrum of compounds, and, indeed, that probably depends on the individual consumer *(101)*.

3. ABSORPTION, CIRCULATION, AND METABOLISM OF WINE COMPOUNDS

Regardless of the mechanism(s) by which the NAC act in vitro, protection in vivo by wine NAC depends on the bioavailability of the disparate molecules in wine and their incorporation into fluids and tissues. There is good evidence that wine NAC are both absorbed and metabolized *(34,35,102,103)*. In fact, it is becoming apparent that wine NAC are rapidly and extensively metabolized into new compounds in the intestine and liver *(104,105)*. Therefore, if wine NAC act in vivo as direct protective molecules, the active protective species are likely to be metabolites of ingested parent molecules. The biological activities of red and white wine NAC metabolites are not well understood, nor are the biological distinctions between wine NAC consumed as wine as opposed to NAC derived from intact grapes or grape juice.

Dose relationships and actual bioactivities among different sources of identical individual phytochemical molecules can develop based on differences in food matrix effects and the response of the body to compounds coingested with phytochemicals. Simply

Table 2

Correlation Coefficients Between Total or Individual Subclasses of the Nonalcoholic
Components of Wine (Wine NAC) and Antioxidant In Vitro or Vasodilation Ex Vivo Activity

Wine NAC	Antioxidant activity in vitro			Vasodilation ex vivo pIC_{50}[a,c]
	ESR[a,c]	$Hydroperoxides$[b,c]	$Hexanal$[b,c]	
Total Folin's phenols	0.96*	0.86*	0.96*	−0.86*
Total HPLC phenols	0.94*	0.63*	0.69*	−0.81*
Gallic acid	0.56*	0.43	0.48*	−0.34
Cinnamates	0.26	0.28	0.29	−0.21
Resveratrols	0.61*	ND	ND	−0.13
Flavan-3-ols	0.60*	0.79*	0.92*	−0.34
Flavonols	0.45	0.69*	0.84*	−0.34
Anthocyanins	0.35	0.79	0.84	−0.53*

[a] See ref. 44 for details of wine sources and phenolic characterization. $N = 19$ wines; *significant correlation coefficient.

[b] See ref. 45 for details of wine sources and phenolic characterization. $N = 16$ wines; *significant correlation coefficient.

[c] ESR, electron spin resonance, Fremy's radicals reduced per L wine × 10^{21}; hydroperoxides (initiation) and hexanal (decomposition) generated during Cu^{2+} initiated oxidation expressed as % inhibition of control sample oxidation.

stated, the effects associated with a single phytochemical compound ingested in isolation may differ from what occurs when the same amount of the same compound is ingested as part of a food, beverage, complex supplement mixture, or meal. Moreover, the effects of wine NAC may not be limited to those compounds themselves but may also include compounds that the body produces in response to a certain level of wine NAC ingestion. For example, Caccetta et al. (102) noted that uric acid, an antioxidant (106) and potentially vasoconstrictive (107) molecule produced in the body, increased in response to ingestion of red wine, phenol-stripped red wine, or dealcoholized red wine. Thus, both alcohol and wine NAC alter metabolic production of CVD-relevant molecules in the body. These effects can be further modified by the foods ingested with wine NAC. Certainly, numerous metabolic and cellular processes that respond to diet can influence LDL oxidation by mechanisms independent of ingested antioxidants (see Section 2.2.) (27). Thus the efficacy of wine NAC may vary depending upon the dietary context in which they are consumed.

As mentioned in Section 2.2 and elsewhere (1), it is likely that one of the strengths of wine as a source of NAC phytochemicals is the complexity and diversity of individual molecular forms that provide both additive and synergistic effects. Serafini et al. (19) also discussed the potential importance of interaction among individual phenolics and between phenolics and other nonphenolics contained in beverages. They pointed out that those mixtures of different phenolics with different redox potentials represent an array of antioxidant compounds that might interact synergistically way. Indeed, there is evidence for this (108). Thus, whereas the total phenolic content correlates with several chemical indices of antioxidant action, it cannot be considered a universal index of in vivo beneficial bioactivity. The extensive postconsumption metabolism of wine NAC phenolics produces metabolites with different antioxidant activities and polarities than the parent compounds, factors that will likely modulate bioactivity. Understanding the actions of individual compounds is requisite but not sufficient to understand the more complex situation evolving from ingestion of phenolic mixtures, such as those present in wine, grapes, or other foods.

4. COMPARATIVE EFFECTS OF GRAPES AND RED AND WHITE WINES ON HEALTH

For some investigators there is controversy about whether there are differences in the potential health effects derived from white and red wines, and specifically whether there are differences between wine and grape juice in their potential to protect against CVD. With respect to the benefits provided by phenolic components from wines, this controversy can only be resolved by determining the bioavailability, bioactivity, and pharmacokinetics of the molecules alone and in combination. The question remains whether wine NAC are identical with respect to bioavailable compounds in unfermented grapes (skin, pulp, and seed) or grape products. If marked differences occur, it must then be determined how important those differences are.

Structural changes occur in phenolics as wine ages (109), and this becomes important when determining the NAC content of aged wines. The pigments initially present in grapes slowly turn into more stable red pigments that are chemically distinct and preclude assumption of identical bioactivities. In contrast, the consumption of grapes or grape products could lead to beneficial effects on human health as a result of the variety and amounts of polyphenols they contain (11), as well as factors such as fiber (110,111) that wine and grape juice do not provide. For example, phenolic extracts from 14 different types of fresh grapes had significant protective actions for human LDL undergoing oxidation in vitro (112). Changes in protective effects for in vitro LDL oxidation when seed crushing and longer extraction times were employed was related to changes in phenolic composition and suggests that chewing seeds could influence the nutritional effect of grape eating. Chemical antioxidant activity has also been related to the phenolic composition of commercial grape juices (113). On the basis of the same total phenolic concentration, the antioxidant activity of grape juices toward LDL oxidation was comparable to that of several red wines. Based on their undiluted total phenolic concentration, however, Concord grape juice and blends of colored grape juices had antioxidant activity comparable to that of the red wines, whereas the white grape juices were less active.

5. CONCLUSION

Will wine consumption continue to be associated with decreased CVD mortality? The breadth of experimental evidence indicates that the positive effects of moderate wine consumption on CVD predominate over the negative. By itself, alcohol in wine can increase HDL cholesterol and inhibit platelet aggregation in vivo. Wine NAC can also improve antioxidant protection, decrease platelet aggregation, and increase vasodilation and through these processes exert positive effects on cardiovascular health. The beneficial effects of red wine should be attributed to the combined effects of several phenolics rather than individual compounds. For this reason, it is currently not possible to say which wine is "best." Recent work suggests that wine effects may be mediated primarily during the postprandial period *(35,92)*, so the traditional pattern of mealtime wine consumption may be important for its maximum health benefit.

Cultures that traditionally drink wine may have other behaviors that directly influence CVD and that are associated with wine consumption. For this reason, although epidemiology has served as an excellent means to generate hypotheses, it also has inherent limitations. For instance, much caution must be exercised before extrapolating to newly wine-drinking populations. Another major limitation of epidemiology is that it provides little mechanistic insight. Care must therefore be extreme for new product formulation so that liability does not develop.

Changes in concentrations of individual molecules or measured antioxidant capacity of plasma after consumption of wine NAC have yet to be related to reduced CVD risk. It is clear that considerable research using validated indices of in vivo oxidant damage are needed to evaluate the nutritional benefits of phytochemical-rich foods or diets. Mechanistic research is essential, especially for phytochemicals for which commercial interests are at stake *(114)*. Nonspecific assays must be considered as screening tools to justify more molecule-specific measurements, and methods for those specific analyses need further improvement. It must be considered highly unlikely that any single assay will accurately reflect the multiplicity of redox biochemistry in human blood and tissues. If the assay is also nonspecific, it will be of questionable clinical utility *(115)*. Therefore, studies generating multiple simultaneous analyses will provide the best mechanistic insight *(116)*. The scientific tools needed to develop this specific information are being developed *(116,117)*.

6. MAIN POINTS FOR PRIMARY AND CLINICAL REVIEW

1. The French Paradox describes the epidemiological relationship between red wine consumption in France and the relatively low incidence of coronary heart disease in that country.
2. Wine nonalcoholic compounds include polyphenolic compounds such as flavonoids, catechins, and cyanidins.
3. These compounds are created by grapes for protection against environmental stressors, such as insects and UV light, and are responsible for the taste and color of wine.
4. These compounds are also responsible for the effects of wine on lipid profile, antioxidant capacity, blood clotting process, and vasodilation.
5. Relative to red wine and fresh grapes, white wines generally contains lesser amounts of the nonalcoholic compounds thought to be protective against heart disease.

REFERENCES

1. German JB, Walzem RL. The health benefits of wine. Ann Rev Nutr 2000;20:561–593.
2. Renaud S, de Lorgeril M. Wine, alcohol, platelets, and the French paradox for coronary heart disease. Lancet 1992;339:1523–1526.
3. Frankel EN, Kanner J, German JB, Parks E, Kinsella JE. Inhibition of oxidation of human low-density lipoprotein by phenolic substances in red wine. Lancet 1993;341:454–457.
4. Frankel EN, Waterhouse AL, Kinsella JE. Inhibition of human LDL oxidation by resveratrol. Lancet 1993;341:1103–1104.
5. Kinsella JE, Frankel EN, German JB. Possible mechanisms for the protective role of antioxidant in wine and plant foods. Food Technol 1993;47:85–89.

6. Kozarevic D, Vojvodic N, Gordon T, Kaelber CT, McGee D, Zukel WJ. Drinking habits and death. The Yugoslavia cardiovascular disease study. Int J Epidemiol 1983;12:145–150.

7. Safer M. The French Paradox. CBS 60 Minutes, November 17, 1991.

8. Shapiro L. To your health? Newsweek, January 22, 1996.

9. Wine Institute. Key facts. Available at website: http//www.wineinstitute.org/communication.statistics/keyfacts_worldpercapitaconsumption.htm. Accessed November 19, 2001.

10. Schramm DD, German JB. Potential effects of flavonoids on the etiology of vascular disease. J Nutr Biochem 1998;9:560–566.

11. Waterhouse AL, Walzem RL. Nutrition of grape phenolics. In: Flavonoids in Health and Disease. vol. 7. Rice-Evans CA, Packer L (eds.). Marcel Dekker, Inc., New York, NY, 1998, pp. 359–385.

12. Soleas GJ, Diamandis EP, Goldberg DM. Wine as a biological fluid: history, production, and role in disease prevention. J Clin Lab Anal 1997;11:287–313.

13. Blanco VZ, Auw JM, Sims CA, O'Keefe SF. Effect of processing on phenolics of wines. In: Process Induced Changes in Food. Shahidi F (ed.). Plenum Press, New York, NY, 1998, pp. 327–340.

14. Hertog MG, Feskens EJ, Hollman PC, Katan MB, Kromhout D. Dietary antioxidant flavonoids and risk of coronary heart disease: the Zutphen Elderly Study. Lancet 1993;342:1007–1011.

15. Mar MH, Zeisel SH. Betaine in wine: answer to the French paradox? Med Hypotheses 1999;53:383–385.

16. Dupuy P. Analytical evidences of sugar added to wine. Ann Nutr Aliment 1978;32:1123–1132.

17. St. Leger AS, Cochrane AL, Moore F. Factors associated with cardiac mortality in developed countries with particular reference to the consumption of wine. Lancet 1979;1:1017–1020.

18. Gronbaek M, Sorensen TI. Alcohol consumption and risk of coronary heart disease. Studies suggest that wine has additional effect to that of ethanol. BMJ 1996;313:365.

19. Serafini M, Laranjinha JAN, Almeida LM, Maiani G. Inhibition of human LDL lipid peroxidation by phenol-rich beverages and their impact on plasma total antioxidant capacity in humans. J Nutr Biochem 2000;11:585–590.

20. Frankel EN, Waterhouse AL, Teissedre PL. Principal phenolic phytochemicals in selected California wines and their antioxidant activity in inhibiting oxidation of human low-density lipoproteins. J Agriculture Food Chem 1995;43:890–894.

21. Fuhrman B, Lavy A, Aviram M. Consumption of red wine with meals reduces the susceptibility of human plasma and low-density lipoprotein to lipid peroxidation. Am J Clin Nutr 1995;61:549–554.

22. Lamuela-Raventos RM, de la Torre-Boronat MC. Beneficial effects of white wines. Drugs Exp Clin Res 1999;25:121–124.

23. Fuhrman B, Volkova N, Suraski A, Aviram M. White wine with red wine-like properties: increased extraction of grape skin polyphenols improves the antioxidant capacity of the derived white wine. J Agriculture Food Chem 2001;49:3164–3168.

24. Klatsky AL, Armstrong MA, Friedman GD. Red wine, white wine, liquor, beer, and risk for coronary artery disease hospitalization. Am J Cardiol 1997;80:416–420.

25. Bolton-Smith C, Woodward M, Smith WC, Tunstall-Pedoe H. Dietary and non-dietary predictors of serum total and HDL-cholesterol in men and women: results from the Scottish Heart Health Study. Int J Epidemiol 1991;20:95–104.

26. German JB, Frankel EN, Waterhouse AL, Hansen RJ, Walzem RL. Wine phenolics and targets of chronic disease. In: Wine Nutritional and Therapeutic Benefits. Watkins T (ed.). American Chemical Society, Washington, DC, 1997, pp. 196–214.

27. Walzem RL, Watkins S, Frankel EN, Hansen RJ, German JB. Older plasma lipoproteins are more susceptible to oxidation: a linking mechanism for the lipid and oxidation theories of atherosclerotic cardiovascular disease. Proc Natl Acad Sci USA 1995;92:7460–7464.

28. Williams KJ, Tabas I. The response-to-retention hypothesis of early atherogenesis. Arterioscler Thromb Vasc Biol 1995;15:551–561.

29. Ross R. The pathogenesis of atherosclerosis: a perspective for the 1990s. Nature 1993;362:801–809.

30. Steinberg D, Parthasarathy S, Carew TE, Khoo JC, Witztum JL. Beyond cholesterol. Modifications of low-density lipoprotein that increase its atherogenicity. N Engl J Med 1989;320:915–924.

31. Navab M, Berliner JA, Watson AD, et al. The Yin and Yang of oxidation in the development of the fatty streak. A review based on the 1994 George Lyman Duff Memorial Lecture. Arterioscler Thromb Vasc Biol 1996;16:831–842.

32. Libby P. Atherosclerosis: the new view. Sci Am 2002;286:46–55.
33. Sattar N, Petrie JR, Jaap AJ. The atherogenic lipoprotein phenotype and vascular endothelial dysfunction. Atherosclerosis 1998;138:229–235.
34. Bell JR, Donovan JL, Wong R, et al. (+)-Catechin in human plasma after ingestion of a single serving of reconstituted red wine. Am J Clin Nutr 2000;71:103–108.
35. Donovan JL, Bell JR, Kasim-Karakas S, et al. Catechin is present as metabolites in human plasma after consumption of red wine. J Nutr 1999;129:1662–1668.
36. de Whalley CV, Rankin SM, Hoult JR, Jessup W, Leake DS. Flavonoids inhibit the oxidative modification of low density lipoproteins by macrophages. Biochem Pharmacol 1990;39:1743–1750.
37. Mangiapane H, Thomson J, Salter A, Brown S, Bell GD, White DA. The inhibition of the oxidation of low density lipoprotein by (+)-catechin, a naturally occurring flavonoid. Biochem Pharmacol 1992; 43:445–450.
38. Carbonneau MA, Leger CL, Monnier L, et al. Supplementation with wine phenolic compounds increases the antioxidant capacity of plasma and vitamin E of low-density lipoprotein without changing the lipoprotein Cu(2+)-oxidizability: possible explanation by phenolic location. Eur J Clin Nutr 1997; 51:682–690.
39. Lotito SB, Fraga CG. (+)-Catechin as antioxidant: mechanisms preventing human plasma oxidation and activity in red wines. Biofactors 1999;10:125–130.
40. Maxwell SRJ. Wine antioxidants and their impact on antioxidant function in vivo. Watkins T (ed.), American Chemical Society, Washington, DC, 1997, pp. 150–165.
41. de Vries JHM, Holloman PCH, van Amersfoort I, Olthof MR, Katan MB. Red wine is a poor source of bioavailable flavonols in men. J Nutr 2001;131:745–748.
42. Gardner PT, McPhail DB, Crozier A, Duthie GG. Electron spin resonance spectroscopic assessment of the contribution of quercetin and other flavonols to the antioxidant capacity of red wines. J Sci Food Agriculture 1999;79:1004–1011.
43. Goldberg DM, Karumanchiri A, Tsang E, Soleas GJ. Catechin and epicatechin concentrations of red wines: regional and cultivar-related differences. American Journal of Enology Viticulture 1998;49: 317–322.
44. Goldberg D, Karumanchiri A, Yan J, et al. A global survey of trans-resveratrol concentration in commercial wines. American Journal of Enology Viticulture 1995;46:159–165.
45. McDonald MS, Hughes M, Burns J, Lean ME, Matthews D, Crozier A. Survey of the free and conjugated myricetin and quercetin content of red wines of different geographical origins. J Agriculture Food Chem 1998;46:368–375.
46. Lamuela-Raventos R, Waterhouse AL. Occurrence of resveratrol in selected California wines by a new HPLC method. J Agriculture Food Chem 1993;41:521–523.
47. Gorinstein S. Comments on "Potential Explanation for the French Paradox." Nutr Res 1999;19: 1599–1602.
48. Burns J, Gardner PT, O'Neil J, et al. Relationship among antioxidant activity, vasodilation capacity, and phenolic content of red wines. J Agriculture Food Chem 2000;48:220–230.
49. Sanchez-Moreno C, Satue-Gracia MT, Frankel EN. Antioxidant activity of selected Spanish wines in corn oil emulsions. J Agriculture Food Chem 2000;48:5581–5587.
50. Fremont L. Biological effects of resveratrol. Life Sci 2000;66:663–673.
51. Soleas GJ, Diamandis EP, Goldberg DM. Resveratrol: a molecule whose time has come? And gone? Clin Biochem 1997;30:91–113.
52. Rice-Evans CA, Miller NJ, Bolwell PG, Bramley PM, Pridham JB. The relative antioxidant activities of plant-derived polyphenolic flavonoids. Free Radic Res 1995;22:375–383.
53. Bertelli AA, Giovannini L, Bernini W, et al. Antiplatelet activity of cis-resveratrol. Drugs Exp Clin Res 1996;22:61–63.
54. Schramm D, Pearson D, German JB. Endothelial cell basal PGI, 2 release is stimulated by wine in vitro: one mechanism that may mediate the vasoprotective effects of wine. J Nutr Biochem 1997;8:647–651.
55. Gehm BD, McAndrews JM, Chien PY, Jameson JL. Resveratrol, a polyphenolic compound found in grapes and wine, is an agonist for the estrogen receptor. Proc Natl Acad Sci USA 1997;94:14,138–14,143.
56. Chen CK, Pace-Asciak CR. Vasorelaxing activity of resveratrol and quercetin in isolated rat aorta. Gen Pharmacol 1996;27:363–366.

57. Subbaramaiah K, Chung WJ, Michaluart P, et al. Resveratrol inhibits cyclooxygenase-2 transcription and activity in phorbol ester-treated human mammary epithelial cells. J Biol Chem 1998;273:21,875–21,882.
58. Laden BP, Porter TD. Resveratrol inhibits human squalene monooxygenase. Nutr Res 2001;21:747–753.
59. Chan WK, Delucchi AB. Resveratrol, a red wine constituent, is a mechanism-based inactivator of cytochrome P450 3A4. Life Sci 2000;67:3103–3112.
60. Wilkinson GR. The effects of diet, aging and disease states on presystemic elimination and oral drug bioavailability in humans. Adv Drug Deliv Rev 1997;27:129–159.
61. Wilson T, Knight TJ, Beitz DC, Lewis DS, Engen RL. Resveratrol promotes atherosclerosis in hypercholesterolemic rabbits. Life Sci 1996;59:L15–L21.
62. Singleton VL, Kratzer F. Plant phenolics. In: Committee on Food Protection, Food and Nutrition Board, National Research Council. Toxicants Occurring Naturally in Foods. National Academy of Sciences, Washington, DC, 1973, pp. 309–345.
63. Xu R, Yokoyama WH, Irving D, Rein D, Walzem RL, German JB. Effect of dietary catechin and vitamin E on aortic fatty streak accumulation in hypercholesterolemic hamsters. Atherosclerosis 1998;137:29–36.
64. Aviram M, Fuhrman B. Polyphenolic flavonoids inhibit macrophage-mediated oxidation of LDL and attenuate atherogenesis. Atherosclerosis 1998;137(Suppl):45S–50S.
65. Ruf JC, Berger JL, Renaud S. Platelet rebound effect of alcohol withdrawal and wine drinking in rats. Relation to tannins and lipid peroxidation. Arterioscler Thromb Vasc Biol 1995;15:140–144.
66. Mizutani K, Ikeda K, Kawai Y, Yamori Y. Extract of wine phenolics improves aortic biomechanical properties in stroke-prone spontaneously hypertensive rats (SHRSP). J Nutr Sci Vitaminol (Tokyo) 1999;45:95–106.
67. Hayek T, Fuhrman B, Vaya J, et al. Reduced progression of atherosclerosis in apolipoprotein E-deficient mice following consumption of red wine, or its polyphenols quercetin or catechin, is associated with reduced susceptibility of LDL to oxidation and aggregation. Arterioscler Thromb Vasc Biol 1997; 17:2744–2752.
68. Demrow HS, Slane PR, Folts JD. Administration of wine and grape juice inhibits in vivo platelet activity and thrombosis in stenosed canine coronary arteries. Circulation 1995;91:1182–1188.
69. Andriambeloson E, Kleschyov AL, Muller B, Beretz A, Stoclet JC, Andriantsitohaina R. Nitric oxide production and endothelium-dependent vasorelaxation induced by wine polyphenols in rat aorta. Br J Pharmacol 1997;120:1053–1058.
70. Cishek MB, Galloway MT, Karim M, German JB, Kappagoda CT. Effect of red wine on endothelium-dependent relaxation in rabbits. Clin Sci (Lond) 1997;93:507–511.
71. da Luz PL, Serrano Junior CV, Chacra AP, et al. The effect of red wine on experimental atherosclerosis: lipid-independent protection. Exp Mol Pathol 1999;65:150–159.
72. Wollny T, Aiello L, Di Tommaso D, Bellavia V, Rotilio D, Donati MB, et al. Modulation of haemostatic function and prevention of experimental thrombosis by red wine in rats: a role for increased nitric oxide production. Br J Pharmacol 1999;127:747–755.
73. Morton LW, Abu-Amsha Caccetta R, Puddey IB, Croft KD. Chemistry and biological effects of dietary phenolic compounds: relevance to cardiovascular disease. Clin Exp Pharmacol Physiol 2000; 27:152–159.
74. Serafini M, Maiani G, Ferro-Luzzi A. Alcohol-free red wine enhances plasma antioxidant capacity in humans. J Nutr 1998;128:1003–1007.
75. van der Gaag MS, van den Berg R, van den Berg H, Schaafsma G, Hendriks HF. Moderate consumption of beer, red wine and spirits has counteracting effects on plasma antioxidants in middle-aged men. Eur J Clin Nutr 2000;54:586–591.
76. Duthie GG, Pedersen MW, Gardner PT, et al. The effect of whisky and wine consumption on total phenol content and antioxidant capacity of plasma from healthy volunteers. Eur J Clin Nutr 1998;52: 733–736.
77. Ivanov V, Carr AC, Frei B. Red wine antioxidants bind to human lipoproteins and protect them from metal ion-dependent and -independent oxidation. J Agriculture Food Chem 2001;49:4442–4449.
78. de Rijke YB, Demacker PN, Assen NA, Sloots LM, Katan MB, Stalenhoef AF. Red wine consumption does not affect oxidizability of low-density lipoproteins in volunteers. Am J Clin Nutr 1996;63: 329–334.
79. Nigdikar SV, Williams NR, Griffin BA, Howard AN. Consumption of red wine polyphenols reduces the susceptibility of low-density lipoproteins to oxidation in vivo. Am J Clin Nutr 1998;68:258–265.

80. Schwarz K, Huang SW, German JB, Tiersch B, Hartmann J, Frankel EN. Activities of antioxidants are affected by colloidal properties of oil-in-water and water-in-oil emulsions and bulk oils. J Agriculture Food Chem 2000;48:4874–4882.

81. Agewall S, Wright S, Doughty RN, Whalley GA, Duxbury M, Sharpe N. Does a glass of red wine improve endothelial function? Eur Heart J 2000;21:74–78.

82. Maxwell S, Thorpe G. Impact of red wine on antioxidant status in vivo. Eur Heart J 2000;21:1482–1483.

83. Combs GFJ. The Vitamins: Fundamental Aspects in Nutrition and Health. Academic Press, New York, NY, 1998.

84. Freedman JE, Parker C 3rd, Li L, et al. Select flavonoids and whole juice from purple grapes inhibit platelet function and enhance nitric oxide release. Circulation 2001;103:2792–2798.

85. Osman HE, Maalej N, Shanmuganayagam D, Folts JD. Grape juice but not orange or grapefruit juice inhibits platelet activity in dogs and monkeys. J Nutr 1998;128:2307–2312.

86. Russo P, Tedesco I, Russo M, Russo GL, Venezia A, Cicala C. Effects of de-alcoholated red wine and its phenolic fractions on platelet aggregation. Nutr Metab Cardiovasc Dis 2001;11:25–29.

87. Pignatelli P, Pulcinelli FM, Celestini A, et al. The flavonoids quercetin and catechin synergistically inhibit platelet function by antagonizing the intracellular production of hydrogen peroxide. Am J Clin Nutr 2000;72:1150–1155.

88. Johansen KM, Skorpe S, Olsen JO, Osterud B. The effect of red wine on the fibrinolytic system and the cellular activation reactions before and after exercise. Thromb Res 1999;96:355–363.

89. Ruf JC. Wine and polyphenols related to platelet aggregation and atherothrombosis. Drugs Exp Clin Res 1999;25:125–131.

90. van de Wiel A, van Golde PM, Kraaijenhagen RJ, von dem Borne PA, Bouma BN, Hart HC. Acute inhibitory effect of alcohol on fibrinolysis. Eur J Clin Invest 2001;31:164–170.

91. Simopoulos AP. n-3 fatty acids and human health: defining strategies for public policy. Lipids 2001;36(Suppl):83S–89S.

92. Ceriello A, Bortolotti N, Motz E, et al. Red wine protects diabetic patients from meal-induced oxidative stress and thrombosis activation: a pleasant approach to the prevention of cardiovascular disease in diabetes. Eur J Clin Invest 2001;31:322–328.

93. Keevil JG, Osman HE, Reed JD, Folts JD. Grape juice, but not orange juice or grapefruit juice, inhibits human platelet aggregation. J Nutr 2000;130:53–56.

94. Diebolt M, Bucher B, Andriantsitohaina R. Wine polyphenols decrease blood pressure, improve NO vasodilatation, and induce gene expression. Hypertension 2001;38:159–165.

95. Flesch M, Schwarz A, Bohm M. Effects of red and white wine on endothelium-dependent vasorelaxation of rat aorta and human coronary arteries. Am J Physiol 1998;275:H1183–H1190.

96. Hashimoto M, Kim S, Eto M, et al. Effect of acute intake of red wine on flow-mediated vasodilatation of the brachial artery. Am J Cardiol 2001;88:1457–1460.

97. Rendig SV, Symons JD, Longhurst JC, Amsterdam EA. Effects of red wine, alcohol, and quercetin on coronary resistance and conductance arteries. J Cardiovasc Pharmacol 2001;38:219–227.

98. Stanley LL, Mazier MJP. Potential explanations for the French paradox. Nutr Res 1999;19:3–15.

99. Hsieh TC, Juan G, Darzynkiewicz Z, Wu JM. Resveratrol increases nitric oxide synthase, induces accumulation of p53 and p21 (WAF1/CIP1), and suppresses cultured bovine pulmonary artery endothelial cell proliferation by perturbing progression through S and G2. Cancer Res 1999;59:2596–2601.

100. Satue-Gracia MT, Andres-Lacueva C, Lamuela-Raventos RM, Frankel EN. Spanish sparkling wines (Cavas) as inhibitors of in vitro human low-density lipoprotein oxidation. J Agriculture Food Chem 1999;47:2198–2202.

101. Watkins SM, Hammock BD, Newman JW, German JB. Individual metabolism should guide agriculture toward foods for improved health and nutrition. Am J Clin Nutr 2001;74:283–286.

102. Caccetta RA, Croft KD, Beilin LJ, Puddey IB. Ingestion of red wine significantly increases plasma phenolic acid concentrations but does not acutely affect ex vivo lipoprotein oxidizability. Am J Clin Nutr 2000;71:67–74.

103. Miyagi Y, Miwa K, Inoue H. Inhibition of human low-density lipoprotein oxidation by flavonoids in red wine and grape juice. Am J Cardiol 1997;80:1627–1631.

104. Donovan JL, Crespy V, Manach C, et al. Catechin is metabolized by both the small intestine and liver of rats. J Nutr 2001;131:1753–1757.

105. Andlauer W, Kolb J, Siebert K, Furst P. Assessment of resveratrol bioavailability in the perfused small intestine of the rat. Drugs Exp Clin Res 2000;26:47–55.
106. Frei B, Stocker R, Ames BN. Antioxidant defenses and lipid peroxidation in human blood plasma. Proc Natl Acad Sci USA 1988;85:9748–9752.
107. Anker SD, Leyva F, Poole-Wilson PA, Kox WJ, Stevenson JC, Coats AJ. Relation between serum uric acid and lower limb blood flow in patients with chronic heart failure. Heart 1997;78:39–43.
108. Saucier CT, Waterhouse AL. Synergetic activity of catechin and other antioxidants. J Agriculture Food Chem 1999;47:4491–4494.
109. Brouillard R, George F, Fougerousse A. Polyphenols produced during red wine aging. Biofactors 1997; 6:403–410.
110. Igartuburu JM, Pando E, Rodriguez-Luis F, Gil-Serrano A. Structure of a hemicellulose B fraction in dietary fiber from the seed of grape variety Palomino (*Vitis vinifera* cv. palomino). J Nat Prod 1998;61: 881–886.
111. Bolton RP, Heaton KW, Burroughs LF. The role of dietary fiber in satiety, glucose, and insulin: studies with fruit and fruit juice. Am J Clin Nutr 1981;34:211–217.
112. Meyer AS, Yi O-S, Pearson DA, Waterhouse AL, Frankel EN. Inhibition of human low-density lipoprotein oxidation in relation to composition of phenolic antioxidants in grapes (*Vitis vinifera*). J Agriculture Food Chem 1997;45:1638–1643.
113. Frankel EN, Bosanek CA, Meyer AS, Silliman K, Kirk LL. Commercial grape juices inhibit the in vitro oxidation of human low-density lipoproteins. J Agriculture Food Chem 1998;46:834–838.
114. Waterhouse AL, German JB, Walzem RL, Hansen RJ, Kasim-Karakas SE. Is it time for a wine trial? Am J Clin Nutr 1998;68:220–221.
115. Woodford FP, Whitehead TP. Is measuring serum antioxidant capacity clinically useful? Ann Clin Biochem 1998;35:48–56.
116. Roberts M, Geiger W, German JB. The revolution in microanalytic chemistry: a macro-opportunity for clinical nutrition. Am J Clin Nutr 2000;71:434–437.
117. Watkins SM, German JB. Metabolomics and biochemical profiling in drug discovery and development. Curr Opin Mol Ther 2002;4:224–228.

III   HEALTH EFFECTS OF FRUIT
AND TOMATO JUICES

4   Cranberry Juice Effects on Health

Ted Wilson

1. INTRODUCTION

Cranberries (*Vacciunium macrocapron*) for millenia have been a part of the diet of North Americans and used for medicinal purposes in folk medicine *(1)*. Although cranberries are most familiar to consumers in North America, close relatives of the cranberry are also consumed in Northern Europe and Asia. In North America and Europe, cranberries are primarily processed and consumed in the form of cranberry juices, cranberry juice cocktails, and cranberry fruit drinks, with the oldest cranberry juice recipe dating back to 1683 *(1)*. Cranberries have only been cultivated for the last 150 yr; therefore, relative to grapes and other cultivated fruits, there is little genetic diversity *(2)*. The typical annual crop size is approx 500 million pounds, with 60% being used directly in beverages, 35% being processed into sauces and concentrates that are mostly made into beverages, and 5% being consumed fresh *(3)*. Cranberries are popular with consumers because of their bitter-tart taste, and because of their positive implication for health as a functional food, they are one of the first functional foods in America. As a functional food, cranberry juice is associated with protection from urinary tract infections (UTIs). Cranberry juice may also be useful for promoting cardiovascular health and inhibiting cancer development, and suggestions have also been made regarding cranberry applications for improving oral and gastric health.

2. CRANBERRY JUICE CONSUMPTION PREVENTS URINARY TRACT INFECTIONS

2.1. Urinary Tract Infections Represent a Major Health Problem

UTIs occur when bacteria (primarily *Escherichia coli* or *E. coli*) adhere to the uro-epithelial cells that line the bladder, kidney, or urethra and then multiply. Bacterial adhesion to uroepithelial cells requires the production of a set of structures called p-fimbriae on the cell walls of the colonizing bacteria. P-fimbria are proteinaceous fibers that form adhesions to carbohydrates on the surface of uroepithelial cells, thereby allowing the bacteria to adhere. Any bacteria present but unable to adhere to the epithelium are normally flushed out of the urinary tract during urination. Adhesion leads to colonization of the urinary tract epithelium and destruction of the lining of the bladder, as well as

From: *Beverages in Nutrition and Health*
Edited by: T. Wilson and N. J. Temple © Humana Press Inc., Totowa, NJ

inflammation and rupturing of the underlying blood vessels, causing blood in the urine in some cases. The resultant inflammation promotes a painful burning sensation; persistent, untreated UTI can lead to cystitis and pyelonephritis *(4)*, which can ultimately lead to the loss of one or both kidneys.

UTIs are common, with approx 60% of American women being affected in their lifetime *(5)*. Persistent infections often require ongoing treatment with expensive antibiotics that necessitate visits to a physician and immense costs to the health care system. In 1995, there were an estimated 11.3 million women affected, with those requiring prescriptions incurring an estimated cost of $1.6 billion *(5)*. UTIs are most typically found in women but also occur in men. Persons at high risk for developing a UTI include the elderly, those who are parapalegic and quadrapalegic. Folk medicine has long supported the use of cranberry juice for the treatment of UTIs, although the mechanism for this effect has been difficult to determine. Consumption of cranberry juice provides a way for affected persons to cost-effectively treat their disease independently of the health care system.

2.2. Early Hypotheses About Urinary Tract Infection Prevention

There has been much speculation about the mechanism by which cranberry products protect against UTIs. In the early 1900s, Blatherwick *(6,7)* observed that consumption of 300–600 g of cranberry sauce/d could promote short-term changes in urine pH. It was hypothesized that this acidification prevented bacterial colonization of the urinary tract epithelium. Although this was the popular theory, subsequent studies were unable to demonstrate that urinary pH was always acidified postconsumption *(8,9)*. However, because urinary hippuric acid excretion also increased after cranberry consumption, that substance was suggested as being responsible for the protective effects. By the 1960s, it was determined that cranberry juice altered urine pH for only a short time, that the degree of acidification was not sufficient to provide bacteriocidal or bacteriostatic effects, and that neither acidification nor hippuric acid could be the primary mechanism *(10)*.

In 1984, Sabota used *E. coli* isolates from people with UTIs to determine that cranberry juice contains a nondialyzable material that specifically inhibits the expression of the p-fimbria of bacteria, hence preventing their attachment to and colonization of the urinary tract *(11)*. Given the large body of evidence showing that cranberry juice does not modify urine pH and UTI incidence, it is surprising that acidification is still mentioned in current news reports and occasionally still taught as such in universities.

2.3. Cranberry Juice Prevents Urinary Tract Infections

As mentioned, for many years cranberry juice has been a popular choice for the treatment and prevention of UTIs. Nevertheless, the first double-blind human clinical trial confirming the effect of cranberry juice was not published until 1994 *(12)*. In this trial, elderly women were randomized to 300 mL/d of a saccharine-sweetened 27% cranberry beverage or a synthetic placebo drink that was indistinguishable in taste, appearance, and vitamin C content but lacked cranberry juice. Cranberry juice consumption led to significant reductions in the numbers of both bacteria and white blood cells in the urine during the 6-mo study period.

Completion of UTI treatment does not always provide permanent protection from reinfection. UTIs reinfect approximately one third of women within 1 yr of initial treatment *(13)*. A recent Finnish Study of UTI recurrence administered a 50 mL daily dose of a cranberry-lingonberry juice mixture to volunteers from a student health facility and an occupational health center *(14)*. Daily cranberry-lingonberry juice consumption for 6 mo was associated with half the risk of UTI recurrence relative to a control group. These studies demonstrate that science does support folklore with regard to using cranberry juice for the treatment of UTIs.

2.4. Theorized Mechanisms of Action on p-Fimbriae

At maturity, cranberries are bright red and richly pigmented with a class of compounds called anthocyanidins *(2)*. Relative to other fruit, cranberries have a low-sugar content and a relatively high polyphenol *(3,15)*. Because these simple polyphenols and benzoic compounds are typically condensed into polymers with a carbohydrate backbone, their isolation and identification with regard to UTI benefits is difficult.

The polyphenolic content of cranberries is the sum of many different compounds, including flavonoids such as quercetin and myrecetin, proanthocyanidins (condensed tannins), and benzoic acid. The presence of large tannin oligomers called proanthocyanidins in cranberry juice is linked to the ability of cranberry juice to prevent UTIs. Although other fruits and vegetables contain proanthocyandins, only the cranberry and its close relative, the blueberry, have the ability to prevent p-fimbriae expression and bacterial adhesion to uroepithelial cells *(16)*.

Proanthocyanidins are produced in plants as part of their natural defense against pests and give plants a somewhat astringent taste. They are called proanthocyanidins because they can be converted to anthocyanidins when heated in acid. Anthocyanidins are also present in plants and provide pigmentation *(17)*. Cranberry proanthocyanidin extracts have been prepared, and their consumption by mice is associated with their gastrointestinal absorption. Furthermore, the mice then produce urine that prevents *E. coli* from producing p-fimbriae required for uroepithelial adhesion. This resembles the situation that occurs when humans consume cranberry juice *(18)*.

Human pharmacokinetic investigations of proanthocyanidins have not been reported. However, studies in rats of proanthocyanidins derived from grapes demonstrate that these compounds are eliminated in both the urine and feces. Oral studies in mice of proanthocyanidins isolated from hawthorn (*Crataeguc sp.*) demonstrate that they are 87% absorbed within 7 h of administration *(17)*. Pharmacokinetic studies and urinary excretion studies are plagued by the problem created by the extensive metabolism of these compounds in the gut before absorption and in the body after absorption. It is possible that the compound in cranberry juice that is responsible for its biological effect is produced as a result of these modifications.

2.5. Other Bacterial Interactions With Cranberry Juice

Several recent reports have suggested that cranberry juice consumption may also have the capacity to affect bacterial populations outside the urinary tract. Adhesions similar to those produced on the p-fimbria of uropathogenic *E. coli* are also required by bacteria that cause disease in the stomach and mouth. Gastric ulcers are largely caused by *Helicobacter pylori*, which require adhesion to the gastric epithelium for pathogenicity. In vitro studies by Burger et al. suggest that a high molecular weight constituent in cranberry juice inhibits the production of adhesions in *H. pylori* and cranberry juice consumption may help prevent gastric ulcers *(19)*. Cranberries are also believed to promote good gum health *(20)* by preventing bacterial adhesion within the oral epithelium and by preventing dental plaque build-up.

3. POSSIBLE EFFECTS OF CRANBERRIES ON CARDIOVASCULAR DISEASE

The French Paradox popularized the consumption of red wine and Concord grape juice for the prevention of coronary heart disease (CHD) *(21)*, a topic discussed in Chapter 3 by Walzem and German. Grape beverages reduce CHD risk by providing antioxidants to protect low-density lipoprotein (LDL) cholesterol particles from oxidative injury, by providing vasodilators that may open up blood vessels in the heart, and by inhibiting platelet aggregation and blood clotting.

Wine and Concord grape juice consumption is problematic for some people. Consumption of wine is not appropriate for alcoholics and is often not consumed for reasons of religion or of personal preference. In addition, Concord grape juice has a high sugar content (160 kcal/8 oz glass), and this is problematic for those who are diabetic attempting to control their blood glucose. In those who are not diabetic, consuming 4 mL Concord grape juice per kg body weight twice daily, Stein et al. *(22)* observed a nearly threefold increase in fasting insulin levels after 14 d of consumption.

Regularly sweetened cranberry cocktails typically have approx 140 kcal/8 oz. However, the caloric content of pure (100%) cranberry juice is 60 kcal/8 oz, and the calorie content of a popular artificially sweetened/reduced-calorie 30% cranberry juice (Sam's Choice Reduced Calorie Cranberry Juice Cocktail) is 25 kcal/8 oz. Cranberry juice represents a nonalcoholic and low-calorie alternative for reducing CHD risk.

Cranberry juice promotes vasodilation in a manner similar to that associated with red wine and Concord grape juice *(22,23)*. Using rat vessels, we have demonstrated in vitro and in vivo that cranberry juice can vasodilate vessels *(24)* at levels comparable to those of grape products and red wine *(25)*. Vessel diameter and blood flow are largely determined by the production of nitric oxide made by the enzyme nitric oxide synthase in arterial endothelial cells. Like red wine, cranberry juice has the ability to stimulate the endothelium to produce nitric oxide and vasodilate rat aorta that are precontracted with phenylephrine. The contraction is rapidly lost when cranberry juice is administered, and the dilation is lost when the nitric oxide inhibitor L-NAME is administered (Fig. 1). However, human consumption studies of vasodilation using Doppler-ultrasound analysis of blood flow and diameter in the brachial artery of humans consuming cranberry juice have been inconclusive (personal unpublished observations).

Red wine and Concord grape juice have also been demonstrated to inhibit platelet aggregation and blood clotting *(26,27)*. Studies of platelet aggregation in humans suggest that the consumption of a single glass of pure cranberry juice is not able to promote measurable inhibition of platelet aggregation, but a pilot study suggested that consumption of a 27% low-calorie cranberry juice (6 oz; four times daily for 4 d) may lead to inhibited platelet aggregation responses to collagen and adenosine diphosphate *(28)*.

Cranberry juice may also help prevent CHD by lowering the blood cholesterol level. Significant reductions in LDL and total plasma cholesterol levels occurred in familial hypercholesterolemic swine when they were administered a cranberry concentrate-based

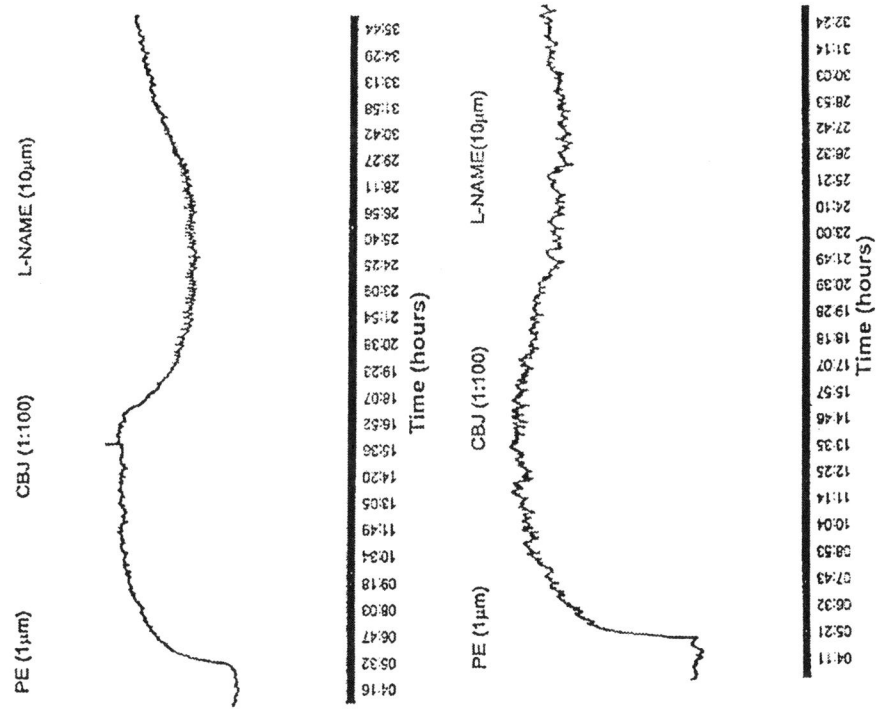

Fig. 1. Cranberry juice (CBJ) vasodilates rat aortic rings that are precontracted with phenylephrine (PE). This vasodilation does not occur if the enzyme nitric oxide synthase is blocked by L-NAME or if the endothelium is removed. Administration of acetylcholine (ACH) verifies that the endothelium is intact. When the endothelium is removed, CBJ is unable to vasodilate the vessel.

Table 1
Physical Characteristics of Cranberry Juice Samples Prepared
in the Laboratory from Cultivars Grown in four Different Locations

Cultivar and location	Gallic acid equivalents (mg GAE/L)	Juice pH when collected from berries	% Soluble solids (Brix) at acidic pH
Stevens–OR	2434 ± 120	2.34	8.98
Crowley–OR	2455 ± 42	2.28	8.13
Stevens–N.WI	2177 ± 66	2.15	8.79
Ben Lear–N.WI	2475 ± 95	2.20	8.89
Stevens–C.WI	2113 ± 119	2.18	9.01
Ben Lear–C.WI	2127 ± 28	2.16	8.96
Stevens–MA	2450 ± 72	2.18	8.88
Ben Lear–MA	2439 ± 88	2.21	8.79

Cranberry (*Vaccinium macrocapron*) cultivars were obtained during September of the 1998 growing season from bogs at the following locations: Brandon, Oregon (Stevens and Crowley cultivars), Manitowash Waters in Northern Wisconsin (Stevens and Ben Lear cultivars), Warrens in Central Wisconsin, and Nantucket, Massachusetts (Stevens and Ben Lear cultivars). The following statistically significant differences ($p < 0.05$) were observed: 1 vs 3, 4, and 6; 2 vs 3, 5, and 6; and 4 vs 5 and 6. Modified from ref. *31*.

powder (90MX) produced by Ocean Spray *(29)*. Comparable studies in humans have not been performed but could be promising.

Antioxidants are hypothesized to slow the rate of LDL oxidation and cholesterol deposition in the arterial wall. Studies in our laboratory have determined that pure, unsweetened *(30–32)* and commercially available cranberry juices *(33)* contain antioxidants that can protect LDL from oxidation in vitro. Consumption of cranberry juice should then lead to a slowing of the rate of cholesterol deposition in the arterial wall in vivo. Pedersen et al. *(34)* recently confirmed that human cranberry juice consumption leads to measurable increases in total plasma antioxidant capacity.

Cranberry juices are rich in polyphenols and have a relatively homogeneous content compared with wines and grape juices. Furthermore, cranberries provide one of the largest amounts of polyphenols available per serving in a fruit or vegetable *(15)*. We recently analyzed the polyphenol content and antioxidant activity of different cranberry cultivars grown in different locations in the United States. The polyphenol contents of the eight cranberry samples tested differed by less than ±9% from the collective mean (2333 mg/L), and a similarly tight clustering of antioxidant activities was also observed (Tables 1 and 2). By comparison, the polyphenol content of white grape and Concord grape juices range from 327 to 1742 mg gallic acid equivalents/L *(35)*, and the polyphenolic content of red wines range from 1800 to 4059 mg/L gallic acid equivalents, with an average of approx 2567 mg/L, while the polyphenol content of white wines was only 239 mg/L *(36)*. Relative to our polyphenol and antioxidant studies, Wang and Stretch *(37)* observed similar but slightly greater variations in their analysis of cranberry polyphenol and antioxidant activities.

4. POSSIBLE EFFECTS OF CRANBERRIES ON CANCER

The development of cancer is linked to deficiencies in antioxidant protection that can result in damage to DNA and other regulatory systems that regulate cellular activity.

Table 2
Effects of Cranberry Juice (CBJ) Dilutions from Eight Sources on the Oxidation of LDL

1:CBJ	Lag-time (min to 1/2-V_{max})			TBARS (ng MDA/100 µL)	
	1:1000	1:5000	1:15,000	1:5000	1:15,000
Control	92.4	92.4	92.4	76.64	76.64
OR					
1-Stevens	347.2	169.2	127.2	19.33	69.04
2-Crowley	342.4	165.8	125.0	14.59	61.04
N. WI					
3-Stevens	345.2	178.4	128.4	10.30	57.55
4-Ben Lear	345.0	186.4	133.4	13.63	58.74
C. WI					
5-Stevens	360.4	180.0	127.8	17.70	60.96
6-Ben Lear	339.8	178.2	130.0	19.33	68.08
MA					
7-Stevens	343.8	173.4	125.6	9.33	60.96
8-Ben Lear	353.4	183.0	124.0	11.85	68.37

Antioxidant effects measured ($n = 5$) using the lag-time and thiobarbituric acid reactive substance (TBARS) tests.

Statistically significant differences ($p < 0.05$): Lag-time at 1:15000 CBJ: (1 vs 2, 3, 4, 5, and 7; 3 vs 6 and 8). TBARS at 1:15000 CBJ: Stevens-OR was not significantly different from control; significant differences between CBJ samples (1 vs 2, 3, 4, 5, and 7; 3 vs 6 and 8; 4 vs 6 and 8).

Data presented as mean ± SD with statistically significant differences indicated below. Modified from ref. *31*.

Cranberries are rich in antioxidant capacity and contain hundreds of compounds that may provide anticancer activities by acting on cellular growth regulators. Using in vitro systems, Bomser et al. *(38)* suggest that extracts from cranberries can inhibit the development of some tumor types *(38)*. In addition, cranberries are a good source of quercetin *(39)*, a substance that may be associated with cancer prevention *(40)*. The association of flavonoids in foods, in general, and cranberries, in particular, with respect to their effect on cancer prevention in humans is poorly understood and warrants further investigation.

5. CRANBERRY BEVERAGE FORMULATIONS AVAILABLE TO THE CONSUMER

One of the problems that clinicians and consumers face regarding the amount of cranberry juice required for health benefits is the considerable variation in the amount of cranberry juice in beverages. The high acidity and polyphenolic content of cranberries limits manufacturers in terms of the formulations that they can prepare that are both palatable and marketable. Polyphenols typically have a somewhat limited water solubility. A high polyphenolic content in a beverage can lead to an unsightly brown precipitation, or what the consumer calls sedimentation, that forms as the product ages on the store shelf. To help prevent this, manufacturers seldom add more than approx 30% cranberry juice to their products, and typically no more than 27%; however, many products actually contain far less than this amount. A list of available over-the-counter products and information about their contents is shown in Table 3.

Table 3

Representative Cranberry Content, Cost, Calorie Content, and Cost of Products
Based on Label Information and Grocer Cost in La Crosse, Wisconsin (August 2002)

Manufacturer	Product name	$/oz	%Cranberry	kcal/8 oz	Comments on sweetening method
Northland Cranberries	Traditional Cranberry	0.059	27	140	Grape and apple (73% v/v other juices)
Sam's Choice	Cranberry Juice Cocktail	0.292	30	140	High-fructose corn syrup (HFCS)
Ocean Spray	Cranberry Juice Cocktail	0.046	27	140	HFCS
Old Orchard	Cranberry Juice Cocktail	0.040	15	140	HFCS
Exceptional Value	Cranberry Apple Juice Cocktail	0.026	Not listed	170	Apple and HFCS (Cranberry + Apple = 15% v/v)
Northland Cranberries	Cranblackberry 100% Juice	0.047	27	140	Grape and blackberry (73% v/v other juices)
Old Orchard	Cranberry Raspberry Juice Cocktail	0.039	Not listed	140	Total cranberry, apple, grape = (20% v/v)
Sam's Club	Reduced Calorie Cranberry Juice Cocktail	0.039	25	25	Aspartame
Mountain Sun	100% Cranberry Juice	0.211	100	60	No added sweeteners
R.W. Knudsen	Just Cranberry	0.203	100	60	No added sweeteners
Ocean Spray	White Cranberry Juice Drink	0.040	Not listed	120	Apple and grape juices

58

The bitter-acidic taste of cranberries also poses a problem for both manufacturers and consumers. The traditional method used to accommodate the taste preferences of consumers has been to use high-fructose corn syrup as a sweetener and also to limit the amount of cranberry juice present in the product, a method pioneered by the Ocean Spray growers cooperative. In the last 10 yr, Northland Cranberries Inc. began improving palatability (sweetness) by adding juices from other fruits; this process has now become popular with other manufacturers. Part of this trend is because of consumer concern about high-fructose corn syrup and their perception of beverages labeled "100% juice" as being more healthy. However, few consumers are likely to be aware that a "100%-juice" product sweetened with grape and apple juices may in fact contain the same concentration of simple sugars as does a beverage sweetened with fructose. Although the sugar content may be approximately the same, the nutrient content of a 27% v/v cranberry juice cocktail that has the remaining 73% volume filled out with grape and apple juice is greater than one with a high content of high-fructose corn syrup and water. This fact has increased the consumer popularity of the "100% juice" cranberry beverages.

Cranberry products can be marketed using several different designations related to the percentage of cranberry juice present in the beverage. Products containing less than 100% of the primary labeled ingredient must contain the words "beverage," "cocktail," or "drink" in the label. As mentioned in Chapter 27 by Krasny:

> For multiple-juice beverages, whether diluted or single-strength, any juices in the product name must be listed in descending order of predominance by weight, unless a characterizing juice is declared as a flavor (e.g., raspberry-flavored apple and grape juice drink). There is also a mandatory percentage juice declaration requirement, based on the soluble solids content of expressed juice (not from concentrate), or minimum Brix levels (for reconstituted juice). When a beverage is made from concentrate, the product name must indicate that fact.

For the consumer, determination of the content of cranberry juice in products available over the counter represents a possible source of confusion. Although the composition of the pure cranberry juice used to prepare the beverage is relatively homogeneous (Tables 1 and 2), the amount of cranberry juice in the product is quite variable (Table 3). For instance, in the clinical trial of Avorn et al. (12) participants consumed 300 mL/d of a product containing 27% cranberry juice. However, if consumers drank a cranberry drink containing only 10% cranberry juice, they would theoretically need to consume more than 800 mL/d to get the same amount of proanthocyanidins and UTI prevention effects.

Another potential source of confusion about the health effects of cranberry juice is related to the possibility that the sweetener used to improve palatability (fructose, saccharine, sucralose, and sugars from noncranberry fruit juices) may also exert health effects. Although pure cranberry juice is available as an over-the-counter product, it is relatively expensive ($0.203/oz for 100% cranberry juice from R.W. Knudsen, vs $0.059/oz for 27% Traditional Cranberry blend from Northland Cranberries Inc.) and its palatability is not appealing to some.

Comparative clinical studies using different over-the-counter cranberry products are difficult to design and carry out and will remain difficult to evaluate. This relates to the nature of cranberry products and their palatability/manufacturing limitations. Moreover, the formulation (content of cranberry juice and of sweetener) changes frequently based on consumer preference and material costs of manufacturing.

Another development of recent interest is an over-the-counter product called "White Cranberry Juice Drink" produced by Ocean Spray. This product uses cranberries that are harvested earlier than usual, before accumulating their pigments that normally give cranberry juice its bright red color. As a result, these beverages are nearly colorless. Studies comparing the health effects of this product to those of the red cranberry juice have not been conducted but may be warranted.

6. CONCLUSIONS

Cranberry juice has been used in folk medicine for millennia. Recent clinical studies have confirmed its usefulness for the prevention of UTIs. The active agents are proanthocyanidins specific to cranberries, which prevent bacterial adhesion to the urinary tract. These antiadhesive effects may also be linked to possible health benefits with respect to oral and gastric health. There is also evidence that cranberries have antioxidant, vasodilatory, and antiplatelet aggregation properties that may make them a viable substitute to red wine and Concord grape juice for protection from CHD. However, consumer and researcher understanding of how cranberries affect human health remains difficult to determine in part because of the large range of product formulations and the differences in the amount of cranberry juice actually present in these beverages.

7. MAIN POINTS FOR PRIMARY AND CLINICAL REVIEW

1. Daily consumption of 300 mL 27% v/v cranberry juice is associated with protection against urinary tract infections.
2. This action is achieved by proanthocyanidins in cranberry juice that prevent bacteria from producing the p-fimbria that permit them to attach to uroepithelial cells, not by acidifying the urine as was once thought.
3. Cranberry juice is rich in polyphenols that may work to protect against heart disease in a manner similar to that associated with wine; cranberry juice may also protect against cancer.
4. Commercially available cranberry products vary widely with respect to cranberry content, caloric content, sweetener type, and cost.
5. Product content variability issues complicate health benefit recommendations.

REFERENCES

1. Henig YS, Leahy MM. Cranberry juice and urinary-tract health: science supports folklore. Nutrition 2000;16:684–687.
2. Roper TR, Vorsa N. Cranberry: botany and horticulture. Horticult Rev 1997;21:215–249.
3. Zuo Y, Wang C, Zhan J. Separation, characterization, and quantification of benzoic and phenolic antioxidants in American cranberry fruit by GC-MS. J Agric Food Chem 2002;50:3789–3794.
4. Dowling KJ, Roberts JA, Kaack MB. P-fimbriated *Escherichia coli* urinary tract infection: a clinical correlation. South Med J 1987;80:1533–1536.
5. Foxman B, Barlow R, D'Arcy H, Gillespie B, Sobel JD. Urinary tract infection: self-reported incidence and associated costs. Ann Epidemiol 2000;10:509–515.
6. Blatherwick ND. The specific role of foods in relation to the composition of urine. Arch Intern Med 1914;14:409–450.
7. Blatherwick ND, Long ML. Studies of urinary acidity—the increased acidity by eating prunes and cranberries. J Biol Chem 1923;57:815–818.
8. Fellers CR, Redmon BC, Parrott EM. Effect of cranberries on urinary acidity and blood alkali reserve. J Nutr 1933;6:455–463.

9. Bodel PI, Cotrain R, Kass EH. Cranberry juice and the antibacterial action of hippuric acid. J Lab Clin Med 1959;54:881—888.

10. Kahn HD, Panareillo VA, Saeji J, Sampson JR, Schwarz E. Effect of cranberry juice on urine. J Am Diet Assoc 1967;52:251–254.

11. Sobota AE. Inhibition of bacterial adherence by cranberry juice: potential use for the treatment of urinary tract infections. J Urol 1984:131:1013–1016.

12. Avorn J, Monane M, Gurwitz JH, Glynn RJ, Choodnovskiy I, Lipsitz LA. Reduction of bacteriuria and pyruria after ingestion of cranberry juice. JAMA 1994;271:751–754.

13. Ikaheimo R, Siitonen A, Heiskanen T, et al. Recurrence of urinary tract infection in a priamry care setting: analysis of a 1-year follow-up of 179 women. Clin Infect Dis 1996;22:91–99.

14. Kontiokari T, Sundquist K, Nuutinen M, Pokka T, Koskela M, Uhari M. Randomized trial of cranberry-lingonberry juice and lactobacillus GG drink for the prevention of urinary tract infections in women. BMJ 2001;322:1571–1584.

15. Vinson JA, Su X, Zubik L, Bose P. Phenol antioxidant quality in foods: fruits. J Agric Food Chem 2001;49:5315–5321.

16. Ofek I, Goldhar J, Sharon N. Anti-*Escherichia coli* adhesion activity of cranberry and blueberry juices. Adv Exp Med Biol 1996;408:179–183.

17. Howell AB. Cranberry proanthocyanidins and the maintenance of urinary tract health. Crit Rev Food Sci Nutr 2002;42(Suppl):273–278.

18. Howell AB, Vorsa N, Marderosian AD, Foo LY. Inhibition of the adherence of p-fimbriated E. coli to uropithelial cell surfaces by proanthocyanidin extracts from cranberries. N Engl J Med 1998;339: 1085–1086.

19. Burger O, Ofek I, Tabak M, Weiss E, Sharon N, Neeman I. A high molecular weight constituent of cranberry juice inhibits *Helicobacter pylori* adhesion to human gastric mucus. FEMS Immunol Med Microbiol 2000;22:1–7.

20. Weiss EI, Lev-Dor R, Kashamn Y, Goldhar J, Sharon N, Ofek I. Inhibiting interspecies coaggregation of plaque bacteria with a cranberry juice constituent. J Am Diet Assoc 1998;129:1719–1723.

21. Renaud S, De Lorgeril M. Wine, alcohol, platelets, and the French paradox for coronary heart disease. Lancet 1992;118:1184–1189.

22. Stein JH, Keevil JG, Wiebe DA, Aeschlimann S, Folts JD. Purple grape juice improves endothelial function and reduces the susceptibility of LDL cholesterol to oxidation in patients with coronary artery disease. Circulation 1999;100:1050–1055.

23. Chou EJ, Keevil JG, Aeschlimann S, Wiebe DA, Folts JD, Stein JH. Effect of ingestion of purple grape juice on endothelial function in patients with coronary heart disease. Am J Cardiol 2000;88:553–555.

24. Maher MA, Mataczynski H, Stephaniak HM, Wilson T. Cranberry juice induces nitric oxide dependent vasodilation and transiently reduces blood pressure. J Med Foods 2000;3:141–147.

25. Flesch M, Schwarz A, Bohm, M. Effects of red wine and white wine on endothelium-dependent vasorelaxation of rat aorta and human coronary arteries. Am J Physiol 1998;275:H1183–H1190.

26. Demrow HS, Slane PR, Folts JD. Administration of wine and grape juice inhibits in vivo platelet activity and thrombosis in stenosed canine coronary arteries. Circulation 1995; 91:1182–1188.

27. Freedman JE, Parker C 3rd, Li L, et al. Select flavonoids and whole juice from purple grapes inhibit platelet function and enhance nitric oxide release. Circulation 2001;103:2792–2798.

28. Wilson T, Marley JC. Effects of cranberry juice consumption on platelet aggregation [abstract]. FASEB J 2001;15:A286.

29. Reed JD, Kreuger CG, Porter ML. Cranberry juice powder decreases low density lipoprotein cholesterol in hypercholesterolemic swine [abstract]. FASEB J 2001;15:54.

30. Wilson T, Porcari JP, Harbin D. Cranberry extract inhibits low density lipoprotein oxidation. Life Sci 1998;62:PL381–PL386.

31. Wilson T, Porcari JP, Maher MA. Cranberry juice inhibits metal- and non-metal initiated oxidation of low density lipoprotein. J Nutra Funct Med Foods 1999;2:5–14.

32. Wilson T, Zoeller WJ, Schaaf PJ, Maher MA. Cultivar and source dependent variation in the ability of cranberry juice to protect human LDL from oxidation in vitro [abstract]. FASEB J 2000;14:A269.

33. Wilson T, Mahoney L, Porcari JP, Maher MA. Polyphenolic content of cranberry juices [abstract]. FASEB J 1998;11:A561.

34. Pederson CB, Kyle J, Jenkinson AM, Gardner PT, McPhail DB, Duthie GG. Effects of blueberry and cranberry juice consumption on the plasma antioxidant capacity of healthy female volunteers. Eur J Clin Nutr 2000;54:405–408.

35. Frankel EN, Meyer AS. Antioxidants in grapes and grape juices and their potential health effects. Pharm Biol 1998;36(Suppl):14–20.

36. Frankel EN, Waterhouse AL, Teissedre PL. Principal phenolic phytochemicals in selected California wines and their antioxidant activity in inhibiting oxidation of low density lipoproteins. J Agric Food Chem 1995;43:890–894.

37. Wang SY, Stretch AW. Antioxidant capacity in cranberry is influenced by cultivar and storage temperature. J Agric Food Chem 2001;49:969–974.

38. Bomser J, Madhavi BL, Singletary K, Smith MA. In vitro anticancer activity of fruit extracts from vaccinium species. Planta Med 1996;62:212–216.

39. Bilyk A, Sapers GM. Varietal differences in the quercetin, kaempferol, and myrecitin contents of highbush blueberry, cranberry, and thornless blackberry fruits. J Agric Food Chem 1986;34:585–588.

40. Weisburger JH. Mechanisms of action of antioxidants as exemplified in vegetables, tomatoes and tea. Food Chem Toxicol 1999;37:943–948.

5 Health Benefits of Citrus Juices

Carla R. McGill, Alissa M. R. Wilson, and Yanni Papanikolaou

The positive outcomes of drinking citrus juice, as well as the biological responses to specific nutrients found in juice, have been researched extensively. This chapter summarizes the role citrus juice plays in providing important nutrients and bioactive compounds to the diet. It also summarizes the relationship of these components to various health benefits.

1. CITRUS JUICES CONTAIN IMPORTANT NUTRIENTS AND OTHER BIOACTIVE COMPOUNDS

1.1. Orange Juice

Orange juice is the most nutrient-dense fruit juice commonly consumed in the United States *(1)*. An 8-oz serving provides 110 cal and contains 72 mg of vitamin C (120% of Daily Value). Orange juice is also a good source of potassium (450 mg, 13% of Daily Value), folate (60 μg, 15% of Daily Value), and thiamin (0.15 mg, 10% of Daily Value). Orange juice is fat free and cholesterol free and is also either sodium free (not-from-concentrate juices) or low in sodium (from-concentrate juices have 15 mg/serving). Other nutrients found in orange juice are vitamin B_6 (6% of Daily Value), niacin (4% of Daily Value), riboflavin (4% of Daily Value), and magnesium (6% of Daily Value). In addition to these nutrients, orange juice contains more than 60 plant phytochemicals, specifically flavonoids, that function as antioxidants, potential anti-inflammatory agents, and may also have other physiological actions. The main flavonoid in orange juice is hesperidin, which occurrs as a glycone, with sugars attached. The sugars are cleaved during digestion, with aglycone as the absorbed form.

Orange juice consumption contributes significantly to the nutrient density of the US diet. It is one of the top three contributors of dietary folate from natural sources *(2)*. Citrus fruit juices also contribute greatly to vitamin C intake. Based on 1994 to 1996 US Department of Agriculture (USDA) survey data, a sample of 2472 men and 2334 women between 25 and 75 yr of age were classified based upon mean daily vitamin C intake as: (1) low (<30 mg), (2) marginal (30–60 mg), or (3) desirable (>60 mg). Overall, 18% of the sample population had low vitamin C intakes, and an additional 24% had marginal

From: *Beverages in Nutrition and Health*
Edited by: T. Wilson and N. J. Temple © Humana Press Inc., Totowa, NJ

vitamin C intakes. For all subjects, the primary contributor to daily vitamin C intake was fruit juice, particularly citrus juices. On average, adults with desirable mean vitamin C intakes consumed at least 1 daily serving of citrus fruit *(3)*. The current adult Dietary Reference Intake for vitamin C recommended by the National Academy of Sciences (NAS) is 90 mg for men and 75 mg for women *(4)*. These values are higher than previous NAS recommendations.

The benefits of consuming orange juice and/or its specific components have been related to risk reduction for cancer *(5–10)*, heart disease *(5,11–15)*, stroke *(14,16–18)*, hypertension *(17,19,20)*, and cataracts *(21–25)*. The ingredients in orange juice that are believed to be responsible for these potential health benefits include vitamin C, folate, potassium, and phytochemicals.

1.2. Grapefruit Juice

Grapefruit juice differs slightly from orange juice in its nutrient profile. An 8-oz serving of grapefruit juice contains fewer than 100 cal and has the same amount of vitamin C as orange juice (72 mg, 120% of Daily Value). One serving also provides approx 300 mg of potassium. Grapefruit juice contains lower concentrations of the B vitamins folate, thiamin, and niacin than does orange juice. Many compounds have been proposed as active components in grapefruit juice, including both flavonoids (naringenin and naringin) and nonflavonoids (6', 7'-dihydroxybergamottin). The principal flavonoid in grapefruit juice is the flavanone glycoside naringin. Red grapefruit juice also contains trace amounts of the carotenoid lycopene. Lycopene has the greatest single oxygen-quenching capacity (in vitro) of the dietary carotenoids. The connection between lycopene from tomato sources and cancer is discussed more completely in Chapter 8 by Hadley et al. The effect of grapefruit juice on drug action is discussed in Chapter 7 by Kane.

2. CITRUS JUICES PROVIDE IMPORTANT NUTRIENTS TO CHILDREN

Citrus juice is an important contributor to total nutrient intakes in children. According to food intake surveys conducted by the USDA, citrus juice and milk intakes have declined during the last two decades, whereas consumption of carbonated soda drinks has increased *(26–28)*. *See* the chapters by Nestle et al. (Chapter 25), Jacobson (Chapter 24), and McBean et al. (Chapter 14) for reviews on these topics. Reports estimate that the percentage of US children achieving the recommended intake for fruit was approx 30% *(28)*. An examination of the 1994–1996 Continuing Survey of Food Intakes by Individuals (children aged 2–17 yr) revealed that the probability of attaining recommended levels of nutrients increased significantly when 100% juice or milk was included in the diet *(26)*. The recent addition of calcium to citrus juice products further enhances the nutritional contribution of these products for children.

Some health care professionals have expressed concern about the contribution of excessive fruit juice intake to failure to thrive and/or childhood obesity *(29)*. Dennison and colleagues *(29)* collected 7-d diet records from 168 children aged 2–5 yr. The researchers determined that 42% of those children who drank more than 12 oz/d of fruit juice (8 out of 19 children) were below the 20th percentile for height for age compared with 14% of those who drank fewer than 12 oz/d (21 out of 149 children). Nearly 32% (6 out of 19) of these children had body mass index (BMI) values above the 90th percentile, compared with 9% (13 out of 149) of those who drank less than 12 oz/d. Because of the cross-sectional nature of this study and the small number of children consuming more than 12 oz of fruit juice per day, it is difficult to conclude that excessive fruit juice intakes caused the short stature and obesity observed. Additionally, Skinner and colleagues (30) conducted a longitudinal study of 105 children aged 2–3 yr. Three days of dietary data were collected twice over a 4-mo period. The researchers found no relationship between consumption of more than 12 oz/d of fruit juice (11% and 14% at interviews 1 and 2, respectively) and BMI or height. Taken as a whole, these data suggest that fruit juices provide important nutrients and should not be limited for fear of obesity or growth stunting.

Therefore, we can conclude that citrus juices are nutrient-dense foods that provide significant levels of important nutrients for children and adults. These juices also contain several other bioactive components. Ongoing and future research will explore the biological effects and potential health benefits of these bioactive components. A large body of evidence already supports the role of citrus juices in providing various health benefits—from helping to reduce the risk of various major chronic diseases (5–7, 10,11,16,17,19,31,32) to improving cognitive function (33,34) and reducing the risk of cataracts (21,22). These data are summarized in the following section.

3. CITRUS JUICES AND CANCER PREVENTION

3.1. Fruits and Vegetables, Including Citrus Juices, May Reduce the Risk of Certain Types of Cancer

Epidemiological evidence indicates that individuals who consume increased amounts of fruits and vegetables have a lowered risk of developing cancer (5,6,35,36). Block and coinvestigators stated in 1992, "Approximately 200 studies that examined the relationship between fruit and vegetable intake and cancers of the lung, colon, breast, cervix, esophagus, oral cavity, stomach, bladder, pancreas, and ovary showed a statistically significant protective effect of fruit and vegetable consumption"(6).

The development of cancer is a complicated biological process that involves distinct phases: (1) Initiation—carcinogenic compounds that produce genetic mutations; (2) Promotion—genetic mutations accumulate, leading to malignant transformation and uncontrolled cell growth; and (3) Metastasis—cancer cells spread beyond natural boundaries to other tissues and organs (7). Research during the 1990s has established the importance of the citrus phytochemicals in preventing initiation and inhibiting the promotion phases of cancer (7).

3.2. Flavonoids in Citrus Juice and Cancer Risk Reduction

Flavonoids are plant phytochemicals (polyphenolic compounds) that have demonstrated antioxidant capabilities in biological models (see Table 1) (5,36). Flavonoids have received considerable interest as key dietary anticarcinogens (8,10,37,38) as a result of their antioxidant (39,40) and antitumor activities (32,41). In vitro and animal studies have shown that flavonoids offer cell protection against ultraviolet-induced DNA damage (42) and γ-ray irradiation (43). Other studies have demonstrated that dietary fla-

Table 1
Select List of Flavonoids in Citrus That Exhibit Anticarcinogenic Activity

Flavonoid	Anticancer activity	Reference
Nobiletin, tangeretin, quercetin	Protects cultured rat liver epithelial-like cells against aflatoxin β-induced cytotoxicity	95
Nobiletin, tangeretin	Induces aryl hydrocarbon hydroxylase activity	96
Tangeretin	Inhibits the invasion of malignant mouse tumor cells into normal tissue	97
Quercetin, kaempferol, tangeretin, rutin, nobiletin	Antioxidant; may reduce cell proliferation; extends actions of vitamin C	35

Source: refs. 7,35.

vonoids lower the incidence of tumors in chemically induced cancer animal models (44–46). In addition, evidence from animal studies suggests that citrus flavonoids may have antimetastatic properties (47).

A recent experiment examined the interactions of naturally occurring flavonoids with human cytochrome P450 enzymes that activate carcinogens. Results verified that the citrus flavonoid hesperetin selectively inhibited P450 cytochromes CYP1A1 and CYP1B1. The researchers noted that hesperetin is a major component of orange juice (>200 mg/L) and concluded that these dietary compounds may offer significant protection from certain cancers (48).

There is also an association between citrus peel and squamous cell carcinoma. In a case-control study conducted by Hakim and colleagues (49), a citrus intake questionnaire was developed to identify citrus consumption in a southern Arizona population. Of those surveyed, 64.3% and 74.5% reported weekly consumption of citrus fruits and citrus juices, respectively. Approximately 35% reported peel consumption as part of their regular diets. Results demonstrated no association between overall fruit and juice consumption and cancer. However, a strong negative relationship was found between citrus peel intake and the risk of squamous cell carcinoma. In fact, this was the first study to document a dose–response relationship between citrus peel consumption and a reduced risk of squamous cell carcinoma. It is believed that limonene, a naturally occurring flavonoid in the peel of oranges, grapefruits, and lemons, may be responsible for the protective effects against cancer. Citrus juices contain small amounts of peel flavonoids extracted during juice processing.

The anticancer activity of flavonoids has attracted interest as a potential breast cancer chemopreventive agent. So and colleagues (50) examined the effects of various flavonoids on cell proliferation and growth of human breast carcinoma cell lines. The studied flavonoids included the citrus flavonoids hesperetin and naringenin and other noncitrus flavonoids. In addition, the researchers tested the capacity of orange juice and grapefruit juice concentrates to inhibit tumor development in a chemically induced animal model with breast cancer. Results showed that orange juice concentrate was the most effective tumor onset inhibitor, and reduced tumor burden (g tumor/rat) (50). Additionally, the citrus flavonoids inhibited the in vitro proliferation of human breast carcinomas.

Miyagi et al. *(51)* conducted an 8-mo study to determine whether feeding pasteurized orange juice inhibits azomethane-induced colon cancer in rats. After a 1-wk washout period, drinking water was replaced with not-from-concentrate orange juice in the experimental group. The control group continued drinking water. Animals in both groups maintained similar body weights throughout the study. Results showed that animals in the orange juice group had a 22% reduction ($p < 0.05$) in tumor incidence. The researchers observed no significant differences in tumor size, suggesting that the anticancer actions of orange juice occurred during the initiation phase. Additionally, these researchers concluded that the anticancer effects were most likely due to hesperidin, limonin, and other phytochemicals present in the orange juice *(51)*.

Clearly, more research is needed to examine the effects of citrus products on the inhibition of cancer development. However, research indicates that the phytochemicals in citrus juices could have a substantial effect on reducing the development of various types of cancer.

3.3. Vitamin C and Folate in Citrus Juice and Cancer Risk Reduction

Vitamin C (ascorbic acid) is an essential water-soluble vitamin that contributes to several metabolic functions due to its capacity as a biologic reducing agent and its strong antioxidant capabilities. Ascorbic acid is needed for neurotransmitter and hormone synthesis, collagen formation, and synthesis of other connective tissues. Additionally, vitamin C enhances iron absorption and protects physiologically active components from oxidative damage. The Panel on Dietary Antioxidants and Related Compounds of the Food and Nutrition Board (an NAS committee) defined an antioxidant as "a substance in foods that significantly decreases the adverse effects of reactive species, such as reactive oxygen and nitrogen species on normal physiological function in humans" *(4)*. Vitamin C meets this definition, because it scavenges reactive oxygen and nitrogen species *(52)*, thus protecting important substrates that are needed for normal function *(53)*. Researchers also believe that ascorbic acid prevents the oxidative degradation of flavonoids and have categorized ascorbic acid as having flavonoid-sparing attributes, which is comparable to flavonoids exhibiting ascorbic acid-sparing traits *(8)*.

Vitamin C's antioxidant capacity may explain its importance in cancer prevention. Research has shown that the risk of developing certain cancers, such as gastric and esophageal, is much lower in people who consume vitamin C-rich foods *(7)*. It is possible that vitamin C reduces the risk of stomach and esophageal cancers by blocking the formation of mutagenic nitrosamines from nitrates and nitrites present in cured meats and in cigarette smoke *(53–55)*.

Carcinogens produce free radicals that initiate damage at the cellular level, often creating a favorable environment for cancer development *(56)*. DNA is highly vulnerable to attacks from free radicals *(57)*. Although cells contain inherent mechanisms for DNA repair, genetic mutations accumulate with age, increasing the likelihood of malignant transformation. With the exception of rare childhood cancers, cancer is therefore a disease of aging *(53)*.

Human trials have shown a reduction in DNA oxidative damage with vitamin C supplementation *(58,59)*. For example, one investigation that studied vitamin C supplementation (60 or 260 mg of vitamin C per day in combination with iron) found a reduction in DNA oxidation subjects who had a lower initial plasma vitamin C concentration but not in subjects with a high initial plasma vitamin C concentration *(58)*. Two other studies demonstrated a decreased susceptibility of lymphocytes to DNA oxidative damage with vitamin C supplementation *(59,60)*. Vitamin C supplementation studies in humans with other specific biomarkers for oxidative damage, however, have presented inconclusive data and require further investigation *(53)*.

Other actions of vitamin C involve immune function modification *(53)*. Although these mechanisms are still unclear, research suggests that vitamin C may be involved in chemotaxis *(61)*, natural killer cell (NKC) activity, and lymphocyte functions *(62)*. Evidence also suggests that vitamin C may affect production of cytokines, antibodies, and compliment components *(62,63)*.

Folate is an essential water-soluble vitamin required for cell division and growth *(33)*, and orange juice is one of the best dietary sources of natural folate *(64,65)*, containing 15% of the Daily Value per 8-oz serving. Folate bioavailability in orange juice is high because it occurs as the well-absorbed monoglutamate form *(64)*.

It is hypothesized that a folate deficiency can increase cancer risk due to a potential obstruction of the DNA repair mechanisms, resulting in cellular mutations and chromosomal damage *(5)*. Tillotson et al. *(5)* conducted an extensive review on the health benefits of citrus, which included a summary of current evidence on folate and cancer. Researchers have observed extensive DNA damage in folate-deficient cells and have reported a reduction in damage during folate supplementation. In addition, folic acid supplementation is associated with positive health benefits in cervical dysplasia and colorectal cancer *(5)*. However, other research suggests weak or no beneficial effects of folic acid supplementation on cancer risk reduction. The authors acknowledge that folate's role in cancer is in the preliminary stages and, as such, must await future findings. These researchers conclude that, "A diet which provides good dietary folate sources on a daily basis is the best recommendation at present, except in cases of genetic diseases which require more aggressive treatment" *(5)*.

4. CITRUS JUICES AND CARDIOVASCULAR DISEASE PREVENTION

Two of the leading causes of morbidity and mortality in the United States are coronary heart disease (CHD) and stroke. One million deaths annually are attributable to cardiovascular disease (CVD). Furthermore, the health care cost and productivity loss have been estimated at $15 billion/yr *(53)*. An elevated blood cholesterol level is a major risk factor for CHD and reductions of total and low-density lipoprotein (LDL) cholesterol decrease the risk of coronary events *(66)*. Low high-density lipoprotein (HDL) cholesterol is also a risk factor for CHD. Thus, the ideal approach to reducing CHD risk is lowering total and LDL cholesterol while increasing HDL cholesterol *(67)*. Typically, diet intervention is the first approach recommended to improve cholesterol levels.

4.1. Orange Juice Consumption Increases HDL Cholesterol Levels

A recently published human intervention trial using not-from-concentrate orange juice has produced promising results concerning HDL cholesterol improvements. Men and women who were hypercholesterolemic who sequentially consumed 250 mL, 500 mL, and then 750 mL orange juice per day during a 12-wk period displayed a 21% elevation in HDL cholesterol. Although LDL levels did not change, the LDL/HDL ratio decreased significantly (16%). The significant HDL cholesterol increase was seen during the 4-wk period of consumption of 750 mL/d orange juice. The researchers suggested that improvements in blood lipids were likely a result of the naturally occurring flavonoids and limonoids in the orange juice; however, because orange juice contains numerous phytochemicals, the exact mechanism of action is still unknown *(11)*.

4.2. Flavonoids in Citrus Juices and CVD Risk Reduction

Some researchers believe that flavonoid-rich diets decrease the CVD risk through mechanisms that reduce inflammatory responses, platelet aggregation, LDL oxidation, and plasma cholesterol concentrations *(40,68)*.

Platelet aggregation inhibition may result from the ability of flavonoids to inhibit the cyclooxygenase pathway, which results in reducing inflammatory mediators, such as prostaglandins and thromboxanes. Flavonoids may also modulate enzymes that regulate cyclic nucleotides (i.e., cAMP, cGMP), compounds involved in promoting platelet aggregation *(5,69)*. Researchers suggest that methoxylated flavonoids (e.g., tangeretin and nobiletin) have increased activity compared with hydroxylated compounds and may operate similarly to acetylsalicylic acid (aspirin), a well-known platelet aggregation inhibitor *(69)*.

Flavonoids have demonstrated antioxidant capabilities in biological models *(36,38)*. A review by Benaventé-Garcia et al. *(69)* stated that flavonoids readily scavenge potentially harmful free radicals such as superoxide anions and peroxy radicals. In vitro evidence suggests that citrus flavonoids suppress LDL oxidation by inhibiting hydroperoxide production and by protecting vitamin E (α-tocopherol), another antioxidant from oxidation *(69)*.

Citrus fruits and juices, which contain biologically relevant amounts of the glycosylated forms of citrus flavonoids (hesperidin and naringin in oranges and grapefruits, respectively *[70]*), share hypocholesterolemic characteristics *(12)*. Kurowska et al. *(12)* demonstrated that rabbits whose drinking water was replaced with either orange or grapefruit juice had a significant reduction in serum LDL cholesterol (43% and 32%, respectively; $p < 0.05$). The authors concluded that the decrease in LDL levels induced by the citrus juices might be related to endogenous effects of the citrus flavonoids *(12)*. In another animal study, Kurowska et al. showed that orange juice administration reduced total plasma cholesterol whereas grapefruit juice decreased both very low-density lipoprotein (VLDL) and LDL in hypercholesterolemic rats *(71)* (as cited in ref. *12*).

Epidemiological evidence suggests that flavonoid intakes are inversely related to death from CHD *(72)*. The Zutphen Elderly study, a longitudinal study of 805 men in the Netherlands, found that CHD mortality risk was 50% lower in those men who had the highest levels of flavonoid intakes compared with the men with the lowest levels.

Based on the current evidence, it is clear that flavonoid intake is associated with reduced CVD risk through a variety of proposed mechanisms. Citrus juices provide a readily available source of flavonoids, also accompanied by other health-promoting phytochemicals. Future research will delineate the specific mechanisms by which flavonoids and other phytochemicals in citrus affect CVD risk.

4.3. Vitamin C and CVD Risk Reduction

Epidemiological data suggest that vitamin C may offer protection against CVD *(13,14,18)*. Vitamin C is a strong antioxidant, possibly explaining its protective effect. To assess vitamin C's antioxidant potential, healthy men consuming a high saturated fat diet took either 50- or 500-mg supplements of vitamin C daily. Results demonstrated a decrease in LDL susceptibility to oxidative damage in individuals consuming 500 mg compared to those with the 50 mg dosage *(73)*. Vitamin C from not-from-concentrate orange juice is well absorbed, as demonstrated by Kurowska et al. *(11)*, which could result in increased antioxidant capacity. Significant increases in plasma vitamin C concentrations with not-from-concentrate orange juice consumption were reported in humans consuming as little as 250 mL/d *(11)*.

A recent review considered several prospective cohort studies examining vitamin C intake and risk of CVD *(53)*. Of the 12 reported studies, 7 demonstrated a significant inverse relationship between vitamin C intake and risk of CVD or cerebrovascular disease. Four studies demonstrated risk reductions with moderate vitamin C intake levels (45–113 mg/d) *(53)*. Plasma vitamin C concentrations, considered to be a more accurate measure of dietary levels of vitamin C than reported dietary intakes, have also been measured by some researchers. One study observed a 30% risk reduction in stroke mortality in study participants with plasma vitamin C levels greater than 28 μmol/L as compared with participants with concentrations less than 12 μmol/L *(18)*. Reduced risk (39–60%) has been reported for CHD, myocardial infarction, and angina pectoris when plasma vitamin C concentrations were greater than 11–57 μmol/L *(74,75)*. It is important to note that observational studies cannot infer causality due to the presence of confounding factors. Relationships most likely exist between vitamin C intake and other health-promoting activities and lifestyle choices, which could affect study results.

4.4. Folate and Cardiovascular Risk Reduction

Folate, as well as vitamins B_6 and B_{12}, are required for methylating homocysteine, a modified amino acid, to less harmful components (methionine and cystathionine). Studies in healthy humans have demonstrated that low serum folate concentrations can lead to elevated blood levels of homocysteine *(76–79)*. Increased serum homocysteine has been associated with a greater risk of CVD *(15,80–82)*.

To assess the contribution of orange juice to serum folate concentrations, healthy volunteers aged 40–82-yr-old consumed 20 oz of not-from-concentrate orange juice along with their normal diet for a 60-d period. Before the experiment, mean dietary folate intakes were 271 μg/d. Orange juice consumption significantly increased dietary folate intakes to 421 μg/d and plasma folate increased by 45% in 30 d. Plasma homocysteine levels decreased significantly by 11%. The authors concluded that folate in orange juice is highly bioavailable and that one serving of orange juice consumed on a daily basis could contribute to a reduction in CVD risk *(83)*.

Recently, Brouwer et al. *(81)* investigated whether dietary folate from citrus fruits and vegetables could improve folate status and reduce total plasma homocysteine levels in healthy subjects. After 4 wk, plasma folate status significantly improved, and total plasma homocysteine concentrations significantly decreased in those subjects consuming a high-folate diet.

4.5. Potassium and Cardiovascular Disease Risk Reduction

Potassium, the most abundant intracellular cation, is important for membrane transport, energy metabolism, and proper cell functioning. Fruits, citrus juices, vegetables, low-fat dairy products, and some whole grains are the best dietary sources of potassium.

Although the mechanisms for the effects of potassium on blood pressure and stroke risk are not fully known, some hypotheses have been proposed. Potassium may directly cause sodium excretion or suppress the renin-angiotensin system. It has also been suggested that potassium could affect vasoconstriction and vascular resistance and inhibit free radical formation *(84)*.

Gillman et al. *(16)* reported data from the Framingham Study, focusing on the dietary intakes of 832 men (mean age of 56 at the start of the study) followed over time. The men averaged 5.1 servings/d of fruits and vegetables at baseline. During the 20-yr follow-up, 97 participants suffered a cerebrovascular event. The researchers found a significant decrease in stroke risk with increasing fruit and vegetable intake. In fact, for every 3 servings/d increase in fruit and vegetable consumption, there was a 22% reduction in risk of stroke. The investigators noted that the protection afforded by fruits and vegetables was possibly related to potassium *(16)*.

Lifestyle changes, including diet counseling, are advised as the first step in treating stage 1 hypertension by the Joint National Committee on Detection, Evaluation and Treatment of High Blood Pressure. This recommendation led to the Dietary Approaches to Stop Hypertension, or DASH study. The DASH diet includes 8–10 servings of fruits, 100% fruit juices, and vegetables, as well as 2 servings/d of low-fat dairy products. Harsha et al. *(19)* reported the findings of the DASH diet study, showing that a diet high in fruits and vegetables can significantly reduce blood pressure in as few as 2 wk.

The DASH study included 459 people, randomized into three diet groups: (1) a control diet (typical American diet, 37% of calories from fat); (2) the control diet, with the addition of 8–10 servings of fruits, 100% fruit juices, and vegetables; and (3) the DASH diet (8–10 servings of fruits, 100% fruit juices, and vegetables, and two servings of low-fat dairy products). The diets were maintained for 8 wk, with all foods prepared by the study centers. After 2 wk the fruits and vegetables and DASH diets resulted in significant reductions in blood pressure that were maintained for the remaining 6 wk of the study. Adding fruits and vegetables to the typical American diet resulted in a 2.8 mmHg drop in systolic blood pressure and a 1.1 mmHg drop in diastolic blood pressure compared to controls. The DASH diet resulted in a 5.5 mmHg drop in systolic blood pressure and a 3.0 mmHg drop in diastolic blood pressure compared with controls. Potassium intakes were significantly greater in the fruits and vegetables and DASH diets compared with the control diet *(19)*.

Ascherio et al. *(17)* followed 43,738 men for 8 yr as part of the Health Professionals Follow-Up Study. A food-frequency questionnaire was administered every 2 yr, with specific questions on potassium supplements. The men were divided into quintiles based on potassium intakes. After 8 yr, 328 cases of stroke were noted. For those men in the highest quintile of potassium intake, risk of stroke was 41% less than those in the lowest group of intake. The authors emphasized the importance of increasing fruit and vegetable intakes to increase daily potassium consumption *(17)*.

Using data from the Nurses' Health Study (14 yr) and the Health Professionals Follow-Up Study (8 yr), Joshipura et al. *(85)* compared fruit and vegetable intake to risk of ischemic stroke. The sample included 75,596 women and 38,683 men; 570 ischemic strokes were recorded during the follow-up period. Each additional serving of fruits or vegetables was associated with a 6% decrease in stroke risk. Cruciferous and green leafy vegetables, as well as citrus fruit and citrus fruit juice, provided the greatest protection *(85)*.

4.6. Food and Drug Administration Approved Health Claim: Potassium and Hypertension and Stroke Risk Reduction

Tropicana Products Inc. led the beverage industry by petitioning the US Food and Drug Administration (FDA) to allow a new health claim communicating the health benefits of potassium-rich foods in reducing the risk of hypertension and stroke. The health claim reads, *"Diets containing foods that are good sources of potassium and low in sodium may reduce the risk of high blood pressure and stroke."* This was only the second new health claim authorized by the FDA through the Food, Drug and Cosmetic Modernization Act (FDAMA) expedited process. This process requires the identification of an authoritative statement by a government public health agency associated with nutrition and health or by one of the relevant divisions of the National Academy of Sciences. This claim was based on two authoritative statements published by the National Academy of Sciences in its *Diet and Health: Implications for Reducing Chronic Disease Risk* report *(84)*:

> *Epidemiological and animal studies indicate that the risk of stroke-related deaths is inversely related to potassium intake over the entire range of blood pressures, and the relationship appears to be dose dependent. The combination of a low-sodium, high-potassium intake is associated with the lowest blood pressure levels and the lowest frequency of stroke in individuals and populations. Although the effects of reducing sodium intake and increasing potassium intake would vary and may be small in some individuals, the estimated reduction in stroke-related mortality for the population is large.*

> *Vegetables and fruits are also good sources of potassium. A diet containing approximately 75 mEq (i.e., approximately 3.5 g of elemental potassium) daily may contribute to reduced risk of stroke, which is especially common among blacks and older people of all races. Potassium supplements are neither necessary nor recommended for the general population.*

Manufacturers of food products that meet certain defined requirements were allowed to convey this new health claim beginning November 2000.

5. CITRUS JUICES MAY IMPROVE COGNITIVE FUNCTION

Cognitive impairment in elderly populations may be related to increased homocysteine levels *(86–88)*. Cognitive performance of an elderly group (aged 65–90) was assessed through various cognitive tests. The highest cognitive performance was observed in participants who consumed higher amounts of fruits, vegetables, carbohydrate, fiber, folate, vitamin C, β-carotene, iron, and zinc and lower intakes of fat. The authors concluded that such a diet not only benefited overall health but also improved cognitive performance *(34)*.

Glucose also improves cognition, particularly memory functions, in both young and elderly subjects. The proposed mechanisms of action may be numerous and, likely, involve more than one pathway. One of the predominant theories is that glucose improves memory through increased acetylcholine production and release in the brain *(89,90)*. Previous work by Messier et al. *(91)* found that poor glucose regulation was associated with a decline in memory performance, which was improved through glucose consumption *(91)*. Orange juice contains approx 22 g of sugar per 8-oz serving, thus providing a source of glucose. A host of nutrients offered by citrus fruit and juices may offer cognitive protective advantages.

6. CITRUS JUICES MAY REDUCE THE RISK
OF CERTAIN BIRTH DEFECTS

It is well established that folate is necessary in the prevention of neural tube defects *(92,93)*. As a result, folic acid supplementation is recommended for women of childbearing age and pregnant women. A statement issued by the Centers for Disease Control and Prevention comments, "The U.S. Public Health Service recommends that all women who could possibly become pregnant get 400 μg (0.4 mg) of folic acid every day—this could prevent up to 70% of some types of serious birth defects" *(94)*. Citrus juices are a readily available source of bioavailable folate and, as such, may help to reduce the risk of neural tube defects.

7. VITAMIN C IN CITRUS JUICES MAY HELP TO PREVENT CATARACTS

Cataracts cause a partial or complete opacity of the eye that leads to visual impairment or blindness. From a dietary perspective, cataract development has been of interest lately. Evidence suggests a possible protective effect with high fruit and vegetable consumption. Adequate levels of antioxidants may significantly reduce the onset of this age-related condition *(23,24)*.

Several epidemiological studies of vitamin C intake and cataract incidence have been reviewed *(53)*. A prospective cohort of 50,828 women reported that vitamin C supplementation of 705 mg/d for more than 10 yr reduced the risk of cataracts by 45%. A cross-sectional study assessing long-term vitamin C intake in women (aged 56–71 yr) without prediagnosed cataracts or diabetes found that vitamin C intakes were associated with a 77% decrease in prevalence of lens opacity. Women who consumed vitamin C supplements for fewer than 10 yr did not show any benefits associated with cataracts. The researchers concluded that high amounts of daily vitamin C substantially lessen the risk of cataract development *(21)*. A case-controlled study conducted in Italy found that supplemental vitamin C was not associated with risk of cataract development. However, a significant inverse relationship was found between citrus fruit and vegetable consumption, folic acid, calcium, and vitamin E and risk of developing cataracts. This led the authors to assert that components within citrus fruits and vegetables, combined with a low-fat diet, may offer protection against cataracts *(22)*.

8. CONCLUSIONS

Citrus juices significantly enhance the diets of both children and adults by providing nutrients, such as carbohydrates, essential vitamins, and minerals. Citrus juices are an excellent source of ascorbic acid and a good source of folate and potassium. Vitamin C is a potent antioxidant, and high vitamin C intake has been associated with decreased risk of certain cancers, especially those of the stomach or esophagus. Folate is a key nutrient responsible for reducing homocysteine levels, an emerging new independent risk factor for heart disease. Further, folic acid plays a role in preventing neural tube defects, stabilizing DNA, and possibly maintaining cognitive function in the elderly. Potassium maintains intracellular fluid balance and, as such, a high intake is associated with reduced blood pressure and a reduced risk of stroke. A diet rich in fruit and vegetables, as well as low-fat dairy products (DASH diet) significantly reduces blood pressure. Recent epidemiological data indicate that for each additional serving of fruit or vegetable, risk of stroke may decrease by 6%. Other research has found that men with high potassium intake had a dramatic reduction (41%) in the risk of stroke compared with men with low potassium intake. Recently, the US FDA authorized a new health claim that allows certain foods to convey information on the association between a diet high in potassium and a reduced risk of both high blood pressure and stroke.

Consumption of a diet rich in fruits and vegetables also results in an increased intake of health-promoting phytochemicals. Citrus juice provides a host of bioactive compounds, namely flavonoids and flavones, that may be important in prevention of chronic diseases. The two main flavonoids in orange juice and grapefruit juice are hespertin and naringin, respectively. Other phytochemicals, including limonene, lutein, quercetin, and lycopene, are also present in citrus juices.

Epidemiological data, clinical investigations, and animal studies provide strong evidence for the health benefits of citrus and citrus juice consumption. These benefits include a reduced risk of several diseases, including heart disease and stroke, some types of cancer, certain birth defects, and cataracts. Citrus products may also help to maintain cognitive function. The evidence suggests a strong association between citrus phytochemicals and antiproliferative, antimetastatic, antitumor, and antioxidant activities. The phytochemicals in citrus products may also influence CVD risk factors. Consumption of orange juice may positively affect the LDL/HDL ratio, and components of citrus juice may also decrease LDL oxidation thus reducing the risk of CVD.

A recommendation to increase consumption of citrus products, particularly citrus juice products, appears to have significant benefits for the human population.

9. MAIN POINTS FOR PRIMARY AND CLINICAL REVIEW

1. Orange juice is one of the most nutrient-dense fruit juices consumed in the United States.
2. Relative to orange juice, grapefruit juice contains fewer calories and vitamins, and has a slightly different flavanoid content, with naringen being the predominant flavonoid.
3. Citrus fruits and juices are rich in ascorbate, folate, and flavonoids that appear to be responsible for reductions in the overall rate of cancer occurence observed in citrus consumers.
4. Regular consumption of citrus products is associated with reduction in the risk for cardiovascular disease.
5. Citrus juices are rich in potassium and the US Food and Drug Administration has approved the following claim for citrus product packaging: "Diets containing foods that are good sources of potassium and low in sodium may reduce the risk of high blood pressure and stroke."

REFERENCES

1. Leibman B, Hurley J. The juice jungle. Nutr Action Health Letter 1999;26:13–15.
2. Subar AF, Block G, James LD. Folate intake and food sources in the US population. Am J Clin Nutr 1989; 50:508–516.
3. Taylor CA, Hampl JS, Johnston CS. Low intakes of vegetables and fruits, especially citrus fruits, lead to inadequate vitamin C intakes among adults. Eur J Clin Nutr 2000;54:573–578.
4. Food and Nutrition Board, Institute of Medicine. Dietary Reference Intakes: Recommended Intakes for Individuals. National Academy of Sciences, Washington, DC, 1998.
5. Tillotson JE, Gershoff SN, Huber AM. Review of the medical and nutritional literature pertaining to the health and nutrition benefits of citrus fruits and juices. School of Nutrition Food Policy Institute, Tufts University, Medford, MA, 1993.

6. Block G, Patterson B, Subar A. Fruit, vegetables, and cancer prevention: a review of the epidemiological evidence. Nutr Cancer 1992;18:1–29.

7. Nagy S, Attaway JA. Anticarcinogenic activity of phytochemicals in citrus fruit and their juice products. Proc Fla Sate Hort Soc 1992;105:162–168.

8. Middleton E, Kandaswami C. Potential health-promoting properties of citrus flavonoids. Food Technol 1994;48:115–119.

9. Steinmetz KA, Potter JD. Vegetables, fruit, and cancer prevention: a review. J Am Diet Assoc 1996;96:1027–1039.

10. Tanaka T, Kawabata K, Kakumoto M, et al. Citrus auraptene exerts dose-dependent chemopreventive activity in rat large bowel tumorigenesis: the inhibition correlates with suppression of cell proliferation and lipid peroxidation and with induction of phase II drug-metabolizing enzymes. Cancer Res 1998;58:2550–2556.

11. Kurowska EM, Spence JD, Jordan J, et al. HDL-cholesterol-raising effect of orange juice in subjects with hypercholesterolemia. Am J Clin Nutr 2000;72:1095–1100.

12. Kurowska EM, Borradaile NM, Spence JD. Hypocholesterolemic effects of dietary citrus juices in rabbits. Nutr Res 2000;20:121–129.

13. Jha P, Flather M, Lonn E, Farkouh M, Yusuf S. The antioxidant vitamins and cardiovascular disease. A critical review of epidemiologic and clinical trial data. Ann Intern Med 1995;123:860–872.

14. Gey KF, Stahelin HB, Eichholzer M. Poor plasma status of carotene and vitamin C is associated with higher mortality from ischemic heart disease and stroke: Basel Prospective Study. Clin Investig 1993;71:3–6.

15. Boushey CJ, Beresford SA, Omenn GS, Motulsky AG. A quantitative assessment of plasma homocysteine as a risk factor for vascular disease. Probable benefits of increasing folic acid intakes. JAMA 1995;274:1049–1057.

16. Gillman MW, Cupples LA, Gagnon D, et al. Protective effect of fruits and vegetables on development of stroke in men. JAMA 1995;273:1113–1117.

17. Ascherio A, Rimm EB, Hernan MA, et al. Intake of potassium, magnesium, calcium, and fiber and risk of stroke among US men. Circulation 1998;98:1198–1204.

18. Gale CR, Martyn CN, Winter PD, Cooper C. Vitamin C and risk of death from stroke and coronary heart disease in cohort of elderly people. BMJ 1995;310:1563–1566.

19. Harsha DW, Lin PH, Obarzanek E, Karanja NM, Moore TJ, Caballero B. Dietary Approaches to Stop Hypertension: a summary of study results. DASH Collaborative Research Group. J Am Diet Assoc 1999;99:S35–S39.

20. Moline J, Bukharovich IF, Wolff MS, Phillips R. Dietary flavonoids and hypertension: is there a link? Med Hypotheses 2000;55:306–309.

21. Jacques PF, Taylor A, Hankinson SE, et al. Long-term vitamin C supplement use and prevalence of early age-related lens opacities. Am J Clin Nutr 1997;66:911–916.

22. Tavani A, Negri E, La Vecchia C. Food and nutrient intake and risk of cataract. Ann Epidemiol 1996;6:41–46.

23. Jacob RA, Burri BJ. Oxidative damage and defense. Am J Clin Nutr 1996;63:985S–990S.

24. Taylor A, Jacques PF, Epstein EM. Relations among aging, antioxidant status, and cataract. Am J Clin Nutr 1995;62:1439S–1447S.

25. Mares-Perlman JA, Lyle BJ, Klein R, et al. Vitamin supplement use and incident cataracts in a population-based study. Arch Ophthalmol 2000;118:1556–1563.

26. Ballew C, Kuester S, Gillespie C. Beverage choices affect adequacy of children's nutrient intakes. Arch Pediatr Adolesc Med 2000;154:1148–1152.

27. Harnack L, Stang J, Story M. Soft drink consumption among US children and adolescents: nutritional consequences. J Am Diet Assoc 1999;99:436–441.

28. Munoz KA, Krebs-Smith SM, Ballard-Barbash R, Cleveland LE. Food intakes of US children and adolescents compared with recommendations. Pediatrics 1997;100:323–329.

29. Dennison BA, Rockwell HL, Baker SL. Excess fruit juice consumption by preschool-aged children is associated with short stature and obesity. Pediatrics 1997;99:15–22.

30. Skinner JD, Carruth BR, Moran J, III, Houck K, Coletta F. Fruit juice intake is not related to children's growth. Pediatrics 1999;103:58–64.

31. Tanaka T, Makita H, Kawabata K, et al. Chemoprevention of azoxymethane-induced rat colon car-
    cinogenesis by the naturally occurring flavonoids, diosmin and hesperidin. Carcinogenesis 1997;18:
    957–965.
32. Miller EG, Fanous R, Rivera-Hidalgo F, Binnie WH, Hasegawa S, Lam LK. The effect of citrus limonoids
    on hamster buccal pouch carcinogenesis. Carcinogenesis 1989;10:1535–1537.
33. Economos C, Clay WD. Nutritional and health benefits of citrus fruits. Twelfth Session of the Intergov-
    ernmental Group on Citrus Fruit, Valencia, Spain, 1998.
34. Ortega RM, Requejo AM, Andres P, et al. Dietary intake and cognitive function in a group of elderly
    people. Am J Clin Nutr 1997;66:803–809.
35. Van Duyn MA, Pivonka E. Overview of the health benefits of fruit and vegetable consumption for the
    dietetics professional: selected literature. J Am Diet Assoc 2000;100:1511–1521.
36. Salah N, Miller NJ, Paganga G, Tijburg L, Bolwell GP, Rice-Evans C. Polyphenolic flavanols as
    scavengers of aqueous phase radicals and as chain-breaking antioxidants. Arch Biochem Biophys 1995;
    322:339–346.
37. Murakami A, Wada K, Ueda N, et al. In vitro absorption and metabolism of a citrus chemopreventive
    agent, auraptene, and its modifying effects on xenobiotic enzyme activities in mouse livers. Nutr Cancer
    2000;36:191–199.
38. Wood AW, Smith DS, Chang RL. Effects of flavonoids on the metabolism of xenobiotics. In: Plant
    Flavonoids in Biology and Medicine: Biochemical, Pharmacological and Structure-Activity Relation-
    ships. Cody V, Middleton E, Harborne JB (eds.). Alan R. Liss, Inc., New York, NY, 1986.
39. Middleton E, Jr., Kandaswami C. Effects of flavonoids on immune and inflammatory cell functions.
    Biochem Pharmacol 1992;43:1167–1179.
40. Middleton E, Jr. Effect of plant flavonoids on immune and inflammatory cell function. Adv Exp Med
    Biol 1998;439:175–182.
41. Hirano T, Gotoh M, Oka K. Natural flavonoids and lignans are potent cytostatic agents against human
    leukemic HL-60 cells. Life Sci 1994;55:1061–1069.
42. Kootstra A. Protection from UV-B-induced DNA damage by flavonoids. Plant Mol Biol 1994;26:
    771–774.
43. Shimoi K, Masuda S, Furugori M, Esaki S, Kinae N. Radioprotective effect of antioxidative flavonoids
    in gamma-ray irradiated mice. Carcinogenesis 1994;15:2669–2672.
44. Deschner EE, Ruperto JF, Wong GY, Newmark HL. The effect of dietary quercetin and rutin on AOM-
    induced acute colonic epithelial abnormalities in mice fed a high-fat diet. Nutr Cancer 1993;20:199–204.
45. Elangovan V, Sekar N, Govindasamy S. Chemopreventive potential of dietary bioflavonoids against 20-
    methylcholanthrene-induced tumorigenesis. Cancer Lett 1994;87:107–113.
46. Fujiki H, Horiuchi T, Yamashita K. Inhibition of tumor promotion by flavonoids. In: Plant Flavonoids
    in Biology and Medicine: Biochemical, Pharmacological and Structure-Activity Relationships. Cody V,
    Middleton E, Harborne JB (eds.). Alan R. Liss, Inc., New York, NY, 1986.
47. Bracke M, Vyncke B, Opdenakker G, Foidart JM, De Pestel G, Mareel M. Effect of catechins and citrus
    flavonoids on invasion in vitro. Clin Exp Metastasis 1991;9:13–25.
48. Doostdar H, Burke MD, Mayer RT. Bioflavonoids: selective substrates and inhibitors for cytochrome
    P450 CYP1A and CYP1B1. Toxicology 2000;144:31–38.
49. Hakim IA, Harris RB, Ritenbaugh C. Citrus peel use is associated with reduced risk of squamous cell
    carcinoma of the skin. Nutr Cancer 2000;37:161–168.
50. So FV, Guthrie N, Chambers AF, Moussa M, Carroll KK. Inhibition of human breast cancer cell
    proliferation and delay of mammary tumorigenesis by flavonoids and citrus juices. Nutr Cancer 1996;26:
    167–181.
51. Miyagi Y, Om AS, Chee KM, Bennink MR. Inhibition of azoxymethane-induced colon cancer by orange
    juice. Nutr Cancer 2000;36:224–229.
52. Halliwell B. Vitamin C: antioxidant or pro-oxidant in vivo? Free Radic Res 1996;25:439–454.
53. Carr AC, Frei B. Toward a new recommended dietary allowance for vitamin C based on antioxidant and
    health effects in humans. Am J Clin Nutr 1999;69:1086–1107.
54. Hecht SS. Approaches to cancer prevention based on an understanding of N-nitrosamine carcinogenesis.
    Proc Soc Exp Biol Med 1997;216:181–191.
55. Tannenbaum SR, Wishnok JS. Inhibition of nitrosamine formation by ascorbic acid. Ann NY Acad Sci
    1987;498:354–363.

56. Comstock GW, Alberg AJ, Huang HY, et al. The risk of developing lung cancer associated with anti-oxidants in the blood: ascorbic acid, carotenoids, alpha-tocopherol, selenium, and total peroxyl radical absorbing capacity. Cancer Epidemiol Biomarkers Prev 1997;6:907–916.

57. Lindahl T. Instability and decay of the primary structure of DNA. Nature 1993;362:709–715.

58. Rehman A, Collis CS, Yang M, et al. The effects of iron and vitamin C co-supplementation on oxidative damage to DNA in healthy volunteers. Biochem Biophys Res Commun 1998;246:293–298.

59. Green MH, Lowe JE, Waugh AP, Aldridge KE, Cole J, Arlett CF. Effect of diet and vitamin C on DNA strand breakage in freshly-isolated human white blood cells. Mutat Res 1994;316:91–102.

60. Panayiotidis M, Collins AR. Ex vivo assessment of lymphocyte antioxidant status using the comet assay. Free Radic Res 1997;27:533–537.

61. Johnston CS, Martin LJ, Cai X. Antihistamine effect of supplemental ascorbic acid and neutrophil chemotaxis. J Am Coll Nutr 1992;11:172–176.

62. Heuser G, Vojdani A. Enhancement of natural killer cell activity and T and B cell function by buffered vitamin C in patients exposed to toxic chemicals: the role of protein kinase-C. Immunopharmacol Immunotoxicol 1997;19:291–312.

63. Haskell BE, Johnston CS. Complement component C1q activity and ascorbic acid nutriture in guinea pigs. Am J Clin Nutr 1991;54:1228S–1230S.

64. Rouseff RL, Nagy S. Health and nutritional benefits of citrus fruit components. Food Technol 1994; 48:125–132.

65. Fellers PJ, Nikdel S, Lee HS. Nutrient content and nutrition labeling of several processed Florida citrus juice products. J Am Diet Assoc 1990;90:1079–1084.

66. National Center for Health Statistics, American Heart Association. Facts about cardiovascular disease [abstract]. Circulation 1992;85:A103.

67. Summary of the second report of the National Cholesterol Education Program (NCEP) Expert Panel on Detection, Evaluation, and Treatment of High Blood Cholesterol in Adults (Adult Treatment Panel II). JAMA 1993;269:3015–3023.

68. Cook NC, Samman S. Flavonoids—chemistry, metabolism, cardioprotective effects, and dietary sources. J Nutr Biochem 1996;7:66–76.

69. Benavente-Garcia O, Castillo J, Marin FR. Uses and properties of citrus flavonoids. J Agric Food Chem 1997;45:4505–4515.

70. Montanari A, Widmer W, Nagy S. Health promoting phytochemicals in citrus fruit and juice products. In: Functionality of Food Phytochemicals. Romeo J (ed.) Plenum Press, New York, NY, 1997.

71. Kurowska EM, Borradaile NM, Meade M. Cholesterol-lowering effects of dietary citrus juices and their flavonoids. Studies in rats, mice and rabbits [abstract]. Atherosclerosis 1997;134:330.

72. Hertog MG, Feskens EJ, Hollman PC, Katan MB, Kromhout D. Dietary antioxidant flavonoids and risk of coronary heart disease: the Zutphen Elderly Study. Lancet 1993;342:1007–1011.

73. Harats D, Chevion S, Nahir M, Norman Y, Sagee O, Berry EM. Citrus fruit supplementation reduces lipoprotein oxidation in young men ingesting a diet high in saturated fat: presumptive evidence for an interaction between vitamins C and E in vivo. Am J Clin Nutr 1998;67:240–245.

74. Singh RB, Ghosh S, Niaz MA, et al. Dietary intake, plasma levels of antioxidant vitamins, and oxidative stress in relation to coronary artery disease in elderly subjects. Am J Cardiol 1995;76:1233–1238.

75. Riemersma RA, Wood DA, Macintyre CC, Elton RA, Gey KF, Oliver MF. Risk of angina pectoris and plasma concentrations of vitamins A, C, and E and carotene. Lancet 1991;337:1–5.

76. Bates CJ, Mansoor MA, van der PJ, Prentice A, Cole TJ, Finch S. Plasma total homocysteine in a representative sample of 972 British men and women aged 65 and over. Eur J Clin Nutr 1997;51:691–697.

77. Pancharuniti N, Lewis CA, Sauberlich HE, et al. Plasma homocyst(e)ine, folate, and vitamin B-12 concentrations and risk for early-onset coronary artery disease. Am J Clin Nutr 1994;59:940–948.

78. Ubbink JB, Vermaak WJ, van der MA, Becker PJ. Vitamin B-12, vitamin B-6, and folate nutritional status in men with hyperhomocysteinemia. Am J Clin Nutr 1993;57:47–53.

79. Loria CM, Ingram DD, Feldman JJ, Wright JD, Madans JH. Serum folate and cardiovascular disease mortality among US men and women. Arch Intern Med 2000;160:3258–3262.

80. Refsum H, Ueland PM, Nygard O, Vollset SE. Homocysteine and cardiovascular disease. Annu Rev Med 1998;49:31–62.

81. Brouwer IA, van Dusseldorp M, West CE, et al. Dietary folate from vegetables and citrus fruit decreases plasma homocysteine concentrations in humans in a dietary controlled trial. J Nutr 1999;129:1135–1139.

82. Nygard O, Nordrehaug JE, Refsum H, Ueland PM, Farstad M, Vollset SE. Plasma homocysteine levels and mortality in patients with coronary artery disease. N Engl J Med 1997;337:230–236.
83. McGill C, Lawrence SL. Dietary folate increases serum folate and decreases homocysteine concentrations in healthy adults [abstract]. J Am Coll Nutr 1998;17:A-133.
84. Food and Nutrition Board, National Academy of Sciences. Diet and Health: Implications for Reducing Chronic Disease Risk. National Academy Press, Washington, DC, 1989.
85. Joshipura KJ, Ascherio A, Manson JE, et al. Fruit and vegetable intake in relation to risk of ischemic stroke. JAMA 1999;282:1233–1239.
86. Miller JW. Homocysteine, Alzheimer's disease, and cognitive function. Nutrition 2000;16:675–677.
87. Riggs KM, Spiro A, III, Tucker K, Rush D. Relations of vitamin B-12, vitamin B-6, folate, and homocysteine to cognitive performance in the Normative Aging Study. Am J Clin Nutr 1996;63:306–314.
88. Lehmann M, Gottfries CG, Regland B. Identification of cognitive impairment in the elderly: homocysteine is an early marker. Dement Geriatr Cog Disord 1999;10:12–20.
89. Messier C, Gagnon M. Glucose regulation and brain aging. J Nutr Health Aging 2000;4:208–213.
90. Messier C, Gagnon M. Glucose regulation and cognitive functions: relation to Alzheimer's disease and diabetes. Behav Brain Res 1996;75:1–11.
91. Messier C, Desrochers A, Gagnon M. Effect of glucose, glucose regulation, and word imagery value on human memory. Behav Neurosci 1999;113:431–438.
92. Stevenson RE, Allen WP, Pai GS, et al. Decline in prevalence of neural tube defects in a high-risk region of the United States. Pediatrics 2000;106:677–683.
93. Cuskelly GJ, McNulty H, Scott JM. Effect of increasing dietary folate on red-cell folate: implications for prevention of neural tube defects. Lancet 1996;347:657–659.
94. Acuna J, Yoon P, Erickson D. The Prevention of Neural Tube Defects with Folic Acid. Centers for Disease Control and Prevention, Atlanta, GA, 1999.
95. Schwartz AG, Rate WR. Inhibition of aflatoxin B1-induced cytotoxicity and binding to DNA in cultured rat liver cells by naturally occurring flavones. J Environ Pathol Toxicol 1979;2:1021–1028.
96. Wattenberg LW. Effects of dietary constituents on the metabolism of chemical carcinogens. Cancer Res 1975;35:3326–3331.
97. Bracke ME, Vyncke BM, Van Larebeke NA, et al. The flavonoid tangeretin inhibits invasion of MO4 mouse cells into embryonic chick heart in vitro. Clin Exp Metastasis 1989;7:283–300.

6

Orange Juice

*Are the Health Benefits
of Oranges Lost During Processing?*

Carol S. Johnston

Citrus fruits are believed to have originated in the Ancient Orient. In the United States, citrus cultivation began in Florida in the early 1800s and later spread to Texas, Arizona, and California. By the 1930s, the citrus fruit production surpassed the demand for fresh fruit, stimulating the development of several of citrus products, and, by 1976, more than 90% of Florida's orange crop was used for orange juice production. Today, orange juice is Americans' most frequently consumed fruit serving *(1)*.

1. ORANGE JUICE CONSUMPTION BY AMERICANS

Diets rich in fruits and vegetables are associated with a decreased risk of cancer and chronic disease *(2–4)*. Most Americans are aware of the health benefits of fruits and vegetables and have increased their consumption of these foods by as much as 80% since the early 1980s (2.9 to 5.2 total servings daily) *(1)*. However, although nearly half of Americans are consuming 5 fruits and vegetables daily, only 18% are consuming the recommended 2 servings of fruit and 3 servings of vegetables. Nearly 40% of Americans consume 3 or more servings of vegetables daily, but only approx 25% are consuming 2 or more fruit servings daily *(1)*. Fruit juice accounts for 35–50% of the fruit consumed in the United States *(5,6)*, and citrus juices are the most commonly consumed juices, representing 70% of juices consumed *(6)*. Orange juice ranks first and is consumed regularly by 23% of Americans *(1)*.

The health effects afforded by fruits and vegetables are attributed to the many biologically active phytochemicals present in these foods *(3)*. These phytochemicals, including nutrient and nonnutrient compounds, possess detoxification, immunostimulating, antiviral, anticancer, and antioxidant properties. Much research has focused on fruits and vegetables antioxidant capacity, particularly because it is believed that oxidative damage plays a key role in cardiovascular disease, cancer initiation, cataract formation, inflammatory diseases, neurologic disorders, and the aging process. Antioxidants protect against oxidative damage by neutralizing the highly reactive chemical species that propagate the oxidative damage. The total antioxidant potential of plant extracts is

From: *Beverages in Nutrition and Health*
Edited by: T. Wilson and N. J. Temple © Humana Press Inc., Totowa, NJ

Table 1
Ascorbic Acid Content and ORAC Score of Oranges and Several Varieties of Orange Juice

	Ascorbic acid	ORAC score[a]
Orange, navel, 131 g without peel	80	983
Orange juice, fresh, 8 fl oz	124	1637
Commercial orange juice		
Reconstituted from frozen concentrate, 8 fl oz	97	—
Chilled, packaged in plastic, 8 fl oz	86	720
Chilled, packaged in carton, 8 fl oz	44	

[a]Adapted from Wang et al. (7).

determined in assay systems that use various radical generators in vitro to quantitate the free radical scavenging capacity of the extracts, e.g., the oxygen radical absorbance capacity (ORAC) assay or the ferric reducing-antioxidant power (FRAP) value.

Fruits and vegetables possess similar antioxidant capacities (7,8), yet one investigation reported that fruits provided twice the antioxidant activity of vegetables per serving (9). Among the different fruits, berries, plums, grapes, and oranges show the highest antioxidant capacity per serving (7,9). Fewer than 9% of Americans consume berries and grapes regularly, whereas approximately one third of Americans consume orange juice or oranges daily; thus, these latter items are likely the major source of fruit-based dietary antioxidant protection for Americans.

2. THE VITAMIN C CONTENT OF ORANGE JUICE

There are many bioactive components present in citrus fruits, including vitamins, ascorbic acid (vitamin C), and folic acid; phytochemicals, flavonoids, and limonoids; citric acid; and dietary fiber. The antioxidant capacity of citrus is attributed to vitamin C and flavonoids. The vitamin C content of orange juices and oranges can be compared using food composition tables, and published ORAC values provide an indication of the potential antioxidant benefit of oranges and orange juice (see Table 1). Fresh orange juice (8 fl oz or 248 mL) is a concentrated source of vitamin C, containing 50% more than a single orange. Similarly, the antioxidant capacity of fresh orange juice is higher than that of a single orange. Orange juice processing (pasteurization and storage), however, reduces its vitamin C content (frozen reconstituted juice > chilled juice in plastic jugs > chilled juice in cartons), as well as its antioxidant capacity. This is an important consideration because chilled juices account for a majority of the orange juice purchased by Americans (6). In fact, the popularity of chilled orange juice caused a marked shift in the industry in the early 1990s causing a decrease in the number of factories producing frozen concentrates and an increase in the number producing chilled orange juices. In 1977, 75% of Florida oranges were processed into frozen concentrate and 14% into chilled juice (10); by 2001, 41% of oranges used for juice production were processed into chilled juice (11).

Orange juice is the leading dietary source of vitamin C for Americans (1,12); hence, the consumption of highly processed orange juice may affect Americans' vitamin C status. Interestingly, the prevalence of vitamin C deficiency in Americans has increased from 5% to 11–16% during the last 20 yr *(13–15)*. Because Americans consume more fruits and vegetables today than they did 20 yr ago, the increased prevalence of vitamin C deficiency is likely a reflection of food choices and, perhaps, food processing, notably orange juice processing. As a side note, orange juice is also an important source of folic acid, and, similar to vitamin C, folic acid levels in chilled orange juice are reduced 50% compared to fresh orange juice. However, as of 1998, grain products in the United States have been fortified with folic acid; these foods include enriched flours, breads, rolls, buns, rice, and noodle products. Therefore, a serving of these grain products provides approx 10% of the recommended daily intake for folic acid (40 μg/serving). Thus, Americans' folic acid status has improved significantly in the past 4 yr, and the prevalence of folate deficiency has decreased 60%, from 4.9% to 1.9% *(16)*, demonstrating the widespread effect of food fortification programs.

3. VITAMIN C LOSSES IN CHILLED ORANGE JUICE: EFFECT OF EXTENSIVE PROCESSING AND STORAGE

The vitamin C molecule quickly degrades when exposed to light, oxygen, and heat; thus, the vitamin is easily lost during food processing and preparation. Fruit salad, prepared by cutting bananas, kiwi, and oranges, had no detectable vitamin C in its reduced active form, ascorbic acid, when analyzed immediately after preparation *(17)*. Rather, most of the vitamin C was detected as dehydroascorbic acid, the oxidized form indicative of vitamin C destruction. (Dehydroascorbic acid is not efficiently absorbed across the intestinal mucosa and cannot be considered a dietary source of vitamin C *[18,19]*). Most chilled orange juice sold in the United States is heat treated, or pasteurized, to reduce spoilage by microbial and enzymatic activities. For heat pasteurization, orange juice is heated to 94.6°C for 30 s, a process that reduces its vitamin C content *(20)*. Furthermore, paperboard cartons and plastic containers that allow the passage of oxygen are commonly used as packaging materials for chilled orange juice.

Freshly squeezed orange juice retains 98% of its vitamin C content in the active form *(17)*. In our laboratories, we also observed a low rate of vitamin C oxidation in freshly squeezed orange juice, approx 11% of the total vitamin C content. Immediately upon reconstitution, frozen orange juice concentrate had a higher content of oxidized vitamin C, approx 30%; however, 76% of the vitamin C in chilled orange juice (packaged in cartons) analyzed 4 wk before expiration, was oxidized (*see* Fig. 1). Chilled orange juice packaged in resealable plastic jugs had intermediate levels of oxidized vitamin C, 51–54% of the total vitamin C content.

Others have reported similar data. More than 25 yr ago, Horowitz et al. *(21)* noted that chilled ready-to-drink orange juice contained 40% less active vitamin C (ascorbic acid) per cup when compared with freshly squeezed or frozen reconstituted orange juice. These researchers warned that the new food processing technologies may affect the vitamin C content of the American diet and that the use of processed foods must be considered when evaluating a patient's diet for vitamin C adequacy *(21)*. Moreover, we, and others, have documented considerable ascorbic acid losses in chilled juices during the storage life in both opened and sealed containers: approx 2% of the ascorbic acid per container is lost per day *(22,23)*. Because chilled orange juice packaged in nonresealable gable-top cartons has low levels of ascorbic acid initially, approx 25–30 mg/8 fl oz, this juice contains little active vitamin C (approx 15 mg/8 fl oz) after 3–4 wk of storage, even if left sealed *(22)*.

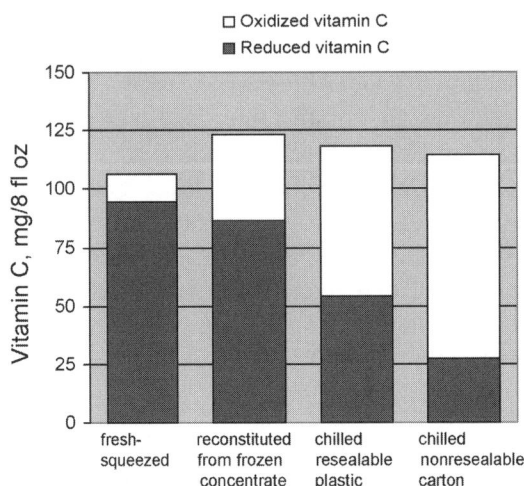

Fig. 1. Levels of oxidized and reduced vitamin C in orange juice: freshly squeezed juice from whole oranges or various varieties of commercially purchased orange juice. Chilled ready-to-drink juices were unsealed and tested immediately at 4 wk before expiration.

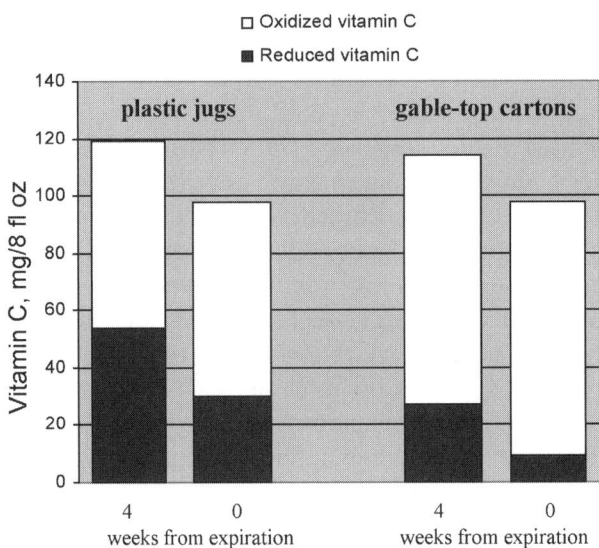

Fig. 2. Levels of oxidized and reduced vitamin C in chilled ready-to-drink commercially purchased orange juice packaged in plastic jugs or gable-top cartons. Each juice was unsealed at 4 wk from expiration and immediately tested. Juices were then stored at 4°C in the resealed original containers and tested at expiration.

Chilled orange juices packaged in plastic jugs also exhibit ascorbic acid losses (2%/d), but represent a better source of vitamin C because ascorbic acid levels are high initially (55–65 mg/8 fl oz initially, falling by half after 4 wk of storage) (*see* Fig. 2).

Together, these data show that the processing and packaging of ready-to-drink chilled orange juice adversely affects its ascorbic acid, or active vitamin C, content. Freshly squeezed orange juice and orange juice reconstituted from frozen concentrates contain approximately the recommended daily intake for adult men and women per 1 cup serving, 75–90 mg. *Note:* The US Food Pyramid classes 0.75 cups juice as 1 serving, yet US food labels classify 1 cup of orange juice as 1 serving. Chilled ready-to-drink orange juices packaged in cartons provide only 20–30% of the recommended daily intake per 1 cup serving. Thus, even regular consumption of orange juice may not protect individuals from vitamin C depletion.

4. INTERVENTION TRIALS USING CHILLED ORANGE JUICE: ARE THE POTENTIAL HEALTH BENEFITS NOT FULLY REALIZED?

In a recent clinical trial, middle-aged men and women with moderately elevated plasma total and low-density lipoprotein (LDL) cholesterol incorporated 1, 2, and 3 cups of orange juice each day into their low-fat diets for 4 wk, with each dosage in a sequential manner *(24)*. The orange juice was chilled, commercially available, and packaged in cartons. The investigators did not analyze the ascorbic acid content of the juice; rather, the manufacturer provided the vitamin C content information, 74.9 mg/8 fl oz. Based on diet analysis using food composition tables, the subjects' daily vitamin C intake increased from 128 mg in the initial 4-wk diet period to 191 mg and 260 mg in the second and third 4-wk diet periods, respectively. Plasma vitamin C concentrations, however, were remarkably low throughout the entire trial. The mean concentration at baseline, 8.5 ± 3.3 μmol/L, was indicative of vitamin C deficiency (<11 μmol/L). Concentrations increased 125% to 19.1 ± 4.8 μmol/L, after the initial diet period when dietary vitamin C averaged 128 mg, but this level of plasma vitamin C falls within the marginal range (11–28 μmol/L). The mean plasma concentration was still marginal (26.8 ± 11.6 μmol/L) after the completion of the second diet period in which subjects reportedly consumed 191 mg d. It was only after the final diet period, dietary vitamin C reportedly averaging 260 mg daily, that subjects' vitamin C status was normalized (32.5 ± 16.3 μmol/L) *(24)*. Tightly controlled vitamin C depletion-repletion pharmacokinetic trials in men and women clearly show that plasma vitamin C concentrations range from 25–45 μmol/L on vitamin C intakes approximating 60 mg/d *(25,26)*. At intakes near 100 mg/d, plasma vitamin C concentrations range from 55 to 60 μmol/L. Thus, it is evident, although not addressed by the investigators of the trial, that the orange juice used did not contain the reported vitamin C level.

Based on our data, commercially available chilled orange juice packaged in cartons contains 15–30 mg/8 fl oz. Thus, the subjects' vitamin C intakes in the previous trial was likely much lower, only 70–80 mg throughout the entire trial. This is a critical detail. The purpose of the orange juice trial was to determine the cardioprotective effects of orange juice, notably the effect of orange juice on high-density (HDL) cholesterol. The investigators reported a significant improvement in HDL cholesterol only in the final diet period; there was no improvement in HDL cholesterol with the regular daily consumption of 1 or 2 cups of orange juice *(24)*. Jacques et al. *(27,28)* estimated that for each 60 μmol/L increase in plasma vitamin C concentrations, there was an associated HDL cholesterol increase of 0.15 mmol/L. Thus, it is likely that if the orange juice had supplied approx 75 mg of ascorbic acid per cup, as claimed, plasma vitamin C concentrations should have changed from approx 8 μmol/L to approx 60 μmol/L after the first diet period, and 1 cup of orange juice might have significantly affected HDL cholesterol concentrations. Future orange juice intervention trials should use fresh orange juice or orange juice reconstituted from frozen concentrates because these forms maintain a high ascorbic acid content; moreover, the ascorbic acid content of the juice should be analyzed directly.

Harats et al. *(29)* conducted an intervention trial to determine the effects of daily orange juice consumption on cardiovascular risk factors in healthy young men. Freshly squeezed orange juice, consumed within 10 min of preparation, was used. As in the previous trial, juice was not analyzed for vitamin C content, rather it was estimated that the juice provided approx 500 mg vitamin C daily. This is unlikely, however, because 500 mg of vitamin C from orange juice represents an added 750 kcal/d. The difference in energy intake between the control and juice groups was, at most, only approx 120 kcal, which equals approx 1 cup of orange juice. After 3 mo, plasma vitamin C concentrations averaged 13.1 ± 2.5 and 51.7 ± 3.1 μmol/L in the control and juice groups, respectively. This indicates that the juice drinkers were consuming approx 100 mg vitamin C daily based on the pharmacokinetic trials mentioned *(25,26)*. This level of juice intake did significantly reduce in vitro susceptibility of lipoproteins to oxidation but did not significantly affect HDL cholesterol concentrations *(29)*. This trial used freshly squeezed orange juice with high vitamin C content, which may have accounted for the observed beneficial effect.

We recently compared the effect of dietary vitamin C in supplement form (approx 70 mg ascorbic acid) vs a serving of commercially available orange juice (approx 70 mg ascorbic acid) on plasma concentrations of lipid peroxides, a marker of oxidative stress *(30)*. Eleven healthy young women restricted fruit and vegetable consumption to approx 1 serving/d during the 12-wk trial and were instructed not to consume either vitamin C-fortified or vitamin E-fortified foods (notably fortified breakfast cereals). After the initial 2-wk washout, subjects were randomly divided into three intervention groups: 1 cup orange juice daily, 2 cups/d orange juice, or a vitamin C supplement daily. The treatment period was 2 wk. This 4-wk design was repeated twice so that each subject received each experimental treatment preceded by a 2-wk washout period. The orange juice was commercially available ready-to-drink chilled juice, and new supplies were provided to subjects weekly. The juice was analyzed at the beginning and end of each week, and the average ascorbic acid concentration (determined analytically) was 70 mg/8 fl oz and 57 mg/8 fl oz at the beginning and end of each week, respectively. Thus, the overall average vitamin C intake of subjects receiving the juice intervention was 64 mg/8 fl oz. The vitamin C supplement was prepared in our laboratories, and each capsule contained, on average, 69 mg ascorbic acid.

Baseline plasma vitamin C and total lipid peroxide concentrations were significantly altered after the 2-wk fruit and vegetable restriction: plasma vitamin C levels fell 16% (p = .016), and plasma total lipid peroxides rose 61% (p < .001) (*see* Fig. 3). These data alone demonstrate the protective role of fruits and vegetables in the diet. Both the vitamin C supplement (approx 70 mg ascorbic acid) and 1 cup of orange juice (approx 70 mg ascorbic acid) lowered plasma total lipid peroxides 45–50%; thus, these sources of vitamin C were equally effective at reducing oxidative stress in vivo, as indicated by plasma lipid peroxide levels. Although the 2-cup orange juice intervention (approx 140 mg ascorbic acid) raised plasma vitamin C concentrations 20% above that noted for the vitamin C supplement, lipid peroxide concentrations were similar after each intervention protocol (*see* Fig. 4). These data indicate that 1 cup of orange juice containing approx 70 mg ascorbic acid does significantly reduce markers of oxidative stress in vivo

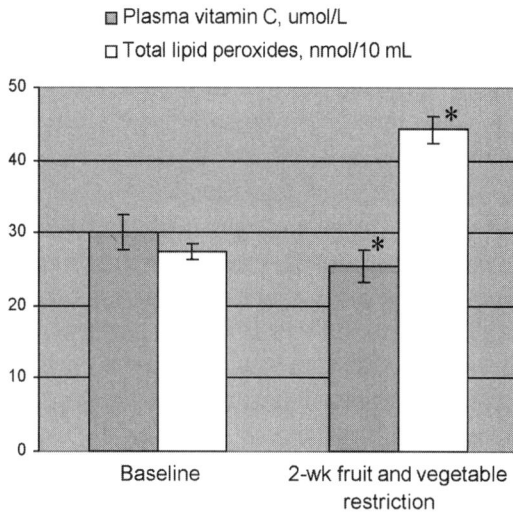

Fig. 3. Plasma concentrations of vitamin C and total lipid peroxides in free-living subjects ($n = 8$) at baseline and after 2 wk of fruit and vegetable restriction. An asterisk denotes a significant change from baseline ($p < 0.05$).

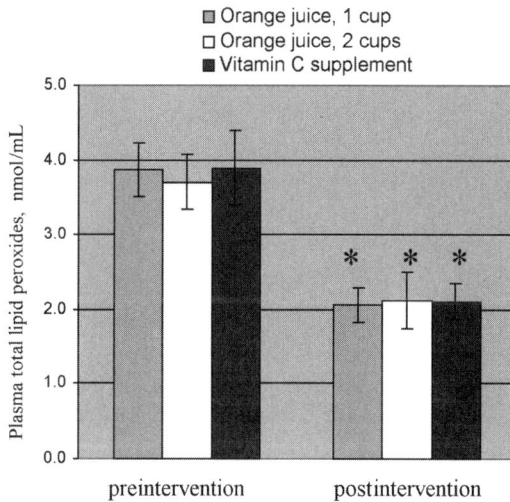

Fig. 4. Plasma total lipid peroxides in free-living subjects ($n = 8$) before and after 2-wk diet intervention: 1 cup/d orange juice (64 mg ascorbic acid/cup); 2 cups/d orange juice (128 mg ascorbic acid/2 cups); and 1 vitamin C supplement/d (69 mg ascorbic acid/capsule). All subjects received each 2-wk treatment proceeded by a 2-wk washout period in a randomized crossover fashion. An asterisk denotes a significant change from preintervention ($p < 0.05$).

and that much of this effect is related to the juice's vitamin C content. Hence, consumption of vitamin C-poor orange juices, e.g., chilled ready-to-drink orange juices purchased 1–2 wk from expiration date or packaged in nonresealable cartons, is not likely to provide the same health benefits as vitamin C-rich orange juice, freshly squeezed orange juice, or orange juice reconstituted from frozen concentrates.

Others agree that the vitamin C content of fruits and vegetables is an important component of the protective effect of fruit and vegetables. Szeto et al. *(31)* measured the total antioxidant and the total ascorbic acid contents of fresh fruits and vegetables. In vitamin C-rich fruits and vegetables (e.g., orange, grapefruit, kiwi, mango, cabbage, turnip greens, and cauliflower), vitamin C accounted for 35–75% of the food's antioxidant power. Yet, several vitamin C-poor foods, most notably plums, had high total antioxidant power, with < 1% accounted for by vitamin C. Using the ORAC assay, Cao et al. *(32)* demonstrated that a single oral dose of vitamin C (1250 mg) increased serum total antioxidant capacity 21% during the next 4 h. In comparison, three servings of strawberries (240 g) and 5 servings of cooked spinach (294 g) raised serum total antioxidant capacity 12% and 24%, respectively *(32)*. The vitamin C content of the strawberries (approx 140 mg) and spinach (approx 40 mg) was far lower than the amount supplied by the vitamin C supplement; thus, fruit and vegetable constituents other than vitamin C also provide antioxidant protection to serum, notably the carotenoids, flavonoids, and hydroxycinnamates *(33)*. However, it is clear that vitamin C alone is a powerful antioxidant at high intakes.

5. PROCESSING AFFECTS PHYTOCHEMICALS, NOTABLY THE FLAVANONES, IN CHILLED ORANGE JUICE

Citric acid and the flavanones hesperidin and naringin in orange juice also possess antioxidant activity. Citric acid chelates metal ions, preventing oxidative reactions, and is widely used for blood *(34)* and food *(35)* preservation and as a therapeutic agent to reduce corneal inflammation *(36,37)*. In subjects who are vitamin C depleted (plasma vitamin C, 19.3 ± 3.4 µmol/L), 150 mg citric acid daily as a supplement reduced plasma lipid peroxide levels significantly after 3 wk (3.93 ± 0.53 nmol/mL pre-citric acid and 2.93 ± 0.28 nmol/ml post-citric acid, p = .045) but did not alter the plasma vitamin C concentration *(38)*. Improving the vitamin C status in these subjects (500 mg/d ascorbic acid for 3 wk) raised plasma vitamin C concentrations significantly (52.6 ± 4.0 µmol/L) but had no further effect on plasma lipid peroxides (3.02 ± 0.69 nmol/mL).

Together, the flavanones hesperidin and naringin represent approx 50% of the total flavonoids in orange juice (approx 50 mg/8 fl oz) and account for approx 25% of the antioxidant capacity of orange juice in vitro *(39)*. However, there is considerable variation in the concentrations of hesperidin and naringin in different commercial juices *(40)*. In nine commercial brands of grapefruit juice, the concentrations of these two compounds ranged from 0.58 to 7.49 and 34.94 to 153.12 mg/cup, respectively. Thus, it is essential in intervention trials investigating the physiological benefits of orange juice consumption that the flavanone content of the juice, as well as the ascorbic acid content (as discussed above), be analyzed directly.

Oral administration of hesperidin reduced oxidative stress in patients with type 1 diabetes *(41)*. This treatment had no side effects and was related to an increase in glutathione peroxidase activity and an increase in the lag time of the copper-induced in vitro oxidizability of non-HDL. These changes were accompanied by a decrease in HbA1c, a long-term indicator of glucose control, particularly in those patients whose initial level of HbA1c was high *(41)*. Diabetic rats fed a hesperidin-enriched diet exhibited less oxidative stress, as indicated by decreased concentrations of lipid peroxides in serum and decreased levels of urinary 8-hydroxydeoxyguanosine, a marker of oxidatively damaged DNA *(42)*. Hesperidin and naringin also possess anticancer activity in vivo. After chemical induction of mammary tumorigenesis, rats that were fed double-strength orange juice or comparable levels of naringin had a lower tumor incidence and tumor burden compared to control subjects *(43)*. In murine fibroblast cell culture, hesperidin was among the most potent flavonoids in preventing chemically induced neoplastic transformation *(44)*.

Orange juice is also a rich source of limonoids, which are responsible for the bitter taste of citrus juices. These substances exhibit cancer chemopreventive properties and inhibit the proliferation of several human cancer cell lines in vitro, including leukemia, ovary, cervix, stomach, liver, and breast *(45)*. In hamsters, chemically induced carcinogenesis was inhibited by topical application of limonin *(46)*, and dietary exposure to limonin significantly reduced the incidence of chemically induced colonic adenocarcinomas in rats *(47)*. The limonoids' anticancer effect has been attributed to their enhancement of glutathione S-transferases, enzymes that detoxify numerous potentially carcinogenic compounds and toxins.

The antioxidant potential of freshly prepared orange juice has been attributed, in part, to constituents other than vitamin C, namely the flavanones and other flavonoids *(39)*, but, as with vitamin C, the processing and storage of orange juice alters its flavonoid content. Hence, the degree of antioxidant protection afforded by orange juice consumption is likely lessened with processing. Hand-squeezed navel orange juice contains approx 750 mg flavanones/L (180 mg/cup), but 15% of the flavanones are precipitated in the cloud fraction of the juice and are unavailable for absorption *(48)*. During refrigerated storage of fresh juice (4°C), 50% of the soluble flavanones precipitate and integrate into the cloud fraction. Because of industrial processing and storage, commercial orange juices contain only 80–200 mg/L (20–50 mg/cup) of soluble flavanones *(48)*. Consequently, flavanone bioavailability from commercial orange juice is < 25% *(49)*, and the total antioxidant capacity of orange juice in vitro may not correlate with antioxidant protection in serum after orange juice consumption.

An additional consideration is the effect of the packaging material used for chilled orange juice. Researchers have reported high losses of limonene from orange juice in contact with polyethylene, the product contact layer used in cartons and plastic containers *(50)*. These investigations were conducted to examine flavor changes due to packaging materials, but loss of limonene from juice may also affect the health benefits associated with orange juice consumption.

6. PROMOTION OF ORANGE JUICE CONSUMPTION FOR HEALTH BENEFITS

Fresh orange juice is an excellent source of vitamins and other compounds, namely vitamin C, flavanones, and lemonoids, which are potent antioxidant and anticancer agents. Thus, ideally, regular consumption of fresh orange juice should be associated with reduced disease risk; however, highly processed orange juice may have a lower content of the biologically active agents, as discussed and may not provide users with the same benefits as fresh orange juice or oranges. Epidemiologic data consistently show a health benefit of fruit and vegetable consumption, but most reports combine fruit and fruit juices into a single category and do not specifically examine potential benefits associated with oranges or orange juice. Several epidemiologic reports that looked specifically at citrus fruit (fruit and fruit juices combined) demonstrated only weak reductions in cancer risk *(51,52)*.

Recently, Hakim et al. *(53)* specifically examined usual citrus consumption patterns and risk for squamous cell carcinoma of the skin in a population at high risk for skin cancer. Interestingly, there was no association between orange juice consumption and skin cancer; yet, orange consumption, and more specifically, citrus peel consumption, reduced skin cancer risk by 11% and 34%, respectively *(53)*. The authors believe that this benefit was related to the high concentrations of limonene in the citrus peel. This research supports the contention that whole-fruit consumption has greater health benefits than fruit juice consumption.

More research delineating the health benefits specific to whole-fruit consumption vs juice consumption is needed. Much of the current research focuses on identifying the compounds in fruits and vegetables that are responsible for the cancer risk reduction. However, most epidemiologic studies have not considered the physical characteristics of foods or the effects of food processing on food constituents, both of which are important determinants of the physiological responses to food ingestion *(54)*.

Should commercial orange juice consumption be encouraged? Yes, of course it should. However, consumers should be advised to purchase frozen concentrates and to drink the juice within a week of its preparation. As discussed, this form of orange juice maintains a high vitamin C concentration, and this likely is an indicator of the overall quality of the juice. Preferably, individuals should make an effort to eat whole fruits in addition to juice for a total of 3–5 servings/d.

One serving of juice daily (8 fl oz), not two or three servings daily, is probably prudent advice. Subjects who are hypercholesterolemic who consumed 3 servings/d of orange juice exhibited a significant increase in fasting blood triglycerides *(23)*, a risk factor for cardiovascular disease. In comparison, in a randomized intervention trial, blood triglycerides were not significantly affected in subjects who increased fruit consumption by 3.5 servings/d (+1 serving juice and +2.5 servings whole fruit) *(55)*. Whole-fruit consumption is advocated also for its dietary fiber. Berries, apples, bananas, pears, and oranges provide approx 5–8 g fiber per serving, and dried fruit provides as much as 18 g fiber per serving. In comparison, fruit juices contain only trace amounts of dietary fiber.

7. MAIN POINTS FOR PRIMARY AND CLINICAL REVIEW

1. Only a quarter of Americans receive the nutritional benefits of consuming more than the USDA recommended two fruit servings per day.
2. Storage methods, packaging methods, and shelf-life vary widely and can be associated with reductions in the nutrient content of the juice relative to the fresh fruit.
3. Chilled orange juice in a plastic jug loses 2% of its ascorbic acid content per day, and orange juice stored in sealed gable-top containers will have lost most of its ascorbic acid by the time the expiration date is reached.
4. Appreciating these reductions in ascorbate content is important for consumers and for those conducting research studies.
5. For optimal intake of ascorbate it is to best to consume either freshly prepared juice or frozen juice prepared just prior to consumption.

REFERENCES

1. Johnston CS, Taylor CA, Hampl JS. More Americans are eating "5 A Day" but intakes of dark green and cruciferous vegetables remain low. J Nutr 2000;130:3063–3067.

2. Steinmetz KA, Potter JD. Vegetables, fruit, and cancer prevention: a review. J Am Dietet Assoc 1996;96: 1027–1039.

3. Lampe JW. Health effects of vegetables and fruit: assessing mechanisms of action in human experimental studies. Am J Clin Nutr 1999;70(Suppl):475S–490S.

4. Joffe M, Robertson A. The potential contribution of increased vegetable and fruit consumption to health gain in the European Union. Public Health Nutr 2001;4:893–901.

5. Krebs-Smith SM, Cook A, Subar AF, Cleveland L, Friday J. US adults' fruit and vegetable intakes, 1989–1991: a revised baseline for the *Healthy People 2000* objective. Am J Pub Health 1995;85:1623–1629.

6. Third Report on Nutrition Monitoring in the United States, vol. 2. Washington, DC, US Government Printing Office, 1995, p. VA-56.

7. Wang H, Cao G, Prior RL. Total antioxidant capacity of fruits. J Agricultur Food Chem 1996;44:701–705.

8. Cao G, Sofic E, Prior RL. Antioxidant capacity of tea and common vegetables. J Agricultur Food Chem 1996;44:3426–3431.

9. Miller HE, Rigelhof F, Marquart L, Prakash A, Kanter M. Antioxidant content of whole grain breakfast cereals, fruits and vegetables. J Am Coll Nutr 2000;19:312S–319S.

10. Nagy S. Vitamin C contents of citrus fruit and their products: a review. J Agricultur Food Chem 1980; 28:8–18.

11. Florida Agricultural Statistics Service. Citrus Summary 2000–01. Florida Department of Agriculture and Consumer Services, Orlando, FL, 2002, p. 17.

12. Taylor CA, Hampl JS, Johnston CS. Low intakes of vegetables and fruits, especially citrus fruits, lead to inadequate vitamin C intakes among adults. Eur J Clin Nutr 2000;54:573–578.

13. Simon JA, Hudes ES. Serum ascorbic acid and cardiovascular disease prevalence in U.S. adults: The Third National Health and Nutrition Examination Survey (NHANES III). Ann Epidemiol 1999;9:358–365.

14. U.S. Department of Health and Human Services. Hematological and Nutrition Biochemistry Reference Data for Persons 6 Months—74 years of age: United States, 1976–80. Advance Data from Vital and Health Statistics, No. 83-1682. National Center for Health Statistics, Hyattsville, MD, 1982, pp. 124–139.

15. Hampl JS, Taylor CA, Johnston CS. NHANES III data indicate that American subgroups have a high risk of vitamin C deficiency [abstract]. J Am Dietet Assoc 2000;100:A59.

16. Choumenkovitch SF, Jacques PF, Nadeau MR, Wilson PW, Rosenberg IH, Selhub J. Folic acid fortification increases red blood cell folate concentrations in the Framingham study. J Nutr 2001;131: 3277–3280.

17. Severi S, Bedogni G, Zoboli GP, et al. Effects of home-based food preparation practices on the micronutrient content of foods. Eur J Cancer Prev 1998;7:331–335.

18. Malo C, Wilson JX. Glucose modulates vitamin C transport in adult human small intestinal brush border membrane vesicles. J Nutr 2000;130:63–69.

19. Ogiri Y, Sun F, Hayami S, et al. Very low vitamin C activity of orally administered L-dehydroascorbic acid. J Agricultur Food Chem 2002;50:227–229.

20. Yeom HW, Streaker CB, Zhang H, Min DB. Effects of pulsed electric fields on the quality of orange juice and comparison with heat pasteurization. J Agricultur Food Chem 2000;48:4597–4605.

21. Horowitz I, Fabry EM, Gerson CD. Bioavailability of ascorbic acid in orange juice. JAMA 1976;235: 2624–2625.

22. Johnston CS, Bowling DL. Stability of ascorbic acid in commercially available orange juices. J Am Diet Assoc 2002;102:525–529.

23. Squires SR, Hanna JG. Concentration and stability of ascorbic acid in marketed reconstituted orange juice. J Agricultur Food Chem 1979;27:639–641.

24. Kurowska EM, Spence JD, Jordan J, et al. HDL-cholesterol-raising effect of orange juice in subjects with hypercholesterolemia. Am J Clin Nutr 2000;72;1095–1100.

25. Levine M, Conry-Cantilena C, Wang U, et al. Vitamin C pharmacokinetics in healthy volunteers: evidence for a recommended dietary allowance. Proc Natl Acad Sci USA 1996;93:3704–3709.

26. Levine M, Wang Y, Padayatty SJ, Morrow J. A new recommended dietary allowance of vitamin C for healthy young women. Proc Natl Acad Sci USA 2001;98:9842–9846.

27. Jacques PF, Hartz SC, McGandy RB, Jacob RA, Russell RM. Vitamin C and blood lipoproteins in an elderly population. Ann NY Acad Sci 1987;498:100–109.

28. Jacques PF, Hartz SC, McGandy RB, Jacot RA, Russell RM. Ascorbic acid, HDL, and total plasma cholesterol in eth elderly. J Am Coll Nutr 1987;6:169–174.

29. Harats D, Chevion S, Nahir M, Norman Y, Sagee O, Berry EM. Citrus fruit supplementation reduces lipoprotein oxidation in young men ingesting a diet high in saturated fat: presumptive evidence for an interaction between vitamins C and E in vivo. Am J Clin Nutr 1998;67:240–245.

30. Johnston CS, Dancho C, Strong G. Antioxidant effects in vivo are similar for supplemental vitamin C and orange juice [abstract]. FASEB J 2002;16:A270.

31. Szeto YT, Tomlinson B, Benzie IFF. Total antioxidant and ascorbic acid content of fresh fruits and vegetables: implications for dietary planning and food preservation. Br J Nutr 2002;87:55–59.

32. Cao G, Russell RM, Lischner N, Prior RL. Serum antioxidant capacity is increased by consumption of strawberries, spinach, red wine or vitamin C in elderly women. J Nutr 1998;128:2383–2390.

33. Paganaga G, Miller N, Rice-Evans CA. The polyphenolic content of fruit and vegetables and their antioxidant activities. What does a serving constitute? Free Rad Res 1999;30:153–162.

34. Suttnar J, Masova L, Dyr JE. Influence of citrate and EDTA anticoagulants on plasma malondialdehyde concentrations estimated by high-performance liquid chromatography. J Chromatogr B Biomed Sci Appl 2001;751:193–197.

35. Almeida ME, Nogueira JN. The control of polyphenol oxidase activity in fruits and vegetables. A study of the interactions between the chemical compounds used and heat treatment. Plant Foods Human Nutr 1995;47:245–256.

36. Pfister RR, Haddox JL, Dodson RW, German VP. The effect of citrate and other compounds on PMN incubated in vitro: further studies on the site and mechanism of action of citrate. Cornea 1984–1985;3: 240–249.

37. Pfister RR, Haddox JL, Yuille-Barr D. The combined effect of citrate/ascorbate treatment in alkali-injured rabbit eyes. Cornea 1991;10:100–104.

38. Deodati C. Hypovitaminosis C and oxidant defense in adult men and women [master's thesis]. Arizona State University, Tempe, AZ, 1996.

39. Rapisarda P, Tomaino A, Lo Cascio R, Bonina F, Pasquale AD, Saija A. Antioxidant effectiveness as influenced by phenolic content of fresh orange juices. J Agricultur Food Chem 1999;47:4718–4723.

40. Ross SA, Ziska DS, Zhao K, ElSohly MA. Variance of common flavonoids by brand of grapefruit juice. Fitoterapia 2000;71:154–161.

41. Manuel Y, Keenoy B, Vertommen J, De Leeuw I. The effect of flavonoid treatment on the glycation and antioxidant status in Type 1 diabetic patients. Diabetes Nutr Metab 1999;12:256–263.

42. Miyake Y, Yamamoto K, Tsujihara N, Osawa T. Protective effects of lemon flavonoids on oxidative stress in diabetic rats. Lipids 1998;33:689–695.

43. So FV, Guthrie N, Chambers AF, Moussa M, Carroll KK. Inhibition of human breast cancer cell proliferation and delay of mammary tumorigenesis by flavonoids and citrus juices. Nutr Cancer 1996;26: 167–181.

44. Franke AA, Cooney RV, Custer LJ, Mordan LJ, Tanaka Y. Inhibition of neoplastic transformation and bioavailability of dietary flavonoid agents. Adv Exp Med Biol 1998;439:237–248.

45. Tian Q, Miller EG, Ahmad H, Tang L, Patil BS. Differential inhibition of human cancer cell proliferation by citrus limonoids. Nutr Cancer 2001;40:180–184.

46. Miller EG, Fanous R, Rivera-Hidalgo F, Binnie WH, Hasegawa S, Lam LK. The effect of citrus limonoids on hamster buccal pouch carcinogenesis. Carcinogenesis 1989;10:1535–1537.

47. Tanaka T, Maeda M, Kohno H, et al. Inhibition of azoxymethane-induced colon carcinogenesis in male F344 rats by the citrus limonoids obacunone and limonin. Carcinogenesis 2000;22:193–198.

48. Hil-Izquierdo A, Gil MI, Ferreres F, Tomas-Barberan FA. In vitro availability of flavonoids and other phenolics in orange juice. J Agricultur Food Chem 2001;49:1035–1041.

49. Ameer B, Weintraub RA, Johnson JV, Yost RA, Rouseff RL. Flavanone absorption after naringin, hesperidin, and citrus administration. Clin Pharmacol Ther 1996;60:34–40.

50. Pieper G, Borgudd L, Ackermann P, Fellers P. Absorption of aroma volatiles of orange juice into laminated carton did not affect sensory quality. J Food Sci 1992;57:1408–1411.

51. Levi F, Pasche C, LaVecchia C, Lucchini F, Franceschl S. Food groups and colorectal cancer risk. Br J Cancer 1999;79:1283–1287.

52. Bueno DE, Mesquita HB, Maisonneuve P, Runia S, Moerman CJ. Intake of foods and nutrients and cancer of the exocrine pancreas: a population-based case-control study in the Netherlands. Int J Cancer 1991;48:540–549.

53. Hakim IA, Harris RB, Ritenbaugh C. Citrus peel use is associated with reduced risk of squamous cell carcinoma of the skin. Nutr Cancer 2000;37:161–168.

54. Riboli E, Slimani N, Daaks R. Identifiability of food components for cancer chemoprevention. IARC Sci Publ 1996;139:23–31.

55. Smith-Warner SA, Elmer PJ, Tharp TM, et al. Increasing vegetable and fruit intake: randomized intervention and monitoring in an at-risk population. Cancer Epidemiol Biomarkers Prev 2000;9: 307–317.

7

How Can the Consumption of Grapefruit Juice and Other Beverages Affect Drug Action?

Garvan C. Kane

1. INTRODUCTION

For practical purposes, every oral medication must be coconsumed with a beverage. Most physicians and pharmacists admit that, ideally, medications should be taken with a glass of water. However, for many reasons, usually patient preference or convenience, this is often not the case. Occasionally, patients will be instructed by their physicians to take their medication with a certain food or beverage to aid palatability (and hence, compliance), minimize local irritation to the gastrointestinal (GI) tract, or aid in drug absorption.

Unfortunately, there are instances when the consumption of certain beverages in combination with certain medications presents problems. At times, a beverage may interfere with the metabolism of a drug, leading to a reduction in the amount of drug absorbed or by inhibiting drug metabolism, resulting in increased drug blood concentrations, which may predispose the patient to dose-dependent side effects. Perhaps the biggest culprit in this regard is grapefruit juice.

This chapter discusses some of the principles that govern drug–beverage interactions, both only those that increase and those that decrease the quantity of drug absorbed. Also discussed is how, in some instances, these interactions are used by physicians to aid in the management of certain problems faced in the caring for their patients.

2. HOW A DRUG GETS FROM THE MOUTH TO THE BLOODSTREAM

To understand how grapefruit juice, red wine, and caffeine-containing beverages may interact with medications, we must first briefly review one of the major processes of drug metabolism by the body. By affecting drug metabolism, these beverages impart their effect.

Cytochrome P450 is the name given to a large family of proteins that is located in the endoplasmic reticulum of cells throughout the body. The largest concentration of these enzymes is in the liver and the enterocytes, which form the lining of the intestinal wall.

From: *Beverages in Nutrition and Health*
Edited by: T. Wilson and N. J. Temple © Humana Press Inc., Totowa, NJ

Here, they are responsible for the oxidative metabolism of many xenobiotics, including many medications. Within this enzyme family, there are several subfamilies that display different properties. These enzyme subfamilies can be divided on the basis of their structure, specificity of substrates, or response to various compounds that increase enzyme activity, so-called enzyme inducers. Many of these inducers are, in themselves, medications. The CYP3A subfamily is the predominant enzyme subfamily, comprising, on average, 30% of CYP content in the liver and up to 70% in enterocytes of the small intestine *(1)*.

To get from the lumen of the small intestine into the systemic circulation, a medication must pass through the intestinal wall and enter the portal venous system. This conduit then carries the medication to the liver and on to the heart, where it can be propelled to its ultimate site of action. Typically, the majority of a drug is absorbed within a few hours of oral administration. This process can be affected by many factors, including motility of the GI tract, the size and formulation of the drug, the intestinal (splanchnic) blood flow, and various biochemical factors, including pH level. Even after the drug is absorbed, much, if not all, of the drug may be inactivated in either the intestine or the liver by these CYP enzymes of metabolism. This combined process is referred to as first-pass metabolism. Generally, only a portion of the drug ingested reaches the systemic circulation; that proportion is termed the oral bioavailability. This term takes into account the processes of absorption across the intestinal mucosa, as well as the extent of first-pass metabolism.

The CYP3A4 enzyme in the intestine is the same as that in the liver; however, different medications may be preferentially metabolized at one site over another. For example, drugs that are less soluble remain locally in the intestine longer, increasing the time that they are exposed to the intestinal enzymes.

In addition to being metabolized by or inducing CYP enzymes, some medications actually inhibit them. Medications such as itraconazole, ketoconazole, cyclosporine, diltiazem, and erythromycin inhibit both intestinal and hepatic CYP3A4. As a result, the reduced presystemic drug metabolism increases the quantity of drug absorbed (oral bioavailability) *(2–4)*. In fact, inhibition of this enzyme system is the cause of many drug–drug interactions. In recent years, terfenadine, mibefradil, cisapride, and cerivastatin have been withdrawn from the US market, because of deaths as a result of drug–drug interactions involving the hepatic CYP3A4 system.

3. HOW BEVERAGES MAY PREVENT DRUG ABSORPTION

Tetracycline is an antibiotic whose absorption is significantly impeded by calcium. Many studies have shown that coadministration with milk (which is calcium rich) severely diminishes tetracycline absorption, even in small volumes, such as those that may accompany tea or coffee *(5,6)*. One would assume that calcium-enriched citrus juices would have the same effect.

4. HOW A BEVERAGE IS USED TO AID DRUG ABSORPTION

Ketaconazole and itraconazole are medications with a broad spectrum of antifungal action. Ketaconazole is active against several yeast, dimorphic fungal, and dermatophytic infections. It is commonly used in the treatment of mucocutaneous fungal infections (e.g., candidiasis) that are common in patients with acquired immune deficiency syndrome (AIDS) or are immunosuppressed from cancer chemotherapy. Itraconazole is

Table 1
pH of Selected Commercially Available Beverages[a]

Beverage	pH
Coca-Cola Classic	2.5
Pepsi	2.5
Canada Dry ginger ale	2.7
Diet Coca-Cola	3.2
Diet Pepsi	3.2
Tropicana grapefruit juice	3.4
7-Up	3.4
Tropicana orange juice	3.8

[a] *Source*: ref. *9* and unpublished data.
[b] Those medications above the dashed line are expected to aid in ketaconazole absorption; those below the line likely do not.

active against aspergillosis and is commonly given as prophylaxis in patients who have undergone organ transplantation. However, these medications are weak alkalis that dissolve poorly in water unless it is acidic, with a pH < 3, or a surrounding pH < 5. Normally, this does not present a problem because the highly acidic gastric juices are responsible for a low pH in the proximal small intestine, thereby facilitating moderate absorption of the drug. However, if the gastric acid production is low (achlorhydria), insufficient drug is absorbed. The resulting low drug level in the blood is insufficient to eradicate the fungal infection. Patients with AIDS commonly have decreased acid production as a manifestation of AIDS gastropathy, a complication of their disease *(7)*. Also, many immunosuppressed patients are at risk of developing gastroesophageal reflux and peptic ulcer diseases. They are therefore frequently treated with acid-suppressing therapy, such as histamine (H_2) antagonists or protein-pump inhibitors, rendering them medically achlorhydric. Malabsorption of both ketaconazole and itraconazole has been seen in patients with achlorhydria *(8)*. In addition, drug failure in such patients is well established. Therefore, coadministering ketaconazole or itraconazole with an acidic beverage is attractive and is now well established. Several acidic beverages have been used. Dilute acids (e.g., hydrochloric acid) were initially tried but must be dispensed and have poor palatability *(8)*. In 1995, Chin et al. *(9)* studied the coadministration of Coca-Cola to aid in ketaconazole absorption in patients with achlorhydria. They found that this increased mean bioavailability of the drug by nearly 50%. Patients are now commonly recommended to take ketaconazole with one of several beverages (Table 1).

5. GRAPEFRUIT JUICE INHIBITS DRUG METABOLISM

Grapefruit juice is consumed by one fifth of American families *(10)*, endorsed by the American Heart Association, rich in vitamin C, and often fortified with supplemental calcium. However, unlike other citrus juices, grapefruit juice interacts with many prescription medications, leading to increased drug levels and the potential for dose-dependent side effects *(11–13)*.

Evidence suggests that certain substances in grapefruit juice are metabolized locally in the intestinal wall to reactive intermediates that then combine with the enzyme CYP3A4. The enzyme is then irreversibly inactivated, likely by a change in its conformation. This process is termed "suicide inhibition." The quantity of grapefruit juice that is typically consumed (200–250 mL) decreases the enterocyte CYP3A4 concentration in the lining of the small bowel without affecting the concentration of the enzyme in the liver. This indicates that grapefruit juice's effect is localized to the intestinal wall when it is consumed in typical quantities. 6',7'-Dihydroxybergamottin and naringin are some of the constituents of grapefruit that may impart this drug interaction. These constituents are also present in the whole fruit, the pulp, and the peel, all of which may impart a similar drug interaction as the juice (14).

There are inherent interindividual differences in the concentration of CYP3A4 in the intestine, which is predetermined by the genetics of the individual. There is evidence that the CYP3A4 enterocyte concentration varies between members of different ethnicities, likely due to the differences in frequencies of genetic polymorphisms between ethnic groups. Grapefruit juice imparts a greater interaction in African Americans than with Caucasians (15). Because of these genetic-based differences in CYP3A4 content, the effect of grapefruit juice on drug action also varies between individuals. Those patients who have the highest CYP3A4 concentrations in enterocytes have the greatest increases in drug levels after coadministration of grapefruit juice (16).

5.1. Cardiovascular Medications

1,4-Dihydropyridine calcium antagonists are lipid-soluble drugs used in the treatment of hypertension and angina pectoris. They are metabolized in vivo by CYP3A4 and interact, to varying degrees, with grapefruit juice. Of all medication classes, this one has probably been the best studied regarding its interaction with grapefruit juice. Indeed, the grapefruit juice effect on drug metabolism was first noticed in studies with the calcium channel antagonist felodipine. In the late 1980s, Bailey et al. (17) observed an interaction between felodipine and grapefruit juice in a study of felodipine and ethanol that used grapefruit juice to mask the taste of ethanol. Subsequent studies confirmed that grapefruit juice significantly increased the oral bioavailability of felodipine (18,19).

Consistent with the interaction mechanism discussed above, grapefruit juice has the most marked effect on those calcium antagonists with the lowest oral bioavailabilities. One glass of grapefruit juice more than doubles the bioavailability of both standard-release (19–21) and extended-release felodipine, albeit in a variable manner amongst individuals (22). Indeed, some patients, perhaps those with the highest intestinal expression of CYP3A4, experience a much greater grapefruit juice interaction. Such an increase in drug levels increases dose-dependent effects (both desirable and undesirable), with studies showing enhanced blood pressure reduction, increased heart rate, and increased vasodilatory adverse effects when felodipine is taken with grapefruit juice (19,20,23). Less commonly prescribed agents, pranidipine, nisoldipine, and nimodipine, have shown 1.5-fold increased bioavailabilities when given with a single glass of grapefruit juice (24–26). Amlodipine and nifedipine have better inherent oral bioavailabilities and hence are less affected by grapefruit juice. However, studies have shown increased blood drug levels (20–30% increases) but much less in altered hemodynamic responses or adverse effects *(18,27,28)*. Surprisingly, although metabolized in vivo by CYP3A4, small clinical studies have not shown an interaction between the nondihydropyridine calcium antagonists diltiazem and verapamil and grapefruit juice *(29)*.

Cilostazol, which is used in the treatment of intermittent claudication (leg pain associated with arterial occlusive disease of the lower extremities), is extensively metabolized in vivo by CYP3A4. No studies evaluating the effect of grapefruit juice on cilostazol pharmacokinetics have been published; however, other CYP3A4 inhibitors, such as erythromycin and diltiazem, have shown increased cilostazol plasma concentrations *(30,31)*. Therefore, the manufacturers of cilostazol suggest that patients receiving the drug avoid grapefruit juice consumption until this interaction is evaluated further *(30)*.

Losartan, an angiotensin II antagonist, is converted to its active metabolite E3174 by CYP3A4 metabolism. Grapefruit juice thus leads to a reduction of conversion of losartan to its active component *(32)*. Thus, if patients taking losartan drink grapefruit juice, the efficacy of their losartan may diminish. This decrease likely has less clinical impact than some of the other interactions discussed in this chapter.

5.2. HMG-CoA Reductase Inhibitors (Statins)

The statins are a family of drugs that act by inhibiting 3-hydroxy-3-methylglutaryl coenzyme A (HMG-CoA) reductase, leading to reduction in plasma cholesterol. This family of medications is one of the most widely prescribed in clinical practice. Lovastatin, simvastatin, and atorvastatin undergo considerable intestinal metabolism by the CYP3A4 system and, to varying degrees, are affected by coadministered grapefruit juice. This is also the case with cerivastatin, a drug recently removed from the market. The other statins, fluvastatin and pravastatin, do not undergo significant interaction with grapefruit juice, because they undergo little CYP3A4 metabolism.

There are conflicting data on the magnitude of the statin drug level increase seen with grapefruit juice which is, in part, due to the quantities of grapefruit juice used in these studies and the timing of their administration. The Area Under the plasma concentration-time Curve (AUC; an excellent measure of the body's exposure to a drug) increased between 2- and 16-fold and that of the active metabolite by 35–350% *(33–36)*. Statins can cause serious adverse effects, including myopathy (muscle inflammation) and rhabdomyolysis (skeletal muscle injury often associated with renal failure). Although the mechanism by which this occurs is unknown, it is not related to high plasma levels of HMG-CoA reductase inhibitors. Rhabdomyolysis has been reported when simvastatin or lovastatin is coadministered with other CYP3A4 inhibitors, such as cyclosporine, diltiazem, erythromycin, itraconazole, or mibefradil *(37–41)*. It therefore, is prudent that patients taking these statins should minimize or avoid consuming grapefruit juice.

5.3. Immunosuppressants

Cyclosporine is a potent T-cell immunosuppressant widely used as first-line therapy in the care of patients after solid organ and bone marrow transplantation. Its absorption is highly variable, ranging from < 5% to 90%, and it is metabolized by the CYP3A4 system. Given the importance of therapeutic cyclosporine levels to transplant function and the many potential drug-cyclosporine interactions, cyclosporine drug levels are routinely monitored.

Many studies have shown a significant elevation of cyclosporine drug levels by grapefruit juice consumption *(42–45)*. Several studies have attempted to boost cyclosporine levels and reduce costs by coadministering grapefruit juice. However, even in the controlled conditions of a clinical study, the increase in cyclosporine levels was variable both between patients (likely explained by different intestinal CYP3A4 intestinal expression) and with time in an individual patient (perhaps explained by changes in the constituents of grapefruit with different crops and preparations) *(46–49)*. We may, in the future, harness the benefits of increases in drug bioavailability by grapefruit juice through either standardizing the constituents or isolating the active ingredients. This might then lead to a safe, effective, and cost-saving means to enhance the absorption of many therapeutic agents, including cyclosporine. Based on its pharmacokinetic characteristics, it would be expected that tacrolimus, used now extensively for immunosuppression in transplant patients, would also interact with grapefruit juice.

5.4. Antihistamines

The antihistamine terfenadine was widely used to treat hay fever and other allergic conditions. It undergoes extensive first-pass metabolism in the gut wall by CYP3A to active carboxylic metabolites, including fexofenadine, so that normal terfenadine levels are not measurable in the plasma. The parent compound has considerable potential to inhibit the delayed rectifier potassium channel in the heart (whereas the metabolites do not). This predisposes to prolongation of the QT interval on the electrocardiogram and an increased risk of ventricular tachycardia and torsades de pointes, potentially lethal cardiac arrhythmias *(50)*. The effects of several CYP3A4 inhibitors (erythromycin, ketoconazole) on causing torsades de pointes by increasing the circulating levels of terfenadine are well recognized. Grapefruit juice also alters the presystemic metabolism of terfenadine, to a degree similar to the changes that occur with itraconazole and erythromycin, leading to the accumulation of a greater amount of terfenadine and QT prolongation (presumably increasing the risk of torsades de pointes) *(51,52)*. Of the other antihistamines, ebastine and loratadine are metabolized by CYP3A4 and may also potentially interact with grapefruit juice.

5.5. Cisapride

In 2000, after causing more than 80 deaths, cisapride was withdrawn from the market and is now only prescribed on a carefully controlled limited-access basis. When present in the blood at high levels, cisapride, like terfenadine, may lead to QT interval prolonged and torsades de pointes. Although it is not associated with any of these 80 reported deaths, grapefruit juice increases cisapride levels *(53,54)* and, therefore, predisposes patients taking the drug to toxicity. Given its potent effects on GI motility and the lack of effective alternatives, it will continue to be prescribed with more careful monitoring. Grapefruit juice should be avoided in all patients taking cisapride.

5.6. Antimicrobial Agents

Although many commonly used antimicrobial agents are metabolized by CYP3A4, few undergo significant intestinal first-pass metabolism. Hence, few are significantly affected by grapefruit juice. Of those that are, artemether is a member of the artemisin family of drugs, which is being used increasingly for treating of malaria in endemic areas, particularly Malaria *falciparum*. The oral bioavailability of artemether is doubled when taken with a glass of grapefruit juice *(55)*.

Members of one particular class of antiviral agents, the protease inhibitors, developed for the treatment of human immunodeficiency virus (HIV) infection, are almost universally substrates for CYP3A4. However, most have high oral bioavailabilities and hence are unlikely to be affected by grapefruit juice. An exception to this is saquinavir, a potent protease inhibitor whose effectiveness is limited by low bioavailability (approx 4%) because of extensive intestinal first-phase metabolism. Grapefruit juice doubles the oral bioavailability of saquinavir *(56)*. A newer formulation of saquinavir mesylate with a softer gel coating provides increased drug exposure. It has improved bioavailability, with levels three to four times higher than conventional capsules. Although it has not yet been formally studied with grapefruit juice, these soft gel capsule is expected to interact also, but perhaps to a lesser degree.

5.7. Neuropsychiatric Medications

The fields of neurology and psychiatry have many medications that undergo significant intestinal and hepatic first-pass metabolism and are commonly involved in drug-drug interactions. Three members of the benzodiazepine family (anxiolytics) interact with grapefruit juice; these are diazepam, midazolam, and triazolam *(57–59)*. No data exist for other commonly prescribed benzodiazepines, such as alprazolam, chlordiazepoxide, clonazepam, flurazepam, and lorazepam. However, they are all likely safe to take with grapefruit juice because their high oral bioavailability leaves little room for elevation. Buspirone is an azapirone anxiolytic agent that produces less sedation and impairment of psychomotor performance than do benzodiazepines. It has poor bioavailability due to extensive first-pass metabolism. When coadministered with buspirone, grapefruit juice has led to an increase in the maximum concentration between 2- and 16-fold (mean, approx 4-fold) *(60)*. Sertraline, a selective serotonin reuptake inhibitor (SSRI) used to treat depression, panic disorder, and obsessive-compulsive disorder, undergoes first-pass metabolism by CYP3A4. A small study has shown both in vitro and in vivo evidence of grapefruit juice inhibiting this metabolism *(61)*. Four of the study's five patients had sertraline levels increased by approx 1.5-fold when one glass of grapefruit juice was consumed daily. The clinical implications of these findings are unclear. Carbamazepine, an anticonvulsant used to treat epilepsy, undergoes an interaction with grapefruit juice. Clomipramine is a tricyclic antidepressant also used in the treatment of obsessive-compulsive disorder. Oesterheld and Kallepalli *(62)* reported their experience using grapefruit juice to elevate the levels of this drug and improve efficacy in two children with obsessive-compulsive disorder. The authors postulated that in some patients demethylation of clomipramine may be largely mediated by the intestinal CYP3A4 system. These data support a considerable interaction between grapefruit juice and clomipramine, and coadministration should probably be done only in a controlled setting.

Haloperidol, trazodone, and zolidem are medications used commonly in neurology and psychiatry and are metabolized in vivo by CYP3A4. However, they all have high oral bioavailabilities ranging from 60% to 70%, and any intestinal CYP3A4 metabolism and possible inhibition by grapefruit juice is probably clinically insignificant. Zaleplon, recently approved by the US Food and Drug Administration for use in the management of insomnia, is at least partially metabolized by CYP3A4, and, given its low oral bioavailability, may interact with grapefruit juice. Methadone, a long-acting oral narcotic used for its analgesic properties but used more commonly in the management of narcotic withdrawal, is metabolized by CYP3A4 in the intestine and also likely interacts with grapefruit juice. However, to the author's knowledge, there have been no studies addressing this.

Finally, sildenafil oral therapy for erectile dysfunction has rapid absorption after oral administration with an absolute bioavailability of 40% and is extensively metabolized by the CYP3A4 system. Drugs that inhibit this enzyme system (e.g., erythromycin, itraconazole, and some protease inhibitors) increase sildenafil plasma levels (63,64). Jetter et al. (65) have shown that grapefruit juice elevates sildenafil levels when concurrently administered.

5.8. Summary of Grapefruit Juice–Drug Interactions

To summarize, grapefruit juice inhibits the metabolism of many medications spanning several clinical fields. In general, the subset of patients in whom grapefruit juice gives the greatest effect are those who at baseline display the greatest amounts of intestinal metabolism and hence the lowest rates of drug bioavailability. In day-to-day practice, this group remains hard to identify and this inhibition of metabolism can lead to many-fold increases in circulating drug levels and place these patients at risk for dose-dependent side effects. Unfortunately, because of several patient and grapefruit factors, this effect is unpredictable and cannot be used clinically. Until these issues are defined, it is prudent to dissuade patients from combining grapefruit juice with any of the medications listed in Table 2, particularly when they are taking these drugs for the first time or in high doses.

6. THE EFFECT OF ALCOHOL ON DRUG ACTION

The effects of alcohol consumption on health are described elsewhere in this book (Chapter 2). Alcohol imparts many effects on drug therapy, both acutely and chronically (66). Alcohol may delay gastric emptying and, thus, slow the onset of absorption of many medications. With time, heavy alcohol consumption may also lead to chronic altered bowel motility. Chronic consumption of excessive quantities of alcohol may result in a cirrhotic liver that functions poorly, impairing drug metabolism (67). Like caffeine and grapefruit juice, alcohol can also acutely and directly affect the metabolism of certain medications. CYP2E1 is one of the enzymes that is responsible for alcohol metabolism. In the acute setting, alcohol, by competing for this enzyme, may reduce metabolism of medications normally metabolized by it (e.g., warfarin, phenytoin, and rifampicin). With prolonged excessive drinking, the expression of this enzyme is increased and, as a result, these medications may be metabolized sooner. A different phenomenon is seen with acetaminophen. One of the minor pathways of its metabolism is by CYP2E1; however, the metabolite of this oxidative reaction is toxic to the liver. Chronic alcohol consumption, by inducing a 5–10-fold increase in CYP2E1 levels, may therefore increase the hepatotoxicity experienced after an overdose of acetaminophen. Hence, much smaller amounts of acetaminophen may be dangerous in someone who chronically drinks excessive quantities of alcohol. Also of significance, the effects of alcohol on the central nervous system include grogginess and altered judgment and reaction time. This can exacerbate the effects of medications, such as tricyclic antidepressants, benzodiazepines, and the older more sedating antihistamines (e.g., diphenylhydramine).

Table 2
Medications With Which Grapefruit Juice Should Not Be Taken in an Unsupervised Manner

Calcium channel blockers	*HMG-CoA reductase inhibitors*
Felodipine	Atorvastatin
Nimodipine	Lovastatin
Nisoldipine	Simvastatin
Pranidipine	*Neuropsychiatric medications*
Antimicrobial agents	Buspirone
Artemether	Carbamazepine
Saquinavir	Clomipramine
	Diazepam
Antihistamines	Methadone
Ebastine	Midazolam
Loratadine	Sertraline
Terfenadine	Triazolam
	Zaleplon
Immunosuppressants	*Others*
Cyclosporine	Cilostazol
Tacrolimus	Sildenafil

Table 3
Medications With Which Dietary Caffeine May Cause
a Clinically Significant Pharmacokinetic Interaction

Drug	Effect on drug by caffeine	Potential clinical effect
Clozapine	50% Increase in plasma levels	Toxicity
Lithium	25% Decrease in plasma levels	Therapeutic failure
Theophylline	25% Reduction in clearance	Toxicity

7. SPECIFIC EFFECTS OF RED WINE ON DRUG ACTION

Red wine also inhibits intestinal CYP3A4, albeit to a lesser extent than grapefruit juice *(68,69)*. However, a clinically significant effect of red wine on medications normally metabolized in the intestine by CYP3A4 would likely be uncommon. It would be localized only to those patients with the highest intestinal CYP3A4 concentrations. Occasionally, red wine could also carry the same risks as grapefruit juice in placing the patient at risk for dose-dependent side effects.

8. THE EFFECT OF CAFFEINE ON DRUG ACTION

Caffeine is widely consumed through coffee, tea, and many carbonated beverages. Acting as a central nervous system stimulant, caffeine elevates mood, reduces fatigue, and increases facility for work. In addition to these stimulant effects and its effects on the cardiovascular system, caffeine interacts with the CYP1A2 enzyme system responsible for the metabolism of many drugs *(70)*. However, it is likely that there are only a few medications in which a clinically significant interaction between them and dietary caffeine occurs, particularly medications with a narrow margin between when they are therapeutic and toxic (*see* Table 3). Dietary caffeine consumption should be minimized in patients taking these medications. Clozapine, an atypical antipsychotic used in the treatment of schizophrenia, is one such medication. There are several reported cases of the presence of dose-dependent clozapine side effects in patients consuming large quantities of caffeine (5–10 cups of coffee/d). It should be noted that this psychiatric population is one in which caffeine consumption is frequently high.

9. CONCLUSION

This chapter reviewed the common drug–beverage interactions. Acting on gastric motility, pH, and drug metabolism, beverages can have several effects on medications. The clinical significance of these interactions range from passing interest to the worries of the potential for significant toxicity. Particularly for those medications, such as grapefruit juice, that affect drug metabolism, there is huge variability from one person to the next and the risks of dangerous interactions are only present in a few. With further understanding and perhaps profiling of patients for their gene expression of metabolic enzymes, it may be possible to identify those most at risk for both beverage-drug and drug–drug interactions. In the meantime, it is best to take your medication with a glass of water.

10. MAIN POINTS FOR PRIMARY AND CLINICAL REVIEW

1. Consumption of acidic beverages, such as colas, is used to increase gut acidity and improve the absorption of some drugs, such as ketaconazole.
2. 6'7'-dihydroxybergamottin is a polyphenolic compound specific to grapefruit that acts as a suicide inhibitor of the intestinal P450 enzyme CYP3A4, such that some absorbed drugs are less metabolized following absorption leading to excess plasma concetrations.
3. Grapefruit juice consumption causes alterations in the bioavailability and plasma concentrations of some calcium channel blockers, HMG-CoA inhibitors, immunosuppressants, antihistamines, antibiotics, and some neuropsychotic medications.
4. Alcohol consumption can alter drug absorption by modifying gut motility, liver function, and the production of toxic secondary drug metabolites as occurs when acetaminophen is coadministered with alcohol.
5. Caffeine from beverages may act as a stimulant that alters some drug responses and may also modify the metabolic rates of some drugs.

ACKNOWLEDGMENT

This chapter is dedicated to my mentor James J. Lipsky, MD.

REFERENCES

1. Zhang QY, Dunbar D, Ostrowska A, Zeisloft S, Yang J, Kaminsky LS. Characterization of human small intestinal cytochromes P-450. Drug Metab Dispos 1999;27:804–809.
2. Kivisto KT, Lamberg TS, Kantola T, Neuvonen PJ. Plasma buspirone concentrations are greatly increased by erythromycin and itraconazole. Clin Pharmacol Ther 1997;62:348–352.
3. Kivisto KT, Kantola T, Neuvonen PJ. Different effects of itraconazole on the pharmacokinetics of fluvastatin and lovastatin. Br J Clin Pharmacol 1998;46:49–53.
4. Azie NE, Brater DC, Becker PA, Jones DR, Hall SD. The interaction of diltiazem with lovastatin and pravastatin. Clin Pharmacol Ther 1998;64:369–377.

5. Leyden JJ. Absorption of minocycline hydrochloride and tetracycline hydrochloride. Effect of food, milk, and iron. J Am Acad Dermatol 1985;12:308–312.

6. Jung H, Peregrina AA, Rodriguez JM, Moreno-Esparza R. The influence of coffee with milk and tea with milk on the bioavailability of tetracycline. Biopharm Drug Dispos 1997;18:459–463.

7. Lake-Bakaar G, Quadros E, Beidas S, et al. Gastric secretory failure in patients with the acquired immunodeficiency syndrome (AIDS). Ann Intern Med 1988;109:502–504.

8. Lake-Bakaar G, Tom W, Lake-Bakaar D, et al. Gastropathy and ketoconazole malabsorption in the acquired immunodeficiency syndrome (AIDS). Ann Intern Med 1988;109:471–473.

9. Chin TW, Loeb M, Fong IW. Effects of an acidic beverage (Coca-Cola) on absorption of ketaconazole. Antimicrob Agents Chemother 1995;39:1671–1675.

10. Lesser PF. Florida grapefruit-juice developments, Presented at: FoodNews Second International Fruit-Juice Conference. Amsterdam, Netherlands, October 7,1997.

11. Bailey DG, Malcolm J, Arnold O, Spence JD. Grapefruit juice-drug interactions. Br J Clin Pharmacol 1998;46:101–110.

12. Kane GC, Lipsky JJ. Drug-grapefruit juice interactions. Mayo Clin Proc 2000;75:933–942.

13. Aronson JK. Forbidden fruit. Nat Med 2001;7:29–30.

14. Bailey DG, Dresser GK, Kreeft JH, Munoz C, Freeman DJ, Bend JR. Grapefruit-felodipine interaction: effect of unprocessed fruit and probable active ingredients. Clin Pharmacol Ther 2000;68:468–477.

15. Lee M, Min DI, Ku YM, Flanigan M. Effect of grapefruit juice on pharmacokinetics of microemulsion cyclosporine in African American subjects compared with Caucasian subjects: does ethnic difference matter? J Clin Pharmacol 2001;41:317–323.

16. Lown KS, Bailey DG, Fontana RJ, et al. Grapefruit juice increases felodipine oral availability in humans by decreasing intestinal CYP3A protein expression. J Clin Invest 1997;99:2545–2553.

17. Bailey DG, Spence JD, Edgar B, Bayliff CD, Arnold JM. Ethanol enhances the hemodynamic effects of felodipine. Clin Invest Med 1989;12:357–362.

18. Bailey DG, Spence JD, Munoz C, Arnold JM. Interaction of citrus juices with felodipine and nifedipine. Lancet 1991;337:268–269.

19. Edgar B, Bailey D, Bergstrand R, Johnsson G, Regardh CG. Acute effects of drinking grapefruit juice on the pharmacokinetics and dynamics of felodipine—and its potential clinical relevance. Eur J Clin Pharmacol 1992;42:313–317.

20. Lundahl J, Regardh CG, Edgar B, Johnsson G. Relationship between time of intake of grapefruit juice and its effect on pharmacokinetics and pharmacodynamics of felodipine in healthy subjects. Eur J Clin Pharmacol 1995;49:61–67.

21. Bailey DG, Arnold JM, Munoz C, Spence JD. Grapefruit juice—felodipine interaction: mechanism, predictability, and effect of naringin. Clin Pharmacol Ther 1993;53:637–642.

22. Bailey DG, Arnold JM, Bend JR, Tran LT, Spence JD. Grapefruit juice—felodipine interaction: reproducibility and characterization with the extended release drug formulation. Br J Clin Pharmacol 1995;40:135–140.

23. Lundahl J, Regardh CG, Edgar B, Johnsson G. Effects of grapefruit juice ingestion—pharmacokinetics and haemodynamics of intravenously and orally administered felodipine in healthy men. Eur J Clin Pharmacol 1997;52:139–145.

24. Bailey DG, Arnold JM, Strong HA, Munoz C, Spence JD. Effect of grapefruit juice and naringin on nisoldipine pharmacokinetics. Clin Pharmacol Ther 1993;54:589–594.

25. Hashimoto K, Shirafuji T, Sekino H, et al. Interaction of citrus juices with pranidipine, a new 1,4-dihydropyridine calcium antagonist, in healthy subjects. Eur J Clin Pharmacol 1998;54:753–760.

26. Fuhr U, Maier-Bruggemann A, Blume H, et al. Grapefruit juice increases oral nimodipine bioavailability. Int J Clin Pharmacol Ther 1998;36:126–132.

27. Rashid TJ, Martin U, Clarke H, Waller DG, Renwick AG, George CF. Factors affecting the absolute bioavailability of nifedipine. Br J Clin Pharmacol 1995;40:51–58.

28. Josefsson M, Zackrisson AL, Ahlner J. Effect of grapefruit juice on the pharmacokinetics of amlodipine in healthy volunteers. Eur J Clin Pharmacol 1996;51:189–193.

29. Zaidenstein R, Dishi V, Gips M, et al. The effect of grapefruit juice on the pharmacokinetics of orally administered verapamil. Eur J Clin Pharmacol 1998;54:337–340.

30. Plental [package insert]. Otsuka America Pharmaceutical Inc., Rockville, MD, 1999.
31. Suri A, Forbes WP, Bramer SL. Effects of CYP3A inhibition on the metabolism of cilostazol. Clinical Pharmacokinet 1999;37(Suppl):61–68.
32. Zaidenstein R, Soback S, Gips M, et al. Effect of grapefruit juice on the pharmacokinetics of losartan and its active metabolite E3174 in healthy volunteers. Ther Drug Monit 2001;23:369–373.
33. Rogers JD, Zhao J, Liu L, et al. Grapefruit juice has minimal effects on plasma concentrations of lovastatin-derived 3-hydroxy-3-methylglutaryl coenzyme A reductase inhibitors. Clin Pharmacol Ther 1999;66: 358–366.
34. Kantola T, Kivisto KT, Neuvonen PJ. Grapefruit juice greatly increases serum concentrations of lovastatin and lovastatin acid. Clin Pharmacol Ther 1998;63:397–402.
35. Lilja JJ, Kivisto KT, Neuvonen PJ. Grapefruit juice-simvastatin interaction: effect on serum concentrations of simvastatin, simvastatin acid, and HMG-CoA reductase inhibitors. Clin Pharmacol Ther 1998;64: 477–483.
36. Lilja JJ, Kivisto KT, Neuvonen PJ. Grapefruit juice increases serum concentrations of atorvastatin and has no effect on pravastatin. Clin Pharmacol Ther 1999;66:118–127.
37. Corpier CL, Jones PH, Suki WN, et al. Rhabdomyolysis and renal injury with lovastatin use. Report of two cases in cardiac transplant recipients. JAMA 1988;260:239–241.
38. Spach DH, Bauwens JE, Clark CD, Burke WG. Rhabdomyolysis associated with lovastatin and erythromycin use. West J Med 1991;154:213–215.
39. Ahmad S. Diltiazem myopathy. Am Heart J 1993;126:1494–1495.
40. Lees RS, Lees AM. Rhabdomyolysis from the coadministration of lovastatin and the antifungal agent itraconazole. N Engl J Med 1995;333:664–665.
41. Schmassmann-Suhijar D, Bullingham R, Gasser R, Schmutz J, Haefeli WE. Rhabdomyolysis due to interaction of simvastatin with mibefradil. Lancet 1998;351:1929–1930.
42. Ioannides-Demos LL, Christophidis N, Ryan P, Angelis P, Liolios L, McLean AJ. Dosing implications of a clinical interaction between grapefruit juice and cyclosporine and metabolite concentrations in patients with autoimmune diseases. J Rheum 1997;24:49–54.
43. Ku YM, Min DI, Flanigan M. Effect of grapefruit juice on the pharmacokinetics of microemulsion cyclosporine and its metabolite in healthy volunteers: does the formulation difference matter? J Clin Pharmacol 1998;38:959–965.
44. Yee GC, Stanley DL, Pessa LJ, et al. Effect of grapefruit juice on blood cyclosporin concentration. Lancet 1995;345:955–956.
45. Proppe DG, Hoch OD, McLean AJ, Visser KE. Influence of chronic ingestion of grapefruit juice on steady-state blood concentrations of cyclosporine A in renal transplant patients with stable graft function. Br J Clin Pharmacol 1995;39:337–338.
46. Taniguchi S, Kobayashi H, Ishii M. Treatment of psoriasis by cyclosporine and grapefruit juice. Arch Dermatol 1996;132:1249.
47. Emilia G, Longo G, Bertesi M, Gandini G, Ferrara L, Valenti C. Clinical interaction between grapefruit juice and cyclosporine: is there any interest for the hematologists? Blood 1998;91:362–363.
48. Brunner LJ, Munar MY, Vallian J, et al. Interaction between cyclosporine and grapefruit juice requires long-term ingestion in stable renal transplant recipients. Pharmacotherapy 1998;18:23–29.
49. Brunner LJ, Pai KS, Munar MY, Lande MB, Olyaei AJ, Mowry JA. Effect of grapefruit juice on cyclosporin A pharmacokinetics in pediatric renal transplant patients. Pediatric Transplant 2000;4: 313–321.
50. Bauman JL. The role of pharmacokinetics, drug interactions and pharmacogenetics in the acquired long QT syndrome. Eur Heart J 2001;3:K93–K100.
51. Lundahl JU, Regardh CG, Edgar B, Johnsson G. The interaction effect of grapefruit juice is maximal after the first glass. Eur J Clin Pharmacol 1998;54:75–81.
52. Benton RE, Honig PK, Zamani K, Cantilena LR, Woosley RL. Grapefruit juice alters terfenadine pharmacokinetics, resulting in prolongation of repolarization on the electrocardiogram. Clin Pharmacol Ther 1996;59:383–388.
53. Gross AS, Goh YD, Addison RS, Shenfield GM. Influence of grapefruit juice on cisapride pharmacokinetics. Clin Pharmacol Ther 1999;65:395–401.
54. Kivisto KT, Lilja JJ, Backman JT, Neuvonen PJ. Repeated consumption of grapefruit juice considerably increases plasma concentrations of cisapride. Clin Pharmacol Ther 1999;66:448–453.

55. van Agtmael MA, Gupta V, van der Graaf CA, van Boxtel CJ. The effect of grapefruit juice on the time-dependent decline of artemether plasma levels in healthy subjects. Clin Pharmacol Ther 1999;66:408–414.
56. Kupferschmidt HH, Fattinger KE, Ha HR, Follath F, Krahenbuhl S. Grapefruit juice enhances the bioavailability of the HIV protease inhibitor saquinavir in man. Br J Clin Pharmacol 1998;45:355–359.
57. Hukkinen SK, Varhe A, Olkkola KT, Neuvonen PJ. Plasma concentrations of triazolam are increased by concomitant ingestion of grapefruit juice. Clin Pharmacol Ther 1995;58:127–131.
58. Kupferschmidt HH, Ha HR, Ziegler WH, Meier PJ, Krahenbuhl S. Interaction between grapefruit juice and midazolam in humans. Clin Pharmacol Ther 1995;58:20–28.
59. Ozdemir M, Aktan Y, Boydag BS, Cingi MI, Musmul A. Interaction between grapefruit juice and diazepam in humans. Eur J Drug Metab Pharmacokinet 1998;23:55–59.
60. Lilja JJ, Kivisto KT, Backman JT, Lamberg TS, Neuvonen PJ. Grapefruit juice substantially increases plasma concentrations of buspirone. Clin Pharmacol Ther 1998;64:655–660.
61. Lee AJ, Chan WK, Harralson AF, Buffum J, Bui BC. The effects of grapefruit juice on sertraline metabolism: an in vitro and in vivo study. Clin Ther 1999;21:1890–1899.
62. Oesterheld J, Kallepalli BR. Grapefruit juice and clomipramine: shifting metabolitic ratios. J Clin Psychopharm 1997;17:62–63.
63. Hall MCS, Ahmad S. Interaction between sildenafil and HIV-1 combination therapy [letter]. Lancet 1999;353:2071–2072.
64. Merry C, Barry MG, Ryan M, et al. Interaction of sildenafil and indinavir when co-administered to HIV-positive patients. Aids 1999;13:F101–F107.
65. Jetter A, Kinzig-Schippers M, Walchner-Bonjean M, et al. Effects of grapefruit juice on the pharmacokinetics of sildenafil. Clin Pharmacol Ther 2002;71:21–29.
66. Fraser AG. Pharmacokinetic interactions between alcohol and other drugs. Clin Pharmacokinet 1997;33:79–90.
67. Morgan DJ, McLean AJ. Clinical pharmacokinetic and pharmacodynamic considerations in patients with liver disease. Clin Pharmacokinet 1995;29:370–391.
68. Chan WK, Nguyen LT, Miller VP, Harris RZ. Mechanism-based inactivation of human cytochrome P450 3A4 by grapefruit juice and red wine. Life Sci 1998;62:L135–L142.
69. Offman EM, Freeman DJ, Dresser GK, Munoz C, Bend JR, Bailey DG. Red wine-cisapride interaction: comparison with grapefruit juice. Clin Pharmacol Ther 2001;70:17–23.
70. Carrillo JA, Benitez J. Clinically significant pharmacokinetic interactions between dietary caffeine and medications. Clin Pharmacokinet 2000;39:127–153.

8 Tomato-Based Beverages

Implications for the Prevention of Cancer and Cardiovascular Disease

Craig W. Hadley, Steven J. Schwartz, and Steven K. Clinton

1. INTRODUCTION

Observational and experimental evidence strongly implicate dietary variables as critical determinants of human health and disease risk. Among the many dietary variables implicated in the promotion of optimal health, a diet rich in several fruits and vegetables is a major contributing factor. Much of the evidence derived from human epidemiological studies suggests that an increased fruit and vegetable intake is associated with a low risk of cardiovascular disease *(1)* and many types of cancer *(2)*. Modern epidemiologic techniques employing detailed diet assessment tools have allowed investigators to further define the potential health benefits of specific fruits and vegetables suggested by observational epidemiologic studies and laboratory investigations. Our research program has been particularly interested in the accumulating evidence focusing upon tomatoes and processed tomato products in disease prevention. An accumulating body of evidence from human epidemiologic studies has associated an increased consumption of tomato products with a reduction in the risk for several cancers *(3)*. There are numerous phytochemicals in tomatoes, such as carotenoids and several polyphenols, that are believed to be responsible for the potential health benefits observed in these studies. For example, an inverse correlation between tissue and serum lycopene, the predominant carotenoid in tomatoes, and the risk for both prostate cancer *(4–7)* and cardiovascular disease *(8–12)* has been observed.

This chapter briefly reviews some of the recent research focusing upon tomato products, with a particular focus upon the role of tomato beverages and the risk for cardiovascular disease and cancer. The presence and potential role of the biologically active phytochemicals in tomato products and a possible reduction in the risk for these diseases is also discussed.

From: *Beverages in Nutrition and Health*
Edited by: T. Wilson and N. J. Temple © Humana Press Inc., Totowa, NJ

Table 1
Production of Principal Vegetables in the United States for 2001[a]

Vegetable Processing	Production (millions of tons)	Vegetable Fresh market	Production (millions of tons)
Tomatoes	9.248	Lettuce, head	3.626
Sweet corn	3.143	Onions[b]	3.354
Snap beans	0.699	Tomatoes	1.848
Cucumbers	0.592	Sweet corn	1.383
Carrots	0.437	Cabbage	1.310
Green peas	0.387	Broccoli	1.021
Cabbage	0.174	Celery	0.941
Spinach	0.142	Bell peppers	0.740
Beets	0.111	Cucumbers	0.545
Lima beans	0.067	Cauliflower	0.403
Broccoli	0.072	Snap beans	0.301
Cauliflower	0.039	Spinach	0.207
Asparagus	0.035	Asparagus	0.104

[a] Data from the US Department of Agriculture, National Agricultural Statistics Service 2001 Summary (13).
[b] Dual usage crops included in total.

2. TOMATOES AND TOMATO PRODUCTS

2.1. Consumption

Tomatoes comprise a substantial portion of the agricultural industry devoted to fruits and vegetables and have become a common food for people in many parts of the world. According to the US Department of Agriculture's Vegetables 2001 Summary, the production of tomatoes for processing and fresh market ranks first and fourth, respectively (see Table 1). Based on the production figures in the United States, approx 11 million tons of tomatoes were available for consumption in 2001. More than 83% of these tomatoes (i.e., 9.2 million tons) were processed into products such as paste, puree, sauce, and juice.

2.2. Nutrient and Phytochemical Content

Tomatoes and tomato-based products are a source of important nutrients (Table 2) and contain numerous phytochemicals that may influence health. Tomatoes contain major minerals, including calcium and magnesium, trace minerals, including copper, iron, manganese, selenium, and zinc, and ultratrace elements, including aluminum, boron, chromium, and molybdenum. Tomatoes provide a small amount of vitamin E and substantial amounts of folate, vitamin C, and potassium (16). In addition to these important nutrients, tomatoes are a rich source of carotenoids. The carotenoids phytofluene, phytoene, neurosporene, lycopene, β-carotene, γ-carotene, and ζ-carotene are among the most abundant phytochemicals in tomatoes (16). Lycopene is the predominant carotenoid in tomatoes (31–77 mg/kg of fresh tomatoes) and is the source of the brilliant red color (17). Although lycopene is present in guava (54 mg/kg), watermelon (41 mg/kg), and pink grapefruit (34 mg/kg), tomatoes and tomato products provide the majority of lycopene

Table 2
Nutrient and Carotenoid Content of Tomatoes and Tomato Products

	Nutrient content (per 100 g)					Carotenoids (mg/100 g edible portion)				
	Vitamin A (IU)	Vitamin C (mg)	Vitamin E (mg, ATE)[a]	Folate (µg)	Potassium (mg)	α-car	β-car	β-cryp	Lut + Zea	Lyc
Tomatoes, crushed, canned	699	9.2	0.532	13	293	NA	NA	NA	NA	NA
Tomatoes, red, ripe, raw, year-round average	623	19.1	0.380	15	222	0.112	0.393	0	0.130	3.02
Tomato juice, canned, without salt	556	18.3	0.910	20	220	0	0.428	0	0.060	9.32
Catsup	1016	15.1	1.465	15	481	0	0.730	0	0	17.01
Sauce, pasta, spaghetti/marinara, ready-to-serve	375	8	1.252	10	295	0	0.440	0	0.160	15.99
Sauce, ready-to-serve, salsa	602	13.9	0.600	16	213	NA	0.398	NA	NA	NA
Tomato products, canned, paste, with salt	2445	42.4	4.300	22	937	0.029	1.242	0	0.170	29.33
Tomato products, canned, puree, with salt	1275	10.4	2.520	11	426	0	0.410	0	0.090	16.67
Tomato products, canned sauce	979	13.1	1.400	9	371	0	0.410	0	0.001	15.92
Tomatoes, red, ripe, cooked, boiled, without salt	743	22.8	0.380	13	279	0	0.300	0	0.150	4.40
Tomatoes, red, ripe, canned, whole, regular pack	595	14.2	0.320	8	221	0	0.186	0	0.040	9.71
Pizza with pepperoni, cheese and sauce, thin crust, frozen	NA	NA	NA	NA	NA	0	0.264	0	0.015	4.45
Pasta in tomato sauce with cheese, canned	NA	NA	NA	NA	NA	0	0.127	0	0	3.16

Source: refs. 14,15.
[a]α-Tocopherol equivalents.

consumed in the American diet *(17)*. Tomatoes are also a source of several phytochemicals, including flavonols (i.e., quercetin and kaempferol), phytosterols, and phenylpropanoids (phenolic acids) *(16,18)*. In a recent study, tomato juice was found to contain numerous phenolic compounds, including chlorogenic acid, caffeic acid, p-coumaric acid, naringenin, and rutin *(19)*. The physiological significance of these compounds and their effects on health and disease at levels provided in the diet by tomatoes and tomato products are the subject of much speculation and forms the basis for many ongoing investigations.

2.3. Effect of Processing on Phytochemical Stability and Bioavailability

Consumption of tomatoes in the form of processed products, such as tomato juice, sauce, paste, puree, catsup, and salsa, accounts for more than 80% of tomatoes produced *(13)*. Thermal or mechanical treatments are often involved in tomato processing and may affect the stability of certain tomato phytochemicals. Early studies found that hydrocarbon carotenoids, such as lycopene, α-carotene, and β-carotene, in processed fruits and vegetables were fairly heat resistant *(20,21)*. In a recent study, no major changes in phytofluene, phytoene, and ζ-carotene were observed during tomato processing *(22)*. However, thermally induced isomerization of β-carotene occurs during the processing of fresh tomatoes to canned tomatoes *(23)*. In addition, a recent evaluation on the effect of processing of different tomato varieties showed ascorbic acid, α-tocopherol, quinone, and β-carotene to be the components most susceptible to thermal degradation *(24)*. Changes in lycopene structure and content during tomato processing result from isomerization and oxidation *(22,25–27)*. In contrast, others have reported that food processing does not affect lycopene stability *(28)*. In addition, it was recently reported by Nguyen et al. *(29)* that during typical cooking of tomato products, common factors such as genotypic differences in overall carotenoid composition and physical changes to tomato tissues did not result in the thermal isomerization of all-*trans*-lycopene, all-*trans*-δ-carotene, all-*trans*-γ-carotene, or prolycopene. Additional information must be gathered on the thermal behavior of carotenoids before definitive conclusions can be offered regarding the physical state and stability of lycopene during processing and cooking.

Phytochemicals present in tomatoes and tomato products must be readily bioavailable for absorption to mediate their hypothesized beneficial health effects. Bioavailability is defined as the fraction of an ingested nutrient that is accessible to the body through absorption for use in normal physiological functions and for metabolic processes *(27)*. Several studies have evaluated the bioavailability of the lipophilic carotenoids found in tomatoes and tomato products. Lipids are required to achieve optimal carotenoid absorption and transport. Consumption of tomato juice in the presence of supplemental fat increases lycopene absorption *(25)*. β-Carotene absorption is considerably higher after consumption of pureed or finely chopped vegetables when compared to sliced or whole raw vegetables *(30,31)*. Mild thermal processing can denature or weaken the protein–carotenoid complexes and/or rupture cell walls, thereby increasing the availability of carotenoids for absorption *(32)*. Heating tomato juice improved the lycopene uptake in humans *(25)*. Thermal processing may also improve the dispersion of crystalline carotenoid aggregates into the lipophilic component of the food matrix. Gartner et al. *(33)* reported that tomato paste provided a more bioavailable source of lycopene compared to fresh tomatoes when both were consumed with corn oil. Recent data from a pilot clinical trial in our laboratory focusing upon women who were lactating showed a greater concentration of lycopene in human milk in those consuming tomato sauces when compared to those consuming fresh tomatoes *(34)*. In a separate pilot clinical trial of healthy men and women, our research group reported an increased lycopene uptake from condensed tomato soup and V8 Vegetable Juice when compared to ready-to-serve tomato soup *(35)*. Additionally, various food-processing operations, such as chopping and pureeing, which result in a reduction in physical size of the food particle, enhance carotenoid bioavailability *(32,36,37)*. Certain types of dietary fiber, particularly pectin, lowered the absorption of β-carotene in both animals and humans *(38)*. Similarly, drugs that interfere with cholesterol absorption *(39)* and nonabsorbable fat analogs, such as sucrose polyesters *(40)*, reduce carotenoid absorption. Therefore, various processing conditions, the amount and type of lipids in the product or meal, and the amount of fiber in the meal are important factors in influencing carotenoid absorption *(41)*.

3. TOMATOES, TOMATO-BASED PRODUCTS, AND CANCER RISK

It has been widely postulated that oxidative damage may contribute to the damage of cellular DNA, proteins, and lipids that initiate or enhance cancer progression. Recent research has focused on the role of reactive oxygen species (ROS) or free radicals that are produced from exogenous and endogenous factors. Dietary antioxidants are believed to be important complements to other cellular systems, such as antioxidant enzymes (glutathione peroxidase, catalase, CuZn- and Mn-superoxide dismutase) and antioxidant quenchers (ceruloplasmin, transferrin, ferritin, Cd/Hg/Zn/Cu metallothioneins), that participate in the free radical defense system and provide protection against oxidative damage. Many of the proposed biological effects and health benefits of tomatoes and tomato products are hypothesized to be associated with the ability of certain phytochemicals, such as lycopene, to enhance the endogenous defense system by protecting against in vivo oxidative damage. However, definitive rodent and human studies have not yet established this relationship. Selection of appropriate markers of oxidation and characterization of their validity present a problem in assessing the association between antioxidants and disease processes *(42)*.

3.1. Cancer Epidemiology

Several studies published in the past 10 yr have suggested a beneficial relationship between tomato product consumption and several types of cancer. Epidemiologic investigations have reported a significant inverse association between dietary consumption of tomatoes and tomato products or serum carotenoid concentrations and the incidence of several cancers including oral/laryngeal/pharyngeal, pancreatic, lung, esophageal, stomach, colon, rectal, prostate, breast, and cervical *(3)*. Several study designs have been used by epidemiologists to examine these relationships. Typically, a comprehensive diet assessment using a food-frequency questionnaire is provided to a population. The intake of various tomato products are quantitated, which then allows the investigator to calculate carotenoid intake using published data regarding the carotenoid content of food items. This calculation does not consider variations in bioavailability or stability. Another commonly employed design is based on measuring concentrations of carotenoids in blood samples as a biomarker of exposure to the food product from which the phytochemical is derived.

A comprehensive review of the epidemiologic evidence regarding tomato products and cancer risk was recently published (3). Nearly 80% of the 72 studies reported in the review revealed evidence of a protective association between consumption of tomatoes, tomato products, or carotenoids provided by these foods and the risk of cancer at several sites. In more than 60% of these studies, the inverse associations were statistically significant. The observed inverse relationship was strongest for lung, stomach, and prostate cancers and was supportive for cervical, breast, oral cavity, pancreatic, colorectal, and esophageal cancers. One study evaluated the effect of tomato juice consumption on the risk for mesothelioma (i.e., cancer of the pleura or peritoneum). A 40% reduction in risk was observed for those consuming tomatoes or tomato juice 16 or more times a month compared to nonconsumers. More case subjects reported not consuming tomatoes or tomato juice compared with controls (9% vs < 2%), implying an elevated risk for low consumers of tomato products (43). In addition, more recent epidemiologic investigations of colon cancer (44), upper aerodigestive cancer (45), prostate cancer (7,46–48), and lung cancer (49) further support the concept that tomato products have cancer-preventive properties.

3.1.1. Prostate Cancer Focus—Diet Studies

Our laboratory is particularly interested in the relationship between tomato product consumption and prostate cancer (PCa) incidence and/or progression. Several case-control studies have reported this potential association. Although not statistically significant, a small study in 1982 reported a reduction in prostate cancer risk in men who consumed large amounts of tomato products (50). A study conducted in Greece showed a significantly lower intake of cooked tomatoes and slightly lower consumption of raw tomatoes for men with prostate cancer compared to those without the disease (46). In the Auckland Prostate Study, Norrish et al. (47) reported a small reduction in prostate cancer risk in men who had a high intake of lycopene from tomato-based foods. Several case-control studies, however, did not detect the relationship (51–55). In summary, the case-control studies are intriguing but alone do not provide strong evidence for a relationship. Issues of study size and power, diet assessment methodology, and reporting bias must also be considered when interpreting these data.

Two prospective cohort studies investigated the relationship between tomato product intake and prostate cancer risk. In a cohort of 14,000 Seventh-Day Adventist Men, Mills et al. (56) corrected data from food-frequency questionnaires and found that only tomato product, bean, lentil, and pea intake was significantly associated with a reduction in prostate cancer risk. In one of the largest and most comprehensive ongoing epidemiologic studies in adult men, Giovannucci et al. (57) investigated the relationship between prostate cancer risk and estimated intake of various fruits, vegetables, retinol, and carotenoids in the Health Professionals Follow-up Study (HPFS). Dietary intake for a 1-yr period was estimated using a validated 131-item food-frequency questionnaire in 47,894 American male health professionals initially free of cancer in 1986. Follow-up questionnaires were sent to all participants in 1988, 1990, and 1992 to renew exposure data and to record new cases of numerous diseases. A total of 812 new cases of prostate cancer were diagnosed in these men between 1986 and 1992. Prostate cancer risk was not associated with retinol, α-carotene, β-carotene, β-cryptoxanthin, or lutein intake. In contrast, dietary lycopene intake was related to a statistically significant reduction (age and energy adjusted RR = 0.79; 95% CI = 0.64–0.99 for high vs low quintile of intake; p for trend = 0.04) in the risk of prostate cancer. The food items that contributed to the majority of the various dietary carotenoids were also measured in these men. A reduced risk for prostate cancer was associated with 4 of the 46 fruits and vegetables or related products. Three of the four foods—tomatoes, pizza, and tomato sauce—were the main sources of lycopene. Other than tomato-based products, none of the major carotenoid-rich foods were associated with prostate cancer risk. Combined consumption of tomatoes, tomato sauce, tomato juice, and pizza, comprising 82% of dietary lycopene intake, was related to a reduced prostate cancer risk. A 35% lower risk was observed in men who consumed > 10 vs < 1.5 servings/wk. When more advanced or aggressive prostate cancers were evaluated, the apparent protective effect was even stronger (RR = 0.47; 95% CI = 0.22–1.00; p for trend = 0.03). The strongest inverse relationship to risk for prostate cancer of any one specific food item was seen with tomato sauce (RR = 0.66, 95% CI = 0.49–0.90; p for trend = 0.001). No association between tomato juice consumption and prostate cancer risk was reported in this study. However, the authors suggest that this null association might be related to the overall lower consumption of juice compared to other products, poor reporting of tomato juice consumption, or possibility of reduced bioavailability of certain phytochemicals and carotenoids from the juice matrix. Although fruit and vegetable consumption may lower the risk for several cancers, tomato-based product intake was highly associated with a lower risk of prostate cancer in the HPFS cohort *(57)*. Recently updated data from the HPFS for 1992 through 1998 confirmed the previous findings. Lycopene intake was associated with a decreased risk for prostate cancer (RR for high compared to low quintiles = 0.84; 95% CI = 0.73–0.96; p for trend = 0.003). An even greater reduction in the risk for prostate cancer was correlated with consumption of tomato sauce (RR for two or more servings/wk vs < 1 serving/mo = 0.77; 95% CI = 0.66–0.90; p for trend = 0.001) *(48)*. Although these results support a relationship between a reduced risk of prostate cancer with an increased consumption of tomato products, no such association was reported in the Netherlands Cohort Study *(58)*.

3.1.2. Prostate Cancer Focus—Blood Biomarker Studies

Several reports have investigated the relationship between blood concentrations of various carotenoids found in tomatoes and prostate cancer risk. In a study of plasma samples obtained in 1982 from men enrolled in the Physicians' Health Study, slight inverse associations were found with higher plasma levels of lycopene in all cases *(6)*. Significant inverse trends for greater concentrations of plasma lycopene and lower overall risk for prostate cancers and aggressive cancers were reported *(6)*. In a study conducted at Memorial Sloan-Kettering Cancer Center from 1993 to 1997, Lu and coworkers *(7)* showed that when plasma carotenoid levels from men in the highest and lowest quartiles were compared, inverse associations for PCa risk were statistically significant for plasma lycopene and zeaxanthin concentrations. In addition, plasma lutein and β-cryptoxanthin levels were associated with a significant reduction in PCa risk. Hsing et al. *(4)* evaluated serum obtained in 1974 from 25,802 persons in Washington County, MD, and reported lower mean serum lycopene concentrations in PCa cancer cases compared to controls. A 50% reduction in the relative risk for PCa was observed when cases in the highest serum lycopene quartile were compared to the lowest quartile. A study conducted by Nomura and colleagues *(59)* in a cohort of 6860 Japanese-American Men examined from 1971 to 1975, however, showed no association between several plasma micronutrients, carotenoids, and prostate cancer risk.

3.1.3. Prostate Cancer Focus—Apparent Inconsistencies

Giovannucci et al. *(48)* outlined several possible explanations for the apparent inconsistencies seen in the literature. Lycopene intake may not be high enough to mediate a beneficial effect in some groups. Consumption and bioavailability of lycopene-containing foods may not be adequately accounted for by dietary questionnaires. Because prostate cancer develops during many decades, single dietary measurements may, therefore, not provide an appropriate indication of the influence of diet on the carcinogenic process. In addition, lycopene may be more effective in aggressive compared to less aggressive stages of PCa. Finally, it is possible that confounding factors contribute to the association between PCa and lycopene. If we consider some of these issues, coupled with the inherent difficulties of precisely defining human intake in epidemiologic studies and the relatively modest changes in risk associated with single dietary components (compared to high risk exposures such as tobacco), we can appreciate that all studies may not provide uniform findings.

3.2. Animal Studies of Carcinogenesis

Few studies have investigated the effects of tomato juice or other tomato products on carcinogenesis in experimental models. One study evaluating urinary bladder carcinogenesis reported that tomato juice consumption significantly reduced the number of transitional cell carcinomas of the urinary bladder in male F344 rats treated with *N*-butyl-*N*-(4-hydroxybutyl)nitrosamine *(60)*. A significantly lower incidence of colon cancer induced by *N*-methylnitrosourea (NMU) was observed in female F344/NSIc rats with free access to tomato juice *(61)*. Two different doses of a lycopene-rich tomato oleoresin were fed to *lacZ* mice to study the effects on short-term benzo[*a*]pyrene (BaP)-induced and long-term spontaneous in vivo mutagenesis in the colon, prostate, and lungs *(62)*. Spontaneous mutagenesis was inhibited in prostate and colon tissue at the higher dose of tomato oleoresin. In addition, BaP-induced mutagenesis in the prostate was also slightly inhibited in mice fed tomato oleoresin *(62)*. We have recently observed a reduced risk of NMU-induced prostate carcinogenesis in rats fed diets supplemented with tomato powder but not pure lycopene *(63)*.

3.3. Clinical Investigations

Carefully designed human clinical intervention trials can provide valuable insight into the biological effects induced by the phytochemicals in tomatoes and tomato products. Furthermore, clinical trials allow investigators to understand how different types of processing can influence the absorption and metabolism of tomato-derived phytochemicals that may be involved in carcinogenesis and other disease processes. Tomato phytochemicals are hypothesized to influence cancer by several mechanisms, although the major focus has been on lycopene and its potential to function as an antioxidant, thus reducing the risk of DNA damage and genetic instability. Investigators are beginning to evaluate biomarkers of oxidative stress or damage in humans fed various tomato products.

Pool-Zobel et al. *(64)* reported a significant decrease in endogenous levels of lymphocyte DNA strand breaks in 23 healthy male volunteers after either tomato juice, carrot juice, or spinach powder supplementation. Although the antioxidant activity of the many phytochemicals present in the tomato products consumed may contribute to the endogenous protection, it was concluded that multiple mechanisms may be involved in the overall protection against DNA damage. In particular, researchers suggested that the induction of numerous different proteins (e.g., cytosolic proteins, GSTP1, and DNA-repair enzymes) might also contribute to the reduced genetic damage reported *(65)*. A study in 10 stable patients with type II diabetes by Lean et al. *(66)* reported a significant decrease in oxidative damage to lymphocyte DNA in subjects consuming a high-flavonol diet that included onions, tomato sauce, and tea. In a study of healthy women, primary lymphocyte resistance to oxidative stress was enhanced following tomato puree consumption *(67,68)*. Lymphocyte DNA damage was significantly reduced in the treatment group *(67,68)*. Rehman et al. *(69)* recently reported that the consumption of a single serving of tomatoes reduced blood levels of the mutagenic oxidized purine base 8-hydroxyguanine within 24 h, suggesting a protective effect against DNA damage. Consumption of tomato sauce-based pasta dishes for 3 wk in men with localized prostate adenocarcinoma significantly reduced leukocyte and prostate tissue 8-OHdG levels *(70)*.

The antioxidant hypothesis is only one of many currently being considered regarding tomato products and carcinogenesis. Carotenoids and other phytochemicals can influence growth factor, hormone, and cytokine networks influencing cell replication, apoptosis, tumor cell invasion, metastasis, and angiogenesis. A detailed mechanistic understanding of how these compounds may influence cancer has not been elucidated.

4. TOMATOES, TOMATO-BASED PRODUCTS, AND CARDIOVASCULAR DISEASE

In past decades, most of the research concerning diet, nutrition, and cardiovascular disease (CVD) focused upon cholesterol concentrations and lipoprotein patterns. Recently we witnessed the emergence of new theories of acute and chronic vascular disease focusing on the complex biology that occurs within the blood vessel wall. Current concepts view vascular disease as an inflammatory response that involves the interactions between oxidatively damaged lipids, endothelial cells, smooth muscle cells, and infiltrating immune cells such as macrophages and lymphocytes *(71,72)*. Lipoprotein oxidation, particularly low-density lipoprotein (LDL), is considered to be an important step in accelerating vascular injury that can ultimately culminate in acute events and chronic vascular disease. Thus, the prevention of LDL oxidation is postulated to be a potential beneficial health effect of dietary antioxidants such as vitamins E and other phytochemicals *(73)*. Diet and nutrition, along with other lifestyle variables, are certainly key factors in defining CVD risk. The Nurses' Health Study examined women who developed CVD and found that those who adhered to specific dietary and lifestyle patterns (i.e., not currently smoking, consumed a minimum of half a drink of an alcoholic beverage daily, had a BMI < 25, participated in moderate-to-vigorous physical activity for at least 30 min/d, and scored in the upper 40% of the cohort for consumption of a diet high in cereal fiber, folate, marine *n*-3 fatty acids, low in trans fat and glycemic load, and a high ratio of polyunsaturated to saturated fat) had a relative risk of coronary events of 0.17 (95% CI = 0.07–0.41) when compared to the other women in the cohort *(74)*. In comparison, nonconclusive evidence from randomized and blinded studies showing a benefit for specific supplemental antioxidant nutrients for the prevention of cardiovascular events has yet to be demonstrated. In addition to an influence on oxidative stress and lipoprotein damage, it is likely that numerous dietary components may influence the function of endothelial cells, smooth muscle cells, and associated immune cells interacting with the vessel wall *(75–78)*. How the specific phytochemicals in tomato products may influence inflammatory processes in the vessel wall and the risk of acute and chronic vascular events will be the subject of extensive investigation in the near future.

4.1. EPIDEMIOLOGY

Epidemiologic studies investigating the relationship between tomato product consumption or lycopene exposure and the risk for vascular diseases are beginning to emerge. Tissue and serum concentrations of lycopene, the major carotenoid in tomatoes, are correlated with a reduced risk for coronary heart disease (CHD) in several case-control studies. A multicenter case-control study was recently conducted to evaluate the relationship between adipose tissue concentration of antioxidants (i.e., α- and β-carotene and lycopene) and acute myocardial infarction *(8)*. Cases and control subjects were recruited from 10 European countries to ensure maximum variability in exposure. Upon simultaneous analyses of the carotenoids and adjustment for other variables, lycopene was the only carotenoid found to be protective (OR = 0.52 when the 10th and 90th percentiles were compared, 95% CI = 0.33–0.82, p for trend = 0.005) *(8)*. Similarly, lower serum lycopene concentrations were related to an increased risk and mortality from CVD in a concomitant cross-sectional study evaluating Swedish and Lithuanian populations displaying diverging mortality rates from CHD ($n = 210$) *(9)*. Klipstein-Grobusch et al. *(10)* investigated the relationship between serum concentrations of the major carotenoids—α-carotene, β-carotene, β-cryptoxanthin, lutein, lycopene, and zeaxanthin—and aortic atherosclerosis as determined by the presence of calcified plaques of the abdominal aorta. A subsample of the elderly population of the Rotterdam Study consisting of 108 subjects with aortic atherosclerosis and controls was used for the case-control analysis. A 45% reduction (OR = 0.55, 95% CI = 0.25–1.22, p for trend = 0.13) in the risk of atherosclerosis was observed for the highest vs the lowest quartile of serum lycopene. When adjustments for smoking status were made, the inverse association was greatest for current and former smokers (OR = 0.35, 95% CI = 0.13–0.94, p for trend = 0.04). No associations were observed with any of the other serum carotenoids studied. A recent report in men (aged 46–64 yr; $n = 725$) from the Kuopio Ischaemic Heart Disease Risk Factor Study (KIHD) indicated that men in the lowest serum lycopene quarter had a 3.3-fold (95% CI = 1.7–6.4; $p < 0.001$) increased risk of acute coronary events or stroke when compared to the others *(11)*. In addition, men in the lowest quarter of serum lycopene had a significant increment in both mean intima-media thickness of common carotid artery wall (CCA-IMT) ($p < 0.006$ for difference) and maximal CCA-IMT ($p = 0.002$) as compared with other men *(12)*. In a cross-sectional analysis of 520 men and women from the Antioxidant Supplementation in the Atherosclerosis Prevention Study (ASAP), low plasma lycopene levels were associated with an 18% increase in IMT in men when compared to men with plasma lycopene levels higher than the median ($p = 0.003$ for difference) *(12)*.

4.2. Animal Studies

Studies in experimental models have evaluated the effect of tomato consumption on biomarkers associated with the risk for CHD. A study of hypercholesterolemic Wistar rats fed a diet with 0.3% supplemental cholesterol assessed the effect of dried tomato, grape, or apple pomace (5% in diet) on cholesterol concentrations in serum and selected organs. Liver cholesterol content was significantly lowered by 15% and 11% in the tomato and apple pomace groups, respectively. An 18–21% reduction in the concentration of cholesterol in the heart was observed for tomato and other types of pomace. Tomato pomace was the only treatment that lowered the triglyceride concentration in the heart. In addition, all tested pomace interventions reduced plasma levels of conjugated dienes, a product of lipoprotein oxidation *(79)*. Suganuma et al. *(80)* investigated the effect of tomato consumption on hypercholesterolemic mice fed atherogenic diets. Mice fed an atherogenic diet containing 20% (w/w) lyophilized tomato powder showed lower plasma lipid peroxide concentrations than mice fed only the atherogenic diet. In addition, tomato-fed hypercholesterolemic mice maintained acetylcholine-induced vaso-relaxation levels similar to that seen in normal mice. Protection from lipid oxidation, as measured by lipid peroxides, and blood vessel vasorelaxation may contribute to the putative protective effect of tomatoes on atherosclerosis *(80)*.

4.3. Clinical Investigations

A clinical study investigated the effect of 7 d of dietary intervention with tomato juice, spaghetti sauce, or tomato oleoresin on LDL oxidation. Serum thiobarbituric acid-reactive substances (TBARS) and conjugated dienes (CD) were measured to estimate LDL oxidation. Both LDL-TBARS and LDL-CD were significantly lowered after treatment with each tomato product. The average decrease for the tomato product treatment over placebo was 25% and 13% for LDL-TBARS and LDL-CD, respectively *(81)*. More recently, an intervention trial was performed to study how dietary intake of carotenoid-rich vegetables, including tomato juice, carrot juice, and spinach powder, affect lipid peroxidation in men ($n = 23$). Both plasma TBARS and ex vivo oxidation of LDL were used as a measure of lipid peroxidation. A significant 12% reduction in plasma TBARS and an 18% improvement in lipoprotein oxidation lag time, indicating a protective effect, were observed for men who consumed tomato juice, whereas the consumption of carrot juice or spinach powder had no effect *(82)*. A study of 57 patients with type II diabetes was conducted to assess the effects of tomato juice, vitamin E, and vitamin C supplementation on LDL susceptibility to oxidation as well as other parameters. LDL oxidation lag time increased by 42% ($p = 0.001$) in subjects who consumed tomato juice. Similar protection was observed for the vitamin E treatment group (54% increased lag time; $p = 0.001$) *(83)*. A recent study by Maruyama et al. *(84)* investigated the oxidative modification of LDL by tomato juice in 31 female Japanese students. Although the lipoprotein oxidation lag time was not prolonged after intervention, a decrease in the propagation rate was observed. A significant decrease in the propagation rate was seen when a large amount (480 g, providing 45 mg of lycopene) of the juice was given but not with a smaller amount (160 g, providing 15 mg lycopene, plus 320 g of the control drink) *(84)*. Our laboratory recently reported an increase in ex vivo Cu^{2+}-mediated lipoprotein oxidation lag time in subjects who consumed tomato soup or tomato juice for a 3-wk period *(85)*. In summary, the data support a continued effort to

all-trans-lycopene

5-*cis*-lycopene

β-carotene

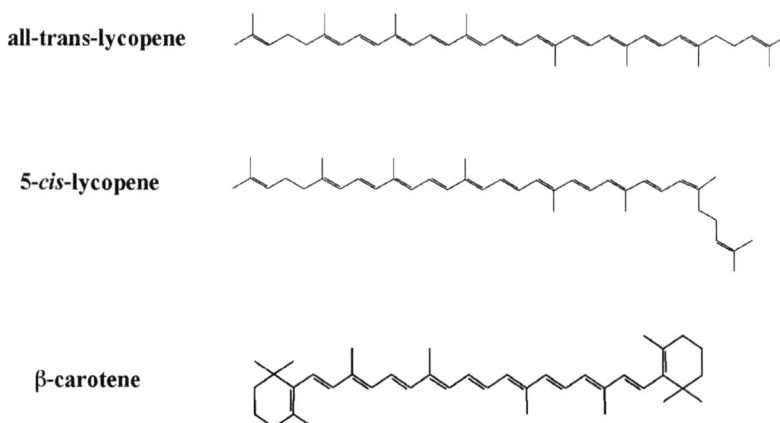

Fig. 1. Representative lycopene and β-carotene structures.

examine how lycopene and other tomato-derived phytochemicals may influence oxidative stress in the vascular wall and its response to injury.

5. THE FOCUS ON LYCOPENE

Lycopene, the predominant carotenoid in tomatoes, has been the focus of many recent studies because it is found in high concentrations in tomato products but in a limited range of other foods. Lycopene, a 40 carbon ($C_{40}H_{56}$) acyclic carotenoid, contains 13 double bonds, 11 of which are linearly arranged in conjugation (*see* Fig. 1). Its structural characteristics contribute to the chemical reactivity of lycopene toward free radicals and oxidizing agents. As a result of having an extensive chromophore system of conjugated carbon-carbon double bonds, lycopene can accept energy from various electronically excited species. Singlet oxygen ($^1O_2$) is a highly reactive high-energy and short-lived oxygen species produced in biological systems that can react with and cause damage to biomolecules. Among the common dietary carotenoids, lycopene is the most efficient quencher of singlet oxygen and free radicals in vitro *(86)*. Lycopene may also interact with reactive oxygen species, such as hydrogen peroxide and nitrogen dioxide *(87–89)*. Lycopene's ability to act as an antioxidant and scavenger of free radicals is postulated to be one of the key mechanisms for its beneficial effects on human health and disease *(90–92)*. However, other biological effects of lycopene that may be independent of its influence on oxidative stress should also be considered. Furthermore, it is premature to assume that the beneficial effects of tomato products are exclusively related to lycopene. The array of other phytochemicals in tomato products must be the focus of additional research.

6. SUMMARY

Nutritional factors are clearly critical in defining the risk for the major diseases that plague economically developed nations. Epidemiologic studies provide overwhelming evidence indicating that diets rich in fruits and vegetables are inversely related to the overall rates of CVD and cancer. More recently, evidence has been accumulating from human epidemiologic studies, in vitro cell culture studies, rodent experiments, and human clinical trials suggesting that tomato products and phytochemicals found in tomato products may influence human health and reduce disease risk. Additional studies are clearly needed, and readers should understand that a causal relationship has not yet been established for tomato products and the prevention of any disease process. Tomato-based beverages, such as tomato juice or V8 Vegetable Juice, may play an important role in future clinical trials of disease prevention. Beverages can be provided in convenient-to-use containers of precise volume that contain a desired concentration of lycopene or other phytochemicals. Furthermore, novel beverages can be prepared with a tomato base and serve as a vehicle for the delivery of other phytochemicals or agents (e.g., soy). Beverages are easy to incorporate into a typical diet, as either a between-meal snack or a component of meals. V8 Vegetable Juice is an example in which numerous phytochemicals from fruit and vegetables can be provided simultaneously in a clinical trial. However, investigators should be aware that the concentrations of sodium in many tomato-based juices can reach more than 500 mg per serving. Sodium is added to tomato-based juices to improve the sensory characteristics of the product but is otherwise not essential. Several companies offer a low-sodium variety of their tomato-based juices, which can provide the health benefits of fruits and vegetables without the concern of excess dietary salt. We expect that new combinations may be developed in the future to target specific disease processes. We are encouraged by the data that are already available, and expect that answers to many questions concerning the relationships between tomatoes, CVD, and cancer should be forthcoming.

7. MAIN POINTS FOR PRIMARY AND CLINICAL REVIEW

1. Tomatoes and tomato products are rich sources of nutrients that are relatively stable during processing.
2. Lycopene is the predominant carotenoid in tomatoes, tomato sauce, and tomato juice, but is found in only limited quantities in other fruits and vegetables.
3. Relative to the consumption of less than 1 serving of tomato sauce per week, the relative risk of prostate cancer in males consuming 2 servings of tomato sauce/week is 0.77.
4. Consumption of tomato products may also protect men and women from cardiovascular disease, although the evidence is less strong for this correlation.
5. Because large amounts of sodium are added to tomato products, low-sodium versions may be preferable, especially for those with hypertension.

REFERENCES

1. van't Veer P, Jansen MC, Klerk M, Kok FJ. Fruits and vegetables in the prevention of cancer and cardiovascular disease. Public Health Nutr 2000;3:103–107.
2. World Cancer Research Fund and American Institute for Cancer Research. Food, Nutrition and the Prevention of Cancer: A Global Perspective. American Institute for Cancer Research, Washington, DC, 1997.
3. Giovannucci E. Tomatoes, tomato-based products, lycopene, and cancer: review of the epidemiologic literature. J Natl Cancer Inst 1999;91:317–331.
4. Hsing AW, Comstock GW, Abbey H, Polk BF. Serologic precursors of cancer. Retinol, carotenoids, and tocopherol and risk of prostate cancer. J Natl Cancer Inst 1990;82:941–946.
5. Rao AV, Fleshner N, Agarwal S. Serum and tissue lycopene and biomarkers of oxidation in prostate cancer patients: a case-control study. Nutr Cancer 1999;33:159–164.

6. Gann PH, Ma J, Giovannucci E, Willet W, Sacks FM, Hennekens CH, Stampfer MJ. Lower prostate cancer risk in men with elevated plasma lycopene levels: results of a prospective analysis. Cancer Res 1999;59:1225–1230.

7. Lu QY, Hung JC, Heber D, et al. Inverse associations between plasma lycopene and other carotenoids and prostate cancer. Cancer Epidemiol Biomarkers Prev 2001;10:749–756.

8. Kohlmeier L, Clark JD, Gomez-Gracia E, et al. Lycopene and myocardial infarction risk in the EURAMIC study. Am J Epidemiol 1997;146:618–626.

9. Kristenson M, Zieden B, Kucinskiene Z, et al. Antioxidant state and mortality from coronary heart disease in Lithuanian and Swedish men: concomitant cross sectional study of men aged 50. Br Med J 1997;314:629–633.

10. Klipstein-Grobusch K, Launer LJ, Geleijnse JM, Boeing H, Hofman A, Witteman JCM. Serum carotenoids and atherosclerosis. The Rotterdam Study. Atherosclerosis 2000;148:49–56.

11. Rissanen TH, Voutilainen S, Nyyssonen K, et al. Low serum lycopene concentration is associated with an excess incidence of acute coronary events and stroke: the Kuopio Ischaemic Heart Disease Risk Factor Study. Br J Nutr 2001;85:749–754.

12. Rissanen TH. Lycopene and cardiovascular disease [abstract]. 13th International Carotenoid Symposium 2002;45.

13. US Department of Agriculture. Agricultural Statistics Board. Vegetables 2001 Summary, National Agricultural Statistics Service (NASS), USDA, Washington, DC, 2002.

14. US Department of Agriculture. Agricultural Research Service. USDA Nutrient Database for Standard Reference, Release 14. Retrieved from Website: http://www.nal.usda.gov/fnic/foodcomp. Accessed May, 2002.

15. USDA-NCC Carotenoid Database for U.S. Foods. Retrieved from Website: http://www.nal.usda.gov/fnic/foodcomp/Data/car98/car98.html. Accessed May, 2002.

16. Beckstrom-Sternberg SM, Duke JA. The phytochemical database. Retrieved from Website: http://www.probe.nalusda.gov:8300/cgi-bin/browse/phytochemdb. Accessed May, 2002.

17. Nguyen ML, Schwartz SJ. Lycopene. In: Natural Food Colorants: Science and Technology. Lauro GJ, Francis FJ (ed.). Marcel Dekker, New York, NY, 2000, pp. 153–192.

18. Stewart AJ, Bozonnet S, Mullen W, Jenkins GI, Lean MEJ, Crozier A. Occurrence of flavonols in tomatoes and tomato-based products. J Agric Food Chem 2000;48:2663–2669.

19. Bremner PD, Blacklock CJ, Paganga G, Mullen W, Rice-Evans CA, Crozier A. Comparison of the phenolic composition of fruit juices by single step gradient HPLC analysis of multiple components versus multiple chromatographic runs optimized for individual families. Free Rad Res 2000;32:549–559.

20. Khachik F, Goli MB, Beecher GR, et al. Effect of food preparation on qualitative and quantitative distribution of major carotenoid constituents of tomatoes and several green vegetables. J Agric Food Chem 1992b;40:390–398.

21. Tonucci LH, Holden JM, Beecher GR, Khachik F, Davis C, Mulokozi G. Carotenoid content of thermally processed tomato-based food products. J Agric Food Chem 1995;43:579–586.

22. Takeoka GR, Dao L, Flessa S, et al. Processing effects on lycopene content and antioxidant activity of tomatoes. J Agric Food Chem 2001;49:3713–3717.

23. Lessin WJ, Catigani GL, Schwartz SJ. Quantification of *cis*-trans isomers of provitamin A carotenoids in fresh and processed fruits and vegetables. J Agric Food Chem 1997;45:3728–3732.

24. Abushita AA, Daood HG, Biacs PA. Change in carotenoids and antioxidant vitamins in tomato as a function of varietal and technological factors. J Agric Food Chem 2000;48:2075–2081.

25. Stahl W, Sies H. Uptake of lycopene and its geometrical isomers is greater from heat-processed than from unprocessed tomato juice in humans. J Nutr 1992;122:2161–2166.

26. Schierle J, Bretzel W, Buhler I, et al. Content and isomeric ratio of lycopene in food and human blood plasma. Food Chem 1997;96:459–465.

27. Shi J, Le Maguer M. Lycopene in tomatoes: chemical and physical properties affected by food processing. Crit Rev Biotechnol 2000;20:293–334.

28. Nguyen ML, Schwartz SJ. Lycopene stability during food processing. Proc Soc Exp Biol Med 1998;218:101–105.

29. Nguyen ML, Francis D, Schwartz SJ. Thermal isomerisation susceptibility of carotenoids in different tomato varieties. J Sci Food Agric 2001;81:910–917.

30. Hume EM, Krebs HA. Vitamin A Requirement of Human Adults. Medical Research Council Special Report Series #264, 1-145. His Majesty's Stationery Office, Great Britain, 1949.

31. Erdman JW, Jr. The physiologic chemistry of carotenes in man. Clin Nutr 1988;7:101–106.

32. Erdman JW, Jr., Bierer TL, Gugger ET. Absorption and transport of carotenoids. In: Carotenoids in Human Health. Canfield LM, Krinsky NI, Olson JA (eds.). New York Academy of Sciences, New York, NY, pp. 1993:76–85.

33. Gartner C, Stahl W, Sies H. Lycopene is more bioavailable from tomato paste than from fresh tomatoes. Am J Clin Nutr 1997;66:116–122.

34. Allen CM, Smith AM, Clinton SK, Schwartz SJ. Tomato consumption increases lycopene isomer concentration in breast milk and plasma of lactating women. J Am Diet Assoc, 2002;102:1257–1262.

35. Hadley CW, Clinton SK, Schwartz SJ. Lycopene-free diets and tomato product consumption significantly alter plasma lycopene-isomer profiles [abstract]. 13th International Carotenoid Symp 2002;140.

36. Erdman JW, Poor CL, Dietz JM. Factors affecting the bioavailability of vitamin A, carotenoids, and vitamin E. Food Technol 1988;42:214–221.

37. Rock CL, Lovalvo JL, Emenhiser C, Ruffin MT, Flatt SW, Schwartz SJ. Bioavailability of beta-carotene is lower in raw than in processed carrots and spinach in women. J Nutr 1998;128:913–916.

38. Rock CL, Swendseid ME. Plasma β-carotene response in humans after meals supplemented with dietary pectin. Am J Clin Nutr 1992;55:96–99.

39. Elinder LS, Hadell K, Johansson J, Holme JM, Olsson AG, Walldius G. Probucol treatment decreases serum concentrations of diet-derived antioxidants. Arterioscler Thromb Vasc Biol 1995;15: 1057–1063.

40. Westrate JA, van het Hof K. Sucrose polyester and plasma carotenoid concentrations in healthy subjects. Am J Clin Nutr 1995;62:591–597.

41. Williams AW, Boileau TWM, Erdman JW. Factors influencing the uptake and absorption of carotenoids. Proc Soc Exp Biol Med 1998;218:106–108.

42. Bray TM. Dietary antioxidants and assessment of oxidative stress. Nutrition 2000;16:578–581.

43. Muscat JE, Huncharek M. Dietary intake and the risk of malignant mesothelioma. Br J Cancer 1996;73: 112–115.

44. Slattery ML, Benson J, Curtin K, Ma K, Schaeffer D, Potter JD. Carotenoids and colon cancer. Am J Clin Nutr 2000;71:575–582.

45. De Stefani E, Oreggia F, Boffetta P, Deneo-Pellegrini H, Ronco A, Mendilaharsu M. Tomatoes, tomato-rich foods, lycopene and cancer of the upper aerodigestive tract: a case-control in Uruguay. Oral Oncol 2000;36:47–53.

46. Tzonou A, Signorello LB, Lagiou P, Wuu J, Trichopoulos D, Trichopoulou A. Diet and cancer of the prostate: a case-control study in Greece. Int J Cancer 1999;80:704–708.

47. Norrish AE, Jackson RT, Sharpe SJ, Skeaff CM. Prostate cancer and dietary carotenoids. Am J Epidemiol 2000;151:124–127.

48. Giovannucci E, Rimm EB, Liu Y, Stampfer MJ, Willet WC. A prospective study of tomato products, lycopene, and prostate cancer risk. J Natl Cancer Inst 2002;94:391–398.

49. Brennan P, Fortes C, Butler J, et al. A multicenter case-control study of diet and lung cancer among non-smokers. Cancer Causes Control 2000;11:49–58.

50. Schuman LM, Mandel JS, Radke A, Seal U, Halberg F. Some selected features of the epidemiology of prostate cancer: Minneapolis—St. Paul, Minnesota case-control study, 1976–1979. In: Trends in Cancer Incidences: Causes and Practical Implications. Magnus K (ed.). Hemisphere Publishing, Washington, DC, 1982, pp. 345–354.

51. Le Marchand L, Hankin JH, Kolonel LN, Wilkens LR. Vegetable and fruit consumption in relation to prostate cancer risk in Hawaii: a reevaluation of the effect of dietary beta-carotene. Am J Epidemiol 1991;133:215–219.

52. Key TJ, Silcocks PB, Davey GK, Appleby PN, Bishop DT. A case-control study of diet and prostate cancer. Br J Cancer 1997;76:678–687.

53. Hayes RB, Ziegler RG, Gridley G, et al. Dietary factors and risks for prostate cancer among black and whites in the United States. Cancer Epidemiol Biomarkers Prev 1999;8:25–34.

54. Kolonel LN, Hankin JH, Whittemore AS, et al. Vegetables, fruits, legumes and prostate cancer: a multi-ethnic case-control study. Cancer Epidemiol Biomarkers Prev 2000;9:795–804.

55. Cohen JH, Kristal AR, Stanford JL. Fruit and vegetable intakes and prostate cancer risk. J Natl Cancer Inst 2000;92:61–68.
56. Mills PK, Beeson WL, Phillips RL, Fraser GE. Cohort study of diet, life-style, and prostate cancer in Adventist men. Cancer 1989;64:598–604.
57. Giovannucci E, Ascherio A, Rimm EB, Stampfer MJ, Colditz GA, Willett WC. Intake of carotenoids and retinol in relation to risk of prostate cancer. J Natl Cancer Inst 1995;87:1767–1776.
58. Schuurman AG, Goldbohm RA, Dorant E, van den Brandt PA. Vegetable and fruit consumption and prostate cancer risk: a cohort study in the Netherlands. Cancer Epidemiol Biomarkers Prev 1998;7: 673–680.
59. Nomura AM, Stemmermann GN, Lee J, Craft NE. Serum micronutrients and prostate cancer in Japanese Americans in Hawaii. Cancer Epidemiol Biomarkers Prev 1997;6:487–491.
60. Okajima E, Tsutsumi M, Ozono S, et al. Inhibitory effect of tomato juice on rat urinary bladder carcinogenesis after N-butyl-N-(4-hydroxybutyl)nitrosamine initiation. Jpn J Cancer Res 1998;89: 22–26.
61. Narisawa T, Fukaura Y, Hasebe M, et al. Prevention of N-methylnitrosourea-induced colon carcinogenesis in F344 rats by lycopene and tomato juice rich in lycopene. Jpn J Cancer Res 1998;89: 1003–1008.
62. Guttenplan JB, Chen M, Kosinska W, Thompson S, Zhao Z, Cohen LA. Effects of a lycopene-rich diet on spontaneous and benzo[a]pyrene-induced mutagenesis in prostate, colon and lungs of the lacZ mouse. Cancer Lett 2001;164:1–6.
63. Boileau TW, Clinton SK, Liao Z, Erdman JW, Jr. Tomato phytochemicals and diet restriction increase survival of rats with N-methyl-N-nitrosourea (NMU)-testosterone-induced prostate cancer [abstract]. FASEB J 2001;494.9:A618.
64. Pool-Zobel BL, Bub A, Muller H, Wollowski I, Rechkemmer G. Consumption of vegetables reduces genetic damage in humans: first results of a human intervention trial with carotenoid-rich foods. Carcinogenesis 1997;18:1847–1850.
65. Pool-Zobel BL, Bub A, Liegibel UM, Treptow-van Lishaut S, Rechkemmer G. Mechanisms by which vegetable consumption reduces genetic damage in humans. Cancer Epidemiol Biomarkers Prev 1998;7: 891–899.
66. Lean MEJ, Noroozi M, Kelly I, et al. Dietary flavonols protect diabetic human lymphocytes against oxidative damage to DNA. Diabetes 1999;48:176–181.
67. Riso P, Pinder A, Santangelo A, Porrini M. Does tomato consumption effectively increase the resistance of lymphocyte DNA to oxidative damage? Am J Clin Nutr 1999;69:712–718.
68. Porrini M, Riso P. Lymphocyte lycopene concentration and DNA protection from oxidative damage is increased in women after a short period of tomato consumption. J Nutr 2000;130:189–192.
69. Rehman A, Bourne LC, Halliwell B, Rice-Evans CA. Tomato consumption modulates oxidative DNA damage in humans. Biochem Biophys Res Commun 1999;262:828–831.
70. Chen L, Stacewicz-Sapuntzakis M, Duncan C. Oxidative DNA damage in prostate cancer patients consuming tomato sauce-based entrees as a whole-food intervention. J Natl Cancer Inst 2001;93: 1872–1879.
71. Libby P, Geng YJ, Aikawa M, et al. Macrophages and atherosclerotic plaque stability. Curr Opin Lipidol 1996;7:330–335.
72. Libby P. Atherosclerosis: the new view. Sci Am 2002;286:46–55.
73. Diaz MN, Frei B, Vita JA, Keaney JF. Mechanisms of disease: antioxidants and atherosclerotic heart disease. N Engl J Med 1997;337:408–416.
74. Stampfer MJ, Hu FB, Manson JE, Rimm EB, Willett WC. Primary prevention of coronary heart disease in women through diet and lifestyle. N Engl J Med 2000;343:16–22.
75. Fleet JC, Clinton SK, Salomon RN, Loppnow H, Libby P. Atherogenic diets increase endotoxin-stimulated cytokine gene expression in rabbit aorta. J Nutr 1992;122:294–305.
76. Clinton SK, Underwood R, Sherman ML, Kufe DK, Libby P. Macrophage-colony stimulation factor gene expression in vascular cells and in experimental and human atherosclerosis. Am J Pathol 1992;140: 301–316.
77. De Caterina R, Cybulsky MI, Clinton SK, Gimbrone Jr MA, Libby P. The omega-3 fatty acid docosahexaenoate reduces cytokine-induced expression of pro-atherogenic and pro-inflammatory proteins in human endothelial cells. Arterioscler Throm 1994;14:1829–1836.

78. Lipton BA, Parthasrathy S, Ord VA, Clinton SK, Libby P, Rosenfeld ME. Components of the protein fraction of oxidized low-density lipoprotein stimulate interleukin-1 production by rabbit arterial macrophage-derived foam cells. J Lipid Res 1995;36:2232–2242.
79. Bobek P, Ozdin L, Hromadova M. The effect of dried tomato, grape and apple pomace on the cholesterol metabolism and antioxidative enzymatic system in rats with hypercholesterolemia. Nahrung 1998;42:317–320.
80. Suganuman H, Inakuma T. Protective effect of dietary tomato against endothelial dysfunction in hypercholesterolemic mice. Biosci Biotechnol Biochem 1999;63:78-82.
81. Agarwal S, Rao AV. Tomato lycopene and low density lipoprotein oxidation: a human dietary intervention study. Lipids 1998;33:981–984.
82. Bub A, Watzl B, Abrahamse L, et al. Moderate intervention with carotenoid-rich vegetable products reduces lipid peroxidation in men. J Nutr 2000;130:2200–2206.
83. Upritchard JE, Sutherland WHF, Mann JI. Effect of supplementation with tomato juice, vitamin E, and vitamin C on LDL oxidation and products of inflammatory activity in type 2 diabetes. Diabetes Care 2000;23:733–738.
84. Maruyama C, Imamura K, Oshima S, et al. Effects of tomato juice consumption on plasma and lipoprotein carotenoid concentrations and the susceptibility of low density lipoprotein to oxidative modification. J Nutr Sci Vitaminol 2001;47:213–221.
85. Hadley CW, Clinton SK, Craft NE, et al. The consumption of processed tomato products enhances plasma lycopene concentrations and reduces oxidative damage to lipoproteins in humans [abstract]. FASEB J 2001;252.12:A297.
86. Di Mascio P, Kaiser S, Sies H. Lycopene as the most efficient biological carotenoid singlet oxygen quencher. Arch Biochem Biophys 1989;274:532–538.
87. Bohm F, Tinkler JH, Truscott TG. Carotenoids protect against cell membrane damage by the nitrogen dioxide radical. Nat Med 1995;1:98–99.
88. Lu Y, Etoh H, Watanabe N, et al. A new carotenoid, hydrogen peroxide oxidation products from lycopene. Biosci Biotech Biochem 1995;59:2153–2155.
89. Woodall AA, Lee SW, Weesie RJ, et al. Oxidation of carotenoids by free radicals: relationship between structure and reactivity. Biochem Biophys Acta 1997;1336:33–42.
90. Clinton SK. Lycopene: chemistry, biology, and implications for human health and disease. Nutr Rev 1998;56:35–51.
91. Rao AV, Agarwal S. Role of antioxidant lycopene in cancer and heart disease. J Am Coll Nutr 2000;19: 563–569.
92. Bohm V, Puspitasari-Nienaber NL, Ferruzzi MG, Schwartz SJ. Trolox equivalent antioxidant capacity of different geometrical isomers of alpha-carotene, beta-carotene, lycopene, and zeaxanthin. J Agric Food Chem 2002;50:221–226.

IV   EFFECT OF CONSUMPTION OF COFFEE, TEA, AND COCOA

9 Coffee Consumption and the Risk of Cancer and Coronary Heart Disease

Alessandra Tavani and Carlo La Vecchia

1. COFFEE AND THE RISK OF CANCER

The possible relationship between coffee and cancer risk was extensively reviewed in 1990 by a Working Group of the International Agency for Research on Cancer (IARC) *(1)*, which concluded that: "In humans there is limited evidence that coffee drinking is carcinogenic to the urinary bladder, lack of evidence for the breast and large bowel and inadequate evidence for the pancreas, ovary and other sites," and gave the overall evaluation that: "Coffee is possibly carcinogenic to the human urinary bladder." Coffee was thus evaluated as a "group B2" substance, which is defined as "the exposure circumstance entails exposure that are possibly carcinogenic to humans." It also added that: "There is some evidence of an inverse relationship between coffee drinking and cancer of the large bowel."

Since then, several epidemiologic studies have been published. This chapter restates the conclusions reached by the IARC Working Group *(1)* for each specific cancer or group of cancers and extends the information to more recent findings.

1.1. Cancer of the Bladder and Lower Urinary Tract

The IARC Monograph summarized the results of 26 studies published before 1990, 22 of which were used to make evaluations *(1)*. Sixteen studies found a moderately increased risk of bladder cancer in coffee drinkers compared to nondrinkers; in seven of these, the association was significant and in three there was also evidence of a dose–risk relation. No relationship was observed in the other six studies. Because smoking is an important risk factor for bladder cancer, lifelong nonsmokers were also considered separately to obtain information on the potential distorting effect of tobacco. The relationship with coffee was still observed, although it was less clear, in part because of the smaller numbers.

The IARC Monograph also considered data on decaffeinated coffee from six case-control studies, which found results similar to those on coffee containing caffeine.

After the publication of the IARC Monograph, at least four cohort *(2–5)* and several case-control studies *(6–18)* provided information on the relationship between coffee and bladder cancer.

From: *Beverages in Nutrition and Health*
Edited by: T. Wilson and N. J. Temple © Humana Press Inc., Totowa, NJ

Three cohort studies found moderately increased risk of bladder cancer in coffee drinkers, in the absence of a dose–risk relationship. In the Californian Seventh-Day Adventists cohort, which included 52 cases, the smoking-adjusted relative risk (RR) was 1.99 (nonsignificant) for ≥ 2 cups/d of coffee compared with nondrinkers, with a stronger relationship in those who never smoked *(2)*. In a cohort of 96 Japanese-Americans living in Hawaii, a high consumption of coffee nonsignificantly increased risk *(3)*, and, in a Norwegian cohort of 43,000 men and women, the RR for drinking ≥ 7 cups/d of coffee was 1.5 in men (based on 40 cases) and 2.4 in women (based on 13 cases) *(4)*. In the Netherlands Cohort Study based on 569 cases, the RR for an increment of 1 cup/d of coffee was 1.03 in men and 0.84 in women *(5)*.

The results from case-control studies agree with those of cohort studies: most found a slightly elevated risk of bladder cancer in coffee drinkers. A weak positive association (RR 2.94) was found in a French study among men, but not women; however, after allowance for smoking, the risk estimate declined and the trend in risk was no longer significant in men *(6)*. No overall association was found in a study of lower urinary tract cancers in both Caucasians and Japanese living in Hawaii (RR 1.0 in men and 0.5 in women) *(7)*, whereas in a German study, a significant twofold increase in risk was found in men drinking ≥ 5 cups of coffee per day after controlling for smoking *(8)*. An Italian study found a nonsignificant 40% increased risk of bladder cancer among drinkers of ≥ 4 cups/d, with a borderline significant trend in risk with duration; in never smokers, the risk was higher, but there was no trend in risk with dose *(9)*. A multicenter Spanish study found no association between coffee consumption and bladder cancer risk in either gender (RR 1.02 in men and 0.71 in women) or in nonsmokers *(10)*. Conversely, daily coffee consumption of > 4 cups/d was associated with a significant increased bladder cancer risk in an American study after controlling for smoking (RR 3.3) *(11)*. In another American study, coffee consumption was associated with an increased risk of bladder cancer among the heaviest coffee drinkers after adjustment for cigarette smoking and dietary factors (RR 2.1); the risk was higher among drinkers of decaffeinated (RR 2.8, nonsignificant) than regular coffee (RR 0.25, nonsignificant) *(12)*. In a French study, drinking > 7 cups/wk for longer than 1 yr was associated with a nonsignificant 60% increase in risk, whereas lifelong consumption of > 60,000 cups significantly increased bladder cancer risk (RR 4.1) *(13)*. No association emerged in two American studies *(14,15)*; in one study, the RR for ≥ 21 cups/wk was 1.0, in the other it was 1.2 in men and 0.6 in women drinking more than 6 cups/d. An Italian study found a significantly increased risk in current coffee drinkers (RR 2.6 in men and 5.2 in women), with a significant trend in risk with dose only in men, after allowance for several covariates, including cigarette smoking *(16)*. A German study found an increased risk of cancer at the higher levels of coffee consumption, but the risk estimates were drastically reduced after allowance for smoking *(17)*. A French study based on 765 cases found an increased risk in men with no dose relation and no association in women *(18)*.

In a pooled analysis of 10 European studies of 564 subjects, there was no excess risk in ever coffee drinkers (OR 1.0); a significantly excess risk was seen in subjects drinking ≥ 10 cups/d, with no linear relation with dose or duration and a small excess risk in nonsmokers who were also heavy coffee drinkers *(19)*. Another meta-analysis, which included 3 cohort and 34 case-control studies, most of which considered bladder cancer, estimated that coffee consumption increased urinary tract cancer risk by approx 20%: the RR, adjusted for age, gender, and smoking for ever vs never drinkers, was 1.18 (95% CI 1.03–1.36) for coffee and 1.18 (95% CI 0.99–1.40) for decaffeinated coffee, in men and women *(20)*.

Thus, the overall data on the coffee–bladder cancer risk relationship allow to exclude a strong association. It is not clear whether the weak association reported in many studies is causal. Caffeine and other substances in coffee have a spectrum of direct and indirect metabolic activities and might induce changes in the carcinogen or anticarcinogen levels in the bladder epithelium, because most substances or metabolites are secreted through the urinary tract and are consequently in direct contact with the bladder mucosa *(1)*. An important confounding factor in the quantification of the coffee–bladder cancer risk relationship is cigarette smoking, which is related to both coffee consumption and bladder cancer risk; however, misclassification of smoking status or residual confounding are unlikely to completely explain the association. Other possible sources of residual confounding might include diet or occupational exposure, although for the latter the similar associations found in men and women suggest that it cannot completely account for the positive results.

1.2. Cancer of the Kidney

The relationship of coffee drinking with cancer risk of transitional cells of the renal pelvis and ureter is similar to that of bladder cancer *(1)*. Published data on adenocarcinoma of the kidney were scarce, but they indicate no consistent association with coffee *(1)*. After the IARC evaluation, no association was found in a Norwegian cohort with a RR of 0.7 in men for ≥ 7 and 1.2 in women for > 6 cups/d *(4)*. A population-based case-control study, conducted in the Boston area and based on 410 cases of renal-cell adenocarcinoma, found slightly elevated risks, with RR of 1.4 for moderate vs low coffee drinking and of 1.2 for high vs low intake; none of these estimates was statistically significant *(21)*. Four case-control studies, 1 American *(21)*, 1 Italian *(22)*, 1 French *(23)*, and 1 Canadian *(24)*, based on 203, 240, 196, and 518 cases respectively, found no association.

Most information on renal-cell cancer, however, comes from the International Renal-Cell Cancer Study, a population-based case-control study conducted in Australia, Denmark, Sweden, and the United States that included 1185 cases *(25)*. The RR was 0.72 in men and 2.11 (significant) in women drinking ≥ 42 cups of coffee/wk, with no significant trend in risk. The positive finding in one gender only and the lack of dose–response relationship argues against a causal role for coffee. Possibly some confounding by a correlate of coffee consumption is responsible for the increased risk in women.

Overall, therefore, epidemiologic data on the relationship between coffee consumption and kidney cancer risk are reassuring to those who chose to drink coffee.

1.3. Cancer of the Pancreas

In the early 1980s, a large case-control study showed a strong association between coffee consumption and pancreatic cancer risk *(26)*. Since then, 21 case-control studies considered the coffee–pancreatic cancer relationship and were reviewed in the IARC Monograph *(1)*. Among them, 10 found moderate positive associations, which were weaker after allowance for smoking, and the remaining studies found no association.

When the results of nine studies, published before 1987 and comprising 1883 cases, were pooled, the overall RR was 1.3 (95% CI 1.1–1.6) for moderate drinkers and 1.6 (95% CI 1.3–2.0) for heavy drinkers compared to nondrinkers *(27)*; when the data from the study that first observed the association *(26)* were excluded from the pooled analysis, the RR was reduced to 1.2 (95% CI 1.0–1.5) for moderate drinkers and 1.4 (95% CI 1.1–1.8) for heavy drinkers compared to nondrinkers. The pooled risk estimates were adjusted for gender and smoking, but at least part of the association depends on residual confounding on account of the rather gross adjustment. Thus, the IARC Working Group recognized a modest association between elevated coffee consumption and pancreatic cancer, which might reflect bias or confounding *(1,28)*. Data on decaffeinated coffee were more scanty and, overall, considered negative *(1,28)*.

Since then, the results of at least six cohort studies have been published. No association emerged in a cohort of 17,633 American men (RR 0.9 for intake of ≥ 7 cups/d, based on 56 cases) *(29)*; in a Norwegian cohort of 43,000 men and women (RR 0.6 in men for ≥ 7 cups/d and 1.2 in women for > 6 cups/d, based, respectively, on 26 and 13 cases) *(4)*; in a cohort of nearly 14,000 residents of a retirement community (RR 0.88 for ≥ 4 cups/d, based on 65 cases) *(30)*; in the Health Professional Follow-up Study (RR 0.37 for coffee and 0.99 for decaffeinated coffee for > 3 cups/d, based on 130 cases) *(31)*; and in the Nurses' Health Study (RR 0.88 for coffee and 0.85 for decaffeinated coffee for > 3 cups/d, based on 158 cases) *(31)*. Conversely, in the cohort study in Iowa based on nearly 34,000 women and 66 incident cases of pancreatic cancer, there was a significant elevated risk for drinkers of more than 17.5 cups/wk of coffee (RR 2.15, 95% CI 1.08–4.30); the association was positive but not significant in never smokers *(32)*.

Most case-control studies published after the IARC Monograph found no significant association between coffee intake and pancreatic cancer risk *(33–42)*, although one study found an inverse association *(43)*. Only two studies found a positive association: an American study based on 149 cases found a RR of 2.38 (95% CI 1.54–3.67), with similar estimates in smokers and nonsmokers and a higher risk for men and for users of decaffeinated coffee *(44)*, and the other, an Italian study based on 570 cases, found a statistically significant dose-response relationship, with a RR of 2.53 (95% CI 1.53–4.18) for consumption of > 3 cups/d *(45)*.

It is possible that the association inconsistently found in a few studies is not causal but explainable through selection bias, residual confounding with cigarette smoking (the major single recognized risk factor for pancreatic cancer) *(46)*, or other sources of bias, including recall bias or occupational history. A strong association between coffee and pancreatic cancer can, therefore, be excluded, but a moderate association remains a possibility.

1.4. Cancer of the Colon and Rectum

The four cohort studies addressing the relationship between coffee and colorectal cancer and considered in the IARC Monograph showed no appreciable association *(1)*. Of the 12 case-control studies, 11 indicated inverse associations, 5 of which were significant. In one of these, a significant inverse dose–response relation was also observed. The IARC Monograph, therefore, concluded that although bias and confounding cannot be excluded, the overall evidence was compatible with a protective effect of coffee on colorectal cancer *(1)*.

Since then, several studies have been published on this issue (4,47–60). Three cohort studies considered colon and rectal cancer separetely, and included a total of 517 cases of colon and 307 cases of rectal cancer. Among case-control studies, six considered colon cancer and included a total of 5912 cases; two studies analyzed rectal cancer and included 1581 cases, and five studies analyzed colorectal cancer and included 687 cases.

In a cohort of Norwegian men and women (4), in a cohort of Finnish male smokers enrolled in the Alpha-Tocopherol Beta-Carotene Cancer Prevention Study trial (47), and in a cohort of Swedish women (48), no association was found between coffee consumption and risk of either colon or rectal cancer.

Of the case-control studies, a small investigation of a selected population of Utah Mormons with low coffee intake found a RR for colon cancer of 2.0 for men drinking more than approx 3 cups/d, with a significant dose–risk relationship, but no relationship in women (49). This finding, however, should be interpreted with caution because of the correlates of coffee consumption in that unusual population. Some of the recent studies that examined colorectal cancer found no association with coffee intake (51,57,58), whereas an Italian study (53) and a Swiss one (59) found an inverse association with a RR of 0.38 and 0.44, respectively, in the highest category of coffee consumption. Some larger studies considering colon and rectal cancer separately found a significant inverse association of coffee intake with colon cancer but a less consistent association with cancer of the rectum (52,55); the RR of colon cancer for the highest category of intake was 0.48 in the Swedish study (52), and 0.77 in men and 0.65 in women in the Italian study (55). However, no association with colon cancer emerged in two American studies (50,54). In another large American study, compared to nondrinkers, low coffee intake in men was associated with an increased risk of colon cancer (RR 1.30), whereas at higher consumption there was an inverse association (RR 0.79) (60).

A meta-analysis of coffee consumption and risk of colorectal cancer found a RR of 0.72 (95% CI 0.61–0.84) for the high vs low category of coffee consumption, combining the results of 12 case-control studies; the findings were similar in population- and hospital-based studies (61). The RR was 0.97, combining the results of five cohort studies, and 0.76 (95% CI 0.66–0.89) combining all studies. The results were similar in men and women and in studies conducted in Asia, Northern and Southern Europe, and North America. This meta-analysis concluded that the results remain open to discussion because of inconsistencies between cohort and case-control studies, although the overall results suggest an inverse relationship between coffee consumption and colorectal cancer risk.

The information on the relationship between decaffeinated coffee and colon cancer comes from three case-control studies and is based on 4905 cases, and the data on rectal cancer derive from a single Italian study comprising 1364 cases. In an American population-based case-control study, based on more than 700 cases of colon cancer, the crude RR for increasing consumption of 10 cups/mo was 0.97 in men and 1.02 in women (50). An Italian hospital-based case-control study, including more than 2000 cases of colon and more than 1300 of rectal cancers, found a RR of 0.92 (95% CI 0.72–1.18) for colon and of 0.88 (95% CI 0.65–1.20) for rectal cancer, based, respectively, on only 94 and 54 cases of drinkers drinking decaffeinated coffee (55). Another American population-based case-control study, including nearly 2000 cases of colon cancer, 380 of whom drank decaffeinated coffee, found a RR of 0.91 (95% CI 0.63–1.31) among the 56 colon cancer cases drinking more than 4 cups/d of decaffeinated coffee (60). Thus, the information for the relationship between decaffeinated coffee and risk of colorectal cancer is inconclusive, because it is based on only a few case-control studies and on a relatively small proportion of drinkers generally reporting moderate consumption.

A constant methodologic bias or residual confounding in case-control studies is unlikely to account for the relative consistency of the results in different countries and settings. A biologic interpretation of the potential protection of coffee against large bowel cancer is provided in terms of a reduction of bile acid and neutral sterol secretion in the colon by substances in coffee, because bile acids are potent promoters of colon carcinogenesis in animals (62–64). This would also be consistent with the association being stronger for (or restricted to) the colon rather than the rectum. Another mechanism is related to the potential antimutagenic properties of some coffee components against heterocyclic amines and other mutagenic agents (1). Finally, coffee intake increases colon motility, which is related to colon cancer risk by influencing the exposure of the epithelia to carcinogens (65). Nevertheless, the biologic interpretation is open to discussion. It is also unclear whether caffeine itself or other substances in coffee beans (including selected antioxidants) (1) are responsible for the apparent protective effect on colon cancer. This is a difficult subject to investigate because the results concerning decaffeinated coffee intake are not informative. This problem derives from the low prevalence of decaffeinated coffee consumption and the limited quantities consumed (65).

1.5. Cancers of the Stomach, Upper Respiratory and Digestive Tracts, Liver, and Gallbladder

The IARC Monograph included data on coffee and gastric cancer risk from five case-control studies (1). There was no evidence of association in any of them. More recently, a Norwegian cohort study observed no association between coffee intake and gastric cancer risk (RR 0.5 in men and in women, not significant, based on 78 cases) (4), although a cohort study of Japanese residents of Hawaii, based on 108 cases, found that men who drank one cup of coffee per day had a significantly elevated risk of gastric cancer compared to nondrinkers (RR 2.5, 95% CI 1.0–6.1) (66). No association between coffee drinking and gastric cancer risk was found in four case-control studies: a Spanish study based on 354 cases (67), a Swedish study based on 338 cases (68), a Japanese study based on 893 cases (56), and a Polish study based on 464 cases (69). Thus, the overall evidence indicates that coffee is unlikely to have any major effect on gastric carcinogenesis.

Six studies providing data on cancers of the oral cavity, pharynx, and osophagus were considered in the IARC Monograph (1). There was no evidence of association with coffee consumption in any of them. Since then, at least one cohort (4) and five case-control studies (70–74) found no association for these cancers, whereas a case-control study based on 598 cases of oral and pharyngeal cancer found that risk approximately halved in the highest compared to the lowest quintile of coffee intake (75).

Coffee intake was not associated with risk of hepatocellular carcinoma in a Greek hospital-based case-control study based on 333 cases (RR 0.7, 95% CI 0.4–1.2 for drinkers of ≥ 20 cups/wk compared to nondrinkers) (76), confirming the conclusions of the IARC Monograph (1). As for gallbladder cancer risk, a Polish case-control study found no association (77), whereas a Canadian study found lower risks in coffee drinkers (RR 0.26, 95% CI 0.07–0.95), which is consistent with some role of coffee on bile acid metabolism (78).

Thus, meaningful associations between coffee and cancer of the stomach, upper respiratory and digestive tracts, liver, and gallbladder can now be excluded.

1.6. Cancer of the Breast

Of the seven case-control studies considered in the IARC Monograph, none found an association between breast cancer risk and coffee consumption *(1)*. More recently, three cohort *(4,79,80)* and four case-control studies *(81–84)*, including an Italian one with nearly 6000 cases *(84)*, found no association. However, a Finnish case-control study reported a protection in postmenopausal women *(85)*. We may conclude, therefore, that there is no relationship between coffee and cancer of the breast.

1.7. Cancer of the Ovary and Female Genital Tract

At the time of the IARC Monograph, of the seven case-control studies on ovarian cancer and coffee, two found significantly elevated risks and five a slightly increased risk *(1)*. Since then, a Norwegian cohort study based on 93 cases reported a nonstatistically significant increase in risk (RR 2.0 for ≥ 7 cups/d) *(4)*, and a hospital-based case-control study from greater Athens, based on 189 cases, found no consistent association between coffee intake and ovarian cancer risk *(86)*. More recently, one American population-based case-control study that included 549 women found an increased risk in premenopausal women only (RR 2.24, 95% CI 1.32–3.78 for ≥ 4 cups/d compared to never drinkers) *(87)*, whereas an Italian hospital-based study, including 1031 cases, found no association between either coffee or decaffeinated coffee and ovarian cancer risk *(88)*. Thus, although a slight elevated risk cannot be completely excluded, the overall evidence suggests no meaningful association of coffee intake with ovarian cancer risk.

Some association with coffee intake was found in a case-control study of cancer of the vulva and in a cohort study of cervical cancer reported in the IARC Monograph *(1)*. A possible association of coffee consumption with cancer of the vulva was also observed in a case-control study based on 201 cases, which found that risk increased irregularly with the number of cups *(89)*. No association between coffee intake and endometrial cancer was seen in a Norwegian cohort *(4)* or in a Swiss-Italian case-control study *(90)*.

1.8. Cancer at Other Sites

The IARC Monograph reported no association in coffee consumption for two cohort and one case-control study of lung cancer, and in a cohort study on Hodgkin's disease, non-Hodgkin's lymphomas, lymphatic and myeloid leukemia, and malignant melanoma *(1)*. The information published since then has further supported the lack of association of coffee drinking with non-Hodgkin's lymphoma *(4,91,92)*, Hodgkin's disease *(4,92)*, myeloma *(92)*, and soft tissue sarcomas *(92)*. Concerning cancer of the lung, a Norwegian cohort study found an elevated risk with coffee intake in men but not in women *(4)*, one case-control study conducted in Uruguay found no association *(93)*, and a Japanese hospital-based case-control study found an elevated risk *(94)*. Coffee drinking in women was associated with significantly lower risk of cutaneous malignant melanoma in a cohort of Norwegian men and women *(95)*. No association was found in a Norwegian cohort *(4)* and four case-control studies of prostate cancer *(96–99)*. An inverse association of borderline significance (RR 0.7 in the highest tertile of intake compared to the lowest) was found in a case-control study of thyroid cancer *(100)*.

1.9. Conclusions

Overall, epidemiological evidence shows the absence of any appreciable association of coffee intake with most common neoplasms, including cancers of the stomach, upper respiratory and digestive tracts, hepatocellular, gallbladder, breast, vulva, endometrium, prostate, lung, non-Hodgkin's lymphoma, Hodgkin's disease, myelomas, soft tissue sarcomas, melanoma, and thyroid. Most recent studies on bladder cancer allow to exclude a strong association with coffee intake; the inconsistent findings in the two genders in several studies, the lack of dose–response relationships, and the similar findings for regular and decaffeinated coffee do not support the hypothesis of causality. A strong association between coffee intake and pancreatic cancer risk can now be excluded; a modest positive association remains possible, although it may be partly due to residual confounding of smoking. For colorectal cancer, four cohort studies reported no association, although most case-control studies reported an inverse association of coffee intake with risk of colon cancer and no association with risk of rectal cancer. Thus, although overall results suggest an inverse relation between coffee consumption and colorectal cancer risk, the results remain open to interpretation, mainly because of inconsistencies between cohort and case-control studies.

2. COFFEE AND RISK OF CORONARY HEART DISEASE

The possibility that high coffee intake enhances the risk of coronary heart disease (CHD) and particularly acute myocardial infarction (AMI) has been debated since the early 1970s, after the reports from a multidisease case-control surveillance program *(101,102)*. Since then, two meta-analyses (including mostly the same studies) have been published, one in 1993 that included 14 cohort and 8 case-control studies *(103)*, and the other in 1994 that included 15 cohort and 8 case-control studies *(104)*. In the latter meta-analysis, the pooled RR from case-control studies for the effect of drinking 5 cups/d of coffee vs none was 1.63 (95% CI 1.50–1.78); the corresponding pooled RR for cohort studies was 1.05 (95% CI 0.99–1.12) *(103)*. Thus, although the prospective studies overall suggest no increased risk of CHD, even with high coffee intake, case-control studies point to an elevated risk.

Recent evidence is also inconsistent. Among cohort studies, one conducted in California found a slightly increased risk of AMI, with a RR of 1.4 (95% CI 1.0–1.9) in drinkers of ≥ 4 cups of coffee per day compared to nondrinkers *(105)*. In a study that included 111 CHD cases, the RR associated with drinking 5 cups/d of coffee was 2.94 (95% CI 1.27–6.81) if computed at baseline, 5.52 (95% CI 1.31–23.18) for average intake, and 1.95 (95% CI 0.86–4.40) for most recent intake *(106)*. In the Primary Prevention Study based on 7495 subjects followed for 27 yr, and including 937 subjects with heart failure, the RR was 1.17 (95% CI 1.05–1.30) for ≥ 5 cups/d *(107)*. Conversely, no association was found in the NHANES II study on CHD *(108)*, in the Copenhagen Male Study based on 184 patients with CHD *(109)*, in the Nurses' Health Study based on 712 women with CHD *(110)*, in a prospective Norwegian study that included 139 CHD deaths *(111)*, in a cohort of Scottish men based on 308 CHD deaths *(112)*, in the Scottish Heart Health Study based on 156 coronary deaths or on 397 patients with CHD *(113)*, and in a Finnish cohort based on 891 CHD events in men and 319 in women *(114)*.

Among case-control studies, one population-based study comprising 340 cases of AMI found no association, with a RR of 0.84 for ≥ 4 cups/d of coffee and 1.25 for more than 1 cup of decaffeinated coffee *(115)*. Conversely, at least eight other case-control studies found a somewhat elevated risk. One study was based on 362 cases of primary cardiac arrest and found a RR of 1.44 (95% CI 0.82–2.53) for a usual caffeine consumption of ≥ 687 mg/d (corresponding to approx ≥ 5 cups/d of coffee); an elevated risk was restricted to high consumption in never smokers (RR 3.2, 95% CI 1.3–8.1) *(116)*. Of the six studies considering AMI, a hospital-based Greek study, based on 329 patients, found a RR of 2.07 (95% CI 1.18–3.61) for ≥ 3 cups/d compared to less than 1 cup *(117)*. A hospital-based Italian study, comprising 801 men, found a RR of 2.6 (95% CI 1.6–4.2) for ≥ 5 cups/d of regular coffee compared to nondrinkers *(118)*, and another based on 433 women found a RR of 2.1 (95% CI 1.1–3.9) for ≥ 2 cups/d of decaffeinated coffee *(119)*. Among the 858 women included in a population-based American study, no increased risk of AMI was found for drinking < 5 cups/d of coffee, but the RR was 2.5 (95%CI 1.0–6.5) in drinkers of ≥ 10 cups/d, with no difference among smokers and nonsmokers *(120)*. Of two other hospital-based Italian studies, one based on 513 cases of AMI found a RR of 3.8 (95% CI 1.8–7.9) for ≥ 5 cups/d *(121)*, and the other, based on 153 cases, found a fourfold elevated risk among smokers and nonsmokers who drank ≥ 4 cups/d *(122)*. In another Italian case-control study, based on 507 cases, the RR for coffee intake was around unity up to 3 cups/d and rose to 1.9 (95% CI 1.1–3.3) for ≥ 6 cups/d; the risk was much higher in smokers because compared to nonsmokers, drinking ≤ 3 cups/d of coffee, the RR was 3.3 (95% CI 2.1–5.0) among current smokers drinking > 3 cups/d *(123)*. Moderate decaffeinated coffee intake was not associated with AMI risk.

Overall, positive associations are more common in case-control than in prospective studies and occur more frequently in studies considering categories of habitual drinkers of large amount of coffee *(103)*. A possible explanation for the different results from prospective and case-control studies is the temporal relationship between exposure to caffeine and the effect on the cardiovascular system. In prospective studies, the reported exposure typically occurs years before the diagnosis of a cardiac event, whereas in case-control studies, more recent habits are considered. Considering our incomplete understanding of the mechanisms of caffeine action on the cardiovascular system, it is not possible to determine the most appropriate exposure time, and this might lead to an underestimation of the strength of the association in cohort studies.

Among potential confounding factors, cigarette smoking, the most important correlate of coffee drinking that might contribute to the positive association in case-control studies, has been almost always allowed for in the estimation of risk, but some residual confounding is still possible. Other potential confounders are dietary fat, vitamin C, alcohol intake, body mass index, and stress *(124)*. Another source of bias may be the inclusion in the multiple logistic analyses of terms for cholesterol, hypertension, and other cardiovascular disorders, which might be intermediate steps of the relationship between coffee and CHD rather than confounding factors. In fact, among the proposed biologic mechanisms through which coffee may increase CHD risk, there are the coffee-dependent rise in blood pressure *(125)*, LDL cholesterol concentration *(126)*, and plasma total homocysteine concentrations *(127)*. The lack of a strong relationship between acute coffee consumption and angina pectoris would, however, be inconsistent with a major effect of coffee on blood pressure and other hemodynamic factors *(125)*.

Another source of error is inaccurate estimation of coffee consumption due to such factors as the size of the container, the habit of refilling the cup, the variability of coffee drinking between weekdays and weekends, and the different intake in different seasons. Another important variable is caffeine concentration, which depends on the method of brewing the coffee, the type of coffee (American coffee, expresso, mocha), and the amount of coffee used. Five surveys using a high-performance liquid chromatography procedure to measure caffeine concentration indicated considerable variations between coffee brands as well as day-to-day variation in coffee samples from commercial shops (128). Caffeine is contained in other beverages (tea, cola, and energy drinks), in foods, and in nonprescription drugs, and these sources may not always be correctly estimated.

Thus, although it is not possible to completely exclude an effect of coffee and caffeine in the CHD etiology, it is reasonable to believe that low to moderate coffee consumption (≤ 3 cups/d) is not a relevant public health problem because it should not increase the risk of CHD.

3. CONCLUSIONS

Epidemiologic studies on the relationship between coffee consumption and cancer risk have mainly focused on cancers of the urinary bladder, pancreas, and colorectum. The relationship between coffee and bladder cancer is still controversial; in most studies, there is a moderate excess risk in coffee drinkers compared to nondrinkers but no clear association with dose or duration. It is, therefore, unclear whether the weak association is causal or nonspecific and the result of some bias or confounding. Most studies suggest that coffee is not materially related to pancreatic cancer risk. Overall, evidence on the coffee–colorectal cancer relation suggests an inverse association, because most case-control studies found risk estimates below unity, particularly for colon cancer; however, the risk pattern is less clear for cohort studies. Possible biological mechanisms for the inverse association include the coffee-related reduction of bile acids and neutral sterol secretion in the colon. Coffee intake is not associated with ovarian cancer risk, although a slight elevated risk cannot be completely excluded. For other cancer sites, including oral cavity, esophagus, stomach, liver, breast, kidney, and lymphoid neoplasms, the relation of coffee drinking with cancer risk has been less extensively investigated, but the evidence is largely reassuring. With reference to CHD, the overall relative risk is approx 1.4 for drinkers of 5 cups/d of coffee vs nondrinkers, with some heterogeneity between cohort and case-control studies. Recent evidence is generally reassuring for low-to-moderate coffee intake (up to 3 cups/d). Higher intakes may increase CHD risk through a coffee-dependent rise in blood pressure and blood levels of LDL cholesterol and total homocysteine.

4. MAIN POINTS FOR PRIMARY AND CLINICAL REVIEW

1. Coffee consumption in excess of 2 cups/d may be weakly associated with an increased risk of bladder cancer.
2. Coffee consumption may provide a slight protective effect with respect to colon cancer.
3. No association has been established between coffee consumption and cancers of the kidney, stomach, rectum, liver, gall bladder, upper respiratory, breast, ovary, prostate, melanoma, thyroid, and lymphoid neoplasms.
4. No consistent associations have been observed between consumption of coffee and coronary heart disease, although more than 3 cups/d may increase the risk.

5. Confounding effects of smoking, diet, and behavior make associations between coffee consumption and cancer and coronary heart disease difficult to interpret and are probably responsible for some of the potentially conflicting results observed in some studies.

ACKNOWLEDGMENTS

This work was supported by a contribution of the Italian Association for Research on Cancer, Milan, Italy, and by the Commission of the European Communities (Contract No. QLK1-CT-2000-00069). The authors thank Mrs. Judy Baggott and Ms. M. Paola Bonifacino for their editorial assistance.

REFERENCES

1. International Agency for Cancer Research. IARC Monographs: Evaluation of Carcinogenic Risks to Humans, vol. 51, Coffee, Tea, Mate, Methylxanthines and Methylglyoxal. International Agency for Cancer Research, Lyon, France, 1991.
2. Mills PK, Beeson WL, Phillips RL, Fraser GE. Bladder cancer in a low risk population: results from the Adventist Health Study. Am J Epidemiol 1991;133:230–239.
3. Chyou P-H, Nomura AMY, Stemmermann GN. A prospective study of diet, smoking, and lower urinary tract cancer. Ann Epidemiol 1993;3:211–216.
4. Stensvold I, Jacobsen BK. Coffee and cancer: a prospective study of 43,000 Norwegian men and women. Cancer Causes Control 1994;5:401–408.
5. Zeegers MPA, Dorant E, Goldbohm RA, van den Brandt PA. Are coffee, tea, and total fluid consumption associated with bladder cancer risk? Results from the Netherlands Cohort Study. Cancer Causes Control 2001;12:231–238.
6. Clavel J, Cordier S. Coffee consumption and bladder cancer risk. Int J Cancer 1991;47:207–212.
7. Nomura AMY, Kolonel LN, Hankin JH, Yoshizawa CN. Dietary factors in cancer of the lower urinary tract. Int J Cancer 1991;48:199–205.
8. Kunze E, Chang-Claude J, Frentzel-Beyme R. Life style and occupational risk factors for bladder cancer in Germany. A case-control study. Cancer 1992;69:1776–1790.
9. D'Avanzo B, La Vecchia C, Franceschi S, Negri E, Talamini R, Buttino I. Coffee consumption and bladder cancer risk. Eur J Cancer 1992;28A:1480–1484.
10. Escolar Pujolar A, Gonzalez CA, Lopez-Abente G. Bladder cancer and coffee consumption in smokers and non-smokers in Spain. Int J Epidemiol 1993;22:8–44.
11. McGeehin MA, Reif JS, Becher JC, Mangione EJ. Case-control study of bladder cancer and water disinfection methods in Colorado. Am J Epidemiol 1993;138:492–501.
12. Vena JE, Freudenheim J, Graham S, et al. Coffee, cigarette smoking, and bladder cancer in western New York. Ann Epidemiol 1993;3:586–591.
13. Momas I, Daures J-P, Festy B, Bontoux J, Gremy F. Relative importance of risk factors in bladder carcinogenesis: some new results about Mediterranean habits. Cancer Causes Control 1994;5: 326–332.
14. Morris Brown L, Hoar Zahm S, Hoover RN, Fraumeni JF. High bladder cancer mortality in rural New England (United States): an etiologic study. Cancer Causes Control 1995;6:361–368.
15. Bruemmer B, White E, Vaughan TL, Cheney CL. Fluid intake and the incidence of bladder cancer among middle-aged men and women in a three-county area of western Washington. Nutr Cancer 1997;29:163–168.
16. Donato F, Boffetta P, Fazioli R, Aulenti V, Gelatti U, Porru S. Bladder cancer, tobacco smoking, coffee and alcohol drinking in Brescia, northern Italy. Eur J Epidemiol 1997;13:795–800.
17. Pohlabeln H, Jockel K-H, Bolm-Audorff U. Non-occupational risk factors for cancer of the lower urinary tract in Germany. Eur J Epidemiol 1999;15:411–419.
18. Geoffroy-Perez B, Cordier S. Fluid consumption and the risk of bladder cancer: results of a multicenter case-control study. Int J Cancer 2001;93:880–887.
19. Sala M, Cordier S, Chang-Claude J, et al. Coffee consumption and bladder cancer in nonsmokers: a pooled analysis of case-control studies in European countries. Cancer Causes Control 2000;11:925–931.

20. Zeegers MPA, Tan FES, Goldbohm RA, van den Brandt PA. Are coffee and tea consumption associated with urinary tract cancer risk? A systematic review and meta-analysis. Int J Epidemiol 2001;30: 353–362.
21. Maclure M, Willett W. A case-control study of diet and risk of renal adenocarcinoma. Epidemiology 1990;1:430–440.
22. Talamini R, Baron AE, Barra S, et al. A case-control study of risk factor for renal cell cancer in northern Italy. Cancer Causes Control 1990;1:125–131.
23. Benhamou S, Lenfant MH, Ory-Paoletti C, Flamant R. Risk factors for renal-cell carcinoma in a French case-control study. Int J Cancer 1993;55:32–36.
24. Kreiger N, Marrett LD, Dodds L, Hilditch S, Darlington GA. Risk factors for renal cell carcinoma: results of a population-based case-control study. Cancer Causes Control 1993;4:101–110.
25. Wolk A, Gridley G, Niwa S, et al. International renal cell cancer study. VII. Role of diet. Int J Cancer 1996;65:67–73.
26. MacMahon B, Yen S, Trichopoulos D, Warren K, Nardi G. Coffee and cancer of the pancreas. N Engl J Med 1981;304:630–633.
27. La Vecchia C, Liati P, Decarli A, Negri E, Franceschi S. Coffee consumption and risk of pancreatic cancer. Int J Cancer 1987;40:309–313.
28. La Vecchia C. Coffee and cancer epidemiology. In: Caffeine, Coffee, and Health. Garattini S (ed.). Raven Press, New York, NY, 1993, pp. 379–398.
29. Zheng W, McLaughlin JK, Gridley G, et al. A cohort study of smoking, alcohol consumption, and dietary factors for pancreatic cancer (United States). Cancer Causes Control 1993;4:477–482.
30. Shibata A, Mack TM, Paganini-Hill A, Ross RK, Henderson BE. A prospective study of pancreatic cancer in the elderly. Int J Cancer 1994;58:46–49.
31. Michaud DS, Giovannucci E, Willett WC, Colditz GA, Fuchs CS. Coffee and alcohol consumption and the risk of pancreatic cancer in two prospective United States cohorts. Cancer Epidemiol Biomarkers Prev 2001;10:429–437.
32. Harnack LJ, Anderson KE, Zheng W, Folsom AR, Sellers TA, Kushi LH. Smoking, alcohol, coffee, and tea intake and incidence of cancer of the exocrine pancreas: The Iowa Women's Health Study. Cancer Epidemiol Biomarkers Prev 1997;6:1081–1086.
33. Farrow DC, Davis S. Risk of pancreatic cancer in relation to medical history and the use of tobacco, alcohol and coffee. Int J Cancer 1990;45:816–820.
34. Baghurst PA, McMichael AJ, Slavotinek AH, Baghurst KJ, Boyle P, Walker AM. A case-control study of diet and cancer of the pancreas. Am J Epidemiol 1991;134:167–179.
35. Ghadirian P, Simard A, Baillargeon J. Tobacco, alcohol, and coffee and cancer of the pancreas. A population-based case-control study in Quebec, Canada. Cancer 1991;67:2664–2670.
36. Jain M, Howe GR, St Louis P, Miller AB. Coffee and alcohol as determinants of risk of pancreas cancer: a case-control study from Toronto. Int J Cancer 1991;47:384–389.
37. Friedman GD, van den Eeden SK. Risk factors for pancreatic cancer: an exploratory study. Int J Epidemiol 1993;22:30–37.
38. Klapothaki V, Tznou A, Hsieh CC, Toupadaki N, Karakatsani A, Trichopoulos D. Tobacco, ethanol, coffee, pancreatitis, diabetes mellitus, and cholelithiasis as risk factors for pancreatic carcinoma. Cancer Causes Control 1993;4:375–382.
39. Zatonski WA, Boyle P, Przewozniak K, Maisonneuve P, Drosik K, Walker AM. Cigarette smoking, alcohol, tea and coffee consumption and pancreas cancer risk: a case-control study from Opole, Poland. Int J Cancer 1993;53:601–607.
40. Partanen T, Hemminki K, Vainio H, Kauppinen T. Coffee consumption not associated with risk of pancreas cancer in Finland. Prev Med 1995;24:213–216.
41. Soler M, Chatenoud L, La Vecchia C, Franceschi S, Negri E. Diet, alcohol, coffee and pancreatic cancer: final results from an Italian study. Eur J Cancer Prev 1998;7:455–460.
42. Villeneuve PJ, Johnson KC, Hanley AJ, Mao Y. Alcohol, tobacco and coffee consumption and the risk of pancreatic cancer: results from the Canadian Enhanced Surveillance System case-control project. Canadian Cancer Registries Epidemiology Research Group. Eur J Cancer Prev 2000;9:49–58.
43. Bueno de Mesquita HB, Maisonneuve P, Moerman CJ, Runia S, Boyle P. Lifetime consumption of alcoholic beverages, tea and coffee and exocrine carcinoma of the pancreas: a population-based case-control study in The Netherlands. Int J Cancer 1992;50:514–522.

44. Lyon JL, Mahoney AW, French TK, Moser R, Jr. Coffee consumption and the risk of cancer of the exocrine pancreas: a case-control study in a low-risk population. Epidemiology 1992;3:164–170.
45. Gullo L, Pezzilli R, Morselli-Labate AM. Coffee and cancer of the pancreas: an Italian multicenter study. The Italian Pancreatic Cancer Study Group. Pancreas 1995;11:223–229.
46. Boyle P, Hsieh CC, Maisonneuve P, et al. Epidemiology of pancreas cancer. Int J Pancreatol 1989; 5:327–346.
47. Hartman TJ, Tangrea JA, Pietinen P, et al. Tea and coffee consumption and risk of colon and rectal cancer in middle-aged Finnish men. Nutr Cancer 1998;31:41–48.
48. Terry P, Bergkvist L, Holmberg L, Wolk A. Coffee consumption and risk of colorectal cancer in a population based prospective cohort of Swedish women. Gut 2001;49:87–90.
49. Slattery ML, West DW, Robinson LM, et al. Tobacco, alcohol, coffee, and caffeine as risk factors for colon cancer in a low-risk population. Epidemiology 1990;1:141–145.
50. Peters RK, Pike MC, Garabrant D, Mack TM. Diet and colon cancer in Los Angeles County, California. Cancer Causes Control 1992;3:457–473.
51. Olsen J, Kronborg O. Coffee, tobacco and alcohol as risk factors for cancer and adenoma of the large intestine. Int J Epidemiol 1993;22:398–402.
52. Baron JA, Gerhardsson de Verdier M, Ekbom A. Coffee, tea, tobacco, and cancer of the large bowel. Cancer Epidemiol Biomarkers Prev 1994;3:565–570.
53. Centonze S, Boeing H, Leoci C, Guerra V, Misciagna G. Dietary habits and colorectal cancer in a low-risk area. Results from a population-based case-control study in southern Italy. Nutr Cancer 1994; 21:233–246.
54. Shannon J, White E, Shattuck AL, Potter JD. Relationship of food groups and water intake to colon cancer risk. Cancer Epidemiol Biomarkers Prev 1996;5:495–502.
55. Tavani A, Pregnolato A, La Vecchia C, Negri E, Talamini R, Franceschi S. Coffee and tea intake and risk of cancers of the colon and rectum: a study of 3,530 cases and 7,057 controls. Int J Cancer 1997;73: 193–197.
56. Inoue M, Tajima K, Hirose K, et al. Tea and coffee consumption and the risk of digestive tract cancers: data from a comparative case-referent study in Japan. Cancer Causes Control 1998;9:209–216.
57. Muñoz SE, Navarro A, Lantieri MJ, et al. Alcohol, methylxanthine-containing beverages, and colorectal cancer in Cordoba, Argentina. Eur J Cancer Prev 1998;7:207–213.
58. Boutron-Ruault MC, Senesse P, Faivre J, Chatelain N, Belghiti C, Meance S. Foods as risk factors for colorectal cancer: a case-control study in Burgundy (France). Eur J Cancer Prev 1999;8: 229–235.
59. Levi F, Pasche C, La Vecchia C, Lucchini F, Franceschi S. Food groups and colorectal cancer risk. Br J Cancer 1999;79:1283–1287.
60. Slattery ML, Caan BJ, Anderson KE, Potter JD. Intake of fluids and methylxanthine-containing beverages: Association with colon cancer. Int J Cancer 1999;81:199–204.
61. Giovannucci E. Meta-analysis of coffee consumption and risk of colorectal cancer. Am J Epidemiol 1998;147:1043–1052.
62. Bjelke E. Colon cancer and blood-cholesterol. Lancet 1974;1:1116–1117.
63. Jacobsen BK, Thelle DS. Coffee, cholesterol, and colon cancer: Is there a link? Br Med J 1987; 294:4–5.
64. La Vecchia C. Epidemiological evidence on coffee and digestive tract cancers: a review. Digestive Dis 1990;8:281–286.
65. Potter JD. Reconciling the epidemiology, physiology, and molecular biology of colon cancer. J Am Dietet Assoc 1992;268:1573–1577.
66. Galanis DJ, Kolonel LN, Lee J, Nomura A. Intakes of selected foods and beverages and the incidence of gastric cancer among the Japanese residents of Hawaii: a prospective study. Int J Epidemiol 1998; 27:173–180.
67. Agudo A, Gonzalez CA, Marcos G, et al. Consumption of alcohol, coffee, and tobacco, and gastric cancer in Spain. Cancer Causes Control 1992;3:137–143.
68. Hansson LE, Nyren O, Bergstrom R, et al. Diet and risk of gastric cancer. A population-based case-control study in Sweden. Int J Cancer 1993;55:181–189.
69. Chow WH, Swanson CA, Lissowska J. Risk of stomach cancer in relation to consumption of cigarettes, alcohol, tea and coffee in Warsaw, Poland. Int J Cancer 1999;81:871–876.

70. La Vecchia C, Negri E, D'Avanzo B, Franceschi S, Decarli A, Boyle P. Dietary indicators of laryngeal cancer risk. Cancer Res 1990;50:4497–4500.

71. Franceschi S, Bidoli E, Baron AE, et al. Nutrition and cancer of the oral cavity and pharynx in North-East Italy. Int J Cancer 1991;47:20–25.

72. Pintos J, Franco EL, Oliveira BV, Kowalski LP, Curado MP, Dewar R. Mate, coffee, and tea consumption and risk of cancers of the upper aerodigestive tract in southern Brazil. Epidemiology 1994; 5:583–590.

73. Bundgaard T, Wildt J, Frydenberg M, Elbrond O, Nielsen JE. Case-control study of squamous cell cancer of the oral cavity in Denmark. Cancer Causes Control 1995;6:57–67.

74. Castellsagué X, Muñoz N, De Stefani E, Victora CG, Castelletto R, Rolón PA. Influence of mate drinking, hot beverages and diet on esophageal cancer risk in South America. Int J Cancer 2000;88: 658–664.

75. Franceschi S, Favero A, Conti E, et al. Food groups, oils and butter, and cancer of the oral cavity and pharynx. Br J Cancer 1999;80:614-620.

76. Kuper H, Tzonou A, Kaklamani E. Tobacco smoking, alcohol consumption and their interaction in the causation of hepatocellular carcinoma. Int J Cancer 2000;85:498–502.

77. Zatonski WA, La Vecchia C, Przewozniak K, Maisonneuve P, Lowenfels AB, Boyle P. Risk factors of gallbladder cancer: a Polish case-control study. Int J Cancer 1992;51:707–711.

78. Ghadirian P, Simard A, Baillargeon J. A population-based case-control study of cancer of the bile ducts and gallbladder in Quebec, Canada. Rev Epidemiol Sante Publique 1993;41:107–112.

79. Hunter DJ, Manson JE, Stampfer MJ, et al. A prospective study of caffeine, coffee, tea, and breast cancer. Am J Epidemiol 1992;136:1000–1001.

80. Folsom AR, McKenzie DR, Bisgard KM, Kushi LH, Sellers TA. No association between caffeine intake and postmenopausal breast cancer incidence in the Iowa Women's Health Study. Am J Epidemiol 1993;138:380–383.

81. McLaughlin CC, Mahoney MC, Nasca PC, Metzger BB, Baptiste MS, Field NA. Breast cancer and methylxanthine consumption. Cancer Causes Control 1992;3:175–178.

82. Levi F, La Vecchia C, Gulie C, Negri E. Dietary factors and breast cancer risk in Vaud, Switzerland. Nutr Cancer 1993;19:327–335.

83. Smith SJ, Deacon JM, Chilvers CE. Alcohol, smoking, passive smoking and caffeine in relation to breast cancer risk in young women. UK National Case-Control Study Group. Br J Cancer 1994;70:112–119.

84. Tavani A, Pregnolato A, La Vecchia C, Favero A, Franceschi S. Coffee consumption and the risk of breast cancer. Eur J Cancer Prev 1998;7:77–82.

85. Mannisto S, Pietinen P, Virtanen M, Kataja V, Uusitupa M. Diet and risk of breast cancer in a case-control study: does the threat of disease have an influence on recall bias? J Clin Epidemiol 1999;52:429–439.

86. Polychronopoulou A, Tzonou A, Hsieh CC, Kaprinis G, Rebelakos A, Toupadaki N, Trichopoulos D. Reproductive variables, tobacco, ethanol, coffee and somatometry as risk factors for ovarian cancer. Int J Cancer 1993;55:402–407.

87. Kuper H, Titus-Ernstoff BL, Cramer DW. Population based study of coffee, alcohol and tobacco use and risk of ovarian cancer. Int J Cancer 2000;88:313–318.

88. Tavani A, Gallus S, Dal Maso L, et al. Coffee and alcohol intake and risk of ovarian cancer: an Italian case-control study. Nutr Cancer 2001;39:29–34.

89. Sturgeon SR, Ziegler RG, Brinton LA, Nasca PC, Mallin K, Gridley G. Diet and the risk of vulvar cancer. Ann Epidemiol 1991;1:427–437.

90. Levi F, Franceschi S, Negri E, La Vecchia C. Dietary factors and the risk of endometrial cancer. Cancer 1993;71:3575–3581.

91. Tavani A, Negri E, Franceschi S, Talamini R, La Vecchia C. Coffee consumption and risk of non-Hodgkin's lymphoma. Eur J Cancer Prev 1994;3:351–356.

92. Tavani A, Pregnolato A, Negri E, et al. Diet and risk of lymphoid neoplasms and soft tissue sarcomas. Nutr Cancer 1997;27:256–260.

93. Mendilaharsu M, De Stefani E, Deneo-Pellegrini H, Carzoglio JC, Ronco A. Consumption of tea and coffee and the risk of lung cancer in cigarette-smoking men: a case-control study in Uruguay. Lung Cancer 1998;19:101–107.

94. Takezaki T, Hirose K, Inoue M, et al. Dietary factors and lung cancer risk in Japanese: with special reference to fish consumption and adenocarciomas. Br J Cancer 2001;84:1199–1206.

95. Veierod MB, Thelle DS, Laake P. Diet and risk of cutaneous malignant melanoma: a prospective study of 50,757 Norwegian men and women. Int J Cancer 1997;71:600–604.

96. Talamini R, Franceschi S, La Vecchia C, Serraino D, Barra S, Negri E. Diet and prostatic cancer: a case-control study in Northern Italy. Nutr Cancer 1992;18:277–286.

97. Slattery ML, West DW. Smoking, alcohol, coffee, tea, caffeine and theobromine: risk of prostate cancer in Utah (United States). Cancer Causes Control 1993;4:559–563.

98. Jain MG, Hislop GT, Howe GR, Burch JD, Ghadirian P. Alcohol and other beverage use and prostate cancer risk among Canadian men. Int J Cancer 1998;78:707–711.

99. Hsieh CC, Thanos A, Mitropoulos D, Deliveliotis C, Mantzoros CS, Trichopoulos D. Risk factors for prostate cancer: a case-control study in Greece. Int J Cancer 1999;80:699–703.

100. Franceschi S, Levi F, Negri E, Fassina A, La Vecchia C. Diet and thyroid cancer: a pooled analysis of four European case-control studies. Int J Cancer 1991;48:395–398.

101. Jick H, Miettinen OS, Shapiro S, Lewis GP, Siskind V, Slone D. Comprehensive drug surveillance. JAMA 1970;213:1455–1460.

102. Coffee drinking and acute myocardial infarction. Report from the Boston Collaborative Drug Surveillance Program. Lancet 1972;2:1278–1281.

103. Greenland S. A meta-analysis of coffee, myocardial infarction, and coronary death. Epidemiology 1993;4:366–374.

104. Kawachi I, Colditz GA, Stone CB. Does coffee drinking increase the risk of coronary heart disease? Results from a meta-analysis. Br Heart J 1994;72:269–275.

105. Klatsky AL, Armstrong MA, Friedman GD. Coffee, tea, and mortality. Ann Epidemiol 1993;3: 375–381.

106. Klag MJ, Mead LA, LaCroix AZ, et al. Coffee intake and coronary heart disease. Ann Epidemiol 1994;4:425–433.

107. Wilhelmsen L, Rosengren A, Eriksson H, Lappas G. Heart failure in the general population of men– morbidity, risk factors and prognosis. J Intern Med 2001;249:253–261.

108. Gartside PS, Glueck CJ. Relationship of dietary intake to hospital admission for coronary heart and vascular disease: the NHANES II national probability study. J Am Coll Nutr 1993;12:676–684.

109. Gyntelberg F, Hein HO, Suadicani P, Sorensen H. Coffee consumption and risk of ischaemic heart disease: a settled issue? J Intern Med 1995;237:55–61.

110. Willett WC, Stampfer MJ, Manson JE, et al. Coffee consumption and coronary heart disease in women. A ten-year follow-up. JAMA 1996;275:458–462.

111. Stensvold I, Tverdal A, Jacobsen BK. Cohort study of coffee intake and death from coronary heart disease over 12 years. Br Med J 1996;312:544–545.

112. Hart C, Davey Smith G. Coffee consumption and coronary heart disease mortality in Scottish men: a 21 year follow up study. J Epidemiol Commun Health 1997;51:461–462.

113. Woodward M, Tunstall-Pedoe H. Coffee and tea consumption in the Scottish Heart Health Study follow up: conflicting relations with coronary risk factors, coronary disease, and all cause mortality. J Epidemiol Commun Health 1999;53:481–487.

114. Kleemola P, Jousilahti P, Pietinen P, Vartiainen E, Tuomilehto J. Coffee consumption and the risk of coronary heart disease and death. Arch Intern Med 2000;160:3393–3400.

115. Sesso HD, Gaziano JM, Buring JE, Hennekens CH. Coffee and tea intake and the risk of myocardial infarction. Am J Epidemiol 1999;149:162–167.

116. Weinmann S, Siscovick DS, Raghunathan TE, et al. Caffeine intake in relation to the risk of primary cardiac arrest. Epidemiology 1997;8:505–508.

117. Kalandidi A, Tzonou A, Toupadaki N, et al. A case-control study of coronary heart disease in Athens, Greece. Int J Epidemiol 1992;21:1074–1080.

118. D'Avanzo B, La Vecchia C, Tognoni G, et al. Coffee consumption and risk of acute myocardial infarction in Italian males. GISSI-EFRIM. Gruppo Italiano per lo Studio della Sopravvivenza nell'Infarto, Epidemiologia dei Fattori di Rischio dell'Infarto Miocardico. Ann Epidemiol 1993;3: 595–604.

119. La Vecchia C, D'Avanzo B, Negri E, Franceschi S, Gentile A, Tavani A. Decaffeinated coffee and acute myocardial infarction. A case-control study in Italian women. Ann Epidemiol 1993;3: 601–604.

120. Palmer JR, Rosenberg L, Rao RS, Shapiro S. Coffee consumption and myocardial infarction in women. Am J Epidemiol 1995;141:724–731.

121. Marchioli R, Di Mascio R, Marfisi RM, Vitullo F, Tognoni G. Coffee intake and death from coronary heart disease. Br Med J 1996;312:1539.

122. Rabajoli F, Martone T, Arneodo D, Balzola F, Leo L, Vineis P. Internal migration, coffee drinking, and nonfatal myocardial infarction in Italy. Arch Environ Health 1997;52:129–133.

123. Tavani A, Bertuzzi M, Negri E, Sorbara L, La Vecchia C. Alcohol, smoking, coffee and risk of nonfatal acute myocardial infarction in Italy. Eur J Epidemiol 2001;17:1131–1137.

124. Schreiber GB, Robins M, Maffeo CE, Masters MN, Bond AP, Morganstein D. Confounders contributing to the reported associations of coffee or caffeine with disease. Prev Med 1988;17:295–309.

125. James JE. Is habitual caffeine use a preventable cardiovascular risk factor? Lancet 1997;349:279–281.

126. Urgert R, Meyboom S, Kuilman M, et al. Comparison of effect of cafetiere and filtered coffee on serum concentrations of liver aminotransferases and lipids: six month randomised controlled trial. Br Med J 1996;313:1362–1366.

127. Olthof MR, Hollman PC, Zock PL, Katan MB. Consumption of high doses of chlorogenic acid, present in coffee, or of black tea increases plasma total homocysteine concentrations in humans. Am J Clin Nutr 2001;73:532–538.

128. Stavric B, Klassen R, Watkinson B, Karpinski K, Stapley R, Fried P. Variability in caffeine consumption from coffee and tea: possible significance for epidemiological studies. Food Chem Toxicol 1988; 26:111–118.

10 Health Benefits of Tea Consumption

Farrukh Afaq, Vaqar M. Adhami,
Nihal Ahmad, and Hasan Mukhtar

1. AN OVERVIEW OF THE ORIGIN
OF TEA AND ITS HEALTH BENEFITS

The tea plant *Camellia sinensis* has been grown in Southeast Asia for thousands of years. According to Chinese mythology, it was the emperor Shen Nung who discovered tea in 2737 BC *(1)*. In ancient China, tea was considered as a medicinal remedy for headaches, body aches and pains, depression, immune enhancement, digestion, and detoxification; as an energizer, and to prolong life. The Japanese population learned the habit of drinking tea from the Chinese in approx 800 AD. Tea consumption has now been adopted and assimilated by many cultures around the world. In the Kamakura era (1191–1333), the monk Eisai stressed the beneficial effect of tea in his book, *Maintaining Health by Drinking Tea*, in 1211 in which he emphasized: "Tea is a miraculous medicine for the maintenance of health."

Of all the beverages consumed today, tea is undoubtedly one of the oldest, most widely known, and most widely consumed. Its consumption was introduced throughout the world by traders and travelers. One thing that makes tea attractive is that it is inexpensive and comes in numerous flavors. Tea drinking is a pleasurable experience that is enjoyed either alone or shared at social gatherings. The Japanese tea ceremony and the English 4 o'clock tea are examples of how important tea has become in the traditions of some cultures.

As we age, a major health issue becomes remaining disease free. Thus, understanding what to eat and drink and what to avoid is important for maintaining a healthy lifestyle. Evidence is accumulating that tea has the potential to help to reduce the incidence of major diseases, especially when combined with a healthy lifestyle. Such a lifestyle includes plenty of exercise and minimizing mental stress. It also includes consuming a diet that possesses health-promoting effects. Nutrition has, therefore, been an area of intense investigation during the past few decades. Some foods and beverages have a beneficial and protective effect. Daily intake of tea, fruit juice, and soy milk is part of a health-promoting dietary tradition. This understanding is based on differences in disease incidence as a function of locally prevailing nutritional habits.

From: *Beverages in Nutrition and Health*
Edited by: T. Wilson and N. J. Temple © Humana Press Inc., Totowa, NJ

Botanicals for medical benefits have played an important role in nearly every culture. Many botanicals and some dietary supplements are good sources of antioxidants *(2,3)*. These botanicals have played an important role in maintaining human health and improving the quality of human life for thousands of years *(2,3)*. Anecdotal evidence has indicated that the tea consumption, especially green tea, is associated with a low incidence of certain diseases *(4,5)*. Recently, this has sparked interest in the possible health-promoting and therapeutic benefits of green tea *(4–6)*. Potentially, green tea might provide humanity with a safe and healthful beverage. Indeed, accumulating research indicates that there are many health benefits related to the intake of green tea. Recent research shows that many of the beneficial effects of tea are probably mediated by a group of chemicals known as polyphenols *(5–7)*. Tea polyphenols are potent antioxidants, substances that have the ability to counteract oxidant radicals.

2. TEA AND ITS CHEMICAL CONSTITUENTS

Tea from the leaves of *C. sinensis*, a plant of the Theaceae family, is consumed by more than two thirds of the world's population and is the most popular beverage, next only to water *(7,8)*. The tea plant is cultivated in more than 30 countries. Approximately 2.5 million metric tons of dried tea are produced annually. Production involves a series of drying and fermenting steps. Green tea is consumed primarily in some Asian countries, such as Japan, China, Korea, and India, and a few countries in North Africa and the Middle East. Black tea is consumed in some Asian countries and Western nations *(7,8)*. Oolong tea is consumed in southeastern China and Taiwan *(7,8)*. There are also many products sold in the market as herbal tea, which are not derived from the plant *C. sinensis*: They are extracts of several herbs.

Teas differ regarding how they are produced. Green tea production involves steaming fresh leaves at elevated temperatures, followed by a series of drying and rolling steps so that the chemical composition essentially remains similar to that of the fresh leaves. Black tea production involves withering plucked leaves, followed by extended fermentation. Thus, depending on the extent of fermentation, the chemical composition of most black teas is different. Oolong tea is made by solar withering of tea leaves followed by partial fermentation.

Tea leaves are unique because they are a rich source of catechins and theanine. These constituents impart flavor and taste to tea beverages. Green tea also contains caffeine, theophylline, and theobromine, the principal alkaloids, and gallic acids and theanine, the phenolic acids. Black tea, in addition to the catechins, also contains thearubigins, theaflavins, and caffeine *(5–7)*. Oolong tea contains monomeric catechins, thearubigins, and theaflavins *(5–7)*. Caffeine is a natural component of all teas. Although a serving of tea usually contains less than half the caffeine of coffee, actual caffeine levels are dependent on specific blends and the brew strength. In general, green tea contains 3–6% and black tea contains 2–4% of dry-weight caffeine. Major green tea catechins are (–)-epigallocatechin-3-gallate (EGCG), (–)-epigallocatechin (EGC), (–)-epicatechin gallate (ECG), (–)-epicatechin (EC), (+)-gallocatechin, and (+)-catechin. EGCG is the major polyphenolic constituent present in green tea and constitutes 25–40% of the total catechin contents that is responsible for these effects in biological model system *(5)*. A brewed cup of green tea contains up to 300 mg of EGCG. Tea contains phenolic acids, mainly caffeic, quinic, and gallic *(5,6)*. Theanine is an amino acid found only in tea leaves, which imparts a pleasantly sweet taste to tea *(5)*. It is degraded to glutamic acid and has relaxation effects in humans. Up to one third of the dry weight of tea comprises catechins and other polyphenols such as quercitin, myricitin, and kaempferol *(6)*.

3. BIOCHEMICAL PROPERTIES OF TEA

According to traditional unscientific claims, some populations consume green tea to improve blood flow, combat cancer and cardiovascular disease, eliminate various toxins, and improve resistance to various diseases *(9)*. Recently, supporting scientific evidence for these claims has emerged. As a result, green tea consumption is increasing. Much emphasis is placed on events at the cellular level, because of the strong antioxidant activity of green tea. Several studies suggest that polyphenols, especially the flavonoids, in green tea possess a high antioxidant activity, which, in turn, protects cells against the adverse effects of damaging reactive oxygen species (ROS) that are constantly produced in the body. ROS, such as superoxide radical, hydroxyl radical, singlet oxygen, hydrogen peroxide, peroxynitrite, and alkoxyradicals, cause cellular injury and cellular dysfunction by damaging lipids, protein, and nucleic acids and cellular components, such as ion channels, membranes, and chromatin. ROS contributes to the etiology of many chronic health problems, such as emphysema, cardiovascular disease (CVD), inflammatory diseases, cataracts, and cancer *(5–8)*. The polyphenolic constituents of tea act as scavengers of ROS and, thereby, prevent damage to cellular macromolecules *(10,11)*. The scavenging activity of the specific catechin molecules is related to the number of o-dihydroxy and o-hydroxyketo groups, C_2-C_3 double bonds, solubility, concentration, accessibility of the active group to the oxidant, and stability of the reaction product *(12)*. Tea catechins, especially EGCG, may also influence cellular mechanisms that are related to the induction of mutagenesis, such as DNA synthesis and repair processes *(13)*.

The effects of tea polyphenols may also result from the chelation of metal ions. Tea manifests chelating activity in vivo, as indicated by tea consumption lowering absorption of dietary iron in controlled feeding studies and decreasing body iron balance *(5)*. This chelating activity is important because it protects iron-loaded hepatocytes from lipid peroxidation by removing iron from these cells *(5)*. EGCG may chelate cations, and this may contribute to its ability to inhibit angiotensin-converting enzyme *(5)*. Polyphenols in all types of tea chelate copper ions, and this mechanism has also been suggested to protect low-density lipoproteins (LDLs) from peroxidation *(14)*. Because of its chelating properties, tea may additionally protect against toxicity due to heavy metals *(5)*. Catechins may also affect signal transduction pathways, modulate many endocrine systems, and alter hormones and other physiologic processes as a result of their binding these metals/enzyme cofactors *(15)*.

4. TEA IN DISEASE CONTROL AND PREVENTION

4.1. Tea and Cancer

Most of the work on cancer chemoprevention by tea has been conducted using green tea or its individual polyphenolic constituents, especially EGCG, which is a major constituent of green tea. Less work has been reported on black tea. In animal studies, the polyphenolic fraction isolated from green tea, the water extract of green tea, or individual polyphenolic antioxidants present in green tea have afforded protection against chemically induced carcinogenesis in the lung, liver, esophagus, forestomach, duodenum, pancreas, colon, and breast *(5–8,16,17)*. This raises the possibility that green tea consumption and its associated catechins may lower cancer risk in humans. Based on recent studies, it is now believed that much of green tea's cancer chemopreventive properties are mediated by EGCG, but other polyphenolic constituents may also be involved *(7,8,16,17)*. However, the mechanisms by which the polyphenolic compounds of green tea achieve this effect are not properly understood. Green tea catechins act as antioxidants and ROS scavengers. EGCG inhibits the enzyme action to prevent the activation of procarcinogens, resulting in their inactivation and, finally, excretion *(18,19)*. Studies have shown that green tea intake increases the excretion of a class of carcinogens known as heterocyclic arylamines formed during the cooking of meat, poultry, and fish; this is expected to reduce DNA adduct formation, in particular, and carcinogenesis, in general *(20)*. Consumption of both green tea and black tea aqueous extracts influences the excretion of mutagens and promutagens in the urine of animals *(21)*.

Tea flavonoids directly neutralize procarcinogens by their strong ROS scavenging action before cell damage occurs. In the Ames test, a measure of DNA damage, and in scavenging superoxide tests, EGCG exhibited substantial protection against DNA scissions and mutations and in nonenzymatic interception of superoxide anions *(22,23)*. Black, green, and oolong teas significantly decreased the reverse mutation induced by different mutagens in cell culture assays; this indicates that the antimutagenic action of these teas is closely associated with their antioxidant action *(23–25)*. Green tea polyphenols reduce the occurrence of chromosome aberrations during mutagen exposure *(26,27)*. Studies show that EGCG and theaflavin-3-3'-digallate block activated protein-1, a signal transducer initiating the development of skin carcinogenesis, and can inhibit the mitotic signal transducers responsible for cell proliferation *(28)*.

Several epidemiological studies suggest that tea and its associated compounds may prevent some, but not all, cancers *(4,5)*. This is understandable, because cancer is a complex disease with multiple etiologies, even for one body site. It is, therefore, a false hope that any nutritional or synthetic agent can prevent or treat all cancer types. However, based on a large volume of cell culture, animal studies, and human observational studies, there is hope that green tea consumption can retard cancer development at selected sites in some populations. The challenge is to elucidate what cancer type can be prevented by tea. This requires extensive research for which considerable resources are required.

Studies conducted in China revealed that green tea users had an approximate 50% reduction in risk for both esophageal cancer *(29)* and stomach cancer *(30)*. Inhabitants of tea-producing districts in Japan have a lower mortality from stomach cancer, possibly the result of regular green tea consumption *(31,32)*. In addition to regular tea drinking, this population consumes green tea in all types of products, including candy, gums, bread, shampoo, lotion, toothpaste, etc. Contrary to the preceding, however, two recent studies found no association between green tea consumption and stomach or colon cancer *(33,34)*. Green tea was linked to a reduced risk of oral cancer in northern Italian and a Chinese population, esophageal cancer in Chinese women, gastric cancer in Swedish adolescents, pancreatic cancer in residents of a retirement community in the United States, and colon cancer in retired male self-defense officials in Japan *(5,35,36)*. Cohort studies suggest that there is a protective effect of green tea for colon, urinary bladder, stomach, pancreatic, and esophageal cancers *(37,38)*. In a Japanese population survey, an overall protection by green tea was observed, together with a slowdown of the increase of cancer incidence with age *(39)*. The effects were more pronounced when the tea consumption was more than 10 cups/d. In another Japanese study, consumption of 7 or more cups per day of green tea significantly decreased the risk of cancer of both the stomach and rectum (by 31% and 54%, respectively) compared with nonusers *(40)*. Regular tea drinkers in China experienced a lower incidence of cancer of the colon, rectum, and pancreas (approx 24%, 35%, and 42%, respectively) compared with non-drinkers of tea *(41)*. A case-control study from Poland reported a significant reduction in risk of pancreatic cancer with increasing lifetime tea consumption *(42)*. An increased green tea consumption was closely associated with a decreased axillary lymph node metastases among patients who were premenopausal with stage I and II breast cancer and overall decreased recurrence of stage I and II breast cancer (17% for individuals drinking more than 5 cups and 24% for those drinking less than 4 cups) *(43)*. There are few human studies examining the relationship between tea consumption and skin cancer. In one such study, ultraviolet-irradiated mice (irradiated for 22 wk) that consumed green or black tea developed 30–42% fewer keratoacanthomas and 26–33% fewer squamous cell carcinomas compared with similarly irradiated mice that consumed water *(44)*.

In vitro studies revealed that catechin gallates selectively inhibit 5-α-reductase. This enzyme is responsible for the conversion of testosterone to 5-α-dihydrotestosterone *(45)*, which, at high levels, has been implicated in the etiology of prostate cancer and male pattern baldness. It was recently suggested that regular consumption of green tea might prolong life expectancy and quality of life in patients with prostate cancer. Consistent with this, our recent studies have shown that green tea polyphenols inhibit the growth and progression of prostate cancer in an animal model. Prostate cancer is an attractive target for prevention by green tea, because the disease is typically diagnosed in older men and, thus, even a modest delay in disease development could produce a substantial benefit (i.e., by delaying the cancer beyond the life expectancy of the man) *(46)*.

The previous studies that were briefly reviewed strongly suggest that drinking tea has cancer chemopreventive effects *(30,36)*. However, a proper understanding of the mechanisms of the biologic effects of tea is essential in the design and improvement of strategies for cancer chemoprevention. Recent studies evaluate the molecular mechanisms involved in the biologic effects of tea polyphenols. The protective effects of these substances have been attributed to the inhibition of enzymes, such as cytochrome P450, which are involved in the bioactivation of some carcinogens *(47)*. EGC also reduced the phosphorylation of many proteins with different molecular weights at the tyrosine site, indicating that EGC may inhibit the protein tyrosine kinase activity or stimulate the protein phosphatase activity. Nitric oxide (NO) is a bioactive molecule that plays an important role in inflammation and carcinogenesis. Gallic acid, EGC, and EGCG inhibited the protein expression of inducible NO synthase, as well as NO generation. Because many studies suggest that the activation of activator protein-1 (AP-1) plays an important role in tumor promotion, the downregulation of this transcription factor has been suggested as a general therapeutic strategy against cancer *(48)*. Recently, it was proposed that the anticancer activity of EGCG is associated with the inhibition of urokinase, which is one of the most frequently expressed enzymes in human cancers *(49)*.

Disruption of the cell cycle is the hallmark of a cancer cell. In recognition of this, there has been much interest in apoptosis (programmed cell death). Because the lifespans of both normal and cancer cells within a living system are determined by the apoptosis rate, chemopreventive agents that can delay apoptosis may affect the steady-state cell population *(50)*. On the one hand, several cancer chemopreventive agents induce apoptosis, whereas, on the other hand, tumor-promoting agents inhibit it *(51,52)*. Therefore, it can be inferred that chemopreventive agents with proven effects in animal tumor bioassay systems and/or human epidemiology and an ability to induce cancer cell apoptosis may have wide potential for the management of cancer. Presently, only a limited number of chemopreventive agents are known to cause apoptosis *(53)*. In our laboratory, we showed that in human epidermoid carcinoma cells, EGCG induces apoptosis and cell cycle arrest and inhibits cell growth *(54)*. Importantly, this apoptotic response was specific for cancer cells because EGCG treatment also resulted in apoptosis induction in three other cancer cells (human carcinoma keratinocytes, human prostate carcinoma cells, and mouse lymphoma cells) but not in normal human epidermal keratinocytes.

4.2. Tea and Cardiovascular Diseases

One of the proposed mechanisms for the possible protective effect of tea against cardiovascular diseases is that tea polyphenols inhibit the oxidation of LDL, which is involved in atherosclerosis development *(55)*. Green tea consumption is associated with decreased serum concentrations of total cholesterol and with a concomitant decrease in LDL proportion *(55)*. In a clinical study, green tea extract containing catechins decreased the plasma phosphatidylcholine hydroperoxide level, a marker of oxidized lipoprotein, suggesting that tea catechins are powerful antioxidants and, therefore, may decrease the risk of heart disease *(56)*. A cross-sectional study revealed that people consuming more than 10 cups of green tea per day had lower levels of serum cholesterol, LDL, very-low-density lipoprotein, and triglycerides; an increase in high-density lipoprotein; and a reduction in the atherogenic index *(57)*. Experiments in rats have indicated that polyphenols in tea (mainly catechins and theaflavins) lower hypercholesterolemia to normal levels, reduce blood pressure, and may decrease the risk of stroke *(58)*. Recent studies by Duffy et al. *(59,60)* indicate that the black tea consumption in patients with coronary heart disease (CHD) did not affect ex vivo platelet aggregation, but short- and long-term tea consumption improved brachial artery dilation in patients with cardiovascular disease (CVD).

Investigations in Japan suggest that consumption of green tea is associated with protection against atherosclerosis *(55)*. In other studies, tea consumption reduced the risk of death from CHD and stroke *(61,62)*. In a long-term study of a Dutch cohort, tea consumption was associated with a low risk of death from CHD and a lower incidence of stroke. In a follow-up study in Rotterdam, an inverse association of tea intake with the severity of aortic atherosclerosis was observed *(63,64)*. The Boston Area Health Study found that subjects who drank 1 or more cups of black tea per day had approximately half the risk of a heart attack compared with those who did not drink tea *(65)*. The risk for developing stroke was 73% lower in the group with the highest intake of flavonoids (> 28.6 mg/d) than in the group with the lowest intake (< 18.3 mg/d) *(66)*.

4.3. Tea and Diabetes

Various tea preparations have been used in Chinese medicine for the treatment of diabetes. Bai-Yu-Cha (BYC) is one such preparation that is made from the catechin-rich tender leaves of old tea trees grown in certain areas in China. An aqueous extract of BYC, orally administered to mice (10 g/kg body weight), protects against experimentally induced damage of pancreatic islets, the major cause of diabetes *(67)*. Orally administered BYC at a dose of 1.5 g/kg also decreases the blood glucose concentration in rabbits without diabetes *(67)*. EC, EGC, GC, and caffeine individually do not have any antidiabetic activity. However, mixtures of the four compounds reconstructed from the isolated compounds, according to the relative levels in BYC, reproduce the protective action against diabetes induced by alloxan in mice *(67)*. The blood-lowering effect of the prescription mixture is comparable to that of clinically used antidiabetic drugs *(67)*.

Tea extracts may be useful as functional foods for patients with diabetes *(68)*. Catechins in tea inhibit the formation of sugars that cause diabetic complications, such as cataracts, retinopathy, neuropathy, and nephropathy *(69)*. EGCG suppresses glucose production and phosphoenolpyruvate carboxykinase and glucose-6-phosphatase gene expression by modulation of the redox state of the cell, suggesting that EGCG may have a beneficial effect in the treatment of diabetes *(70)*.

4.4. Tea and Obesity

In oriental countries, long-term use of green tea is considered to be beneficial for keeping a healthy body weight. However, supporting evidence for this became evident only recently. EGCG given to rats by intraperitoneal injection at a dosage of 50 to 90 mg EGCG/kg body weight daily could reduce body weight by approx 20% to 30% within 2 to 7 d *(71)*. Other structurally related catechins, such as EC, EGC, and ECG, are not effective at the same dose. Reduction of body weight is the result of EGCG-induced reduction in food intake, although the loss of appetite might involve neuropeptide(s) in tea. The effective dose of EGCG is, at first, 30–50 mg EGCG/kg body weight; however, rats gradually adapt, and, within 1 wk, higher doses of EGCG (100 mg/kg) are needed to reduce or prevent weight gain. The weight loss is reversible when EGCG administration is stopped *(72)*. The EGCG effect on food intake is apparently not dependent on an intact leptin receptor. Lean (leptin-receptor positive) and obese (leptin-receptor deficient) male and female rats treated with EGCG lose weight and have lower blood levels of glucose, insulin, and serum levels of sex hormones, leptin, and insulin growth factor-1 *(71,72)*. EGCG may interact specifically with a component of leptin receptor-independent appetite control pathway and reduce food intake. Green tea increases the 24-h energy expenditure, suggesting a role in weight reduction *(73)*. Diminished catechol-*o*-methyl-transferase (COMT) activity delays the metabolism of norepinephrine and epinephrine and may cause subsequent increases in sympathetic thermogenesis. This may explain why humans increase their 24-h energy expenditure after consuming EGCG-containing green tea extracts and why EGCG alone or synergistically with caffeine augments and prolongs sympathetic stimulation of thermogenesis in rat brown adipose tissues *(74)*. Obesity is also often associated with a decreased sympathetic nervous system activity; hence, sympathomimetic agents have been proposed as a possible way to partially correct this situation. One of these agents, caffeine, is present in varied amounts in all teas. Caffeine increases energy expenditure and reduces energy intake under some circumstances and, thus, aids in weight loss *(75,76)*.

4.5. Tea and Longevity

There is some evidence that drinking tea may also promote longevity. For instance, a low mortality rate has been reported among Japanese women who are practitioners of the traditional tea ceremony *(77)*. It has been shown, for example, that the higher the concentration of the antioxidants vitamins E and C in the bodies of animals, the longer they live *(78)*. This suggests that active consumption of agents that are effective antioxidants may slow the aging process. Green tea is rich in antioxidants. It has recently been demonstrated that catechins in green tea are far stronger antioxidants than vitamin E (approx 20 times stronger) *(79)*. Although there is no direct evidence that suggests a relationship between green tea consumption and aging, it contains powerful antioxidants, which is suggestive that it can help slow the aging process. The Saitama Cancer Center in Japan conducted an 8-yr follow-up survey concerning the green tea effects on the prolongation of human life using 8500 participants in Saitama Prefecture. Those who had more than 10 cups of green tea each day had a longer lifespan than those who had 3 or more cups daily (70 vs 66 yr for men and to 74 vs 68 yr for women). In this study, a decreased relative risk of death from CVD was also found for people consuming more than 10 cups/d of green tea, and, importantly, green tea consumption also had life-prolonging effects on cumulative survival *(80)*.

4.6. Tea and Osteoporosis

In osteoporosis, a disease of low bone-mineral density (BMD), the bones and joints become thin and fragile. It is the biggest cause of fractures among elderly women. Hormone deficiencies are the leading cause of the disease. Tea is reported to protect against hip fractures *(81)*. A recent study suggests that drinking 1–6 cups/d of tea may significantly reduce the risk of bone fracture by increasing BMD. Studies suggest that isoflavonoids in tea increase BMD and help reduce the risk of fractures in old age *(82)*. Of the 1256 women between the ages of 65 and 76 yr who were surveyed, 1134 drank at least 1 cup/d of tea. BMD at the base of the spine and at two hip regions was significantly higher in tea drinkers when the data were adjusted to account for age and body weight *(82)*.

4.7. Tea, Arthritis, and Inflammation

In a study in mice, we found that consumption of green tea polyphenols produces a significant reduction in arthritis incidence, with a marked reduction of inflammatory mediators, of neutral endopeptidase activity, of IgG and type II collagen-specific IgG levels in arthritic joints *(83)*. Many published studies suggest that green tea has antiinflammatory properties, and new research is beginning to explain why. Previous animal studies and other laboratory researches found that green tea polyphenols are potent antiinflammatory agents, but the mechanism behind this action is not well understood. EGCG inhibits the expression of the interleukin gene involved in the inflammatory response *(84)*. EGCG blocked the expression of many biologic parameters that are associated with enhanced inflammatory responses.

4.8. Tea and Neurologic Effects

Tea components, such as EGCG and ECG, competitively inhibit tyrosinase, the rate-limiting enzyme in the synthesis of melanin, L-dihydroxyphenylalanine, norepinephrine, and epinephrine *(85)*. EGCG and EGC competitively inhibit COMT, one of the major enzymes in the metabolism of catecholamines, which is associated with Parkinson's disease *(86)*. A high activity of prolylendopeptidase is found in patients with Alzheimer's disease and other neuropathologic disorders, and some studies have shown that this enzyme may be inhibited by EGCG *(87)*.

4.9. Tea Effects on Bacterial Growth

Green tea polyphenols are believed to offer protection against tooth decay by: (1) killing the causative bacteria, such as *Streptococcus mutans (88)*, (2) inhibiting the collagenase activity of the bacteria resident below the gum line *(89)*, and (3) increasing the resistance of tooth enamel to acid-induced erosion *(90)*. All teas are a rich source of fluoride and, thus, strengthen tooth enamel. Even one cup a day can provide a significant amount of fluoride. Tea can also reduce plaque formation on teeth that can lead to gum inflammation and bleeding and eventually lost teeth. On the negative side, tea compounds can discolor teeth.

In Japan, tea flavonoids given to elderly women on feeding tubes favorably altered the gut bacteria and reduced fecal odor *(91)*. The study was repeated in bedridden patients not on feeding tubes, and, again, green tea improved the gut bacteria *(92)*. These studies also raise the possibility of using green tea in other settings where gut bacteria are disturbed, such as after taking antibiotics. In the GI tract, tea polyphenols modulate the microflora composition. A high Clostridia content and a low percentage of bifidobacteria have been observed in the intestinal microflora of patients with colon cancer. Tea polyphenols selectively inhibit the growth of Clostridia and promote bifidobacteria colonization, contributing to a decrease in the pH of feces *(93)*. Viruses, bacteria, and worms have been implicated in the development of cancers; hepatitis viruses, herpes viruses, *Helicobacter pylori*, and parasitic worms are some well-known causes of cancer *(5)*. Tea plays another role in the prevention of cancer through its antimicrobial activity *(94)*. It has been demonstrated that tea can inhibit the growth of *H. pylori*, which is associated with gastric cancer *(95)*. The cellular process involved could be the generation of powerful oxidants to destroy the invaders and protect the cells. Bacteria can also synthesize nitrosating agents endogenously and activate macrophages *(96)*. Nitrosating agents that are potentially carcinogenic can be destroyed by polyphenols.

4.10. Miscellaneous Effects of Tea

Tea is a naturally refreshing drink and, when taken without milk and sugar, has no calories. When taken with milk, which is a popular form of tea consumption globally, 4 cups a day can provide significant amounts of the following nutrients: approx 17% of the recommended intake for calcium, 5% for zinc, 22% for vitamin B_2, 5% for folate, and trace amounts of vitamins B_1 and B_6.

Tea helps to replace fluids that are lost through day-to-day activities, which is why doctors recommend that we drink at least 1.5 L of fluid per day to prevent dehydration. Perhaps the most important reason to drink plenty of tea is how it helps people to maintain enough water in their tissues. This is especially important during the hot summer. Active outdoors people and the elderly are particularly prone to dehydration if they are overly exposed to hot temperatures. Tea, which, on average, accounts for 40% of our daily fluid intake, can help people to reach their daily target of 1.5 L.

5. CONCLUSION

Investigations throughout the past 15 yr have provided a scientific basis for the beneficial effects of tea on health. A major focus of interest in tea stems from its high levels of polyphenols, which are potent antioxidants. Tea polyphenols have a broad spectrum of health benefits, which include prevention and treatment of cancer, cardiovascular diseases, inflammatory conditions, arthritis, asthma, periodontal disease, liver disease, cataracts, and macular degeneration. Tea polyphenols also decrease the rate of cell division, especially of transformed or damaged cells involved in cancer development. Thus, the concept of tea as a cancer chemopreventive agent has gained much attention. All teas—green, black, and oolong—are considered to have health-promoting potential. Among the different types of teas, the beneficial effects of green tea are much clearer. Based on the available data, black tea possesses similar beneficial effects.

Studies of the effect of tea on human populations are complex. Due to our diversity in food habits, lifestyle, heredity, age, gender, and environment, unambiguous interpretation of the data is difficult. In epidemiological studies of the effects of tea consumption on health, the confounding factors are generally more variable than the effect tested and, as a result, the results are not conclusive. This is an issue with most studies in which the beneficial or adverse effects of a single nutrient in a complex diet consumed by humans are examined. However, as elaborated in this chapter, there is good reason to believe that tea consumption may have health-promoting effects in humans. Perhaps the most important reason to drink plenty of tea is that it also helps people to maintain enough water in their tissues. This is especially important during the summer. Active outdoors people are particularly prone to dehydration if they are overly exposed to hot temperatures. The challenge for the future is to decipher what diseases and which populations could reap the most benefits by consuming tea or any of its bioactive components.

6. MAIN POINTS FOR PRIMARY AND CLINICAL REVIEW

1. Tea is rich in polyphenolic compounds that may be responsible for its biological activity.
2. Although there are many forms of tea available, green and black teas remain the two teas most commonly associated with health benefits.
3. Green tea is the type of tea with the strongest protective association against various forms of cancer.
4. Tea consumption is also associated with protection from cardiovascular disease and improvement of lipid profiles.
5. Tea consumption has also been suggested to promote healthy changes in diabetes, obesity, longevity, osteoporosis, inflammation, neural function, and fecal odor.

REFERENCES

1. Harbowy ME, Balentine DA. Tea chemistry. Crit Rev Plant Sci 1997;16:415–480.
2. Ames BN. Dietary carcinogens and anticarcinogens. Science 1983;221:1256–1264.
3. Block G. Micronutrients and cancer: time for action? J Natl Cancer Inst 1993;85:846–848.
4. Trevisanato SI, Kim YI. Tea and health. Nutr Rev 2000;58:1–10.
5. Liao S, Kao YH, Hiipakka RA. Green tea: biochemical and biological basis for healthbenefits. Vitam Horm 2001;62:1–94.
6. Dufresne CJ, Farnworth ER. A review of latest research findings on the health promotion properties of tea. J Nutr Biochem 2001;12:404–421.

7. Katiyar SK, Mukhtar H. Tea in chemoprevention of cancer: epidemiological and experimental studies. Int J Oncol 1996;8:221–238.
8. Yang CS, Wang ZY. Tea and cancer. J Natl Cancer Inst 1993;85:1038–1049.
9. Balentine DA, Wiseman SA, Bouwens LC. The chemistry of tea flavonoids. Crit Rev Food Sci Nutr 1997;37:693–704.
10. Rice-Evans CA, Diplock AT. Current status of antioxidant therapy. Free Rad Biol Med 1993;15:77–96.
11. Wei H, Zhang X, Zhao JF, Wang ZY, Bickers D, Lebwohl M. Scavenging of hydrogen peroxide and inhibition of ultraviolet light-induced oxidative DNA damage by aqueous extracts from green and black teas. Free Rad Biol Med 1996;26:1427–1435.
12. Sergediene E, Jonsson K, Szymusiak H, Tyrakowska B, Rietjens IM, Cenas N. Prooxidant toxicity of polyphenolic antioxidants to HL-60 cells: description of quantitative structure-activity relationships. FEBS Lett 1999;462:392–396.
13. Hayatsu H, Inada N, Kakutani T, et al. Suppression of genotoxicity of carcinogens by (–)-epigallocatechin gallate. Prev Med 1992;21:370–376.
14. Yokozawa T, Dong E, Liu ZW, et al. Magnesium lithospermate B ameliorates cephaloridine-induced renal injury. Exp Toxicol Pathol 1997;49:337–341.
15. Kao YH, Hiipakka RA, Liao S. Modulation of endocrine systems and food intake by green tea epigallocatechin gallate. Endocrinology 2000;141:980–987.
16. Mukhtar H, Ahmad N. Cancer chemoprevention: future holds in multiple agents. Toxicol Appl Pharmacol 1999;158:207–210.
17. Ahmad N, Katiyar SK, Mukhtar H. Cancer chemoprevention by tea polyphenols. In: Nutrition and Chemical Toxicity. Ioannides C (ed.), John Wiley & Sons Ltd., West Sussex, England, 1996, pp. 301–343.
18. Gordon MH. Dietary anti-oxidants in disease prevention. Natural Prod Rep 1996;13:265–273.
19. Lin JK, Liang YC, Lin-Shiau SY. Cancer chemoprevention by tea polyphenols through mitotic signal transduction blockade. Biochem Pharmacol 1999;58:911–915.
20. Embola CW, Weisburger JH, Weisburger MC. Urinary excretion of N-OH-2-amino-3-methyl-imidazo[4,5-f]quinoline-N-glucuronide in F344 rats is enhanced by green tea. Carcinogenesis 2001;22:1095–1098.
21. McArdle NJ, Clifford MN, Ioannides C. Consumption of tea modulates urinary excretion of mutagens in rats treated with IQ. Role of caffeine. Mutat Res 1999;441:191–203.
22. Yoshioka H, Akai G, Yoshinaga K, Hasegawa K, Yoshioka H. Protecting effect of a green tea percolate and its main constituents against gamma ray-induced scission of DNA. Biosci Biotechnol Biochem 1996;60:117–119.
23. Yamada J, Tonita Y. Antimutagenic activity of water extract of black tea and oolong tea. Biosc Biotect Biochem 1994;12:2197–2200.
24. Kuroda Y, Hara Y. Antimutagenic and anticarcinogenic activity of tea polyphenols. Mutat Res 1999;436:69–97.
25. Steele VE, Kelloff GJ, Balentine D, et al. Comparative chemopreventive mechanisms of green tea, black tea and selected polyphenol extracts measured by in vitro bioassays. Carcinogenesis 2000;21:63–67.
26. Weisburger JH, Nagao M, Wakabayashi K, Oguri A. Prevention of heterocyclic amine formation by tea and tea polyphenols. Cancer Lett 1994;83:143–147.
27. Sasaki YF, Yamada H, Shimoi K, Kator K, Kinae N. The aclastogen-suppressing effects of green tea, Polei tea and Rooibos tea in CHO cells and mice. Mutat Res 1993;286:221–232.
28. Chung JY, Huang C, Meng X, Dong Z, Yang CS. Inhibition of activator protein 1 activity and cell growth by purified green tea and black tea polyphenols in H-ras-transformed cells: structure-activity relationship and mechanisms involved. Cancer Res 1999;59:4610–4617.
29. Gao YT, McLaughlin JK, Blot WJ, Ji BT, Dai Q, Fraumeni JF, Jr. Reduced risk of esophageal cancer associated with green tea consumption. J Natl Cancer Inst 1994;86:855–858.
30. Yu GP, Hsieh CC, Wang LY, Yu SZ, Li XL, Jin TH. Green-tea consumption and risk of stomach cancer: a population-based case-control study in Shanghai, China. Cancer Causes Control 1995;6:532–538.
31. Kono S, Ikeda M, Tokudome S, Kuratsune M. A case-control study of gastric cancer and diet in northern Kyushu, Japan. Jpn J Cancer Res 1988;79:1067–1074.
32. Oguni I, Nasu K, Kanaya S, Ota Y, Yamamoto S, Nomura T. Epidemiological and experimental studies on the anti-tumor activity by green tea extracts. Jpn J Nutr 1989;47:93–102.

33. Hoshiyama Y, Kawaguchi T, Miura Y, et al. A prospective study of stomach cancer death in relation to green tea consumption in Japan. Br J Cancer 2002;87:309–313.
34. Cerhan JR, Putnam SD, Bianchi GD, Parker AS, Lynch CF, Cantor KP. Tea consumption and the risk of cancer of the colon and rectum. Nutr Cancer 2001;41:33–40.
35. Kono S, Shinchi K, Ikeda N, Yanai F, Imanishi K. Physical activity, dietary habits and adenomatous polyps of the sigmoid colon: a study of self-defense officials in Japan. J Clin Epidemiol 1991;44: 1255–1261.
36. Schwarz B, Bischof HP, Kunze M. Coffee, tea and lifestyle. Prev Med 1994;23:377–384.
37. Landau JM, Wang ZY, Yang ZY, Ding W, Yang CS. Inhibition of spontaneous formation of lung tumors and rhabdomyosarcomas in A/J mice by black and green tea. Carcinogenesis 1998;19:501–507.
38. Bushman JL. Green tea and cancer in humans: a review of the literature. Nutr Cancer 1998;31: 151–159.
39. Imai K, Suga K, Nakachi K. Cancer-preventive effects of drinking green tea among a Japanese population. Prev Med 1997;26:769–775.
40. Inoue M, Tajima K, Hirose K, et al. Tea and coffee consumption and the risk of digestive tract cancers: data from a comparative case-referent study in Japan. Cancer Causes Control 1998;9:209–216.
41. Ji BT, Chow WH, Hsing AW, et al. Green tea consumption and the risk of pancreatic and colorectal cancers. Int J Cancer 1997;70:255–258.
42. Zatonski WA, Boyle P, Przewozniak K, Maisonneuve P, Drosik K, Walker AM. Cigarette smoking, alcohol, tea and coffee consumption and pancreas cancer risk: a case-control study from Opole, Poland. Int J Cancer 1993;53:601–607.
43. Nakachi K, Suemasu K, Suga K, Takeo T, Imai K, Higashi Y. Influence of drinking green tea on breast cancer malignancy among Japanese patients. Jpn J Cancer Res 1998;89:254–261.
44. Conney AH, Lu Y-P, Lou Y-R, Xie J, Huang M. Inhibitory effect of green and black tea on tumor growth. Proc Soc Exp Biol Med 1999;220:229–233.
45. Shatsung L, Hiipakka RA. Selective inhibition of steroid 5-α-reductase isoenzymes by tea epicatechin 3-gallate and EGC3-gallate. Biochem Biophys Res Commun 1995;214:833–838.
46. Gupta S, Hastak K, Ahmad N, Lewin JS, Mukhtar H. Inhibition of prostate carcinogenesis in TRAMP mice by oral infusion of green tea polyphenols. Proc Natl Acad Sci 2001;98:10,350–10,355.
47. Yu R, Jiao JJ, Duh JL, Gudehithlu K, Tan TH, Kong AN. Activation of mitogen-activated protein kinases by green tea polyphenols: potential signaling pathways in the regulation of antioxidant-responsive element-mediated phase II enzyme gene expression. Carcinogenesis 1997;18:451–456.
48. McCarty MF. Polyphenol-mediated inhibition of AP-1 transactivating activity may slow cancer growth by impeding angiogenesis and tumor invasiveness. Med Hypotheses 1998;50:511–514.
49. Jankun J, Selman SH, Swiercz R, Skrzypczak-Jankun E. Why drinking green tea could prevent cancer. Nature 1997;387:561.
50. Fesus L, Szondy Z, Uray I. Probing the molecular program of apoptosis by cancer chemopreventive agents. J Cell Biochem 1995;22(Suppl):151–161.
51. Boolbol SK, Dannenberg AJ, Chadburn A, et al. Cyclooxygenase-2 overexpression and tumor formation are blocked by sulindac in murine model of familial polyposis. Cancer Res 1996;56:2556–2560.
52. Mills JJ, Chari RS, Boyer IJ, Gould MN, Jirtle RL. Induction of apoptosis in liver tumors by the monoterpene perillyl alcohol. Cancer Res 1995;55:979–983.
53. Jiang MC, Yang-Yen HF, Yen JJY, Lin JK. Curcumin induces apoptosis in immortalized NIH 3T3 and malignant cancer cell lines. Nutr Cancer 1996;26:111–120.
54. Ahmad N, Feyes DK, Nieminen A-L, Agarwal R, Mukhtar H. Green tea constituent epigallocatechin-3-gallate and induction of apoptosis and cell cycle arrest in human carcinoma cells. J Natl Cancer Inst 1997;89:1881–1886.
55. Kono S, Shinchi K, Wakabayashi K, et al. Relation of green tea consumption to serum lipids and lipoproteins in Japanese men. J Epidemiol 1996;6:128–133.
56. Nakagawa K, Ninomiya M, Okuba T, et al. Tea catechin supplementation increases antioxidant capacity and prevents phospholipid hydroperoxidation in plasma humans. J Agric Food Chem 1999;47: 3967–3973.
57. Imai K, Nakachi K. Cross-sectional study of the effects of drinking green tea on cardiovascular and liver diseases. Br Med J 1995;310:693–696.

58. Hara Y. The effect of tea polyphenols on cardiovascular disease [abstract]. Prev Med 1992;21:333.

59. Duffy SJ, Keaney JF, Jr, Holbrook M, et al. Short- and long-term black tea consumption reverses dysfunction in patients with coronary artery disease. Circulation 2001;104:151–156.

60. Duffy SJ, Vita JA, Holbrook M, Swerdloff PL, Keaney JF, Jr. Effect of acute and chronic tea consumption on platelet aggregation in patients with coronary artery disease. Arterioscler Thromb Vasc Biol 2001;21:1084–1089.

61. Young W, Hotovec RL, Romero AG. Tea and atherosclerosis. Nature 1967;216:1015–1016.

62. Hertog MG, Feskens EJ, Hollman PC, Katan MB, Kromhout D. Dietary antioxidant flavonoids and risk of coronary heart disease: the Zutphen elderly study. Lancet 1993;342:1007–1011.

63. Geleijnse JM, Launer LJ, Hofman A, Pols HA, Witteman JC. Tea flavonoids may protect against atherosclerosis: the Rotterdam study. Arch Intern Med 1999;159:2170–2174.

64. Geleijnse JM, Launer LJ, Van der Kuip DA, Hofman A, Witteman JC. Inverse association of tea flavonoid intakes with incident myocardial infarction: the Rotterdam study. Am J Clin Nutr 2002;75: 880–886.

65. Sesso HD, Gazlano JM, Buring JE, Hennekens CH. Coffee and tea intake and the risk of myocardial infarction. Am J Epidemiol 1999;149:162–167.

66. Keli SO, Hertog MGL, Feskens EJM, Kromhout D. Dietary flavonoids, antioxidant vitamins, and incidence of stroke. Arch Intern Med 1996;156:637–642.

67. Zhu DY, Li XY, Jiang FX, et al. Studies on anti-diabetic principles from Bai-Yu-Cha. Planta Med 1990;56:684–685.

68. Murata M, Irie J, Homma S. Aldolase reductase inhibitors from green tea. Food Sci Technol 1994;27: 401–405.

69. Kador PF, Kinoshita JH, Sharpless NE. Aldolase reductase inhibitors: a potential new class of agents for the pharmacological control of certain diabetic complications. J Med Chem 1985;28:841–849.

70. Waltner-Law ME, Wang XL, Law BK, Hall RK, Nawano M, Granner DK. Epigallocatechin gallate, a constituent of green tea, represses hepatic glucose production. J Biol Chem 2002;277:34,933–34,940.

71. Kao YH, Hiipakka RA, Liao S. Modulation of endocrine systems and food intake by green tea epigallocatechin gallate. Endocrinology 2000;141:980–987.

72. Kao YH, Hiipakka RA, Liao S. Modulation of obesity by a green tea catechin. Am J Clin Nutr 2000; 72;1232–1233.

73. Bell SJ, Goodrick GK. A functional food product for the management of weight. Crit Rev Food Sci Nutr 2002;42:163–178.

74. Dulloo AG, Seydoux J, Girardier L, Chantre P, Vandermander J. Green tea and thermogenesis: interactions between catechin-polyphenols, caffeine and sympathetic activity. Int J Obes Relat Metab Disord 2000;24:252–258.

75. Doucet E, Tremblay A. Food intake, energy balance and body weight control. Eur J Clin Nutr 1997; 51:846–855.

76. Astrup A, Breum L, Toubro S. Pharmacological and clinical studies of ephedrine and other thermogenic agonists. Obes Res 1995;(Suppl):537S–540S.

77. Sadakata S. Mortality among female practitioners of Chanyou (Japanese tea ceremony). Tohoku J Exp Med 1995;166:475–477.

78. Cutler RG. Antioxidants and longevity of mammalian species. Basic Life Sci 1985;35:15–73.

79. Rice-Evans C. Implications of the mechanisms of action of tea polyphenols as antioxidants in vitro for chemoprevention in humans. Proc Soc Exp Biol Med 1999;220:262–266.

80. Fujiki H, Suganuma M, Okabe S, et al. Japanese green tea as a cancer preventive in humans. Nutr Rev 1996;54:S67–S70.

81. Kanis J, Johnell O, Gullberg B, et al. Risk factors for hip fracture in men from Southern Europe: the MEDOS study. Mediterranean osteoporosis study. Osteoporos Int 1999;9:45–55.

82. Hegarty VM, May HM, Khaw KT. Tea drinking and bone mineral density in older women. Am J Clin Nutr 2000;71:1003–1007.

83. Haqqi TM, Anthony DD, Gupta S, et al. Prevention of collagen-induced arthritis in mice by apolyphenolic fraction from green tea. Proc Natl Acad Sci 1999;96:4524–4529.

84. Suganuma M, Sueoka E, Sueoka N, Okabe S, Fujiki H. Mechanisms of cancer prevention by tea polyphenols based on inhibition of TNF-alpha expression. Biofactors 2000;13:67–72.

85. No JK, Soung DY, Kim YJ, et al. Inhibition of tyrosinase by green tea components. Life Sci 1999; 65:L241–L246.
86. Akiyama K, Shimizu Y, Yokoi I, Kabuto H, Mori A, Ozaki M. Effects of epigallocatechin and epigallocatechin-3-O-gallate on catechol-o-methyltransferase. Neuroscience 1989;15:262–264.
87. Fan W, Tezuka Y, Komatsu K, Namba T, Kadota S. Prolyl endopeptidase inhibitors from the underground part of Rhodiola sacra S.H. Fu. Biol Pharm Bull 1999;22:157–161.
88. Horiba N, Maekawa Y, Ito M, Matsumoto T, Nakamura H. A pilot study of Japanese green tea as a medicament: antibacterial and bactericidal effects. J Endod 1991;17:122–124.
89. Makimura M, Hirasawa M, Kobayashi K, et al. Inhibitory effect of tea catechins on collagenase activity. J Periodontol 1993;64:630–636.
90. Yu H, Oho T, Xu LX. Effects of several tea components on acid resistance of human tooth enamel. J Dent 1995;23:101–105.
91. Goto K, Kanaya S, Nishikawa T. The influence of tea catechins on fecal flora of elderly residents in long-term care facilities. Ann Long Term Care 1998;6:43–48.
92. Goto K, Kanaya S, Ishigami T, Hara Y. The effects of tea catechins on fecal conditions of elderly residents in a long-term care facility. J Nutr Sci Vitaminol 1999;45:135–141.
93. Yamamoto Y, Juneja LR, Chu DC, Kim M. Chemistry and Applications of Green Tea. CRC Press LLC, Boca Raton, FL, 1997.
94. Weisburger JH. Tea and health: the underlying mechanisms. Proc Soc Exp Biol Med 1999;220:271–275.
95. Ernest P. Review article: the role of inflammation in the pathogenesis of gastric cancer. Aliment Pharmacol Therapeut 1999;13(Suppl):13–18.
96. Lampe JW. Health effects of vegetables and fruits: assessing mechanisms of action in human experimental studies. Am J Clin Nutr 1999;70(Suppl):475S–490S.

11 Effect of Cocoa and Chocolate Beverage Consumption on Human Cardiovascular Health

Harold H. Schmitz, Mark A. Kelm, and John F. Hammerstone

Cocoa and chocolate have a rich history of use as both a medicine and a vehicle to deliver other medicines. This was, and still is in some communities, in the context of a traditional medicine popular in Central America. In addition, many of these uses were transferred and modified for approximately four centuries in Europe after New World contact. Interestingly, chocolate was consumed predominantly as a beverage; its now-familiar solid format appeared later as a result of food manufacturing innovation in Europe during the 19th century. However, the standard cocoa and chocolate beverage formats we are familiar with bear little, if any, resemblance to the recipes developed by ancient Central Americans. Dillinger et al. *(1)* convincingly illustrate the versatility of cocoa and chocolate as medical and nutritional uses in their research. As shown in Table 1, the number of different indications, multiplied by different preparations in the accompanying text, is impressive. Continuing research by Dillinger et al. and others on the use of these products by the native populations before European contact may provide additional and important insights on cocoa's cultural origins and geographical aspects and its medical uses (L. Grivetti and H. Yana-Shapiro, personal communication).

Application of modern food and nutrition sciences during the 1990s has provided evidence that, in some cases, the use of some types of cocoa and chocolate was prudent. Cocoa is relatively rich in magnesium, copper, and manganese; thus chocolates, depending on the cocoa content, may provide a good source of certain essential minerals (*see* Table 2). More recently, some cocoa seeds and derivative products, depending on postharvest and product processing practices, contain a high level of select flavonoids relative to many other plant foods *(2)*. This observation may be important in that epidemiological data suggest that flavonoid-rich diets may confer protection against cardiovascular disease (CVD) risk *(3)*. Indeed, Holt et al. *(4)* recently noted that chocolate manufactured from cocoa rich in specific classes of flavonoids may favorably modulate platelet function, which plays a key role in thrombus formation and cardiovascular health *(5,6)*.

From: *Beverages in Nutrition and Health*
Edited by: T. Wilson and N. J. Temple © Humana Press Inc., Totowa, NJ

Table 1

Cocoa/Chocolate in Medical Treatment: A Historical Summary of Positive Claims and Uses[a]

Indication	Positive claim
Agitation	Lessens/reduces (Quélus, 1730, p. 51)
Anemia	Improves (Villanueva y Francesconi, 1890, p. 329)
Angina/heart pain	Reduces (Lavendan, 1796)
Asthma	Reduces (Hughes, 1672, pp. 153–154; Graham, 1828, p. 231)
Belching	Controls/lessens (Lardizabal, 1788, pp. 16–18)
Blood	Generates/produces (Hughes, 1672, pp. 153–154; Lavendan, 1796; Stubbe 1662, pp. 68–69)
Body	Fortifies/invigorates/nourishing to/refreshes/repairs (Brillat-Savarin, 1825, p. 95; Florentine Codex, 1590, Part 12: 119–120; de Quélus, 1730, p. 46; Hughes, 1672, pp. 153–154; Lavedan, 1796, Linné [Linnaeus] 1741)
Brain	Strengthens (Stubbe, 1662, pp. 53–54)
Breast milk	Milk production/lactation: increases quantity (Debay, 1864, pp. 101–108; Stubbe, 1662, pp. 58–60)
Cancer	Reduces (Villanueva y Francesconi, 1890, p. 329)
Colds	Reduces (Stubbe, 1662, p. 67)
Colic	Reduces (Lavedan, 1796)
Conception	Improves probability (Colmenero de Ledesma, 1631, p. A4)
Consumption/ tuberculosis	Reduces (Colmenero de Ledesma, 1631, p. A4; Donzelli, 1686, pp. 284–287; Hughes, 1672, pp. 146, 153–154; Lavedan, 1796)
Cough	Reduces (Blégny, 1687, pp. 282–285; Colmenero de Ledesma, 1631, p. A4; Florentine Codex, 1590, Part 12: p. 12; Stubbe, 1662, p. 11)
Diarrhea/belly fluxes/dysentery/ griping of the guts	Reduces (Blégny, 1687, pp. 282–285; Donzelli, 1686, pp. 284–287; Dufour, 1685, p. 77; Florentine Codex, 1590, Part 12: p. 170; Hernández, 1577, p. 305; Lavedan 1796; Stubbe, 1662, pp. 58–60; Villanueva y Fransconi, 1890, p. 333)
Digestion	Improves/promotes (Brillat-Savarin, 1825, pp. 95–96; Colmenero de Ledesma, 1631, p. A4; Quélus, 1730, pp. 44, 50; Hurtado, 1645, Vol. 1, 2: p. 13; Panadés y Poblet, 1878, p. 191; Rengade, 1886, p. 91; Saint-Arroman, 1846, p. 86; Savarin, 1825, pp. 95–96)
Energy	Improves (Stubbe, 1662, p. 3)
Exhaustion	Relieves/repairs (Brillat-Savarin, 1825, pp. 95–96; Debay, 1864, pp. 101–108; Quélus, 1730, p. 45)
Fatigue	Reduces (Brillat-Savarin, 1825, pp. 95–96; Debay, 1864, pp. 101–108; Blégny, 1687, pp. 282–285; Stubbe, 1662, p. 3)
Female complaints (general)	Reduces (Saint-Arroman, 1846, p. 86)
Fever	Reduces/relieves (Blégny, 1687, pp. 282–285; Donzelli, 1686, pp. 182, 284–287; Dufour, 1685, p. 77; Florentine Codex, 1590, Part 12: 176, 178; Hernández, 1577, p. 305; Hughes 1672, pp. 153–154, Princeton Codex, 1965; Incantation XIV, pp. 35–37; Stubbe, 1662, p. 79)
Gout/podagre	Reduces (Lavedan, 1796)
Gums	Strengthens (Stubbe, 1662, pp. 53–54)
Hangover	Reduces effects of (Brillat-Savarin, 1825, p. 97)

(continued)

Table 1 *(Continued)*

Indication	Positive claim
Health	Essential to/preserves (Hughes, 1672, p. 124; Quélus, 1730, pp. 44–45; Lavedan, 1796)
Heart	Corroborates/strengthens/vivifies (Dufour, 1685, pp. 90–91; Lavedan 1796; Stubbe, 1662, pp. 53–54, 68–69)
Heart palpitations	Relieves (Blégny, 1687, pp. 282–285)
Hypochondria	Reduces (Linné [Linnaeus], 1741)
Infection (general)	Reduces (Colmenero de Ledesma, 1631, p. A4; Florentine Codex, 1590, Part 12: p. 112)
Inflammation (general)	Reduces (Colmenero de Ledesma, 1631, p.A4; Stubbe, 1662, p. 43)
Intestinal complaints (general distress)	Reduces (Colmenero de Ledesma, 1631, p. A4; Debay, 1864, pp. 60, 101–108; Florentine Codex, 1590, Part 12: p. 112)
Irritation (mental)	Reduces (Brillat-Savarin, 1825, p. 100)
Itch	Reduces (Stubbe, 1662, pp. 58–60)
Jaundice	Reduces (Colmenero de Ledesma, 1631, p. A4)
Kidney complaints (general)	Reduces (Dufour, 1685, pp. 75–76; Gage, 1648, p. 108; Priar Agustín Dávila padilla cited by Torres, 1997, p. 244)
Kidney stone/gravel	Cures/expels (Colmenero de Ledesma, 1631, p. A4; Hughes, 1672, p. 153–154)
Labor/childbirth/ delivery	Facilitates (Buchan, 1792, p. 224; Colmenero de Ledesma, 1631, p. A4)
Life	Improves (Debay, 1864, pp. 101–108)
Liver complaints/ distempers	Reduces (Donzelli, 1686, p. 182; Dufour, 1685, pp. 111–113; Gage 1648, pp. 107–108; Hernández, 1577, p. 305)
Longevity	Improves/lengthens/prolongs (Quélus, 1730, pp. 45, 58; Lavendan, 1796; Stubbe, 1662, pp. 84–86)
Lung inflammation/ irritation	Reduces (Blégny, 1687, pp. 282–285; Quélus, 1730, pp. 76–77)
Nerves (delicate)/nervous distress	Calms/improves (Brillat-Savarin, 1825, p. 100; Debay, 1864, pp. 60, 101–108; Rengade, 1886, p. 91)
Nutrition/nutritious	Improves (Villanueva y Francesconi, 1897, p. 23)
Pain (general)	Eases (Quélus, 1730, pp. 76–77)
Pain (abdominal)	Eases (Aguilera, 1985, p. 119)
Poison	Antidote/counters/expels (Aguilera, 1985, p. 119; Colmenero de Ledesma, 1631, p. A4; Quélus, 1730, pp. 76–77; Dufour, 1685, pp. 90–91)
Pregnancy	Nourishes embryo (Hughes, 1672, pp. 153–154)
Rheumatism	Reduces (Blégny, 1687, pp. 282–285; Hughes, 1672, p. 146)
Seizures	Reduces (Princeton Codex, 1965; Incantation XIV, pp. 35–37)
Sexual appetite/ aphrodisiac properties/desire/ pleasure	Increases (Hernández, 1577, p. 305; Colmenero de Ledesma, 1631, p. A4; Linné [Linnaeus], 1741; Monlau, 1881, p. 238; Aguilera, 1985, p. 119)

(continued)

Table 1 *(Continued)*

Indication	Positive claim
Spirit	Gladdens/invigorates/revives (Florentine Codex, 1590, Part 12: pp. 119–120; Hughes, 1672, pp. 153–154; Stubbe, 1662, pp. 68–69)
Strength	Recovers/repairs (Quélus, 1730, pp. 45, 51)
Teeth	Cleans (Colmenero de Ledesma, 1631, p. A4)
Thinking (tormented)	Soothes (Brillat-Savarin, 1825, p. 97)
Thirst	Quenches (Quélus, 1730, p. 46; Stubbe, 1662, pp. 58–60)
Throat (infected/ inflamed)	Reduces (Blégny, 1687, pp. 282–285; Dufour, 1685, pp. 75–76)
Toothache	Reduces (Stubbe, 1662, pp. 53–54)
Tumors/swellings/ pustules	Reduces (Hughes, 1672, p. 144; Stubbe, 1662, pp. 53–54)
Ulcers	Reduces (Stubbe, 1662, pp. 58–60)
Virility	Increases (Lavedan, 1796)
Violence	Reduces (Debay, 1864, pp. 101–108)

[a]Adapted from ref. *1*.

Thus, the purpose of this chapter is to review briefly the history of cocoa and chocolate uses and to provide a detailed current review of the increasing evidence that suggests a potential cardiovascular health benefit associated with regular consumption of cocoa and chocolate. Although the potential for medical and nutritional uses of cocoa and chocolate stem from their original use in various beverage formats by the ancient Central Americans, the current literature contains reports using both beverage and solid formats as dietary interventions. It is apparent that the bioactive agents are derived from the cocoa seed; thus, the data sets obtained from solid-format interventions (e.g., chocolate bars) are germane to any discussion centered on the potential health benefits of cocoa and chocolate beverages.

1. HISTORY OF USE AS FOOD AND MEDICINE

The relevant literature regarding the use of cocoa and chocolate as food and medicine is sufficiently rich; therefore, this chapter provides only brief overviews. The article by Dillinger et al. *(1)* is the most significant recent literature addition to document the medical uses of cocoa and chocolate. The use of cocoa and chocolate, or *cacahuatl* in Nahuatl (Aztec language), originated in the New World among the Olmec, Mayan, and Aztec civilizations, and was prepared exclusively as a beverage before contact with Europeans in the early 16th century. As noted, the number of uses as a medicine ascribed to this beverage is substantial (Table 1). Interestingly, the number of recipe variations is also substantial, and a better understanding of the other ingredients in chocolate preparations might be important. Some of the indications noted by Dillinger et al. *(1)* from primary Aztec and Spanish references include "to alleviate fever and panting of breath and to treat the faint of heart." These are broad descriptions of conditions that we now know are adversely affected by an imbalance in the inflammatory cascades within our immune system and subsequently affect vascular biology and health *(6)*. In a 1999 issue

Table 2
Composition of Cocoa Dry Powder,
Unsweetened [a]

Mineral	mg/100 g
Calcium	128
Iron	13.8
Magnesium	499
Phosphorous	734
Potassium	1524
Sodium	21
Zinc	6.8
Copper	3.7
Manganese	3.8
Selenium	0.01

[a]Adapted from ref. *35.*

of the *New England Journal of Medicine*, it was stated in a seminal review by Ross *(6)* that "Atherosclerosis is an inflammatory disease." Given the rapid increase in experimental biology publications suggesting that some naturally occurring cocoa compounds may favorably modulate biochemical mechanisms associated with the inflammatory reaction pathways in vascular biology *(7–10)*, it is possible that some of the ancients' beliefs and observations are valid.

After contact with ancient Mexicans, the popularity of cocoa and chocolate spread slowly, but persistently, throughout most of Europe after its introduction to the Spanish court in 1544. Its employment as a strictly culinary agent slowly began to represent an increasing proportion of its uses. However, the purported value of chocolate as a broadranging medicine was quickly embraced and its use in medical practice subsided only in the early 20th century *(1)*. In some Central American regions, chocolate is still used as a nutritional, medicinal, and sacred product. However, the transformation of chocolate preparation induced by Conrad van Houten's invention in the middle of the 19th century radically changed its public health perception. It is amazing that chocolate was once highly valued as a medicine, and now is an indulgent and fun contribution to everyday life.

2. COCOA AND CHOCOLATE COMPOSITION

Theobroma cacao (family Sterculiaceae) is a tree that typically grows in the shade of the higher canopies present in the equatorial rainforests of the world. It originated in South America and spread to Central America and to western Africa and parts of Asia by the Europeans. *T. cacao* produces a fruit, the pod, and the seeds inside this pod are called "cocoa beans." These seeds contain several phytochemicals, and their natural product composition is interesting because they contribute unique sensory attributes to chocolate food and beverage products. The macronutrient and micronutrient composition of *T. cacao* seeds is reasonably well-characterized, as is the presence of the methylxanthine alkaloids theobromine and caffeine. Typical macronutrients and other components of cocoa bean nibs are listed in Table 3. Composition variations result from an array of biotic and abiotic factors. Soil type, precipitation, light exposure, disease, herbivory, and cultural practices influence primary and secondary plant metabolism. As is evident in the levels of albumin and glutenin proteins in Criollo and Nacional varieties (*see* Table 4), the genetics or variety of cocoa cultivated can also affect composition.

As previously mentioned, cocoa and its products contain substantial amounts of essential dietary minerals *(11)*. Minerals found in nonalkalized cocoa powder are shown in Table 2. Mineral composition can vary between different cocoa varieties and within the same variety because of different variables, as discussed. However, cocoa and chocolate can provide significant amounts of the Daily Reference Intake/Recommended Daily Allowance of iron, magnesium, and zinc and the Estimated Safe and Adequate Daily Dietary Intakes for copper and manganese *(12)*.

In addition, several compounds that contribute to the flavor profile of raw and processed cocoa products have been identified. Cocoa contains more than 300 volatile compounds. Important flavor components include aliphatic esters, polyphenols, unsaturated aromatic carbonyls, pyrazines, diketopiperazines, and theobromine *(13)*. During fermentation, enzymatic hydrolysis liberates free amino acids (and reducing sugars), which, during roasting, participate in Maillard reactions to produce 3-methylbutanal, phenylacetylaldehyde, 2-methyl-3(methyldithio)furan, 2-ethyl-3,5-dimethylpyrazine, and 2,3-diethyl-5-methylpyrazine *(14,15)*. Table 5 lists important cocoa aroma compounds and their respective descriptors. Bitter flavors in cocoa come from theobromine, caffeine, and protein thermal degradation products, such as diketopiperazines *(14)*. Cocoa's astringency is due to flavanols such as (+)-catechin, (–)-epicatechin, and their related oligomers, the procyanidins. Similar to red wine, catechins, and, to a lesser extent, procyanidins, also contribute to cocoa's bitterness. Also similar to red wine, astringency is more associated with the procyanidin component *(16)*. Astringency is attenuated during the latter stages of fermentation, when flavonoids become susceptible to oxidation followed by condensation reactions with amino acids to form phlobaphenes.

Focus has been increasingly placed on characterizing the flavonoid components present in raw cocoa and finished cocoa and chocolate products *(17,18)*. Although these investigations have revealed the presence of several types of flavonoids *(19)*; they also show that the most abundant class of flavonoids present in raw cocoa and in finished cocoa and chocolate products is the flavanols, including members of the flavanol oligomer series known as procyanidins (*see* Fig. 1 for chemical structures of (–)-epicatechin and procyanidin dimers B2 and B5).

Raw cocoa contains significantly more (–)-epicatechin than (+)-catechin, and the procyanidins are, therefore, believed to contain a high density of epicatechin subunits. Interestingly, epicatechin and its related dimeric procyanidins are unstable in some thermal and extreme pH environments, and significant conversion of epicatechin to catechin can be observed *(20)*. Thus, it is apparent that many standard postharvest handling and food-processing practices associated with manufacturing cocoa and chocolate products can substantially reduce or eliminate the flavanols and procyanidins originally present in the cocoa seeds at harvest. The most prominent of these practices include fermentation, roasting, and alkalization.

Rigorous fractionation of the procyanidin series has provided the opportunity to learn more about the potential for structure specificity when flavonoids interact with biological

Table 3
Percent Composition of Fermented
and Air-Dried Cocoa Beans (Nibs)[a]

Constituent	Percentage
Moisture	5.0
Fat	54.0
Caffeine	0.2
Theobromine	1.2
Theophylline	Trace
Polyhydroxylphenols	6.0
Crude protein	11.5
Monosaccharides and oligosaccharides	1.0
Starch	6.0
Pentosans	1.5
Cellulose	9.0
Carboxylic acids	1.5
Other compounds	0.5
Ash	2.6

[a]Adapted from refs. *14* and *36.*

Table 4
Cocoa Protein Distribution in Fresh Beans[a]

Protein	Variety	
	Criollo (nonpigmented)	Nacional (pigmented)
Albumin	32%	51%
Globulin	25%	25%
Prolamine	12%	12%
Glutenin	31%	12%
Total	100%	100%

[a]Data shows percent distribution. Adapted from ref. *15.*

systems *(8–10,21)*. However, isomerically pure fractions are not yet available, except through limited synthetic options *(22)*. Additional work elucidating the absolute structure of individual flavanols and procyanidins in cocoa seeds will provide opportunities to understand potentially significant structure–function aspects related to their observed bioactivity in the context of vascular biology.

3. POTENTIAL MECHANISMS OF BIOLOGICAL ACTION

The recent research focus on the biologic actions of flavanols and procyanidins in cocoa and chocolate began in 1996, with the demonstration of the ability of the polyphenolic component of cocoa to inhibit in vitro and ex vivo oxidation of human low-density lipoproteins (LDL) *(23,24)*. Subsequent research has confirmed and extended these

Table 5
Important Odorants of Cocoa Mass,
Results of Aroma Extraction Dilution Analysis[a]

Compound	Odor descriptor	FD-factor[b]
3-methylbutanal	Malty	1024
Ethyl 2-methylbutanoate	Fruity	1024
Hexanal	Green	512
Unknown	Fruity, waxy	512
2-methoxy-3-isopropyl pyrazine	Peasy, earthy	512
(E)-2-Octenal	Fatty, waxy	512
Unknown	Tallowy	512
2-methyl-3(methyldithio)furan	Cooked meat-like	512
2-ethyl-3,5-dimethylpyrazine	Earthy, roasty	256
2,3-diethyl-5-methylpyrazine	Earthy, roasty	256
(E)-2-nonenal	Tallowy, green	256
Unknown	Pungent, grassy	128
Unknown	Sweet, waxy	128
Phenylacetylaldehyde	Honey-like	64
(Z)-4-heptenal	Biscuit-like	64
δ-octenolactone	Sweet, coconut-like	64
δ-decalactone	Sweet peach-like	64

[a] Adapted from ref. *14*.

[b] Flavor dilution factor (FD-factor) is the number of parts of solvent required to dilute the aroma extract until the aroma value is reduced to one.

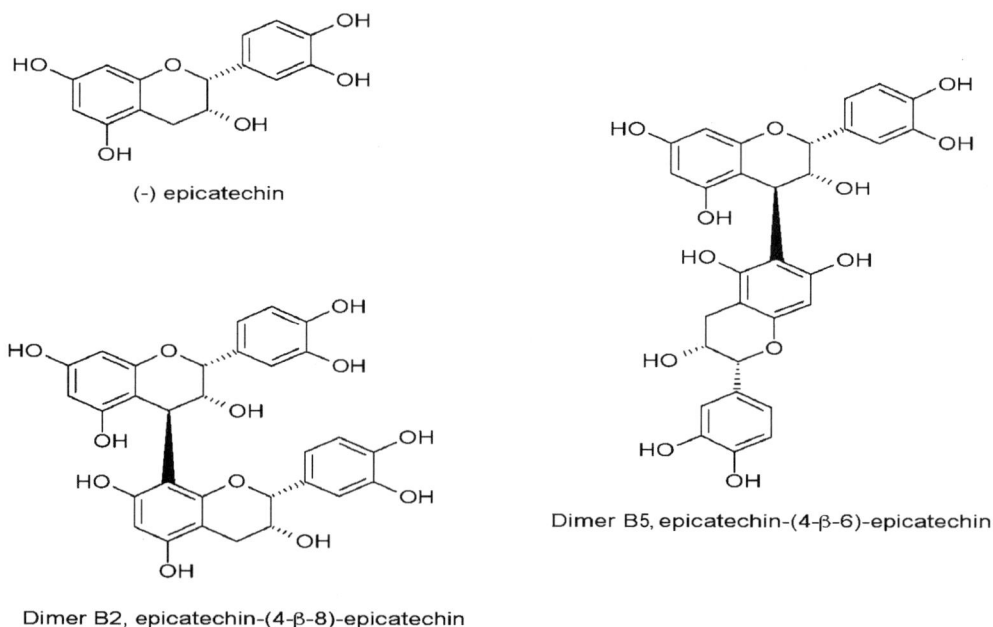

(−) epicatechin

Dimer B2, epicatechin-(4-β-8)-epicatechin

Dimer B5, epicatechin-(4-β-6)-epicatechin

Fig. 1. Chemical structures (−)-epicatechin and procyanidin dimers B2 and B5. Adapted from ref. *17*.

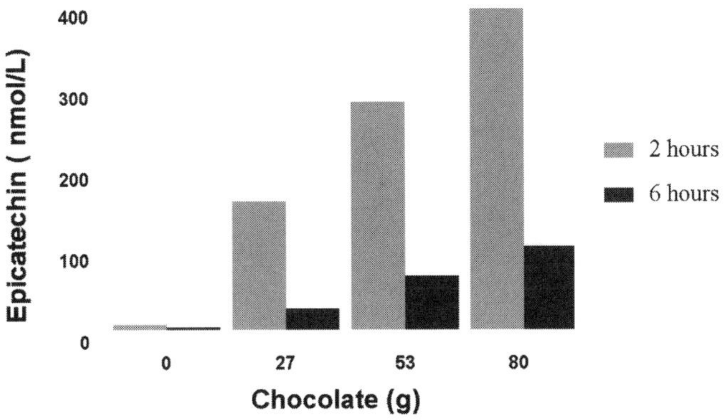

Fig. 2. Absorption of epicatechin in humans after consumption of flavanol-rich chocolate. Adapted from ref. *31.*

observations *(9,18,21,25)* and demonstrated that the redox chemistry of flavanols and procyanidins provides potential for a multiplicity of benefits in reducing local oxidative stress in cellular systems. For example, a recent report by Zhu et al. *(26)* demonstrates that flavanol-rich and procyanidin-rich cocoa can protect red blood cell membranes in vitro and in vivo after exposure to oxidative stress.

The flavanols and procyanidins in cocoa and chocolate have also displayed considerable bioactivity outside the antioxidant realm. Indeed, crude extracts, as well as purified fractions, have demonstrated the potential to modulate nitric oxide synthesis, eicosanoid synthesis, and platelet function *(7,10,27)*. Given the biologic functions attributed to nitric oxide *(28)* and some of the eicosanoids (e.g., prostacyclin), it is speculated that the flavanols and procyanidins act through these pathways to modulate platelet activation and aggregation *(7)*. In addition, in vitro studies have been published suggesting that flavanols and procyanidins in cocoa and chocolate have the potential to modify the secretion of select cytokines, which are potent signaling peptides associated with the immune response *(8,29)*. The data thus far indicate that individual flavanol and procyanidin fractions can have large differences in bioactivity with respect to their role in modulating cytokine secretion. In light of the fundamental importance of cytokine biology to the inflammatory cascade and immune function and the bioactivity suggested by these initial reports, more research should be conducted on the flavanol and procyanidin effects on cytokine secretion.

4. HUMAN INTERVENTION TRIALS AND CHOCOLATE FLAVANOLS

The effects of flavanols and procyanidins on the mechanisms briefly described may have significant implications on cardiovascular health. Indeed, the effects may take on additional significance because heart disease is the number one killer in most of the developed world *(5)*. Therefore, it is critical to gain an understanding of whether the bioactivity observed in vitro is also observed in vivo after ingestion of flavanol- and procyanidin-rich cocoa or chocolate by humans. A paucity of data in this area existed only a short time ago; however, research activity by several groups in the last few years has provided a more robust information base.

Epicatechin and catechin can be absorbed from cocoa and chocolate products, and available kinetic data suggest at least a portion of the absorption curve display a dose–response relationship (see Fig. 2). In addition, the presence of procyanidin dimer B2 in blood after flavanol- and procyanidin-rich cocoa consumption has recently been reported for the first time (30), reinforcing the need to understand if structure-specific differences in function exist in these molecules.

Wang et al. (31) suggest that antioxidant capacity increases and levels of 2-thiobarbituric acid reactive substances (TBARS) decrease in the blood in a dose–response relationship that generally follows the epicatechin absorption curve; however, more data are needed to confirm the pharmacokinetics of this relationship. Beyond TBARS, functional significance for the improved antioxidant capacity conferred by flavanol- and procyanidin-rich cocoa was suggested by Kondo et al. (24), who showed that after its consumption, ex vivo LDL oxidation was inhibited. These data were recently confirmed and extended by Wan et al. (32), who fed flavanol- and procyanidin-rich cocoa and chocolate products to human subjects for approx 4 wk and observed a significant increase in LDL's resistance to ex vivo oxidation.

Flavanol- and procyanidin-rich cocoa and chocolate products have demonstrated impressive potential for modulating platelet activation and function in a manner resembling that of low-dose aspirin (27,33). Consumption of a cocoa beverage containing approx 900 mg of flavanols and procyanidins was shown by Rein et al. (33) to inhibit ex vivo primary hemostasis in humans. In addition, expression of glycoprotein IIb/IIIa was significantly reduced by consumption of the flavanol- and procyanidin-rich cocoa beverage after ex vivo stimulation by either epinephrine or adenosine diphosphate, and expression of P-selectin was similarly reduced after adenosine diphosphate stimulation. Glycoprotein IIb/IIIa and P-selectin are surface proteins that play significant roles in facilitating platelet aggregation and adherence to vascular walls, and significant research programs have been initiated to develop agents capable of modulating the expression of these proteins (5).

Subsequent to the observations on platelet activation and function described, a crossover study was conducted to better understand if modulation of select eicosanoids could be at least partly responsible for these effects (7). Subjects received dark chocolates either rich or deficient in flavanol and procyanidin. After consumption of the flavanol- and procyanidin-rich chocolate, subjects displayed significantly elevated prostacyclin levels in blood compared with their levels after they consumed the chocolate deficient in these compounds. Moreover, the ratio of prostacyclin to leukotrienes was significantly increased after consumption of the flavanol- and procyanidin-rich chocolate vs consumption of the chocolate deficient in these compounds. Importantly, these in vivo findings were comparable to the results obtained in vitro after treatment of human aortic endothelial cells with cocoa-derived flavanols and procyanidins. The relevance of these results to those above focused on platelet activation and function can be found in the literature describing the ability of prostacyclin to inhibit platelet aggregation (7).

A common feature of the published data in this field is the observation that both the absorption and the apparent bioactivity of the flavanols and procyanidins is transient (7,30,31,38). Among other things, this suggests that the mechanism of action(s) associated with these compounds is different from that of aspirin regarding inhibition of platelet activation. Aspirin intervenes to irreversibly inhibit prostaglandin formation at the initial step of the prostaglandin cascade (i.e., the cyclooxygenases) and, thus, limit thromboxane A2 production, which is proaggregatory in nature (33). In contrast, the available data suggest that cocoa-derived flavanols and procyanidins encourage prostacyclin production, which is dependent on prostaglandin H2 synthesis from the cyclooxygenases (7). In addition, it is speculated that cocoa-derived flavanols and procyanidins have the potential to either enhance synthesis (10) of nitric oxide or, perhaps, to modulate favorably kinetics of the free radical reaction environment of nitric oxide in blood and the vascular system based on their antioxidant potential (28). However, further research is needed to test and validate all of these hypotheses associated with the effect(s) of flavanols and procyanidins on platelet function and subsequent effect cardiovascular health.

Another common feature of this research is additional data confirming the results from the original clinical studies by Kris-Etherton's group, demonstrating that chronic consumption of cocoa-derived lipids (i.e., cocoa butter) in the form of chocolate has a neutral effect on blood cholesterol levels (32). Finally, it should also be noted that other beverages containing flavanols and procyanidins (i.e., some teas and purple grape juice) have begun to show similarly promising results in a cardiovascular health context in human intervention trials (28,34). Given the magnitude of the cardiovascular health issues facing public health professionals in much of the world, recommendations for consumption of a range of specific plant-based foods and beverages rich in flavanols and procyanidins may be warranted if research results continue to support the hypothesis that these compounds can yield significant cardiovascular health benefits.

5. CONCLUSION

Cocoa and chocolate have a rich history regarding their medicinal use, both as a medicine and as a vehicle to deliver other medicines. Interestingly, the origin of this use is as a beverage rather than the more familiar solid-food products with which the modern Western European influence has driven. Our increasing understanding of cocoa seed composition suggests that there are indeed several natural products present that may confer some level of bioactivity that is relevant to human health, especially regarding the flavanols and procyanidins. This concept is supported by the findings that much of the potential bioactivity portended by in vitro studies has, in fact, been observed in human intervention studies using flavanol- and procyanidin-rich cocoas and chocolates, including protection against some types of oxidative stress and inhibition of platelet activation. Intervention vehicles for these trials have included flavanol and procyanindin-rich cocoa beverages, as well as chocolate food products, suggesting that numerous formats can deliver the potential bioactivity of these compounds. The nature of this evidence suggests that the most promising area for cocoa-derived food and beverage products to positively influence human health may be in cardiovascular health. Finally, data on the chemical stability of the flavanols and procyanidins demonstrate that it is essential to consider the effects of postharvest handling and processing practices when developing food and beverage products that have the potential to deliver the cardiovascular health benefits to consumers suggested by the research to date.

6. MAIN POINTS FOR PRIMARY AND CLINICAL REVIEW

1. Cocoa originally grew in the equatorial rainforest of the New World where it was used as a beverage, food, and drug by the Olmec, Mayan, and Aztec civilizations prior to its introduction to Europe.
2. Conversion of cocoa into the solid form in Europe in the middle of the 17th century lead to a rapid increase in its consumption.
3. Cocoa contains substantial amounts of minerals, fats, proteins, phenolic compounds, flavonoids, and caffeine that can provide significant contributions to a consumer's intake.
4. Processing of cocoa into chocolate can result in a substantial alteration to the phenolic and flavonoid compounds.
5. Phenolic and flavonoid compounds in cocoa and chocolate may provide consumers with beneficial biological activities related to antioxidant activity, blood clotting, inflammation, endothelial activity, and possibly lipid profile.

ACKNOWLEDGMENT

The authors thank Ms. Laura Plunkett for her help in preparing the manuscript.

REFERENCES

1. Dillinger TL, Barriga P, Escarcega S, Jimenez M, Lowe DS, Grivetti LE. Food of the Gods—cure for humanity? A cultural history of the medicinal and ritual use of chocolate. J Nutr 2000;130:2057S–2072S.
2. Hammerstone JF, Lazarus SA, Schmitz HH. Proanthocyanidin content and variation in some commonly consumed foods. J Nutr 2000;130:2086S–2092S.
3. Hertog MG, Feskens EJ, Hollman PC, Katan MB, Kromhout D. Zutphen elderly study. Lancet 1993; 342:1007–1011.
4. Holt RR, Schramm DD, Keen CL, Lazarus SA, Schmitz HH. Chocolate consumption and platelet function. JAMA 2002;287:2212–2221.
5. Lefkowitz RJ, Willerson JT. Prospects for cardiovascular research. JAMA 2001;285:581–587.
6. Ross R. Mechanisms of disease: atherosclerosis—an inflammatory disease. N Engl J Med 1999;340: 115–126.
7. Schramm DD, Wang JF, Holt RR, et al. Chocolate procyanidins decrease the leukotriene/prostacyclin ratio in humans and human aortic endothelial cells. Am J Clin Nutr 2001;73:36–40.
8. Mao T, van de Water J, Keen CL, Schmitz HH, Gershwin ME. Cocoa procyanidins and human cytokine transcription and secretion. J Nutr 2000;130:2093S–2099S.
9. Arteel G, Sies H. Protection against peroxynitrite by cocoa polyphenol oligomers. FEBS Lett 1999; 462:167–170.
10. Karim M, McCormick K, Kappagoda CT. Effects of cocoa extracts on endothelium dependent relaxation. J Nutr 2000;130:2105S–2108S.
11. Chevaux KA, Jackson L, Villar ME, et al. Proximate, mineral, and procyanidin content of consumed by the Kuna Amerinds of Panama. J Food Comp Anal 2001;14:553–563.
12. Knight I. Minerals in cocoa and chocolate. In: Chocolate and Cocoa—Health and Nutrition. Knight I (ed.). Blackwell Sciences, Malden, MA, 1999, pp. 143–152.
13. Duke JA. Handbook of Medicinal Herbs. CRC Press, Boca Raton, FL, 1985, pp. 479–480.
14. Belitz HD, Grosch W. Coffee, tea, cocoa. In: Food Chemistry, 2nd Ed. Belitz HD, Grosch W (eds.). Springer-Verlag, New York, NY, 1999, pp. 874–904.
15. Wursch P, Finot PA. Carbohydrate and protein. In: Chocolate and Cocoa—Health and Nutrition. Knight I (ed.). Blackwell Sciences, Malden, MA, 1999, pp. 105–115.
16. Gawal R. Red wine astringency: a review. Aust J Grape Wine Res 1998;4:74–95.

17. Hammerstone JF, Lazarus SA, Mitchell AE, Rucker RB, Schmitz HH. Identification of procyanidins in cocoa (*Theobroma cacao*) and chocolate using high-performance liquid chromatography/mass spectrometry. J Agric Food Chem 1999;47:490–496.

18. Adamson GE, Lazarus SA, Mitchell AE, et al. HPLC method for the quantification of procyanidins in cocoa and chocolate samples and correlation to total antioxidant capacity. J Agric Food Chem 1999; 47:4184–4188.

19. Fraga C, Lazarus SA, Hammerstone JF, Schmitz HH, Keen CL. More antioxidants in cocoa [reply]? J Nutr 2001;131:835.

20. Zhu QY, Holt RR, Lazarus SA, et al. pH Stability of the flavan-3-ols epicatechin and catechin and some related dimeric procyanidins derived from cocoa. J Agric Food Chem 2002;50:1700–1705.

21. Pearson DA, Schmitz HH, Lazarus SA, Keen CL. Inhibition of in vitro low-density lipoprotein oxidation by oligomeric procyanidins present in chocolate and cocoas. Meth Enzymol 2001;335:350-360.

22. Kozakowski AP, Tuckmantel W, Hu Y, Romanczyck LJ. Studies in polyphenol chemistry and bioactivity. 3. Stereocontrolled synthesis of epicatechin-4α,8-epicatechin, an unnatural isomer of the B-type procyanidins. J Organ Chem 2001;66:1287-1296.

23. Waterhouse AL, Shirley JR, Donovan JL. Antioxidants in chocolate. Lancet 1996;348:834.

24. Kondo K, Hirano R, Matsumoto A, Igarashi O, Itakura H. Inhibition of LDL oxidation by cocoa. Lancet 1998;348:1514.

25. Lotito SB, Actis-Goretta L, Renart ML, et al. Influence of oligomer chain length on theantioxidant activity of procyanidins. Biochem Biophys Res Comm 2000;276:945–951.

26. Zhu QY, Holt RR, Lazarus SA, Orozco TJ, Keen CL. Inhibitory effects of cocoa flavanols and procyanidin oligomers on free radical-induced erythrocyte hemolysis. Exp Biol Med 2002;227: 321–329.

27. Rein D, Paglieroni TG, Pearson DA, et al. Cocoa and wine polyphenols modulate platelet activation and function. J Nutr 2000;130:2120S–2126S.

28. Freedman JE, Parker C, Li L, et al. Select flavonoids and whole juice from purple grapes inhibit platelet function and enhance nitric oxide release. Circulation 2001;103:2792–2798.

29. Sanbongi C, Suzuki N, Sakane T. Polyphenols in chocolate, which have antioxidant activity, modulate immune functions in humans in vitro. Cell Immunol 1997;177:129–136.

30. Holt R, Lazarus SA, Schmitz HH, Keen CL. Procyanidin dimer B2 (epicatechin-(4β-8)-epicatechin) in human plasma after the consumption of a flavanol-rich cocoa. Am J Clin Nutr 2002;76:798–804.

31. Wang JF, Schramm DD, Holt RR, et al. A dose-response effect from chocolate consumption on plasma epicatechin and oxidative damage. J Nutr 2000;130:2115S–2119S.

32. Wan Y, Vinson JA, Etherton TD, Proch J, Lazarus SA, Kris-Etherton P. Effects of cocoa powder and dark chocolate on LDL oxidative susceptibility and prostaglandin levels in humans. Am J Clin Nutr 2001;74:596–602.

33. Rein D, Paglieroni TG, Wun T, et al. Cocoa inhibits platelet activation and function. Am J Clin Nutr 2000;72:30–35.

34. Duffy SJ, Keaney JF, Holbrook M, et al. Short- and long-term black tea consumption reverses endothelial dysfunction in patients with coronary artery disease. Circulation 2001;104:151–156.

35. US Department of Agriculture, Agriculture Research Service (July 2001). USDA Nutrient Database for Standard Reference, Release 14. Nutrient Data Laboratory home page. Retrieved from http://www.nal.usda.gov/fnic/foodcomp/index.html, accessed July 2002.

36. Apgar JL, Tarka SM. Methylxanthines. In: Chocolate and Cocoa—Health and Nutrition. Knight I (ed.). Blackwell Sciences, Malden, MA, 1999, pp. 153–173.

37. The EPIC Investigators. Use of a monoclonal antibody directed against the platelet glycoprotein IIb/IIIa receptor in high-risk coronary angioplasty. N Engl J Med 1994;330:956–961.

38. Richelle M, Tavazzi I, Enslen M, Offard EA. Plasma kinetics in man of epicatechin from black chocolate. Eur J Clin Nutr 1999;53:22–26.

12 Caffeine and Health

Bennett Alan Weinberg
and Bonnie K. Bealer

1. WHAT ARE OUR CAFFEINE CONSUMPTION PATTERNS?

There have been few field studies of caffeine consumption patterns, especially outside of the United States. However, it is obvious that there is considerable variation in this consumption among individuals and populations. Some overall observations can be reliably made:

Age: Caffeine consumption increases progressively with age until stabilizing in middle age and decreasing slightly in old age *(1)*. This increase of use with age, until middle age, is one of the most bedeviling confounders in long-term studies of the health effects of caffeine consumption.

Gender: There is little or no gender difference in consumption levels, and it is uncertain which gender consumes more *(2)*. Many studies focus on caffeine exposure levels, because women weigh so much less than men, and exposure is a function of body weight.

Abstainers: At least 90% of people surveyed consistently state that they regularly drink coffee or tea. The prevalence of caffeine use is even higher if soft drinks and other dietary sources are considered *(3)*. Fewer than 5% of survey participants are abstainers, because they never consume caffeine from any source. This leaves approx 5% in the category of occasional users. The average daily consumption among caffeine consumers in the United States is approx 280 mg.

Generations: Over the centuries attitudes toward different beverages have varied widely from one era to the next. In America, alcohol consumption, which peaked in 1980, has declined more than 15%, the biggest drop found in distilled spirits and smaller decreases in wine and beer. Caffeine use has exploded in the last few decades, even though industry data indicate that there was a progressive decrease in coffee as a source between 1962 and 1982. However, because of increases in specialty coffee consumption, use is once again increasing and the decline in alcohol consumption continues *(2)*.

This chapter reviews how caffeine consumption, from beverages, affects us. For more complete descriptions of the health and nutritional affects of specific types of beverages, such as coffee, tea, herbal teas, and soft drinks, *see* Chapters 9, 10, 13, 24, and 25.

From: *Beverages in Nutrition and Health*
Edited by: T. Wilson and N. J. Temple © Humana Press Inc., Totowa, NJ

2. CAFFEINE AND CHEMISTRY

Caffeine is a chemical compound built of four of the most common elements on earth: carbon, hydrogen, nitrogen, and oxygen. It is collected as a residue of coffee decaffeination, recovered from waste tea leaves, produced by methylating the organic compounds theophylline or theobromine, or synthesized from dimethylurea and malonic acid. At room temperature, caffeine is odorless and slightly bitter, and consists of a white fleecy powder resembling cornstarch or of long flexible silky prismatic crystals. It is moderately soluble in water at body temperature and freely soluble in hot water.

Caffeine is one of a group of purine alkaloids, sometimes called methylated xanthines, or simply, xanthines. Other methylated xanthines include theophylline, theobromine, and paraxanthine. All three are isomers, or chemical variations, of caffeine, and all three are primary products of caffeine metabolism in human beings. Theobromine is present in pharmacologically significant amounts in cacao and chocolate. Theophylline is present in small quantities in tea. Although purine itself is not found in the human body, chemicals in the purine family are widely present in the body as throughout nature.

3. THE DISTRIBUTION AND METABOLISM OF CAFFEINE

3.1. Caffeine Absorption

Because caffeine is fat soluble, it passes through plasma membranes with relative ease. As a result, it is quickly and completely absorbed from the stomach and intestines into the bloodstream and rapidly distributed to all parts of the body. Caffeine's permeability results in an evenness of distribution that is exceptional when compared with most other pharmacologic agents; because the human body presents no significant physiologic barrier to hinder its passage through tissues, the concentrations attained by caffeine are virtually the same in blood, saliva, breast milk, and semen (1).

Caffeine's stimulating effects largely depend on its power to infiltrate the central nervous system (CNS). This infiltration can only be accomplished by crossing the blood–brain barrier, a defensive mechanism that protects the CNS from biologic or chemical exposure. Caffeine passes through this blood–brain barrier as if the barrier does not exist (1).

The maximum concentration of caffeine in the body is typically attained within 1 h after consumption of a cup of coffee or tea. However, approx 75% of peak levels are attained in approx 15 min. It is important to remember that the caffeine concentration in one's body is a function not only of the amount of caffeine consumed but also of one's weight. After drinking a small cup of coffee with a typical 100 mg of caffeine, a 200-lb man would attain a concentration of approx 1 mg/kg of body weight. A 100-pound woman would attain approx 2 mg/kg and would therefore (all other metabolic factors being considered equal) experience double the effects experienced by the man.

3.2. The Pathway of Caffeine Metabolism

The bloodstream carries caffeine from the stomach and intestines to the liver, where it can be metabolized or pass unmodified to the rest of the body. Caffeine's biotransformation is complex, producing more than a dozen different metabolites. More than 98% of the caffeine a person consumes is metabolized and exits the body in the urine. The study of these transformations in human beings has been impeded by metabolic routes for caffeine that demonstrate a remarkable variation between humans and different animal species.

Because caffeine passes into and out of tissues so easily and completely, it does not accumulate in any body organs. Caffeine does not accumulate in body fat, where it might otherwise be retained for weeks or even months, unlike other psychotropic drugs, such as marijuana.

For most animal species, including humans, the mean elimination half-life of caffeine is from 3 to 7 h, with more than 90% being removed from the body in approx 12 h (1). However, the half-life can be influenced by several factors and, therefore, demonstrates considerable individual and group variation. This causes differences in sensitivity to caffeine, which is a source of confusion in studies of its effects. One cause of these variations in the rate of caffeine metabolism is inherited metabolic differences. Other factors are as follows: Women using oral contraceptives have a rate of caffeine metabolism that is dramatically slowed (4). Similarly, pregnancy results in a considerable increase in the half-life, with a concomitant increase in exposure to the fetus (5). Because caffeine is metabolized in the liver, hepatic impairment also slows caffeine's metabolism. Newborn infants are dramatically less capable of metabolizing caffeine than are adults, probably because their livers are unable to produce the requisite enzymes, an incapacity that extends the drug's half-life in newborn infants to 85 h (6). Many other factors, including the use of certain drugs, can raise or lower caffeine's metabolic rate (7). For example, cigarette smoking doubles the rate at which caffeine is eliminated, which means that smokers can drink more coffee but will feel it for a shorter time than nonsmokers. Conversely, alcohol consumption slows caffeine's elimination rate; therefore, alcohol drinkers feel the caffeine for a longer time (8).

Caffeine's actions may help account for the common attempt to use caffeine to combat the effects of alcohol. Although it is true that the degree of alcohol intoxication depends on the alcohol level in the blood, a level that caffeine cannot alter, caffeine has been shown to mitigate alcohol-induced impairments in reaction time, reasoning, and coordination (1,9).

4. MECHANISMS OF ACTION

Almost everyone would agree that caffeine helps to keep you awake, increase your energy, and improve your mood and your ability to think clearly. To discover how and to what degree caffeine does these and other things, scientists have arguably investigated it more extensively than any other drug. In approaching the question of how caffeine works, scientists are confronted with the complex circumstance that the drug produces an effect and, in certain instances, more than one effect, on the cardiovascular, respiratory, renal, and central and peripheral nervous systems. Partly as a consequence of this complexity, no one has identified caffeine's mechanism of action with any certainty. Particularly unclear are the sources of its psychostimulant and cardiovascular effects.

Many neurotransmitters and hormones function by causing cells to create a second messenger called cyclic adenosine monophosphate (cAMP). cAMP may be responsible for some of the physiological effects of caffeine, such as dilation of airways and increased force of heart contractions. cAMP is destroyed inside the cell by an enzyme called phosphodiesterase, and phsophodiesterase activity is inhibited by the presence of caffeine *(10,11)*. Increased levels of cAMP produced by this mechanism may make cells more sensitive to the neurotransmitter and hormonal messages they receive.

However, caffeine's primary mechanism of action is to act as a competitive antagonist of adenosine; that is, it achieves most of its stimulant effects by blocking the uptake of, and thereby the actions of, adenosine *(12)*. Adenosine is a neurotransmitter with mood-depressing, hypnotic (sleep-inducing), and anticonvulsant properties and induces hypotension (low blood pressure), bradycardia (slowed heartbeat), and vasodilation. It also decreases urination and gastric secretion. Adenosine decreases the rate of spontaneous nerve cell firing and depresses evoked nerve cell potentials in the brain by inhibiting the release of other neurotransmitters that control the excitability, or responsiveness, of central neurons.

The ultimate evaluation of this theory of caffeine's mechanism of action is complicated by the numerous adenosine receptors and their differing roles in different tissues. However, caffeine's complex effects on behavior are probably not fully explicable in terms of this blockade alone *(5)*. The adenosine system also affects the excitablity of the other neurotransmitter systems, and, in any case, chronic caffeine use causes changes in numerous other neurotransmitters, including norepinephrine, dopamine, serotonin, acetylcholine, GABA, and the glutamate systems in the brain *(7)*. Researchers must determine what part, if any, these changes play in the behavioral effects associated with caffeine use.

5. DIETARY SOURCES OF CAFFEINE

Few of us in Western countries today chew the leaves, bark, fruit, or nuts of caffeine-containing plants. We get our caffeine and other methylxanthines from drinks, foods, and pills. In the United States, approx 70% of caffeine comes from coffee beans, approx 14% from tea leaves, more than 12% from soft drinks, nearly 3% from cocoa beans, and the remaining fraction comes from all other sources, including cola nut, maté, and guarana *(2,4)*. The caffeine in cola drinks is not derived from cola nuts but is a super-added extract of caffeine derived from coffee or tea. Caffeine is found in some over-the-counter medications, such as alertness aids (Vivarin) and aspirin compounds, and in prescription medications, such as narcotic pain killers, to which it is added as an adjuvant to their analgesic power. Common dietary and medicinal sources, with the amount of caffeine found in each, are listed in Table 1.

A cup of coffee is generally considered to contain an average of 100 mg of caffeine. This sounds simple and straightforward, suggesting that it is fairly easy to determine how much caffeine we are taking when we have a cup of coffee. But exactly how much liquid is in a "cup of coffee?" The cup itself as a standard liquid measure is 8 oz. A big mug or large paper cup, filled to the brim, may be 10 oz or even 12 oz. If not filled to the brim, a small cup may hold as little as 4 oz. When we speak of a cup, we may be speaking of 4, 5, 6, 8, 10, 12 oz or more of coffee. Another problem is the question of the amount of caffeine in the coffee, ounce for ounce. This number varies widely with such variables as method of preparation, type of coffee bean (robusta beans have twice the caffeine of arabica beans), roasting method, and amount of coffee used.

These uncertainties produce a remarkably wide range for what might constitute the "correct" value for the amount of caffeine in a "cup" of coffee. A small cup of instant coffee that was prepared relatively weak might have as few as 50 mg. A large cup of

Table 1
Caffeine Content of Common Beverages and Foods

Drink	Type	Caffeine content (mg)
Coffee (6-oz cup, arabica beans)	Filter drip	130–189 (average 150)
	Espresso (1.3 to 2 oz)	100
	Instant	50–130
	Decaffeinated (instant)	2–6
	Decaffeinated (as prepared in coffee shops)	5–25
Tea (6-oz cup, 3-min brew)	Green tea	10–15
	Black tea	50
Bottled iced tea (16-oz bottle)	Snapple iced tea (all varieties)	31
	Lipton iced tea (all varieties)	18–40
	Nestea iced tea (all varieties)	16–26
	Arizona iced tea (all varieties)	15–30
Chocolate product	Hot chocolate (mix, 6 oz)	10
	Chocolate milk (6 oz)	4
	Milk chocolate (28 g)	6
	Dark chocolate (28 g)	20
	Baking chocolate (28 g)	35
Miscellaneous	Cocoa Puffs breakfast cereal (4 oz)	2
	Penguin Mints (1 mint)	7
	Dannon Coffee Yogurt (8 oz)	45
	Dannon Light Cappucino Yogurt (8 oz)	< 1
	Yoplait Café Au Lait Yogurt (6 oz)	5
	Stonyfield Farm Cappuccino Yogurt (8 oz)	0
	Häagen Dazs Coffee Ice Cream (1 cup)	58
	Häagen Dazs Coffee Frozen Yogurt, fat-free (1 cup)	40
	Starbucks Coffee Ice Cream, assorted flavors (1 cup)	40–60
	Ben & Jerry's No-Fat Coffee Fudge Frozen Yogurt (1 cup)	85

Most people think that an espresso has more caffeine than an ordinary cup of coffee, but this is a myth. While espresso has much more caffeine per ounce, it is usually served in cups of between 1.5 and 2 oz. Because regular filter drip coffee is usually served in cups that are 6 oz or larger, the amount of caffeine in an espresso is actually smaller than the amount in a cup of regular filter drip coffee.

The table shows that sometimes so-called decaffeinated coffees aren't really as caffeine-free as they pretend to be. Instant decaffeinated coffees, such as Sanka, are reliable and contain only a few milligrams of caffeine at most.

Remember that the caffeine content of robusta beans is twice that of arabica beans.

Sources: Hershey's website: www.hersheys.com; Center for Science in the Public Interest website: www.cspinet.org; and ref. 2 (p. 327).

infused coffee steeped for a long time with a lot of robusta beans might have 350 mg. Admittedly, these are extreme values, but we believe that doses in the range of between 100 mg and 250 mg are common. According to the Food and Drug Administration, a 5-oz cup of coffee contains 40–180 mg of caffeine *(2)*.

Tea is the second largest source of caffeine consumption in the world. As discussed in Chapter 10, all true tea is produced from the leaves of the plant *Camella sinensis*. The leaves are cured differently to produce green, oolong, and black varieties. A cup of green tea has approx 15 mg of caffeine, a cup of black tea has approx 40 mg, and oolong has an amount between the two. The same problems beset an evaluation of how much caffeine is in a cup of tea as beset the evaluation of how much is in a cup of coffee, although, of course, the average caffeine levels in tea are lower than those for coffee.

Maté also is an important source of caffeine, especially in Brazil, but its caffeine content is difficult to determine. Maté is made from the leaves of *Ilex paraguariensis*, and as many as 60 varieties of plants are used in making the drink. To make matters even more confusing, the caffeine content of maté leaves varies widely according to their age at the time of harvesting. Maté leaves aged > 2 yr, 1–2 yr, and < 1 yr at the time of harvest contain, respectively, approx 0.7%, 1.5%, and 2% caffeine by weight.

Guarana is a major source of caffeine for millions of South Americans and is also widely sold in Europe and the United States in herbal teas and energy powders in health food stores.

In Brazil, where Guarana carbonated drinks are popular, some consumers claim the effects are somewhat different from coffee. This difference may be imagined or, as we have seen in other cases of natural drugs, result from the chemical complexity of guarana and from the fact that it contains other active alkaloids that augment or modify the effects of caffeine.

Small amounts of caffeine are found in chocolate and other cocoa products, a topic also discussed in Chapter 11. A 1.58-oz milk chocolate Hershey bar has 12 mg of caffeine and an average 6-oz cup of hot chocolate prepared from a mix has 5 mg of caffeine.

Finally, soft drinks are a major dietary source of caffeine. The amount in each varies widely, as shown in Table 2. Jolt Cola, at or near the top of any list, has 70 mg of caffeine in a 12-oz can, Coca Cola has 38 mg, and Canada Dry Diet Cola has 1 mg.

6. METHODS FOR INDUSTRIAL EXTRACTION OF CAFFEINE

6.1. How Is Extracted Caffeine Used?

The United States imports large quantities of caffeine for medical purposes and for spiking soft drinks, most of which is extracted from low-quality coffee beans or waste tea leaves or collected as a by-product of coffee and tea decaffeination. Two different techniques can be used to accomplish this: bean decaffeination and extract decaffeination.

6.2. How Do Bean and Extract Decaffeination Procedures Differ?

Bean decaffeination is used when the bean moisture level is below 40%. The crucial step is to treat the raw coffee beans in static or rotating drums with a preliminary steam wetting before using solvents to dissolve the caffeine. The solvents once used were benzol, chloroform, and alcohol; today's solvents include dichloromethane or super-critical carbon dioxide.

Table 2
Caffeine Content of Soft Drinks [a]

Drink (12 oz)	Caffeine content (mg)
Jolt Cola	70
Mountain Dew	55
Diet Mountain Dew	55
Surge	52
Tab	47
Diet Coke	45
Shasta Cola	45
Shasta Cherry Cola	45
Shasta Diet Cola	45
RC Cola	43
Diet RC	43
Dr. Pepper	42
Diet Dr. Pepper	42
Sunkist Orange Soda	42
Pepsi-Cola	38
Diet Pepsi	36
Aspen	36
Diet Rite	36
Coca-Cola Classic	34
Canada Dry Cola	30
A&W Cream Soda	29
Diet A&W Cream Soda	22
Barq's Root Beer	22
Canada Dry Diet Cola	1
Diet Barq's Root Beer	0
Minute Maid Orange Soda	0
Sprite	0
Diet Sprite	0
7-Up	0

[a] Most soft drinks contain approx 40 mg of caffeine in a 12-oz serving. Note in the table, however, that Coca-Cola Classic contains only 34 mg, whereas Diet Coke contains 46 mg. For a person drinking several servings or who is unusually sensitive to caffeine, this difference may matter. Also note that Sunkist Orange Soda contains 42 mg of caffeine in a 12-oz serving, whereas Minute Maid Orange Soda has no caffeine. This underscores the importance of checking the labels.
Source: ref. 7.

Extract decaffeination is used when the bean moisture content is more than 60%. In this process, raw coffee beans are usually soaked in nearly boiling water for a few minutes to a few hours, and the resulting liquid is decaffeinated either by liquid–liquid extraction with any of the solvents used in the first method or by selective absorption of caffeine on acid-treated active carbon. Alternative adsorption processes, which do not rely on solvents to recover the caffeine from the extract, are called "water decaffeination" *(5).*

Pure caffeine crystals are toxic and must be handled with hooded ventilation systems, masks, and gloves. Therefore, chemical supply companies are not permitted to sell pure caffeine to individual purchasers.

7. CAFFEINE EFFECTS ON HEALTH

7.1. Health Overview

"What is it in man's devious make-up that makes him round on the seemingly more wholesome and pleasurable aspects of his environment and suspect them of being causes of his misfortunes? Whatever it is, stimulants of all kinds (and especially coffee and caffeine) maintain a position high on the list of suspicion, despite a continuing lack of real evidence of any hazard to health" (13).

Caffeine and, before caffeine was identified, coffee, tea, and chocolate have been believed to cause, exacerbate, palliate, or cure several diseases and have also been believed to confer marvelous benefits, including increases in both intellectual and physical capacities. If, like the great majority of people in the world, you use caffeine regularly, you are faced with a complex, confusing, and often apparently contradictory cacophony of traditional and contemporary claims about its effects on health. In former centuries, caffeine lovers had no guidance, only the often-fanciful discourses of the medical men of their time. We are fortunate that, in the last half of the 20th century, an explosion of general medical knowledge and numerous controlled experiments have shed scientific light on many of caffeine's effects. It has been often and truly said that caffeine is the most studied drug in history. Yet, caffeine is not understood as fully as it ought to be because of its nearly universal use, the variety of its modes of consumption, its presence in and effects on nearly all bodily systems, its occurrence in chemically complex foods and beverages, and the social and psychologic factors that shape its use.

Fetuses that survive to infancy do not have more gross teratology. However, the possibility of more subtle neurologic deficits or other less obvious problems has not been excluded. Moreover, caffeine has been associated with miscarriage and, therefore, pregnant women would be best advised to avoid caffeine *(7)*. Caffeine may be effective as a therapy for neonatal apnea and as a topical treatment of atopic dermatitis *(14)*. Caffeine has long been recognized as an analgesic adjuvant, or enhancer of pain medications. It also increases the length of time that chronic stable angina patients can walk without feeling pain.

7.2. Caffeine, the Cardiovascular System, and Total Mortality

An absence of any relation between caffeine consumption and all or any causes of death was also found in a 1990 study of 45,000 men *(15)* and also by the Framingham study *(16)*, the Evans County study (1960–1969) *(17)*, and a study in Gothenburg, Sweden *(18)*. The relationship between coffee and risk of coronary heart disease (CHD) is reviewed in Chapter 9.

Caffeine can have important acute effects on the cardiovascular system. It is useful in averting acute hypotension (a sudden drop in blood pressure), such as sometimes occurs after breakfast, especially in the elderly. People experiencing this problem are advised to consume 200–250 mg of caffeine or about two cups of coffee, each day *(19)*.

7.3. Caffeine and Cancer and Tumor Activity

In 1990, the International Agency for Research of Cancer (IARC), after performing an extensive review of research on digestive, bladder and urinary tract, breast, and other cancer sites, published a monograph summarizing findings on coffee and cancer. The results specifically excluded any link between caffeine use and the incidence of cancer of the oral cavity, esophagus, stomach, liver, breast, ovaries, kidney, or the lympho-recticular system, including Hodgkin's disease, non-Hodgkin's lymphomas, and lymphatic and myeloid leukemia. The association between coffee intake and cancer risk is reviewed in more detail in Chapter 9.

Studies with rats suggest that caffeine may protect against cancerous tumors generally and indicate that caffeine specifically "decreased the incidence of tumors that developed . . . in mice treated with cigarette smoke condensate, ultraviolet light" and other mutagenic agents in the skin and lungs (20).

7.4. Diuretic Effects

Does a cup of caffeinated coffee cause diuresis, and is the diuresis physiologically significant to the body's fluid electrolytes and physical performance? Nussberg et al. (1990) suggested that consumption of a single cup of caffeinated coffee does promote an increase in urine formation (diuresis) that was not associated with the consumption of decaffeinated coffee (21). A more recent review of 10 studies of caffeine-induced diuresis concluded that caffeine consumption without the fluid media does promote a diuretic effect but the effect is similar to that created by the consumption of a cup of water (22). This diuresis is not associated with fluid electrolyte imbalances in the blood that would be detrimental to physical performance (22) or hydration status (23).

8. DEPENDENCE, TOLERANCE, AND WITHDRAWAL

When certain drugs are used regularly, the body adapts to their presence by requiring increasing dosages to achieve the same effects. This increasing resistance is called "tolerance." Drugs that create tolerance generally exhibit a physical dependence, which means that if a person stops using them abruptly, he or she will experience withdrawal symptoms.

Users of dangerous drugs, such as heroin, barbiturates, and amphetamines, develop extremely large tolerances, a process that forces them to take ever-increasing amounts to maintain the same level of effect. In contrast to the open-ended tolerance of these drugs, only limited tolerance develops to many of caffeine's effects and no tolerance seems to develop to others. Tolerance does not develop to caffeine's ergogenic effects or to its benefits to memory, reasoning, reaction time, attention span, and mood.

However, even though a tolerance does not develop to many of caffeine's effects, there is no denying that continued caffeine use results in mild physical dependence. When we regularly use any substance that supports a physical dependence and then suddenly discontinue its use, we can experience withdrawal symptoms. Such response patterns occur with many drugs, for example, selective serotonin reuptake inhibitors (SSRIs). Caffeine's tolerance and withdrawal properties have been well recognized for more than a century. In 1893, Bridge published a warning that people who terminated their caffeine use abruptly were at risk of developing a severe headache (24). We now know that headaches are, in fact, the most common symptom associated with discontinuing caffeine use too quickly. Other symptoms of caffeine withdrawal in decreasing order of frequency are: fatigue, sleepiness, disphoria, difficulty concentrating, difficulty working, depression, anxiety, irritability, and flu-like symptoms (nausea, muscle aches, hot–cold spells, runny nose). On average, approximately one third of people who suddenly stop caffeine use will experience headaches, and a lower percentage will experience the other symptoms. There also remains considerable disagreement about the prevalence or severity of the other symptoms. However, when a person decides to stop using caffeine, he or she will be advised to do so slowly, by progressively reducing the dose during a period of several days.

It is also fair to ask if caffeine is addictive. Almost all psychiatrists and pharmacologists agree that it is not, using the word "addictive" only to describe a drug that causes serious damage to and disruption of people's lives. Drugs such as heroin, cocaine, and amphetamines clearly fall into this category. In contrast, no one, apparently, has ever lost a job, a spouse, or a house from using too much caffeine or because he or she had to obtain caffeine.

Drug discrimination studies provide evidence for individual differences in sensitivity to caffeine and document that some people can detect remarkably small amounts of the drug. In one report, the lowest oral dose administered in water that was detectable by research subjects ranged from a minimum of 1.8 mg to as much as 178 mg, with approx 70% of them detecting 56 mg or less and approx 35% detecting 18 mg or less *(25)*. Other scientists have purportedly identified more unusual reactions. For example, Hayreh *(26)*, in a 1973 study, gives an account of his own extreme sensitivity to caffeine, which he describes as manifested in "dizziness, weakness, and tremors, lasting two hours, and my pulse-rate went very high," effects he claims are experienced by many others.

9. CAFFEINE AND COGNITIVE PERFORMANCE

9.1. Caffeine Effect on Arousal

Caffeine, when taken by a well-rested person at the height of his or her normal mental powers, increases mental performance in a host of areas, including reasoning ability, reaction time, memory, computational ability, alertness and attention span, and verbal fluency. In recent years, researchers have recognized that the nature and extent of caffeine's effects on cognitive performance are mediated by arousal levels. It is established that caffeine demonstrates a biphasic pattern of effects on the various parameters of mental performance that is a function of total arousal *(7)*. One of the consequences of this is that, all other arousal factors being equal, small doses of caffeine confer some benefits, medium to large doses of caffeine confer more pronounced benefits, but large doses of caffeine do not increase benefits further and may even cause decrements. What is a "small" dose or a "medium" dose of caffeine? It depends on the user's personality type, weight, and state of health; on the activity or kind of work the user engages in; and on the user's individual sensitivity to caffeine.

Many factors contribute to total arousal at any given moment. For example, if you're tired or sick, your arousal level decreases. If you're in a crowded room, surrounded by distracting conversations when you're trying to work, your arousal level increases. Caffeine increases arousal levels, in proportion to the dose taken. Total state of arousal is what governs how much benefit in cognitive performance you can expect to gain from a given dose of caffeine. When your total arousal level is too high, you probably won't get any benefits from larger doses—and might even lose the benefits conferred by smaller doses.

The important factors that contribute to arousal are: dose of caffeine in proportion to body weight, baseline arousal (state of excitation when task performance begins, determined by personality type, gender, state of health, and state of fatigue), relative task complexity (complex tasks increase arousal levels), environmental arousal (loud noises or other harsh stimuli), and individual caffeine sensitivity. It should also be noted that the factors contributing to arousal levels are additive.

Therefore, because high arousal levels reduce mental performance, the dose of caffeine you use must be adjusted to account for all of these arousal factors. It is wrong to simply say that caffeine impairs performance at high arousal levels: lower doses may help more highly aroused people to perform better than they would have without caffeine, even though moderate doses may be too much for them.

9.2. Specific Cognitive Improvements Attributable to Caffeine

Psychometricians, who design IQ tests, have come up with the concept of "g," their name for the general intelligence that underlies achievement at school and success in the workplace. Important components of g include abstract reasoning, rapid information processing (27), verbal fluency, computational ability, and memory. Caffeine improves performance on all of these tests; in other words, caffeine raises the IQ and, by every objective measure, makes a person smarter.

Caffeine offers additional benefits to mental function apart from improving our thinking ability. By improving what is called "vigilance," the ability to sustain attention for a long period of time, and "divided attention," the ability to pay attention to two things at once, caffeine dramatically increases our capacity to focus on our work. As a result, we accomplish more and do it faster and with fewer errors. Adding further to its power as a "brain tonic," caffeine also improves psychomotor performance, enabling us, for example, to use a word processor more adeptly.

Many scientists have demonstrated that caffeine improves both the speed and the accuracy of logical reasoning. A particularly interesting study found that caffeine improved performance on something called a "semantic processing test," in which subjects were shown a series of statements and had to decide, based on general knowledge, which ones were true (28,29).

Caffeine enhances memory functions, such as delayed recall, recognition, semantic and verbal memory, and long-term memory, and improves performance on simple and sometimes on difficult memory tasks. A moderate dose of caffeine in the morning can improve memory for the entire day.

Psychomotor tasks are those that link our decisions about what action to take with executing the action. Everyday tasks that require good psychomotor control include driving and word processing, in which a person must use his brain to continuously direct the motions of his fingers and hands. Caffeine causes a highly significant improvement in most measures of psychomotor performance (30). This benefit does not decline with long-term caffeine use, nor does it require us to keep increasing the amount of caffeine to achieve these benefits.

Finally, even though caffeine sharpens mental performance in all age groups, it improves the performance of older people in reasoning, memory, and reaction time tests more than it does with younger people; in many cases, it closes the gap in performance between the older and younger group *(31)*.

9.3. Caffeine in Complex Real-Life Work Settings

Obviously, the mental challenges arising in real life are far more complex than the demands posed by laboratory experiments in cognition. Typically, laboratory studies employ well-defined tasks that require concentrating on one or two sources of stimuli or information and providing a relatively simple response. In contrast, real-life situations often require decision making in which incomplete or uncertain information must be gathered from many sources before reaching a complex decision and making a complex response. Research on caffeine's contributions to the cognitive processes in the workplace is limited. However, provocative studies do exist, suggesting that managerial performance is improved when either managers or employees are using caffeine *(31–33)*.

Caffeine contributes to other significant workplace benefits in addition to increasing wakefulness and alertness, sharpening reasoning, and improving memory and reaction time. For example, headaches are a common complaint in the workplace, whether caused by job tensions or other problems. One study has shown that workers actually use caffeine to relieve these headaches—one of the proven therapeutic uses of caffeine—which improves their efficiency *(34)*. Another contribution of caffeine to workplace performance depends on its power to relieve boredom. If caffeine is taken before undertaking repetitive work, habituation, that is, the discomforts that accompany repetition, is dramatically slowed, which means the person doesn't become bored as quickly. The result is that work becomes more pleasant, productive, and accurate *(35)*.

10. CAFFEINE AND ATHLETIC PERFORMANCE

Caffeine has always been recognized as an agent that stimulates the release of energy in the body. Among the Aztecs, the energy-giving power of cocoa was so jealously prized that, apart from the nobility, only soldiers on campaign and the pochta, a hereditary class of merchant-adventurers, were permitted to use it *(2)*. Montezuma I even promulgated a law that no one who had not participated in armed conflict, not even the king's son, could enjoy the privilege of consuming it. Similarly, American soldiers in World War II carried ration packs that included caffeine pills to keep them going strong in combat. For many years, athletes, specifically weight lifters and long-distance runners, swimmers, and cyclists, have relied on caffeine's energy-giving powers to boost their performance in training and competition *(36)*.

In the last few decades, scientists have demonstrated caffeine's benefits to muscle activity, physical training, competitive sports, endurance and, more recently, short-term physical activity as well. In his ambitious 2001 metastudy, Graham *(36)* concluded that caffeine improves performance in most, if not all, sports activities and has no detrimental side effects on athletes. Graham also stated that caffeine is a "powerful ergogenic aid" at urinary levels markedly below the permissible limit of the International Olympic Committee (IOC) of 12 mg/L (equivalent to about four 6-oz cups of filter coffee for a 150-lb person) and that it is beneficial in both training and competition *(2)*.

Caffeine enables the athlete to train at a greater power output, with greater speed, and for a longer time. It has also been proven to increase power, speed, and endurance in simulated and actual race conditions. Although old theories held that caffeine benefited only endurance athletics, we know now that caffeine's beneficial effects are operative in activities that last as few as 60 s. Although it is still not clear if caffeine can improve maximal strength, it makes a valuable contribution to strength training and performance by imparting enhanced endurance or resistance to fatigue and also by relieving pain. There is no evidence that caffeine ingestion before exercise leads to dehydration, ion imbalance, upset stomach, or other adverse effects.

Importantly, caffeine tolerance does not affect its ergogenic, or energy-producing, benefits, which means that both nonusers and long-term users will respond to it in the same way and to the same degree. Men and women metabolize caffeine in the same way, and, given the same dose of caffeine in proportion to their body weight, will exhibit the same blood levels and concentrations of metabolites, the substances into which caffeine is transformed by the body. It is unknown how caffeine produces its ergogenic and other athletic benefits, but they may be a result of a combination of its systemic CNS effects and its local effects on muscle tissue (36).

Recent work strongly suggests that there are major differences in the ergogenic benefits from caffeine consumption in the matrix of coffee as compared with taking caffeine pills (37). For example, in one study, high-performance runners ran to exhaustion at a pace approximating their best time on a 10 ki (6 mi) run. Caffeine, approx 4.5 mg/kg (or approx 300 mg for a 150-lb man, about as much as is found in 2 cups of filtered coffee) mixed with water, when taken 1 h before the run, produced a remarkable improvement in endurance of nearly 33%, an increase in running time from 32 min to 41 min. However, surprisingly, the same amount of caffeine delivered in coffee (or in decaffeinated coffee mixed with powdered caffeine) produced no improvement.

The study by Graham et al. (37) concludes that tolerance does not develop to caffeine's ergogenic actions. In other words, all other things being equal, a dose of caffeine will give the same boost to an athlete who never used caffeine and to one who uses it every day, and, moreover, will continue to deliver the same boost indefinitely. This was confirmed by Wiles et al. (38), who administered 2–2.5 mg/kg of caffeine (equivalent to a 6–8 oz cup of filterer coffee for a 150-lb person) to 1500-m runners and "found no relationship between caffeine habits and degree of performance response."

11. CONCLUSIONS

Caffeine is the world's most popular drug, used regularly by approx 90% of the US population. One of a group of purine alkaloids, caffeine is fat soluble and passes readily through plasma membranes and is quickly and completely diffused throughout the body. Caffeine exhibits a complex pattern of biotransformation, producing a dozen different metabolites. More than 98% of ingested caffeine is metabolized and excreted in the urine. Study of this metabolism is impeded by its remarkable variation between humans.

Caffeine's mean elimination half-life is from 3–7 h. However, the half-life exhibits great variation and is influenced by diverse factors, including the use of oral contraceptives and other medications, alcohol consumption, cigarette smoking, and genetic determinants. Caffeine acts as a competitive antagonist of adenosine, and it achieves many of its stimulant effects by blocking adenosine's uptake. Caffeine also exerts its effects by inhibiting the enzyme phosphodiesterase and the destruction of the intracellular second messenger cAMP.

In the United States, most caffeine is consumed in coffee, but significant amounts also are consumed in tea and carbonated soft drinks. In other countries, it is found in several other drinks brewed from plant products, such as maté leaves or cola nuts. The average cup of coffee is often believed to contain 100 mg of caffeine, but this figure is probably too low for most of the large cups of filtered coffees served today. A better estimate is that a 6-oz cup of filter drip coffee contains approx 150 mg of caffeine.

Caffeine users typically demonstrate both a tolerance to some of the effects of the drug and withdrawal symptoms when its use is abruptly discontinued. Caffeine should not be called "addictive," however, because, in today's scientific lexicon, this word is reserved for drugs that can cause serious disruption of people's lives. Furthermore, caffeine does not demonstrate deleterious effects on physical or mental performance and may actually improve performance in this regard.

12. MAIN POINTS FOR PRIMARY AND CLINICAL REVIEW

1. In the United States, approx 70% of caffeine comes from coffee, approx 14% from tea, over 12% is from soft drinks, and nearly 3% is from cocoa beans.
2. A cup of coffee typically has between 100 mg and 250 mg of caffeine with a range of 50–350 mg.
3. Caffeine has no association with overall mortality rate.
4. Caffeine causes mild dependence and, as a result, when its use is suddenly discontinued, there are mild withdrawal symptoms, such as headache.
5. Caffeine itself increases arousal levels, cognitive performance, psychomotor performance, and sports performance.

REFERENCES

1. James JE. Caffeine and Health. Harcourt Brace Javonovich, London, 1991.
2. Weinberg BA, Bealer BK. The World of Caffeine. Routledge, New York, 2001.
3. Shirlow MJ. Patterns of caffeine consumption. Human Nutr Appl Nutr 1983;37a:307–313.
4. Gilbert RM. Caffeine: The Most Popular Stimulant. Chelsea House, New York, NY, 1992.
5. Garattini S. (ed.) Caffeine, Coffee, and Health. Raven Press, New York, NY, 1993.
6. Sewester CS. (ed.) Drug Facts and Comparisons. J. B. Lippincott Company, Philadelphia, PA, 1999.
7. Weinberg BA, Bealer BK. The Caffeine Advantage. Free Press, New York, NY, 2002.
8. James JE. Caffeine and Health. Harcourt Brace Javonovich, London, 1991.
9. Caffeine's ability to antagonize alcohol-induced drowsiness is the one antagonism that James finds the most credible.
10. Howell LL, Coffin VL, Spealman RD. Behavioral and physiological effects of xanthines in non human primates. Psychopharmacology (Berl) 1997;129:1–14.
11. Nehlig A, Daval JL, Debry G. Caffeine and the central nervous system: mechanisms of action, biochemical, metabolic and psychostimulant effects. Brain Res Brain Res Rev 1992;17:139–170.
12. Julien RM. A Primer of Drug Action. W. H. Freeman and Company, New York, NY, 2001.
13. Caffeine, coffee, and cancer [editorial]. Br Med J 1976;1:1031–1032.
14. Curatolo PW, Robertson D. The health consequences of caffeine. Ann Intern Med 1983;98:641–653.
15. Grobbee DE, Rimm EB, Giovannucci E, Colditz G, Stampfer M, Willett W. Coffee, caffeine, and cardiovascular disease in men. N Engl J Med 1990;323:1026–1032.

16. Wilson PW, Garrison RJ, Kannel WB, McGee DL, Castelli WP. Is coffee consumption a contributor to cardiovascular disease? Insights from the Framingham Study. Arch Intern Med 1989;149:1169–1172.

17. Heyden S, Tyroler HA, Heiss G, Hames CG, Bartel A. Coffee consumption and mortality. Total mortality, stroke mortality, and coronary heart disease mortality. Arch Intern Med 1978;138:1472–1475.

18. Wilhelmsen L, Tibblin G, Elmfeldt D, Wedel H, Werko L. Coffee consumption and coronary heart disease in middle-aged Swedish men. Acta Med Scand 1977;201:547–552.

19. Onrot J, Goldberg MR, Biaggioni I, Hollister AS, Kingaid D, Robertson D. Hemodynamic and humoral effects of caffeine in autonomic failure. Therapeutic implications for postprandial hypotension. N Engl J Med 1985;313:549–554.

20. Adamson R. Evaluation of coffee and caffeine for mutagenic, carcinogenic and anticarcinogenic activity. In: Caffeinated Beverages. Parliament TH (ed.). American Chemical Society, Washington, DC, 2000, pp. 75–76.

21. Nussberger J, Mooser V, Maridor G, Juillerat L, Waeber B, Brunner HR. Caffeine-induced diruesis and atrial natruiretic peptides. J Cardiovasc Pharmacol 1990;15:685–691.

22. Armstrong LE. Caffeine, body fluid-electrolyte balance, and exercise performance. Int J Sprot Nutr Exerc Metab 2002;12:189–206.

23. Wemple RD, Lamb DR, McKeever KH. Caffeine vs caffeine-free sports drinks: effects on urine production at rest and during prolonged exercise. Int J Sprots Med. 1997;18:40–46.

24. Bridge N. Coffee drinking as a frequent cause of disease. Transact Assoc Am Physicians 1893;8: 281–288.

25. Schster CR, Kuhar MJ. (eds.) Handbook of Experimental Pharmacology. Springer-Verlag, Berlin, 1996, pp. 315–341.

26. Hayreh SS. Lancet 1973;1:45.

27. Eysenck HJ. A New Look Intelligence. Transaction Publishers, New Brunswick, NJ, 1998.

28. Smith AP, Brockman P, Flynn R, Maben A, Thomas M. Investigation of the effects of coffee on alertness and performance during the day and night. Neuropsychobiology 1993;27:217–223.

29. Smith A, Kendrick A, Maben A, Salmon J. Effects of breakfast and caffeine on cognitive performance, mood and cardiovascular functioning. Appetite 1994;22:39–55.

30. Rogers PJ, Richardson NJ, Dernoncourt C. Caffeine use: is there a net benefit for mood and psychomotor performance? Neuropsychobiology 1995;31:195–199.

31. Streufert S, Satish U, Pogash R, et al. Excess coffee consumption in simulated complex work settings: detriment or facilitation of performance? J Appl Psychol 1997;82:774–782.

32. Streufert S, Pogash R, Miller J, et al. Effects of caffeine deprivation on complex human functioning. Psychopharmacology (Berl) 1995;118:377–384.

33. Cole KJ, Costill DL, Starling RD, Goodpaster BH, Trappe SW, Fink WJ. Effect of caffeine ingestion on perception of effort and subsequent work production. Int J Sport Nutr 1996;6:14–23.

34. Sargeant J, Solbach P. Stress and headache in the workplace: the role of caffeine. Med Psychotherapeutics 1996;1:83.

35. http://knowledge.wharton.upenn.edu/121901_ss6.html. Wharton School of the University of Pennsylvania, PA. Retrieved September 7, 2002 from Caffeine: stimulant to better living or a dangerous and sinful vice?

36. Graham TE. Caffeine and exercise: metabolism, endurance and performance. Sports Med 2001;31: 785–807.

37. Graham TE, Hibbert E, Sathasivam P. Metabolic and exercise endurance effects of coffee and caffeine ingestion. J Appl Physiol 1998;85:883–889.

38. Wiles JD, Bird SR, Hopkins J, Riley M. Effect of caffeinated coffee on running speed, respiratory factors, blood lactate and perceived exertion during 1500-m treadmill running. Br J Sports Med 1992; 26:116–120.

13 The Therapeutic Use and Safety of Common Herbal Beverages

Winston J. Craig

1. INTRODUCTION

Drinking herbal beverages is popular in America for several reasons. Herbal teas provide opportunities to have a low-calorie beverage or a healthy caffeine-free alternative to coffee. Other teas may provide a medicinal effect. These herbal beverages may contain extracts from the bark, roots, seeds, flowers, leaves, or fruits of trees and shrubs. Today, the herbal tea industry has become a multimillion-dollar business. The potential health effect of green and black teas is reviewed in Chapter 10.

It was common for American Indians to use herbal preparations to treat various ailments and illnesses. For example, a tea made from Yarrow leaves was used to cure stomach disorders, to treat hemorrhaging, and break a fever. Bee balm was prepared as a tea by the Oswego Indians to treat colic, colds, fevers, stomachaches, nosebleeds, and insomnia. Witch hazel was used to treat rheumatism, hemorrhoids, backaches, cuts, insect bites, and bruises. Wild yam was used to treat gastrointestinal (GI) problems and to relieve labor pains, and slippery elm was used as a soothing laxative. Various Native-American tribes used motherwort to treat gynecologic disorders, whereas a tea made from goldenseal root was used as a general tonic.

After Europeans came to America, other herbal teas were used for various purposes. For example, hop tea was useful to induce sleep, passionflower was used to treat insomnia, and peppermint tea was successfully used to relieve nausea and indigestion. In addition, willow bark was used for muscle aches and pains and to treat fevers, and white oak bark was used as a gargle for sore throats and to relieve skin problems (1).

To avoid consuming caffeine-containing beverages, some people choose cereal-based beverages. These were originally developed from roasted cereals and molasses. Years ago, these coffee substitutes were popular. Because these beverages stimulate gastric acid secretion (2), persons who develop peptic ulcer should not consume the roasted cereal beverages on an empty stomach.

From: *Beverages in Nutrition and Health*
Edited by: T. Wilson and N. J. Temple © Humana Press Inc., Totowa, NJ

2. NEW TRENDS

Food manufacturers have started adding herbal products to teas, juices, soups, and snack foods to facilitate their marketing as functional foods. *Ginkgo biloba*, St. John's Wort, and Kava kava are herbs typical of those added to foods and beverages. This recent practice raises numerous concerns. Some people may be allergic to the added herbs, and there may be contraindications for women who are pregnant and lactating, as well as safety concerns for small children.

There are limited data available about whether the herbs are effective when taken long-term and regularly as part of a food or beverage. The effects of beverage processing methods on the herb activity are unknown. The risk of a potential interaction between an added herb and a conventional drug is increased when the herb is regularly consumed as part of the diet and is, likewise, a largely uninvestigated area of potential health significance.

3. POTENCY OF HERBAL INGREDIENTS IS VARIABLE

In supermarkets and health food stores today, there are several different herbal beverages with such catchy names as Scarlet Sunrise, Lemon Appeal, Sunburst C, Tangy Autumn, Mint Magic, and Country Peach Passion. These herbal beverages may provide some therapeutic medicinal value. Those herbal beverages for which therapeutic properties are claimed may vary widely in their potency; therefore, a desired effect may be obtained. In addition, reaction to a particular herb can vary greatly from one person to another.

The potency of herbal beverages, and, hence, their effectiveness, cannot be accurately predicted, because the concentration of active ingredients in the plant material can vary enormously. Several factors can influence the potency of a herb, such as age of the plant, growing conditions, growing location, storage and handling procedures, extraction methods, and postharvest processing. Any of these factors may produce a wide variation in the properties associated with an herbal tea.

Poor standardization of herbal teas can produce unreliable effects due to the great variation in the active constituents. The lack of standardization can contribute to the risk of overdose. In a recent study of 25 commercial ginseng preparations, the concentration of marker compounds differed greatly from the label claims *(3)*. There was also significant variability in the concentration of the marker compounds from one brand of product to another. Among *Panax* samples, the level of ginsenosides ranged from 18% to 137% of the label claim. Among the Siberian ginseng samples, the level of eleutherosides ranged from 12% to 328% of label claim. The concentrations of ginsenosides varied by 15-fold in capsules and 36-fold in liquid products, although the concentrations of eleutherosides varied by 43- and 184-fold in capsules and liquids, respectively *(3)*.

Other issues to consider relate to species identification and whether the correct part of the plant is used. Different species of a particular genus may not act similarly. For example, the three species of *Echinacea* have different activities. The oral use of the upper parts of *Echinacea purpurea* are recognized as beneficial for colds and respiratory infections, whereas it is the roots and not the upper parts of *E. pallida* that are useful for the treatment of influenza-like infections. On the other hand, neither the root nor the upper parts of *E. angustifolia* provide any benefit for the treatment of respiratory tract infections *(4)*. Because of the worldwide shortage of Echinacea, some manufacturers have diluted their Echinacea preparations with wild quinine root, a cheaper look-alike substitute, which is inactive.

4. CONCERN REGARDING THE CONTENTS

In 1975, the Food and Drug Administration (FDA) evaluated 171 herbs commonly used for brewing teas. Of these, 27 herbs were classified as unsafe, and 91 were determined to be safe. The safety of the remaining 53 could not be determined conclusively; neither could it be predicted with any certainty what their physiologic effects would be at various concentrations. To alert consumers to the dangers of the unsafe herbs, the FDA compiled a list of those herbs that should not be used in foods, beverages, or drugs *(5)*. Table 1 is a compilation describing the properties of the herbs listed by the FDA.

The FDA also believes that the consumer needs better protection from mislabeling of herbs. Some herbal products may be contaminated with substances other than those declared on the label. For example, a woman who was taking burdock root tea complained of blurred vision, hallucinations, dry mouth, and other anticholinergic symptoms. Analysis of the tea indicated that the commercial product contained a substantial level of atropine *(6)*.

Some ginseng and other herbal preparations contain added substances to provide a desired stimulant property *(7)*. A recent analysis of ginseng suggested that caffeine was present in some ginseng products in varying amounts. Because ginseng does not contain caffeine, the presence of that substance indicates that it was added to some ginseng products, presumably to mimic or potentiate the ginseng effect *(8)*. In another study, 8 out of 21 ginseng brands were contaminated with significant levels of pesticides, whereas others had significant lead levels. Almost one in four Gingko products tested did not have the advertised levels of the active ingredient *Gingko biloba* extract *(9)*.

Although some herbal teas contain physiologically active constituents, they may not necessarily be suitable for regular use. The appropriate use of herbal teas that possess medicinal value is considered safe and may provide useful relief, but the indiscriminate or excessive use of herbal teas is not recommended and could be harmful in some cases *(10)*. Echinacea is likely to lose its effectiveness if taken daily on a continuous basis. It is best taken at the onset of cold or flu symptoms and continued for 2 wk, followed by a resting period of a least 1 wk.

5. BEWARE OF TOXICITIES

Because manufacturers are not required to list potential toxicities on the labels, consumers may be unknowingly exposed to harmful substances. More than 30 herbal teas contain substances that cause serious toxicities, including liver, GI tract, nervous system, and circulatory system disorders *(11)*.

Chaparral, an herbal preparation made from the leaves of the creosote bush (*Larrea tridentata*) of the American southwest desert, is used in teas, capsules, and tablet preparations. Chaparral is promoted for the treatment of cancer, to retard aging, and as a free radical scavenger because of its antioxidant properties. In December 1992, the FDA Center for Food Safety and Applied Nutrition issued a warning suggesting a potential link between chaparral use and liver toxicity after six cases of hepatitis were reported after

Table 1
Unsafe Herbal Tea Ingredients

Common name	Botanical name	Properties
Arnica	*Arnica montana* L.	Produces violent gastroenteritis
Bittersweet	*Solanum dulcamara* L.	Contains the toxic alkaloids solanine, solanidine
Bloodroot	*Sanguinaris canadensis* L.	Contains toxic alkaloids, including sanguinarine.
Calamus (sweet flag)	*Acorus calamus* L.	Oil of calamus causes cancer
Deadly nightshade	*Atropa belladonna* L.	Contains the toxic alkaloids, hyoscyamine, atropine and hyoscine
Heliotrope	*Heliotropium europaeum* L.	Contains alkaloids that cause liver damage
Henbane	*Hyoscyamus niger* L.	Contains the poisonous alkaloids atropine, scopolamine, and hyoscyamine
Jalap	*Ipomoea jalapa* Nutt.	Resin of this vine has powerful purgative properties
Jimson weed	*Datura stramonium* L.	Contains atropine, hyoscyamine, and scopolamine
Lily of the Valley	*Convallaria majalis* L.	Contains toxic cardiac glycosides convallatoxin, convallarin, and convallamarin
Lobelia or Indian tobacco	*Lobelia inflata* L.	Contains lobeline and other pyridine alkaloids
Mandrake	*Mandragora officinarum* L.	A poisonous narcotic containing alkaloids hyoscyamine, scopolamine, and mandragorine
Mayapple	*Podophyllum peltatum* L.	A poisonous plant containing podophyllotoxin; the green fruit causes gastroenteritis and vomiting
Mistletoe	*Phoradendron flavescens* Nutt.	Contains toxic pressor amines
Morning glory	*Ipomoea purpurea* L.	Seeds contain amides of lysergic acid
Periwinkle	*Vinca major* L.	Contains vinblastine and vincristine that have cytotoxic and neurological actions
Poison hemlock	*Conium maculatum* L.	Contains coniine and other toxic alkaloids
Scotch broom	*Cytisus scoparius* L.	Contains the toxic alkaloids sparteine and isosparteine
Wormwood	*Artemisia absinthium* L.	Volatile oil is a narcotic poison

consumption of the herb. Some of the serious liver problems required hospitalization *(12)*. Reports suggest that chaparral has an adverse effect on the liver *(13)*. A 60-yr-old woman who had taken chaparral for 10 mo suffered such serious liver damage that she required a liver transplant *(14)*. Nordihydroguaiaretic acid, an antioxidant in chaparral, is a potent inhibitor of the lipoxygenase pathway, even at low doses. At higher concentrations, it also inhibits the cyclooxygenase pathway.

An herbal tea containing woodruff, melilot, and tonka beans produced abnormal clotting function and mild clinical bleeding due to its high content of natural anticoagulants called coumadins *(15)*. Deaths have also been reported from the use of herbal teas made from oleander leaves (*Nerium oleander*) that are rich in toxic cardiac glycosides *(16)* and mistletoe berries (*Viscum album*) that contain viscotoxin and other toxic principles *(17)*.

A tea made from Pau d'arco (*Tabebuia impetiginosa*), also called lapacho or taheebo, is prepared from the inner bark of Tabebuia trees of South America and is used as a herbal cancer "cure" *(10)*. Research conducted by the National Cancer Institute has not confirmed any anticancer activity in Pau d'arco. Undesirable Pau d'arco side effects reported in human studies include nausea and GI distress. Although it is widely used outside the United States by herbalists to treat viral, fungal, and bacterial infections, it is not recommended due to its mild toxicity.

Using herbal teas in home remedies for common childhood illnesses may trigger serious health problems for the child. Peppermint and chamomile teas are commonly used among Mexican-American populations. Their prolonged use, in the absence of normal food, may result in water intoxication and seizures in young children resulting from an inadequate sodium intake *(18)*.

Furthermore, many herbal beverages are actually a concoction of several herbs. With the lack of comprehensive data on individual herbs, it is difficult to predict the combined effect of a complex mixture of herbs that may act in concert, in conflict, or synergistically with each other.

6. CARCINOGENIC HERBS

Several commonly used herbal teas are potentially carcinogenic, because they contain substances that cause tumors in experimental animals *(19)*. Bayberry tea (*Myrica cerifera*) contains a family of phenolic compounds, comfrey tea (*Symphytum officinale*) contains symphytine and other alkaloids, and sassafras (*Sassafras albidum*) contains safrole. Safrole was used as a flavoring agent for soft drinks, such as root beer, until the FDA banned its use in 1960 after safrole was shown to be a liver carcinogen. Despite the legal restrictions, sassafras is freely available in health food stores throughout the country. A cup of strong sassafras tea may contain up to 200 mg of safrole, more than four times the minimal amount believed hazardous to humans if consumed regularly *(20)*.

In addition to the tumor-causing properties of symphytine in comfrey, the pyrrolizidine alkaloid components are also hepatotoxic and may cause liver failure *(21)*. Serious liver damage has been reported from a daily consumption of comfrey tea and capsules. Although it is toxic, comfrey is widely available in commercial preparations as a tea, a powder, and as capsules. Coltsfoot tea (*Tussilago farfara*) is a popular folk remedy for coughs and bronchial congestion from throat-soothing mucilage. Coltsfoot contains senkirkine, a pyrrolizidine alkaloid, that produces liver tumors *(10)*.

Some herbs may increase the risk of cancer, whereas others may diminish the risk. Rosemary, sage, thyme, and red clover contain terpenoids and phenolic compounds that possibly provide some measure of protection against cancer.

7. NUTRIENT AND DRUG INTERACTIONS

One must be aware of the interactions between herbs and nutrients and between herbs and medications. Many herbal teas are rich in tannins, which can bind with minerals or conventional drugs. Hence, the bioavailability of minerals such as iron and calcium can diminish substantially, and the teas may decrease the effectiveness of administered drugs. Due to the therapeutic components of some herbal beverages, their use with conventional drugs may enhance or negate the medications' effect *(22)*. For example, nonsteroidal antiinflammatory drugs (NSAIDS) negate the effect of feverfew for treating migraines. The activity of anticoagulants, such as warfarin, is enhanced by the use of ginkgo or garlic, which are also blood thinners. Valerian, when ingested concomitantly with barbiturates, can cause excessive sedation.

8. SAFE AND PROPER USE OF HERBS

Some individuals who believe that a certain herb provides a therapeutic effect may experience some medicinal benefit, even though there are no known active components in the herb (a placebo effect). Some herbal products may not be detrimental to one's health, but their use may involve substantial expenditures, with the hope of obtaining some therapeutic benefit. This expectation often results from the exaggerated claims that are made for the products. Although the products may not be harmful themselves, they often deflect people away from choosing a balanced approach to good eating and healthful living.

Physicians and consumers must be made aware of herbal toxicities. Labels warning of potential side effects of herbal tea components are not required by law; therefore, inadvertent exposure to harmful ingredients in herb teas should be expected. The subtle cases of herbal tea toxicity may pass by unnoticed unless the public and physicians are alerted to such issues *(23,24)*.

Self-medication using an herbal product for a serious health condition is not recommended. In such a case, safe and proper medical help may be delayed unnecessarily. For example, using capsules containing yucca to treat rheumatoid arthritis may be harmless and they are also ineffective. To depend upon the saponin-containing yucca extract for therapeutic help may allow the inflammatory disease to progress, causing further disability.

The consumer should be careful in selecting the source of information about herbs and herbal teas, because there are many unreliable sources available. The sales clerk at the local health food store or the salesperson who works for a company based on pyramid marketing should not be considered an expert on supplements or the therapeutic benefit of herbal products. Many books, magazines, newspapers, and talk shows provide unreliable or misleading herbal information. There are, fortunately, numerous books available that contain reliable herbal information *(10,22,25–27)*. Furthermore, there are some guidelines for the safe use of common herbal beverages (*see* Table 2).

Table 2
Guidelines for Safe Use of Herbal Beverages

The following guidelines are recommended to ensure the safe use of herbal beverages *(28)*:

1. Refrain from considering herbal beverages as natural panaceas. They are not a substitute for a healthy lifestyle, which includes a good diet, regular exercise, and adequate rest and relaxation.
2. Be acquainted with the toxicities of certain herbs (*see* Table 1).
3. Read labels carefully. Use only prepackaged teas with safe ingredients.
4. Avoid unlabeled bulk teas.
5. Teas used in a prophylactic fashion should not be used continuously for long periods of time without regular periods of nonuse.
6. Pregnant women should use caution in drinking any herbal tea because few have been thoroughly tested for safety. Pregnant women should consult with their physicians regarding the use of herbal teas. Likewise young children should be restricted in their use of herbal teas.
7. No more than 1–2 cups of tea should be consumed per day on a regular basis. The long-term effect of drinking most herbal teas in large quantities is unknown.
8. The use of a herb tea for a specific medical problem should not be a substitute for competent medical advice.
9. Individuals who regularly use herbal products should discuss with their health-care provider the medicinal effects of such herbs.
10. Individuals who are allergic to ragweed, asters, or chrysanthemums should avoid teas containing yarrow and chamomile.

8.1. Diuretics

Numerous teas and herbal preparations have also been widely used as diuretics to treat premenstrual syndrome and other conditions. Extracts of goldenrod (*Solidago sp.*), juniper (*Juniperus communis*), parsley (*Petroselinum crispum*), bearberry or uva ursi (*Arctostaphylos uva-ursi*), fennel (*Foeniculum vulgare*), and stinging nettle (*Urtica dioica*) are modestly effective diuretics that may be used safely in moderation, either singly or in various combinations *(10)*. Of these, goldenrod is probably the most effective diuretic. It also possesses antiinflammatory and antibacterial activity. The active constituents of goldenrod include flavonoids, tannins, and saponins *(25)*. There are no reports of adverse reactions from its use.

The dried ripe berries of the juniper tree (*J. communis*) function as a diuretic and also provide antiseptic activity for the urinary tract. Juniper's diuretic effect results from its content of terpinen-4-ol, which increases the glomerular filtration rate in the kidney. One must exercise caution when using juniper berries, because large amounts may produce kidney damage characterized by albuminuria or renal hematuria *(25)*. Juniper tea is also contraindicated during pregnancy.

Stinging nettle (*U. dioica*) is feared by many because its leaves and stems are covered with tiny hairs that inject formic acid and release histamine when touched. However, the stinging irritant is tamed by cooking or drying. The dried leaves of *U. dioica* possess diuretic activity, possibly due to its high flavonoid content *(26)*. Stinging nettle preparations are also reported to provide substantial relief for hay fever sufferers *(29)*. Stinging nettle has recently become popular for symptomatic relief of urinary difficulties associated with benign prostate hypertrophy.

Additional herbs that possess weak diuretic activity include the dandelion (*Taraxacum officinale*), hibiscus (*Hibiscus sabdariffa* L.), horsetail (*Equisetum arvense* L.), and rose hips (*Rosa* spp.) *(10,30)*. Parsley is widely used in salads and soups as a garnish. The leaves and roots of parsley are helpful for reducing urinary tract inflammations. Bearberry or uva ursi is also effective against urinary tract infections as a result of its antibacterial action. Its antiseptic action results from the presence of two phenolic glycosides. For bearberry to be effective, the urine must be alkaline *(25)*. Juice made from cranberry (*Vaccinium macrocarpon*) also provides protection against the colonization of *Esherichia coli* bacteria in urinary tract infections *(31)* (*see* Chapter 4).

8.2. Special Herbs for Women

Some women may use herbal teas during pregnancy to get away from caffeine-containing beverages. However, because of the potentially embryotoxic, teratogenic, and abortifacient effects of some herbal teas, pregnant women are advised to exercise moderation in their use of herbal beverages *(32)*. Before using any herbal tea, a pregnant woman should first consult with her physician.

A tea made from the above-ground parts of motherwort (*Leonurus cardiaca* L.), a member of the mint family, has been used to treat amenorrhea and irregular menstruation and to stimulate uterine activity. Motherwort contains the alkaloids stachydrine and leonurine, as well as flavonoids, iridoids, tannins, and terpenoids. Extracts of motherwort have shown antispasmodic, cardiotonic, hypotensive, and sedative properties *(26)*. Motherwort is not recommended during pregnancy.

Shepherd's purse (*Capsella bursa-pastoris*) is a member of the mustard family and grows as a weed in backyards, farmlands, and roadsides nationwide. Its name derives from the purse shape of the seedpods of the plant. The above-ground parts can be prepared into capsules, tablets, or a tea. The plant has been historically used for its antihemorrhagic action. It is used in Europe today for the symptomatic treatment of nosebleeds and mild menorrhagia and metrorrhagia *(26)*.

The fruit of the chaste tree (*Vitex agnus-castus*) has been used for centuries for menstrual difficulties. Today, it is used to treat premenstrual syndrome (PMS) and menstrual irregularities *(26)*. In a recent study, 93% of patients treated with vitex experienced alleviation or elimination of PMS symptoms, such as breast tenderness, bloating, irritability, headache, anger, and depression *(33)*.

Red raspberry (*Rubus idaeus*) is commonly used by women to shorten labor and facilitate an easier childbirth. Red raspberry contains a compound that produces more regular uterine contractions; hence, raspberry is widely used as a childbirth aid *(25)*. An Australian study found raspberry leaves safe and effective for shortening the second stage of labor *(34)*. The study also indicated that women ingesting raspberry leaves might be less likely to experience premature rupture of their membranes or require a Caesarean section, forceps, or vacuum birth than the control group *(35)*. Red raspberry is also used as a mouthwash and gargle for sore throats due to its astringent properties.

8.3. Stimulants

There are several commonly consumed herbal beverages that stimulate the central nervous system (CNS). Guarana (made from the crushed seed of the Brazilian shrub *Paullinia cupana* H.B.K.) and maté (the dried leaves of *Ilex paraguariensis*) are Latin American herbs with stimulatory properties, due to the high levels of caffeine they contain—approx 3.5% and 2% caffeine, respectively *(10)*. A typical 6-oz cup of maté may contain 25–50 mg of caffeine. Green tea (*Camellia sinesis*) may contain approx 35–65 mg of caffeine per cup, whereas lemon-flavored Lipton green tea contains approx 15 mg caffeine per 12-oz can. Each of these beverages provides substantially less caffeine than coffee, which provides approx 60–130 mg/cup (*see* Chapter 10).

Ephedra spp. (*Ma huang*) is commonly used for the treatment of respiratory ailments, such as bronchial asthma. Ephedra contains the alkaloid stimulants ephedrine and pseudoephedrine. Because of its adrenergic properties, ephedrine has been widely used as a nasal decongestant and to treat bronchial asthma *(25)*. Ephedra, combined with caffeine, is also promoted for use as a diet aid to help in weight-loss programs and is also sold as an energy-boosting formula. Ephedra can raise both systolic and diastolic blood pressure and the heart rate.

Side effects of ephedra include insomnia, motor restlessness, nausea, headaches, irritability, dizziness, tachycardia, urination disturbances, and vomiting *(26)*. With such side effects, it is recommended to avoid any indiscriminate or heavy use, especially by persons with heart conditions, hypertension, diabetes, or thyroid disease. The misuse and abuse of ephedra products, especially when combined with caffeine, has led to more than 20 deaths and hundreds of reports of adverse effects, prompting a closer look at such products. The German Commission E recommends that ephedra preparations should only be used short-term because of the danger of addiction and side effects. Presently, the FDA has attempted to impose stricter regulations for ephedra products.

8.4. Ginseng

Asian ginseng (*Panax ginseng*) is sold as a tea, a tea ingredient, or as a powdered beverage additive. It is marketed as a tonic to combat feelings of lassitude and debility, to boost energy and enhance endurance, and to help increase concentration. Ginseng is also considered an adaptogen to help an individual cope with stress *(36)*. The major active ingredients of ginseng root are a group of approx 20 saponins (triterpenoid glycosides) called ginsenosides.

Different ginseng fractions may have conflicting effects. For example, some components may stimulate the CNS, and others may have a sedative action *(22)*. Experiments reveal that ginsenosides have antiinflammatory activity, enhance immune activity, and inhibit blood clotting *(22)*. Earlier reports from various researchers show that Asian ginseng extract increased mental alertness and concentration, increased work efficiency and shortened reaction times, and enhanced adaptation to environmental stresses. Most of these studies were not placebo-controlled or double blind. More recent definitive studies provide little convincing evidence that ginseng affects physical or mental performance or general well-being *(37,38)*.

The popularity of ginseng as a general tonic to improve health and to increase energy, stamina, and endurance is reflected in its enormous annual sales. It has been suggested that for effectiveness, ginseng be used no longer than 3 mo, then discontinued for 2 to 4 wk. Ginseng may also lack effectiveness because its contents vary considerably. As noted, the lack of standardization in the content of ginsenosides may explain the variable results obtained with ginseng *(3,39)*.

8.5. Effective Sedation

Several herbal teas are available that provide some relief from anxiety and insomnia. The dried rhizome and roots of valerian (*Valerianae radix*) is an example of an herb that can be effectively used to treat anxiety and insomnia. Valerian has been used as a mild tranquilizer and sleep aid for more than 1000 yr. It reduces sleep latency and wake time after sleep onset occurs *(40)*. A tea prepared from a teaspoonful of dried rhizome and roots can be safely taken several times daily. There have been no reports of side effects or contraindications to its use *(25)*.

Because of its mild sedative action, passionflower (*Passiflora incarnata*) is widely used in Europe to treat nervous anxiety and restlessness and sleep disturbances. Pharmacological studies show that passionflower acts as a sedative, anxiolytic, and antispasmodic. Its sedative and anxiety-relieving activity is possibly due to several substances that may act synergistically *(26,41)*.

Lemon balm (*Melissa officinalis*) has pleasant tasting citrus-scented leaves that can be brewed into a delicious tea. Melissa is used in Europe as a sedative to treat insomnia caused by nervous conditions and to treat digestive disorders *(26)*. The active principles of lemon balm are found in the terpenoid-rich oil of the leaves—citronellal, geraniol, linalool, citral, limonene, caryophyllene, and eugenol *(42)*. Mixtures of the above herbs (valerian, lemon balm, and passionflower) are often available as an aid to treat anxiety and sleeplessness.

Hops are the fruit of the vine *Humulus lupulus*. Hop teas are commonly used to relieve insomnia, restlessness, nervous tension, sleep disturbances, and other nervous conditions. The active principles of hops include the essential oil components (including humulene, myrcene, beta-caryophyllene, and farnesene) and the resinous bitter principles (including humulone and lupulone). During storage the latter two compounds degrade to 2-methyl-3-buten-2-ol, which has CNS depressing activity *(25,26)*.

8.6. Herbs for Gastrointestinal Problems

German chamomile (*Matricaria recutita*) is marketed in Europe to treat several ailments. It has been used for centuries to settle an upset stomach, to soothe aches and pains, and to heal bruises. Chamomile has been used effectively both internally and externally for its antiinflammatory, antispasmodic, and antibacterial properties *(25,26)*. Chamomile tea is used to relieve GI spasms, indigestion, peptic ulcers, and menstrual cramps. To be effective, chamomile tea should be made from the fresh herb. Rinses or gargles are used to treat inflammations and irritations of the mouth, gums, and respiratory tract.

The blue oil obtained from chamomile contains numerous terpenoids and flavonoids that provide the antiinflammatory and antispasmodic effects. The major activity of chamomile is believed to be provided by alpha-bisabolol, which comprises approx 10% to 15% of the essential oil *(36)*. Unfortunately, much of the commercial chamomile oil available in the United States has been adulterated with cheaper inactive material. People allergic to flowers in the daisy family may suffer allergic reactions with chamomile.

Goldenseal (*Hydrastis canadensis*), a member of the buttercup family, is a commonly used herbal tea. It is widely used as an antiseptic, to stop bleeding, as an antiinflammatory for the mucous membranes, for nasal congestions, and as a general tonic *(1,30)*. Goldenseal can also stimulate IgM antibody production *(30)*. The dried rhizomes and roots of goldenseal contain the alkaloids berberine and hydrastine, which have antibacterial properties. Berberine provides both the yellow color and bitter taste to goldenseal roots and is reported to be effective against influenza viruses *(43)*. Because the alkaloids are poorly absorbed in humans, goldenseal teas are not expected to achieve berberine and hydrastine blood concentrations high enough to be effective *(30)*.

Medicinal rhubarbs (*Rheum palmatum* and *R. officinale*) are members of the buckwheat family and originate from China. Their roots have been used as laxatives for thousands of years. A tea made from the rhubarb root is a useful laxative because of the presence of anthroquinone glycosides. The root extract stimulates intestinal motility and, by virtue of its astringent properties, is especially useful to relieve hemorrhoids *(44)*.

Horehound (*Marrubium vulgare*), a bitter-flavored member of the mint family, has long been used as a stimulant of the appetite and bile production and to treat coughs and catarrhs of the respiratory tract. Although there are no known side effects or contra-indications, the use of the bitter digestive tonic is not as widespread as might be expected *(45)*.

Rosemary tea (*Rosmarinus officinalis*) is recognized for its ability to resolve dyspeptic complaints and flatulence and to improve biliary function. Rosemary is rich in protective phenolic acids and terpenoids *(26)*. A tea made from the leaves of sage (*Salvia officinalis*) is also useful to treat dyspeptic symptoms, excessive sweating, and inflammation of the gums and throat. Sage is also rich in phenolic acids, terpenoids, and tannins *(26)*.

A beverage made from the inner bark of slippery elm (*Ulmus rubra*) is used to soothe irritated mucous membranes of the throat, as well as soothe gastric inflammation and intestinal colitis. Slippery elm contains high levels of mucilage, which provides its soothing properties *(30)*.

Preparations of silymarin (a mixture of flavonolignans) extracted from milk thistle (*Silybum marianum*) are used to treat liver disease and chronic hepatitis, as well as protection of the liver against environmental toxins. A tea made from milk thistle is ineffective, because silymarin is poorly soluble in water. Oral use requires a concentrated product, because silymarin is poorly absorbed from the GI tract *(42)*.

8.7. Respiratory Relief

A tea made from the flowers and leaves of mullein (*Verbascum thapsus* and *V. densiflorum*) is commonly used as an expectorant to treat coughs, sore throats, and catarrhs of the upper respiratory tract. The leaves contain a soothing mucilage. The saponins and tannins of mullein provide mild expectorant and astringent properties, respectively. Extracts of mullein flowers promote antiviral action against herpes simplex type I virus and influenza A and B strains *(26,30)*.

A tea made from the root of marshmallow (*Althaea officinalis*) has been widely used in Europe for centuries to treat sore throat, dry cough, and mild inflammation of the gastric and intestinal mucosa and the upper respiratory tract. Marshmallow root contains mucilages rich in rhamnose and arabinose, several flavonoid glycosides, phenolic acids, and phytosterols. It is the mucilage that acts as a demulcent to relieve irritation of the mucosal lining. The leaves of marshmallow, which contain similar constituents, act similarly as root preparations *(26,30)*.

Common plantain (*Plantago major*) and English plantain (*P. lanceolata*) are widely distributed in Europe and North America and are commonly found in residential lawns. Plantain is effectively used for catarrhs of the respiratory tract. Plantain tea is indicated for breaking up phlegm in the upper respiratory tract and may provide useful treatment of chronic bronchitis. It has mild antibiotic and antiinflammatory activity. Plantain's action is from its rich content of mucilage and iridoid glycosides. The mucilage provides the soothing and softening properties, and the iridoid glycosides provide antibacterial activity *(26,30)*.

Common thyme (*Thymus vulgaris*) is a member of the mint family. In ancient Rome, thyme was added to cheese and alcoholic beverages. Today, the herb is approved by the German Commission E to treat bronchitis, whooping cough, and inflammation of the upper respiratory tract. Thyme activity derives mainly from its flavonoids and essential oil content. Thymol and carvacrol are the major active terpenoids. The tea is not recommended during pregnancy *(26)*.

Teas made from *Echinacea* are used for respiratory infections. *Echinacea* is available in three forms—*E. angustifolia* (narrow-leaved purple coneflower), *E. pallida* (pale purple coneflower), and *E. purpurea* (common purple coneflower). However, only the latter two species are capable of providing protection. A tea made from *E. pallida* or *E. purpurea* stimulates the immune system to fight minor viral and bacterial infections, such as colds and flu. Repeated doses are needed to sustain the action.

Echinacea preparations can help to prevent colds and reduce the severity and duration of flu symptoms *(46,47)*. A measurable effect can be seen within 4 d of starting the treatment. The activity of *Echinacea* is believed to result from the presence of polysaccharides and other compounds that stimulate phagocytosis. Although goldenseal (*Hydrastis canadensis*) is often included with *Echinacea* preparations, it is questionable whether this adds protection, for reasons discussed in Subheading 8.6.

8.8. Herbs With Psychoactive Properties

Approximately 10% of the commercial herbs contain various psychoactive substances *(41)*. Mandrake, nutmeg, periwinkle, yohimbe, mistletoe, and jimsonweed all produce hallucinogenic effects. Wormwood tea (*Artemisia absinthium*) produces a narcotic-analgesic effect. The volatile oil contains a CNS depressant, causing trembling and stupor *(10,30)*. Tansy (*Tanacetum vulgare*) is a plant that grows along roadsides. A tea is made from the leaves and golden flowers of tansy. However, its content of thujone, a fairly toxic substance also found in wormwood, can induce convulsions and psychotic effects *(10)*.

Numerous species of the morning glory family of plants contain hallucinogenic properties, due to the high concentration of LSD-like alkaloids in their seeds *(48)*. Peyote, a small cactus native to northern Mexico and southern Texas, can be eaten fresh or dried or made into a tea. Peyote cactus plays an important role in Indian religious ceremonies of the Southwest *(48)*. Peyote can cause nausea, vomiting, and psychological effects, such as color and auditory hallucinations, feelings of weightlessness, and synesthesia (a confusion of the senses; for example, a sound may produce a mental image). The hallucinogenic properties of peyote result from the presence of the amine, mescaline.

Some patients are reluctant to use conventional antidepressants because of possible side effects. A tea prepared from the leaves and flowering tops of St. John's Wort (*Hyperi-cum perforatum*) is a popular herbal remedy for depression, with few reported side effects. It is widely used as an effective treatment for sleep disorders, anxiety, and depression *(25,49)*. Its content of various flavonoids and xanthones (hypericin and hyperflorin) plays a key role in the antidepressant action of St John's Wort. Several clinical trials have demonstrated the effectiveness of St. John's Wort in the treatment of mild to moderate depressive disorders *(50)*. Recently, randomized controlled trials have failed to show the efficacy of *H. perforatum* in patients with severe depression *(51,52)*. Furthermore, St. John's Wort may diminish the effectiveness of numerous commonly used medications if coadministered with the herbal preparation *(22,53)*.

9. CONCLUSIONS

Although the discriminate use of many herbal beverages is safe and some therapeutic benefits may be derived from their proper usage, the indiscriminate or excessive use of herbs can be unsafe and may even be dangerous. Due to numerous factors, the active components in herbal products may vary considerably, suggesting the need for standardization to ensure quality assurance in the herbal products. There are several herbal beverages that can provide relief for problems of the GI, respiratory, and urinary tracts; gynecologic disorders; and help for numerous other problems, such as sleep disorders, fatigue, depression, fluid retention, and flu symptoms. What remains to be determined is how these potential beverage ingredients will be used in the formulation of beverages in the future.

10. MAIN POINTS FOR PRIMARY AND CLINICAL REVIEW

1. Herbal beverages are consumed for two sometimes separate and interchangeable purposes: taste and claimed health benefits.
2. Very few double-blind clinical trials have been performed on the biological effects of these herbs.
3. The content of active ingredients in herbs is highly variable and this is probably an important reason that results of studies lack consistency.
4. Herbs may have toxic and carcinogenic effects and may interfere in drug action.
5. Although actual fatalities associated with their use are rare, clinicians and consumers should be aware of the potential harmful effects of herbs.

REFERENCES

1. Foster S. 101 Medicinal Herbs: An Illustrated Guide. Interweave Press, Loveland, CO, 1998.
2. Ohnell H, Berg H. Zur frage uber die ventrikelfunktion nach verabreichung verschiedener arten von kaffee. Acta Med Scand 1931;76:491–520.
3. Harkey MR, Henderson GL, Gershwin ME, Stern JS, Hackman RM. Variability in commercial ginseng products: an analysis of 25 preparations. Am J Clin Nutr 2001;73:1101–1106.
4. Percival SS, Turner RE. Applications of herbs to functional foods. In: Handbook of Nutraceuticals and Functional Foods. Wildman REC (ed.). CRC Press, Boca Raton, FL, 2001, pp. 393–406.
5. Larkin T. Herbs are often more toxic than magical. FDA Consumer 1983;17(8):4–11.
6. Bryson PD, Watanabe AS, Rumack BH, Murphy RC. Burdock root tea poisoning. Case report involving a commercial preparation. JAMA 1978;239:2157.

7. Dubick MA. Dietary supplements and health aids: a critical evaluation. Part 3—Natural and miscellaneous products. J Nutr Educ 1983;15:123–129.
8. Bahrke MS, Morgan WR. Evaluation of the ergogenic properties of ginseng: an update. Sports Med 2000;29:113–133.
9. Smith IK. Ginseng surprise. An independent report finds that what's listed on a supplement's label is not always what's inside. Time 2000;156(5):68.
10. Foster S, Tyler VE. Tyler's Honest Herbal. The Haworth Press, Binghamton, NY, 1999.
11. Ridker PM. Toxic effects of herbal teas. Arch Environ Health 1987;42:133–136.
12. FDA. Public warning about herbal product. JAMA 1993;269:328.
13. Katz M, Saibal F. Herbal hepatitis: subacute hepatic necrosis secondary to chaparral leaf. J Clin Gastroenterol 1990;12:203–206.
14. Gordon DW, Rosenthal G, Hart J, Sirota R, Baker AL. Chaparral ingestion. The broadening spectrum of liver injury caused by herbal medications. JAMA 1995;273:489–490.
15. Hogan RP. Hemorrhagic diathesis caused by drinking an herbal tea. JAMA 1983;249:2679–2680.
16. Haynes BE, Bessen HA, Wightman WD. Oleander tea: herbal draught of death. Ann Emerg Med 1985; 114:350–353.
17. Marderosian AD, Liberti L. Natural Product Medicine. A Scientific Guide to Foods, Drugs, Cosmetics. George F. Stickley Company, Philadelphia, PA, 1988.
18. Lipsitz DJ. Herbal teas and water intoxication in a young child. J Fam Practice 1984;18:933–937.
19. Kapadia GJ, Subba Rao G, Morton JF. Herbal tea consumption and esophageal cancer. In: Carcinogens and Mutagens in the Environment, Part 3. Stich HF (ed.). CRC Press, Boca Raton, FL, 1982, pp. 1–10.
20. Selegman AB, Segelman FP, Karliner J, Sofia RD. Sassafras and herb tea. Potential health hazards. JAMA 1976;236:477.
21. Ridker PM, McDermott WV. Comfrey herb tea and hepatic veno-occlusive disease. Lancet 1989;1: 657–658.
22. Jellin JM, Gregory P, Batz F, et al. (eds.). Pharmacist's Letter/Prescriber's Letter Natural Medicine Comprehensive Database, 3rd Ed. Therapeutic Research Faculty, Stockton, CA, 2000.
23. Ridker PM. Health hazards of unusual herbal teas. Am Fam Physician 1989;39:153–156.
24. Eichler I. Cryptic illness from self-medication with herbal remedy. Lancet 1983;1:356.
25. Tyler V. Herbs of Choice. The Therapeutic Use of Phytomedicinals. Haworth Press, Binghamton, NY, 1994.
26. Blumenthal M (ed.). Herbal Medicine. Expanded Commission E Monographs. Integrative Medicine Communications, Newton, MA, 2000.
27. Craig W. The Use and Safety of Common Herbs and Herbal Teas, 2nd Ed. Golden Harvest Books, Berrien Springs, MI, 1996, pp. 1–75.
28. Tyler V. An expert answers questions on herbal teas. Tufts Univ Diet Nutr Letter 1986;4:7–8.
29. Mittman P. Randomized, double-blind study of freeze-dried Urtica dioica in the treatment of allergic rhinitis. Planta Med 1990;56:44–47.
30. Gruenwald J, Brendler T, Jaenicke C (eds.). PDR for Herbal Medicines, 2nd Ed. Medical Economics Comp., Montvale, NJ, 2000.
31. Avorn J, Manone M, Gurwitz JH, Glynn RJ, Choodnovskiy I, Lipsitz LA. Reduction of bacteriuria and pyuria after ingestion of cranberry juice. JAMA 1994;271:751–754.
32. Summary Report. Canada's national guidelines on prenatal nutrition. Nutr Today 1987;22(4):34–35.
33. Loch EG, Selle H, Boblitz N. Treatment of premenstrual syndrome with a phytopharmaceutical formulation containing Vitex agnus castus. J Womens Health Gender Based Med 2000;9:315–320.
34. Simpson M, Parsons M, Greenwood J, Wade K. Raspberry leaf in pregnancy: its safety and efficacy in labor. J Midwifery Womens Health 2001;46:51–59.
35. Parsons M, Simpson M, Ponton T. Raspberry leaf and its effect on labour: safety and efficacy. Aust Coll Midwives Inc J 1999;12(3):20–25.
36. Wichtl M (ed.). Herbal Drugs and Phytopharmaceuticals, 2nd Ed. CRC Press, Boca Raton, FL, 1994.
37. Lieberman HR. The effects of ginseng, ephedrine, and caffeine on cognitive performance, mood and energy. Nutr Rev 2001;59:91–102.
38. Vogler BK, Pittle MH, Ernst E. The efficacy of ginseng. A systematic review of randomized clinical trials. Eur J Clin Pharmacol 1999;55:567–575.

39. Ansley D (ed.). Ginseng. Much ado about nothing? Consumer Rep 1995;60:699.
40. Balderer G, Borbely AA. Effect of valerian on human sleep. Psychopharmacology 1985;87:406–409.
41. Speroni E, Minghetti A. Neuropharmacological activity of extracts from Passiflora incarnata. Planta Med 1988;54:488–491.
42. Tyler VE. Phytomedicines in Western Europe: their potential impact on herbal medicine in the United States. HerbalGram 1994;30:24–30, 67–68, 77.
43. Lesnau A, Hils J, Pohl G, Beyer G, Janka M, Hoa LT. Antiviral activity of berberine salts. Pharmazie 1990;45:638–639.
44. Chirikdjian JJ, Kopp B, Beran H. Laxative action of a new anthraquinone glycoside from rhubarb roots. Planta Med 1983;48:34–37.
45. Sahpaz S, Garbacki N, Tits M, Bailleul F. Isolation and pharmacological activity of phenylpropanoid esters from Marrubium vulgare. J Ethnopharmacol 2002;79:389–392.
46. Melchart D, Linde K, Worku F, Bauer R, Wagner H. Immunomodulation with Echinacea—a systematic review of controlled clinical trials. Phytomedicine 1994;1:245–254.
47. Schoneberger D. The influence of immune-stimulating effects of pressed juice from Echinacea purpurea on the course and severity of colds. Forum Immunologie 1992;8:2–12.
48. Richardson PM. The cactus family. In: Flowering Plants. Magic in Bloom. Snyder SH, Jacobs BL (eds.), Chelsea House Publishers, New York, NY, 1986, pp. 53–59.
49. Linde K, Ramirez G, Mulrow CD, Pauls A, Weidenhammer W, Melchart D. St John's wort for depression—an overview and meta-analysis of randomized trials. Br Med J 1996;313:253–258.
50. Harrer G, Sommer H. Treatment of mild/moderate depression with Hypericum. Phytomedicine 1994; 1:3–8.
51. Shelton RC, Keller MB, Gelenberg A, et al. Effectiveness of St John's wort in major depression. JAMA 2001;285:1978–1986.
52. Hypericum Depression Trial Study Group. Effect of Hypericum perforatum (St. John's wort) in major depressive disorder: a randomized controlled trial. JAMA 2002;287:1807–1814.
53. Bilia AR, Gallori S, Vincieri FF. St. John's wort and depression. Efficacy, safety, and tolerability—an update. Life Sci 2002;70:3077–3096.

V HEALTH IMPACT OF MILK AND MILK ALTERNATIVES

14 Effect of Cow's Milk on Human Health

Lois D. McBean, Gregory D. Miller, and Robert P. Heaney

1. INTRODUCTION

Milk has been a staple of the diet of Old World temperate zone people since the agricultural revolution, approx 8000 BC. Milk is mentioned more than 20 times in the Hebrew scriptures (". . . a land flowing with milk and honey . . .") as a metaphor for abundance and wholesomeness. Also, in one of the Islamic medicine tomes, we read "Drink milk, for it wipes away heat from the heart, strengthens the back, increases the brain, augments the intelligence, renews vision, and drives away forgetfulness" *(1)*. Although they are not supported by contemporary standards, those claims, nevertheless, illustrate the generally high esteem that milk has enjoyed throughout its history. Milk is a thirst-quenching nourishing beverage. For some segments of the population (i.e., nomadic pastoralists) milk became, and is still today, the principal source of almost all nutrients, with daily consumption of approx 5–7 L.

Nutritional science emerged only at the beginning of the 20th century and quickly recognized the value of milk in a balanced diet. Virtually all US government nutrition programs and nutritional policy statements for the last century have emphasized the importance of milk. As nutritional science grew, so also did the understanding of the composition of milk and of its many benefits. However, during the past 30–40 yr particularly, several factors have converged to alter perceptions of the role of milk in the human diet. These include: (1) the emergence and promotion of alternative beverages (and the relative affluence that made their purchase possible), (2) medicine's emphasis on treating nutrients as toxins (e.g., fat, sodium, cholesterol), (3) animal rights activism, and (4) a still-growing technophobia.

In this overview, we review milk's nutrient composition; milk's role in meeting nutritional requirements; milk's health effects, both positive and negative; trends in milk consumption and the forces producing the trends; and changes in the dairy industry and its responses to these forces.

From: *Beverages in Nutrition and Health*
Edited by: T. Wilson and N. J. Temple © Humana Press Inc., Totowa, NJ

2. NUTRITIONAL VALUE OF MILK

The principal value of any food or beverage is that it nourishes and satisfies. Nutritional science scrutinizes this benefit, dissecting individual nutrients for study and characterizing the roles they play in body metabolism. Although this dissection is necessary if we are to understand how nutrition works, we must remember that our bodies need adequate intakes of *all* nutrients for total health, that foods are almost always more than a sum of their parts, and that inadequate intakes of specific nutrients generally affect multiple body systems and organs, not just the ones involved in the index diseases classically connected to single nutrients.

2.1. Nutrient Density

Cow's milk is a nutrient-dense food, providing a high concentration of nutrients in relation to its energy (calorie) content *(2,3)*. This is shown in Table 1. Note that 2 servings/day (a figure that characterized US milk intake through most of the 20th century) provide fewer than 10% of the calories; yet they provide 50% or more of the recommended phosphorus, calcium, vitamin D, riboflavin, and vitamin B_{12} intakes. For all the other nutrients listed, milk provides substantially more per calorie than the average food in the diet. Precisely because of its rich nutrient content, cow's milk improves the overall nutritional quality of any diet into which it is incorporated *(4,5)*.

2.2. Specific Nutrients

Milk is a complex aqueous mixture, containing nutrients in solution, suspension, and emulsion. It is roughly 90% water by weight and, like all complete foods, contains protein, fat, carbohydrates, minerals, and vitamins. The specific quantity and type of each have been optimized throughout evolution to provide all the nutrients needed for the early postnatal growth stages of all mammals.

2.2.1. PROTEIN

The principal proteins of milk are casein and whey proteins (e.g., beta lactoglobulin and alpha lactalbumin). These are high-quality proteins, together containing, in varying amounts, all of the essential amino acids required for human growth and tissue maintenance. Because of its content of the amino acid tryptophan, milk is also an important source of niacin equivalents.

2.2.2. CARBOHYDRATE

The primary carbohydrate in cow's milk is lactose, a disaccharide. However, lactose is a barrier to milk consumption for some people, because some adults lose the mucosal enzyme lactase to a greater or lesser extent as they age (*see* Section 3.1.).

2.2.3. FAT

Fat in cow's milk contributes to its appearance, texture, and flavor. Milk fat is also a source of both energy and essential fatty acids. Furthermore, milk fat carries with it fat-soluble vitamins (A, D, E, and K), and several health-promoting components, such as conjugated linoleic acid (CLA), sphingomyelin, butyric acid, and myristic acid *(3,6,7)*. The fatty acids in milk fat are approx 62% saturated, 30% monounsaturated, and 4% polyunsaturated, with the remaining 4% comprising other minor types of fatty acids *(3)*.

Table 1

Contribution to Recommended Intakes for Various Nutrients
from Two Servings of Milk Per Day (Mature Adult) [a]

Nutrient	Content	% Daily recommended intake[b]
Protein	16 g	25/32
Phosphorus	470 mg	67
Calcium	600 mg	60
Vitamin D	200 IU	50
Potassium[c]	762 mg	38
Magnesium	68 mg	16/21
Riboflavin (B_2)	0.8 mg	62/73
Pyridoxine (B_6)	0.2 mg	12/13
Vitamin B_{12}	1.8 μg	75
Zinc	1.9 mg	13/16
Energy[d]	204 kcal	9

[a] Men or women aged 40–50; as recommendations vary for different ages, so will percent daily recommended intakes (2,8,9).

[b] First value is for men, second for women (where recommendations vary by gender).

[c] Potassium has no intake comparable to an RDA. The estimated minimum requirement is 2000 mg/d.

[d] Assuming 2200 kcal/d.

Milk fat is unique among animal fats because it contains a relatively high proportion of short-chain and medium-chain saturated fatty acids (i.e., those with 4–14 carbons in length). Although cholesterol is a normal milk constituent, its content is relatively low (i.e., < 0.5% of milk fat). One-cup servings (8 oz) of whole, 2%, and nonfat (skim) milk contain 34 mg, 19.5 mg, and 5 mg cholesterol, respectively (2).

Cow's milk is also an important source of numerous vitamins and minerals. Vitamin A in whole milk and added to low-fat and fat-free milk in the United States and Canada, plays a key role in vision, cellular differentiation, and immunity (8). Nearly all fluid milks in the United States and Canada are fortified with vitamin D to obtain the standardized amount of 400 IU/q (9). Fortification is much lower, even nonexistent, in most European countries. Vitamin D enhances the intestinal absorption of calcium and phosphorus and is essential for the maintenance of a healthy skeleton, among other still-emerging effects. In addition to these fat-soluble vitamins, milk contributes appreciable amounts of water-soluble vitamins, such as riboflavin, vitamin B_{12}, and vitamin B_6 to the diet.

Concerning minerals, cow's milk and other dairy foods are major sources of calcium and phosphorus (2,10). All milks (unflavored and flavored), regardless of their fat content—whole, 2% reduced fat, 1% low-fat, and nonfat milks—contain approx 300 mg calcium per 8-oz serving and approx 235 mg phosphorus (2). Without including cow's milk (or other dairy foods) in the diet, it is difficult to meet calcium needs (11–13). In fact, milk and other dairy foods are the preferred source of calcium of several health professional organizations, as summarized by Miller et al. *(14)*.

In addition to calcium and phosphorus, cow's milk contributes other essential minerals to the diet, such as magnesium, potassium, and trace elements, such as zinc *(2)*, each of which supports skeletal and total body health *(15)*. Potassium and magnesium also play a beneficial role in blood pressure regulation *(3)*.

3. HEALTH EFFECTS OF MILK

As noted, the principal health effect of milk, like any food, is nourishment. Its nutritional power is especially evident in its support of growth. Through most of the past 10,000 yr, this benefit has been largely taken for granted. Except for using milk as a vehicle for vitamin D (and with it the specific prevention of rickets), little attention was paid to milk's role in either promoting particular aspects of health or disease causation. This situation changed when medicine linked hypercholesterolemia to heart disease and saturated fat intake to blood cholesterol concentration. Although this connection has always been tenuous and was clearly revealed as such in a recent critical review *(16)*, milk fat has never been directly linked to heart disease. As noted, milk fat consists mainly of short-chain fatty acids. Nevertheless, milk was a victim of the antifat frenzy, and, from a former position of presumed wholesomeness, milk has been recently presumed guilty and has had to prove its innocence.

Adding to this pressure has been the anti-milk campaigns of animal rights groups (most notably the Physicians' Committee for Responsible Medicine [PCRM] and People for the Ethical Treatment of Animals [PETA]). As Jeanne Goldberg noted in a recent review *(17)*, these groups, unable to convince the American public to forgo animal products on ethical grounds, have promoted their agenda instead by questioning the safety of products such as milk, hoping to frighten consumers into using plant-based alternatives, such as soy beverages. Milk is alleged to cause disorders as varied as heart disease, prostate cancer, juvenile onset diabetes, obesity, and asthma. We review specific disease issues in this section of this chapter to negate these allegations.

Also contributing to a cloud of suspicion hovering over milk is a growing technophobia, aided paradoxically by the technology of the Internet, which provides these groups a global platform. The focus has been on milk production practices and the fear that they may affect the wholesomeness of the milk supply. This fear has led, for example, to the emergence of so-called "organic" milks and even a bootleg market in nonpasteurized milk. This concern has caused an increase in the efficiency of milk production, especially during the past 20 yr. Figure 1 shows that milk production has increased from just under 12,000 to approx 20,000 lb per cow per year during this time *(18)*. This increase results from improved animal nutrition (leading to a more efficient conversion of feed to milk), genetic selection of high producers, and better infection control in herd animals. In a small percentage of animals in some herds, bovine somatotrophin (BST) has been used to improve production in cows with low milk output. Although BST is not widely used, it has become a rallying cry for the anti-milk activists. What the public is not told in these campaigns is that BST is naturally produced by all cows to stimulate lactation, that a small amount of it is found in all milks (including those designated "organic"), and that it does not affect humans.

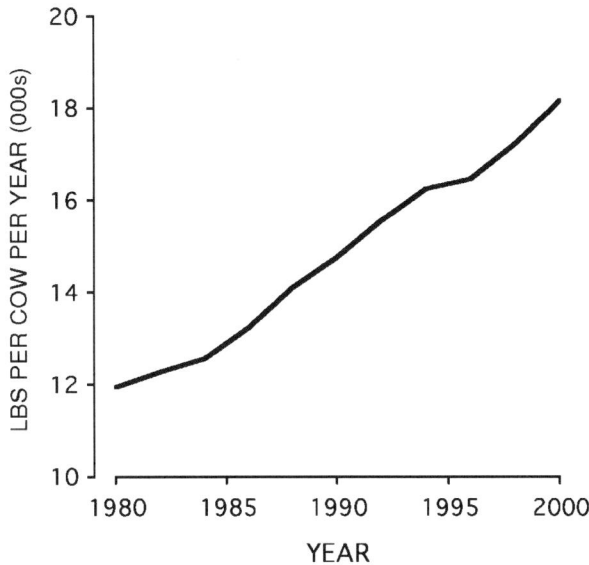

Fig. 1. Milk production efficiency from 1980 to 2000 *(18)*. Values are thousands of pounds per cow per year.

Milk is the most highly regulated food in the human diet. It is constantly monitored for residues of unwanted substances (such as antibiotics), and contaminated batches are weeded out and disposed. Concerns about the safety of North American milks, although understandable, are, nevertheless, groundless.

3.1. Lactose Intolerance

Some individuals have difficulty metabolizing lactose because of reduced lactase levels, a condition called lactase nonpersistence. However, most people with lactase nonpersistence can comfortably consume the amount of lactose in up to 2 or more cups of milk/d, when taken with meals *(3,19)*. Also, gradually increasing milk intake improves lactose tolerance *(20)*, which is due to symbiosis between the intestinal flora and the human host. Just as vegetarians develop a flora that helps them digest the complex carbohydrates of beans, milk drinkers develop a flora with lactase, which digests lactose. Symptomatic lactose intolerance develops only in lactase-nonpersistent individuals who do not regularly consume milk.

3.2. Cardiovascular Disease

Despite allegations that milk, because of its fat and cholesterol content, causes heart disease, there is no persuasive evidence to support this claim *(3,21,22)*. Although milk fat is a source of saturated fatty acids, its stearic acid and short- and medium-chain fatty acids do not raise blood cholesterol levels. Nevertheless, for individuals wishing to reduce their dietary fat intake, reduced-fat/low-fat and nonfat milks are available. Not only does milk make a relatively small contribution to total cholesterol intake, but also dietary cholesterol, regardless of source, has, at most, only a modest effect on blood cholesterol levels. Moreover, individuals vary in their blood cholesterol responses to dietary fat and cholesterol as a result of diet–gene interactions *(3)*. In fact, in some individuals, a low-fat diet increases the risk of cardiovascular disease (CVD) *(23,24)*.

Findings from epidemiological studies of milk-fat consumption and coronary heart disease (CHD) are inconsistent *(21)*. Recent investigations suggest that, rather than leading to heart disease, milk fat may actually have a protective effect on heart disease risk. A 25-yr prospective study of nearly 6000 men in Scotland found that men who drank between 2/3 and 2–2/3 cups/d of milk (most likely whole milk) were 8% less likely to die from CVD or any cause than were those who drank fewer than 2/3 cups of milk per day *(25)*. In a study of adolescents in Sweden, higher intakes of saturated fatty acids derived from milk fat were associated with lower blood levels of cholesterol and apolipoprotein B *(26)*. The findings led the authors to suggest "milk fat contains or is associated with some component ... which counterbalances the expected positive relationships between saturated fat intake and blood lipids." As noted, perhaps the relationship should not have been "expected" for saturated fats consisting mostly of short-chain fatty acids. Laboratory animal and in vitro studies indicate that CLA and sphingolipids, two of the components of milk fat, may protect against heart disease *(3,27–29)*.

Recently, increased attention has focused on the role of nonlipid risk factors in the development of CVD *(30)*. The American Heart Association's (AHAs) dietary guidelines now emphasize healthy eating patterns and behaviors rather than a narrow focus on dietary fat intake *(31)*. Interestingly, although the AHA guidelines of 20 yr ago had virtually eliminated milk from a cardioprotective diet, the guidelines now recommend 2–4 servings of low-fat milk products as part of an overall healthy eating plan *(31)*.

3.3. Hypertension and Stroke

The landmark DASH (Dietary Approaches to Stop Hypertension) study demonstrated that a low-fat diet containing 3 or more servings of dairy foods, predominately low-fat milk, in combination with fruits and vegetables, significantly and quickly reduced blood pressure in persons with high normal blood pressure *(32)* and in patients with isolated systolic hypertension *(33)*. The blood pressure-lowering effect of the DASH combination diet containing dairy foods was significantly more effective in lowering blood pressure than the diet emphasizing fruits and vegetables alone. Nutrients such as calcium, potassium, and magnesium are believed to contribute to milk's blood pressure-lowering effect.

In addition to its beneficial effect on hypertension, the DASH combination diet positively affects other heart disease risk factors. The DASH diet significantly reduced blood total and low density lipoprotein (LDL) cholesterol without affecting blood triacylglycerol levels *(22)* and lowered homocysteine blood levels *(34)*. Abnormally high blood levels of this nonstructural amino acid are associated with increased risk for heart disease and stroke. Based on the reduction in homocysteine levels, researchers estimate that intake of the DASH diet could lower atherosclerotic CVD by 7% to 9% *(34)* in addition to the 15% reduction in heart disease and 27% reduction in stroke estimated by the DASH-induced decrease in blood pressure *(32)*.

Other studies, focusing specifically on stroke, reach the same conclusion. Massey's analysis of 30 studies *(35)* indicates that milk's nutrients, such as calcium, potassium, and magnesium, play a role in reducing the risk for stroke. Additional support for milk's beneficial effect against stroke is provided by an epidemiological study of more than 3000 Japanese men aged 55–68 yr who were followed for 22 yr *(36)*. In this study, nonmilk drinkers experienced twice the rate of stroke as those who consumed two or more 8-oz/d glasses of milk *(36)*. Other studies have associated calcium, potassium, and magnesium with reduced risk for stroke *(3,36)*. Calcium intake from dairy foods, such as milk, has a greater effect on reducing stroke risk than nondairy sources of calcium *(37)*.

3.4. Osteoporosis

Adequate intake of milk and other calcium-rich foods throughout life helps to reduce the risk for osteoporosis, a bone-thinning disease affecting more than 28 million Americans, of whom three fourths are women. Dairy foods constitute the principal source of calcium in the American diet *(2)*. A recent analysis of 139 research papers on calcium intake and bone health found that in 50 of the 52 controlled trials and metabolic studies, augmenting calcium intake increased bone gain during growth, reduced bone loss in later years, or lowered fracture risk *(13)*. Contrary to PCRM claims that the protein and sodium of milk negate its calcium effect, the six trials that used dairy sources of calcium were all positive. Further, a multicenter randomized controlled trial found that drinking 3 servings of fat-free or low-fat milk each day improved indices of skeletal health in older adults *(38)*. Likewise, in a recent 2-yr randomized controlled trial of 200 Chinese women who were postmenopausal, milk supplementation (800 mg calcium/d) reduced bone loss by more than 50%, which is estimated to decrease lifetime fracture risk by 7% to 16% *(39)*.

Americans' low calcium intake is a major public health problem *(12)*. Reduced intake of dairy products, such as milk, and substitution of low-calcium beverages, such as soft drinks, contribute to Americans' low calcium intake *(40,41)*. Whiting et al. *(42)* demonstrated that when low-nutrient beverages replace nutrient-rich milk, bone mass may be adversely affected. Adolescent girls who consumed more nutrient-free or nutrient-poor beverages, including soft drinks, juice drinks, and iced teas, had significantly lower bone mineral content than those whose intake of such beverages was lower *(42)*. Unfortunately, as consumption of nutrient-free or nutrient-poor beverages increased, milk consumption decreased. Because of children's low calcium intake, the American Academy of Pediatrics *(43)* issued a policy statement indicating that pediatricians should recommend that cow's milk (as well as cheese, yogurt, and other calcium-rich foods) be included in children's diets to help build bone mass and prevent rickets.

3.5. Cancer

Despite some reports to the contrary, intake of cow's milk may reduce the risk for certain cancers, such as colon and breast. According to a randomized single-blinded controlled study of 70 patients with a history of developing polyps or noncancerous growths in the colon, increased intake of calcium food sources, specifically dairy foods such as low-fat milk, reduced the risk for colon cancer *(44)*. In a recent case-control study of more than 14,000 men aged 40–84 yr enrolled in the Physician's Health Study, low-fat milk intake was associated with a lower risk for colorectal cancer *(45)*.

Milk consumption is also associated with reduced risk for breast cancer, according to a recent 6-yr prospective study of almost 49,000 Norwegian women who were premenopausal *(46)*. Compared to nonmilk drinkers, women aged 34–39 yr who consumed more than three 8-oz/d glasses of milk had a 44% lower incidence of breast cancer. This relationship did not change after adjusting for other factors that could influence breast cancer, such as age, body mass index, and reproduction and hormonal factors. Whole, low-fat, and skim milks were equally protective against breast cancer *(46)*. The results of this study support earlier research findings that indicate a protective effect of cow's milk on breast cancer *(47,48)*. Although more research is needed to determine how milk consumption may help reduce the risk of developing colon or breast cancer, several nutrients, such as calcium and certain milk fat components (CLA, sphingolipids, and butyric acid), can be identified tentatively as responsible for the benefit *(3,6,29,49,50)*.

The most extensively publicized milk-cancer association linked milk consumption with increased risk of prostate cancer and was the subject of the notorious PETA billboard featuring New York Mayor Rudy Giuliani with a milk mustache and the question "Got prostate cancer?" Such a link was suggested in some, but not all, epidemiologic studies *(51–53)*. The perceived mechanism was that milk (and calcium generally) lowers serum $1,25(OH)_2D_3$ levels. This compound is the active form of vitamin D and in laboratory studies retards hyperplasia of prostatic mucosal cells. However, this hypothetical mechanism is effectively falsified by those African-American males who, with the lowest milk intake in the United States (and the highest serum $1,25(OH)_2D_3$ levels) also have the highest prostate cancer rates. The only clinical trial data bearing on this question indicate, in fact, that high calcium intakes lower the risk of prostate cancer *(54)*. In its recent review of risk factors for prostate cancer, the American Council on Science and Health concludes: "drinking milk is not an established—or even reasonably suggestive—risk factor for prostate cancer. In fact, the evidence for a role of milk is merely speculative" *(55)*.

This example illustrates the disruptive impact of campaigns such as those of PETA and PCRM. It takes little to raise a question about milk safety, whereas proving the allegation groundless takes years of effort and often millions of dollars. Some believe that such activism is unable to establish the correctness of its views on their own merits and, therefore, is designed, to punish nonbelievers.

3.6. Kidney Stones

Consuming milk may help to reduce the risk of kidney stones, specifically calcium oxalate stones (the most common type), according to two prospective observational studies *(56,57)*. In both, calcium food sources (mainly dairy) were protective against kidney stones. A high calcium intake is believed to reduce kidney stone risk by forming an insoluble calcium-oxalate complex in the intestinal lumen, thereby decreasing the intestinal absorption and renal excretion of the oxalate found in foods (such as vegetables and whole grains) or produced by bacterial fermentation of fatty acids. Urinary oxalate levels are more important contributors to kidney stone formation than urinary calcium levels. When adults with a history of calcium oxalate kidney stones and normal urine calcium levels substituted 1.5 cups of skim milk for apple juice (i.e., increasing calcium intake from less than 400 to 800 mg/d) with meals, urine calcium levels increased and urine oxalate levels decreased by an average of 18% *(58)*. To support both the protective effect and the underlying mechanism, a randomized trial of high and low calcium intakes (mostly from dairy sources) in stone-forming men showed both a 50% reduction in stone risk and a reduction in urinary oxalate excretion *(59)*.

3.7. Weight Control

Emerging research supports a potentially beneficial role for cow's milk in weight control *(60–65)*. In transgenic mice expressing the *agouti* gene in adipocytes, increasing

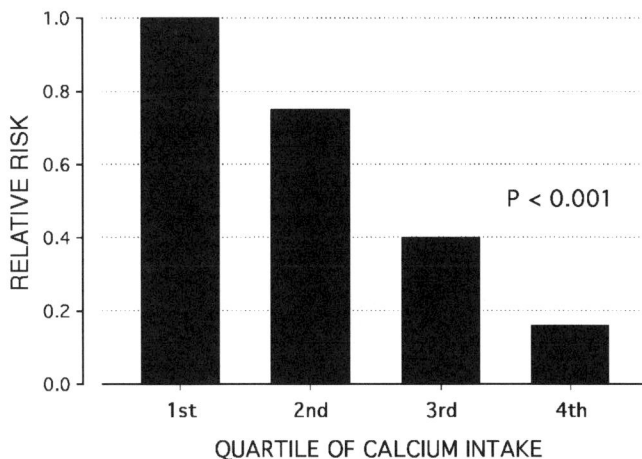

Fig. 2. Relative risk of being in the highest body body mass index quartile, expressed by quartile of calcium intake. Data are from NHANES-III, and are adjusted for age, gender, and energy intake, among other variables *(61)*.

dietary calcium from either supplements (calcium carbonate) or dairy foods (nonfat dry milk) reduced weight gain and body fat *(61)*. Further, weight gain was significantly lower in animals that were fed the high dairy diet. In mice that were fed the diets supplemented with calcium or dairy foods, adipocyte fatty acid synthase expression and activity were inhibited and lipolysis stimulation was increased *(61)*.

Human studies also link calcium/dairy intake to weight control. When data from the National Health and Nutrition Examination Survey (NHANES III) were analyzed, an inverse association was found between intake of calcium/dairy foods and obesity, especially among adult women *(61)* *(see* Fig. 2). Dairy/calcium intake has also been proven beneficial for weight control in young children *(64)*. When the diets of 53 preschool children were analyzed during a 3-yr period, lower body fat was found in children with higher dairy/calcium intakes. Also, when data from previously conducted clinical studies examining calcium and bone health (four observational and one double-blind, randomized, placebo-controlled trial, total $N = 780$) were reevaluated, a lower calcium intake was associated with a higher body fat at baseline and with more weight gain while under observation *(62)*. In the randomized controlled 4-yr trial from this retrospective analysis, increasing calcium intake by 1000 mg/d was associated with a nearly 18-lb lower average body weight. However, there was a great variation in weight in these individuals, and calcium explained only approx 3% of the total variance in body weight *(62)*. In a recent 2-yr prospective study of 54 normal-weight young women aged 18–31 yr, those who consumed high calcium intakes from dairy foods, corrected for total energy intake, gained less weight and body fat during the 2 yr than women with lower calcium intakes *(63)*.

Most recently Zemel et al. *(65)* showed significantly greater weight reduction in subjects on an approx 1300 kcal weight loss regimen when calcium was added, and significantly more when the calcium came from milk. Most impressively, the calcium-supplemented diets produced a much greater reduction in truncal obesity, and the milk (but not the calcium-only) regimen improved glucose tolerance substantially.

Confirmatory of these findings is a report from the Coronary Artery Risk Development in Young Adults (CARDIA) study cohort (more than 3000 black and white adults aged 18–30, followed for 10 yr) showing that dairy consumption was inversely associated with risk of developing each of the components of the insulin resistance syndrome (obesity, insulin resistance, and hyperinsulinemia in individuals who are overweight) (66). Each daily serving of a dairy food was associated with a 21% reduction in risk, and 3 servings/ d reduced risk by more than 60%. The findings were the same for men and women, black and white.

3.8. Other

Because cow milk is a major source of calcium in the diet, its intake may confer beneficial roles in other disorders (e.g., premenstrual syndrome, polycystic ovary syndrome, lead intoxication, periodontal disease) associated with low calcium intakes (14,67).

4. TRENDS IN COW'S MILK CONSUMPTION

Per-capita milk consumption from 1900 to the 1940s was stable, at just under two servings per person per day (see Fig. 3). It rose during World War II, but throughout the last years of the 20th century, total per-capita milk consumption declined. Annual milk consumption dropped from 29.8 gal per capita in 1970–1979 to 23.6 gal in 1999 (from 1.31 to 1.03 servings/d) (68). This decrease in milk consumption is attributed, in large part, to displacement of milk by carbonated soft drinks, as well as by other beverages, such as fruit juices, fruit drinks, and flavored teas. In 1945, Americans' milk intake was more than four times that of carbonated beverages (68) (see Fig. 4). By 1998, that relationship had nearly completely reversed: intake of carbonated beverages was more than twice as great as milk consumption.

Another pronounced trend is the shift away from whole milk to reduced-fat and nonfat milks in the United States (68,69). Between 1970–1979 and 1999, annual consumption of plain whole milk decreased by 62%, to 8 gal per person (less than 3 oz/d). During this same period, 2% low-fat milk consumption increased by 60%; 1% low-fat milk consumption increased by 160%; and skim (nonfat) milk consumption increased by 171% (69). Nevertheless, consumption of plain low-fat (1% and 2%) and skim milks was still relatively low at 13.9 gal/person per year in 1999 (69). Also noteworthy is the recent increase (15%) in flavored milks, especially chocolate milk (69,70).

Recent data for milk sales at supermarkets and supercenters indicate that total fluid milk, total white milk, whole white, reduced-fat white, and particularly flavored milks increased in 2000 when compared to 1999, whereas sales declined for low-fat and particularly fat-free white milks (71). This recent shift away from fat-free unflavored milk and the slight increase in whole milk may reflect consumers' declining concern about dietary fat and their preference for taste over ostensible healthfulness. The 2000 Trends survey conducted for the Food Marketing Institute (72) indicated that, although fat content of foods remains a concern for consumers, the percentage of consumers citing fat content as a concern dropped from a high of 65% in 1995 to 46% in 2000. Also, restrictive diets are less popular, and consumers' concern about nutrition has decreased. In 1994,

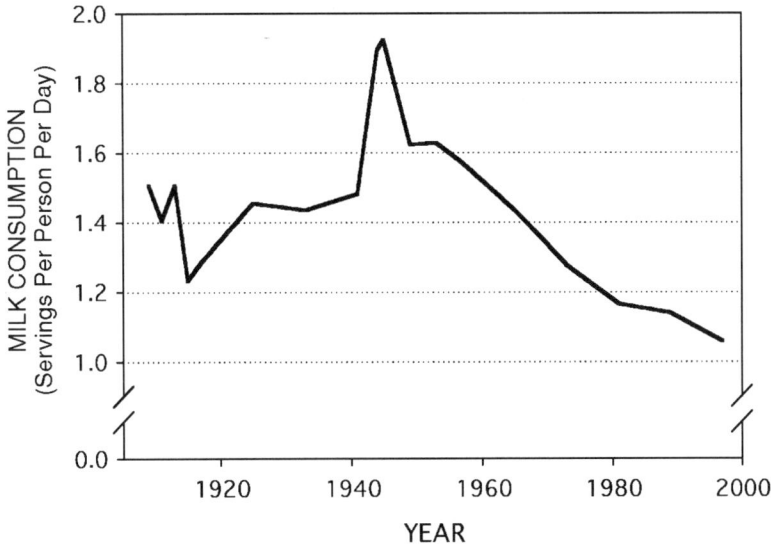

Fig. 3. Per-capita total milk consumption in the United States throughout the 20th century *(10)*.

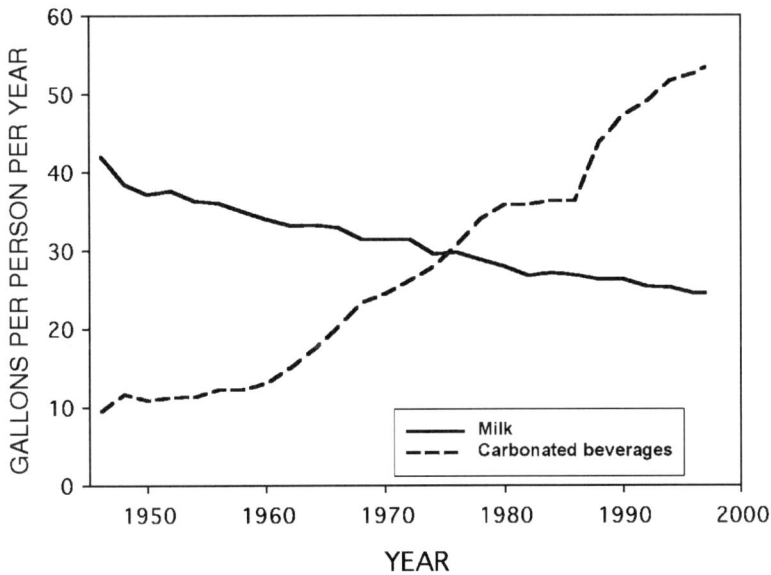

Fig. 4. Pattern of carbonated beverage and total milk consumption for the 50 yr from 1947 through 1997. Redrawn from Putnam *(68)*.

62% of consumers surveyed were "very concerned" about nutrition, whereas in 2000, only 46% were "very concerned" *(72)*. The recent shift away from fat-free milk at retail may also reflect increased use of non-milk beverages, such as fruit juices, fruit drinks, teas, lemonades, and bottled waters.

The growth in flavored milks, predominantly reduced-fat, low-fat, and nonfat chocolate varieties *(9,18)*, may be explained by their taste and increased availability, as well as by an increasing number of consumers viewing flavored milks as a healthy beverage. When choosing food or beverages, consumers consider taste the most important factor influencing their decision *(72)*. A recent telephone survey of 300 pediatricians found that the majority (87%) agreed that chocolate milk is a nutritious beverage option for children *(73)*. Nearly 60% of the pediatricians agreed that low-fat or fat-free chocolate milk is "the best beverage source of calcium," placing it above both calcium fortified orange juice and soy beverage.

5. INDUSTRY EFFORTS TO INCREASE MILK CONSUMPTION

Dairy industry responses to declining per-capita consumption include producing several milk beverages to meet consumers' taste and health demands, making fluid milk more convenient and accessible, and enhancing milk's positive image by innovative marketing strategies *(74)*.

To meet consumers' earlier demands for lower fat foods, the dairy industry developed and promoted numerous reduced-fat and nonfat (skim) milks fortified with nutrients such as vitamin A and vitamin D. For occasional milk drinkers who have lactase non-persistence, lactose-reduced (70% less lactose) and lactose-free (99.5% less lactose) milks were made available. Also, concern about Americans' low calcium intake has led some dairy processors to add calcium to milk, even though this beverage is already calcium rich *(74)*. Fluid milk is also an excellent carrier for probiotic cultures or health-promoting bacteria *(75)* (*see also* Chapter 17). Several health benefits have been attributed to specific strains of lactic acid bacteria (e.g., *Lactobacillus, Bifidobacterium*) or foods such as cultured milks containing these probiotic cultures.

The dairy industry has introduced numerous flavored milks (e.g., chocolate, strawberry, vanilla, mocha, banana, cappuccino) of varied fat content (e.g., whole, low-fat, and nonfat) *(76)*. Chocolate milk in lower and nonfat varieties is the most popular flavored milk *(18,76)*. Survey findings indicate that children will drink more milk if chocolate milk is available *(76)*. Like unflavored milks, flavored milks contain approx 300 mg calcium per 8-oz serving, or one third to one half of children's daily calcium recommendation *(2,9)*.

Increasing children's milk intake is particularly important, given the high percentage of children not meeting their daily calcium recommendations *(9,77)*. As many as 70% of preteen girls and 60% of preteen boys aged 6–11 and nearly 90% of teenage girls and almost 70% of teenage boys aged 12–19 fall short of meeting their calcium needs *(9,77)*. Offering flavored milk as part of the school meal programs has increased milk and nutrient intake *(76,78)*. A recent study of a representative sample ($N = 3888$) of children aged 12–17 found that children who consumed flavored milk drank more milk and had higher calcium intakes than children who did not drink flavored milk *(79)*. Moreover, the flavored milk drinkers did not have higher percentages of fat or sugars in their total diet compared with children who did not consume flavored milk.

A relatively new approach to increase students' milk intake is to provide various in-school milk vending machines *(80)*. Findings from a 5-mo milk vending study in middle and high schools in five major US markets demonstrated students' strong interest in vended milk *(80)*. The study revealed that many students would choose milk over competitive beverages if it were available when, where, and how they wanted it. If school milk vending were widespread, school milk consumption could potentially increase by 16.3 million gallons, or 4% per year, according to this study *(80)*. Each milk vending machine in the study offered at least three flavored milks in a variety of fat levels in 16-oz resealable plastic containers. Chocolate milk was particularly popular, outselling white milk 9 to 1. The students liked the 16-oz serving size, which contained 600 mg calcium. Intake of vended milk replaced soft drinks, fruit drinks, and water, but not school lunch milk *(80)*.

Appealing to consumers' demand for convenience, the dairy industry offers milks in attractive packaging, such as resealable single-serve plastic containers (e.g., 10 oz, 12 oz, 16 oz), with extended shelf life, and in more locations, such as convenience stores and in milk vending machines *(74)*. The availability of single-serve bottles has driven the increase in flavored milk consumption *(74)*. To increase opportunities for fluid milk consumption, dairy processors are also applying new technologies to extend milk's shelf life. These include thermal processing (e.g., high-temperature, short-time pasteurization), packaging (e.g., retort processing), and physical manipulation (e.g., filtration processing) *(74,81)*.

During the past 30 yr, soft drink and noncitrus juice consumption among children aged 11 to 18 yr nearly tripled, whereas their total milk consumption decreased almost 40% *(82)*. If this trend continues, it could lead to a higher risk for osteoporosis and obesity once children reach adulthood. If the availability of milk in vending machines can encourage children to drink milk more often, this may help them meet their needs for calcium and other nutrients at a critical time in their growth and development.

Dairy producers and processors have supported high-profile advertising and promotions such as the "Got Milk?" and "Milk Mustache" campaigns, to improve milk's image or make it "cool" to consume this beverage. For example, the "Milk Mustache" ads, which feature a celebrity sporting a milk mustache and include a message about the nutritional qualities of milk, have contributed to increased sales of fluid milk *(83)*. Some of the promotional campaigns to increase milk consumption target specific groups, such as children, mothers, or African Americans, whereas others focus on the contribution of milk to health (e.g., milk and reduced risk for osteoporosis or hypertension). New findings demonstrating that mothers' milk consumption patterns influence the amount and type of milk consumed by their children *(84,85)* indicate that milk-promotion efforts targeted to one group (e.g., women to prevent osteoporosis) may have a farther reaching effect (e.g., by increasing children's milk consumption).

6. CONCLUSION

Because cow's milk is a nutrient-dense inexpensive food, its consumption improves the overall nutritional quality of the diet. Contrary to allegations from special interest groups, accumulating scientific evidence indicates that cow's milk consumption is associated with numerous health benefits, including reduced risk for osteoporosis, hypertension, some cancers, stroke, and kidney stones, as well as better weight control. Throughout the past 40 yr, cow's milk intake has changed dramatically. Consumption of total and whole milk has decreased, whereas intake of reduced-fat milks has increased. The decline in total milk consumption contributes to the growing problem of Americans' low calcium intake. To help increase cow's milk intake and improve Americans' overall nutritional status and health, the dairy industry has introduced an increasing variety of milks. In addition to milks of varied fat content, flavored milks, fortified milks, specialty milks (e.g., low or reduced in lactose), and milks with extended shelf life are available. Also, milks are being offered in visually attractive resealable single-serve containers and in more settings, such as convenience stores and vending machines. Milk's good taste, nutrition, and health benefits; contemporary "fuel-to-go" image; and increased accessibility, as well as effective advertising and promotional campaigns, are helping to make milk a more competitive beverage.

7. MAIN POINTS FOR PRIMARY AND CLINICAL REVIEW

1. Milk has a high nutrient density relative to most other beverages and foods.
2. Individuals with lactose intolerance can include dairy in their diet, for example, by choosing low-lactose or lactose-free milk and fermented dairy products such as yogurt.
3. Milk has been associated with reduced risk of cardiovascular disease, hypertension, osteoporosis, breast cancer, kidney stones, and overweight.
4. In the last 20 yr, milk consumption has declined whereas intake of soft drinks and fruit juice has increased.
5. Innovative marketing campaigns are beginning to reverse this trend, resulting in increased milk consumption, especially in the area of flavored milks.

ACKNOWLEDGMENTS

The authors thank Mary Pat Anders, Director, Marketing Research, Dairy Management, Inc., Rosemont, IL, for her help in preparing this article.

REFERENCES

1. Anonymous. The medicine of the prophet. Eastern Caliphate, 11th Century.
2. US Department of Agriculture, Agricultural Research Service. USDA Nutrient Database for Standard Reference, Release 14, 2001. Nutrient Data Laboratory Home Page. Retrieved October 2001, from http://www.nal.usda.gov/fnic/foodcomp
3. Miller GD, Jarvis JK, McBean LD. Handbook of Dairy Foods and Nutrition, 2nd Ed. CRC Press Inc., Boca Raton, FL, 2000.
4. Johnson RK, Panely C, Wang MQ. The association between noon beverage consumption and the diet quality of school-age children. J Child Nutr Manage 1998;22:95–100.
5. Barr SI, McCarron DA, Heaney RP, et al. Effects of increased consumption of fluid milk on energy and nutrient intake, body weight, and cardiovascular risk factors in healthy older adults. J Am Dietet Assoc 2000;100:810–817.
6. Parodi PW. Cow's milk components with anti-cancer potential. Aust J Dairy Technol 2001;56:65–73.
7. Molkentin J. Occurrence and biochemical characteristics of natural bioactive substances in bovine milk lipids. Br J Nutr 2000;84(Suppl):47S–53S.
8. Institute of Medicine, Standing Committee on the Scientific Evaluation of Dietary Reference Intakes. Dietary Reference Intakes for Vitamin A, Vitamin K, Arsenic, Boron, Chromium, Copper, Iodine, Iron, Manganese, Molybdenum, Nickel, Silicon, Vanadium, and Zinc. National Academy Press, Washington, DC, 2001.
9. Institute of Medicine, Standing Committee on the Scientific Evaluation of Dietary Reference Intakes. Dietary Reference Intakes for Calcium, Phosphorus, Magnesium, Vitamin D, and Fluoride. National Academy Press, Washington, DC, 1997.
10. Gerrior S, Bente L. Nutrient Content of the US Food Supply, 1909–97. US Department of Agriculture, Center for Nutrition Policy and Promotion. Home Economics Research Report No. 54. March 2001, pp. 130–131.

11. Weaver CM, Proulx WR, Heaney R. Choices for achieving adequate dietary calcium with a vegetarian diet. Am J Clin Nutr 1999;70(Suppl):543S–548S.
12. US Department of Health and Human Services. Healthy People 2010 (Conference Edition, in Two Volumes). Washington, DC, January 2000. www.health.gov/healthypeople
13. Heaney RP. Calcium, dairy products and osteoporosis. J Am Coll Nutr 2000;19(Suppl):83S–99S.
14. Miller GD, Jarvis JK, McBean LD. The importance of meeting calcium needs with foods. J Am Coll Nutr 2001;20:168S–185S.
15. Ilich JZ, Kerstetter JE. Nutrition in bone health revisited: a story beyond calcium. J Am Coll Nutr 2000;19:715–737.
16. Taubes G. The soft science of dietary fat. Science 2001;291:2536–2545.
17. Goldberg JP, Folta SC, Must A. Milk: can a "good" food be so bad? Pediatrics 2002;110:826–832.
18. International Dairy Foods Association. Milk Facts 2000 Edition. International Dairy Foods Association, Washington, DC, 2000.
19. Suarez FL, Savaiano D, Arbisi P, Levitt MD. Tolerance to the daily ingestion of two cups of milk by individuals claiming lactose intolerance. Am J Clin Nutr 1997;65:1502–1506.
20. Pribila BA, Hertzler SR, Martin BR, Weaver CM, Savaiano DA. Improved lactose digestion and intolerance among African-American adolescent girls fed a dairy-rich diet. J Am Dietet Assoc 2000; 100:524–528.
21. Lefevre M. Is milkfat the scapegoat for CHD? Dialogue Dairy Advisory Bureau (New Zealand) 1999; 30:5–9.
22. Obarzanek E, Sacks FM, Vollmer WM, et al. Effects on blood lipids of a blood pressure-lowering diet: the Dietary Approaches to Stop Hypertension (DASH) Trial. Am J Clin Nutr 2001;74:80–89.
23. Williams PT, Krauss RM. Low fat diets, lipoprotein subclasses, and heart disease risk. Am J Clin Nutr 1999;70:949–950.
24. Krauss RM. Atherogenic lipoprotein phenotype and diet-gene interactions. J Nutr 2001;131(Suppl): 340S–343S.
25. Ness AR, Smith GD, Hart C. Milk, coronary heart disease and mortality. J Epidemiol Commun Health 2001;55:379–382.
26. Samuelson G, Bratteby L-E, Mohsen R, Vessby B. Dietary fat intake in healthy adolescents: inverse relationships between the estimated intake of saturated fatty acids and serum cholesterol. Br J Nutr 2001; 85:333–341.
27. Kritchevsky D, Tepper SA, Wright S, Tso P, Czarnecki SK. Influence of conjugated linoleic acid (CLA) on establishment and progression of atherosclerosis in rabbits. J Am Coll Nutr 2000;19(Suppl): 472S–477S.
28. Kobayashi T, Shimizugawa T, Osakabe T, Watanabe S, Okuyama H. A long-term feeding of sphingolipids affected the levels of plasma cholesterol and hepatic triacylglycerol but not tissue phospholipids and sphingolipids. Nutr Res 1997;17:111–114.
29. Vesper H, Schmelz EM, Nikolova-Karakashian MN, Dillehay DL, Lynch DV, Merrill AH Jr. Sphingolipids in food and the emerging importance of sphingolipids to nutrition. J Nutr 1999;129: 1239–1250.
30. McGill HC Jr, McMahan CA, Zieske AW, Malcom GT, Tracy RE, Strong JP for the Pathobiological Determinants of Atherosclerosis in Youth (PDAY) Research Group. Effects of nonlipid risk factors on atherosclerosis in youth with a favorable lipoprotein profile. Circulation 2001;103:1546–1550.
31. American Heart Association, Nutrition Committee. AHA Dietary Guidelines. Revision 2000. A statement for healthcare professionals from the Nutrition Committee of the American Heart Association. Circulation 2000;102:2284–2299.
32. Appel LJ, Moore TJ, Obarzanek E, et al. A clinical trial of the effects of dietary patterns on blood pressure. N Engl J Med 1997;336:1117–1124.
33. Moore TJ, Conlin PR, Ard J, Svetkey LP for the DASH Collaborative Research Group. DASH (Dietary Approaches to Stop Hypertension) diet is effective treatment for stage 1 isolated systolic hypertension. Hypertension 2001;38:155–158.
34. Appel LJ, Miller ER III, Jee SH, et al. Effect of dietary patterns on serum homocysteine. Results of a randomized, controlled feeding trial. Circulation 2000;102:852–857.
35. Massey LK. Dairy food consumption, blood pressure and stroke. J Nutr 2001;131:1875–1878.

36. Abbott RD, Curb JD, Rodriquez BL, Sharp DS, Burchfiel CM, Yano K. Effect of dietary calcium and milk consumption on risk of thromboembolic stroke in older middle-aged men. The Honolulu Heart Program. Stroke 1996;27:813–818.

37. Iso H, Stampfer MJ, Manson JE, et al. Prospective study of calcium, potassium, and magnesium intake and risk of stroke in women. Stroke 1999;30:1772–1779.

38. Heaney RP, McCarron DA, Dawson-Hughes B, et al. Dietary changes favorably affect bone remodeling in older adults. J Am Dietet Assoc 1999;99:1128–1233.

39. Lau EMC, Woo J, Lam V, Hong A. Milk supplementation of the diet of postmenopausal Chinese women on a low calcium intake retards bone loss. J Bone Min Res 2001;16:1704–1709.

40. US Department of Agriculture and US Department of Health and Human Services. Nutrition and Your Health: Dietary Guidelines for Americans, 5th Ed. Home and Garden Bulletin No. 232. US Government Printing Office, Washington, DC, 2000.

41. NIH Consensus Development Panel on Osteoporosis Prevention, Diagnosis, and Therapy. Osteoporosis prevention, diagnosis, and therapy. JAMA 2001;285;785–795.

42. Whiting SJ, Healey A, Psiuk S, Mirwald R, Kowalski K, Bailey DA. Relationship between carbonated and other low nutrient dense beverages and bone mineral content of adolescents. Nutr Res 2001;21: 1107–1115.

43. American Academy of Pediatrics, Committee on Nutrition. Calcium requirements of infants, children, and adolescents. Pediatrics 1999;104:1152–1157.

44. Holt PR, Atillasoy EO, Gilman J, et al. Modulation of abnormal colon epithelial cell proliferation and differentiation by low-fat dairy foods: a randomized controlled trial. JAMA 1998;280:1074–1079.

45. Ma J, Giovannucci E, Pollak M, et al. Milk intake, circulating levels of insulin-like growth factor-1, and risk of colorectal cancer in men. J Natl Cancer Inst 2001;93:1330–1336.

46. Hjartåker A, Laake P, Lund E. Childhood and adult milk consumption and risk of premenopausal breast cancer in a cohort of 48,844 women—the Norwegian women and cancer study. Int J Cancer 2001;93:888–893.

47. Knekt P, Jarvinen R, Seppanen R, Pukkala E, Aromas A. Intake of dairy products and the risk of breast cancer. Br J Nutr 1996;73:687–691.

48. Jarvinen R, Knekt P, Seppanen R, Teppo L. Diet and breast cancer in a cohort of Finnish women. Cancer Lett 1997;114:251–253.

49. Parodi PW. An assessment of the evidence linking calcium and vitamin D to colon cancer prevention. Austr J Dairy Technol 2001;56:38–58.

50. Lipkin M, Newmark HL. Vitamin D, calcium and prevention of breast cancer: a review. J Am Coll Nutr 1999;18(Suppl):392S–397S.

51. Chan JM, Giovannucci EL. Dairy products, calcium, and vitamin D and risk of prostate cancer. Epidemiol Rev 2001;23:87–92.

52. Chan JM, Stampfer MJ, Ma J, Gann PH, Gaziano JM, Giovannucci EL. Dairy products, calcium, and prostate cancer risk in the Physicians' Health Study. Am J Clin Nutr 2001;74:549–554.

53. Tavani A, Gallus S, Franceschi S, La Vecchia C. Calcium, dairy products, and the risk of prostate cancer. Prostate 2001;48:118–121

54. Wallace K, Pearson LH, Beach ML, Mott LA, Baron JA. Calcium supplementation and prostate cancer risk: a randomized analysis. Proceedings AACR 2001;42:poster #2479.

55. Meister K. Risk factors for prostate cancer. American Council on Science and Health, New York, 2000.

56. Curhan GC, Willett WC, Rimm EB, Stampfer MJ. A prospective study of dietary calcium and other nutrients and the risk of symptomatic kidney stones. N Engl J Med 1993;328:833–838.

57. Curhan GC, Willett WC, Speizer FE, Spiegelman D, Stampfer MJ. Comparison of dietary calcium with supplemental calcium and other nutrients as factors affecting the risk for kidney stones in women. Ann Intern Med 1997;126:497–504.

58. Massey LK, Kynast-Gales SA. Substituting milk for apple juice does not increase kidney stone risk in most normocalciuric adults who form calcium oxalate stones. J Am Dietet Assoc 1998;98:303–308.

59. Borghi L, Schianchi T, Meschi T, et al. Comparison of two diets for the prevention of recurrent stones in idiopathic hypercalciuria. N Engl J Med 2002;346:77–84.

60. Summerbell CD, Watts C, Higgins JPT, Garrow JS. Randomised controlled trial of novel, simple, and well supervised weight reducing diets in outpatients. Br Med J 1998;17:1487–1489.

61. Zemel MB, Shi H, Greer B, DiRienzo D, Zemel PC. Regulation of adiposity by dietary calcium. FASEB J 2000;14:1132–1138.
62. Davies KM, Heaney RP, Recker RR, et al. Calcium intake and body weight. J Clin Endocrinol Metab 2000;85:4635–4638.
63. Lin Y-C, Lyle RM, McCabe LD, McCabe GP, Weaver CM, Teegarden D. Dairy calcium is related to changes in body composition during a two-year exercise intervention in young women. J Am Coll Nutr 2000;19:754–760.
64. Carruth BR, Skinner JD. The role of dietary calcium and other nutrients in moderating body fat in preschool children. Int J Obesity 2001;25:559–566.
65. Zemel MB, Thompson W, Zemel P, et al. Dietary calcium and dairy products accelerate weight and fat loss during energy restriction in obese adults. Am J Clin Nutr 2002;75:342S–343S.
66. Pereira MA, Jacobs DR Jr, Van Horn L, Slattery ML, Kartashov AI, Ludwig DS. Dairy consumption, obesity, and the insulin resistance syndrome in young adults. The CARDIA Study. JAMA 2002;287: 2081–2089.
67. Heaney RP. Ethnicity, bone status, and the calcium requirement. Nutr Res 2002;22:153–178.
68. Putnam J. Major trends in US food supply, 1909-99. Food Rev 2000;23:8–15.
69. Putnam J, Kantor LS, Allshouse J. Per capita food supply trends: progress toward dietary guidelines. Food Rev 2000;23:2–14.
70. Fusaro D. A watershed year for fluid milk? Dairy Foods 2001;102:16–17.
71. Information Resources Inc. Retail Scanner Sale Information. Dairy Management Inc. Planning & Research Group, 2001.
72. Food Marketing Institute. Trends in the United States. Consumer Attitudes and the Supermarket 2000. Conducted for the Food Marketing Institute by Research International USA. Food Marketing Institute, Washington, DC, 2000.
73. Pediatrician Attitude Survey. Prepared by Bruskin Research for BSMG Worldwide. January 2001.
74. Modern milk. Beverage Industry 2000;91:38–40.
75. National Dairy Council. Functional foods: an overview. Dairy Council Digest 1999;70:31–36.
76. National Dairy Council. Flavored Milk in Perspective. 2001. Retrieved October 14, 2001, from http://www.nationaldairy council.org
77. US Department of Agriculture, Agricultural Research Service. Data tables: Results from USDA's 1994–96 Continuing Survey of Food Intakes by Individuals and 1994–96 Diet and Knowledge Survey. ARS, USDA, Riverdale, MD, 1999.
78. Guthrie HA. Effect of a flavored milk option on a school lunch program. J Am Dietet Assoc 1997; 71:35–40.
79. Johnson RK, Frary C, Wang MQ. The nutritional consequences of flavored-milk consumption by school-aged children and adolescents in the United States. J Am Dietet Assoc 2002;102:853–856.
80. Milk PEP/DMI School Milk Vending Test—Executive Summary. 2001 Retrieved February 28, 2002, from http://www.idfa.org/mktg/gotmilk.htm
81. Dairy Management Inc. Achieving extended shelf life in fluid milk: creating hurdles for spoilage factors. Innovations in Dairy October 2001. Retrieved October 15, 2001, from http://www.extraordinarydairy.com
82. Cavadini C, Siega-Riz AM, Popkin BM. US adolescent food intake trends from 1965 to 1996. Arch Dis Child 2000;83:18–24.
83. Blisard N. Advertising's influence: the case of dairy products. Food Rev 1998;21:44–45.
84. Fisher JO, Mitchell DC, Smiciklas-Wright H, Birch LL. Maternal milk consumption predicts the tradeoff between milk and soft drinks in young girls' diets. J Nutr 2000;131:246–250.
85. Johnson RK, Panely CV, Wang MQ. Associations between the milk mothers drink and the milk consumed by their school-aged children. Family Econ Nutr Rev 2001;13:27–36.

15 Are Soy-Milk Products Viable Alternatives to Cow's Milk?

Jayne V. Woodside and Michael S. Morton

1. INTRODUCTION

There has been a recent growth in the popularity of cow's milk alternatives. These include milk substitutes manufactured from soy, rice, and almond sources. Little research has been carried out on the health benefits of either rice milk or almond milk, so this chapter concentrates on the health implications of soy beverages, with respect to conditions such as lactose intolerance, osteoporosis, cancer, and heart disease and discusses whether these products are nutritionally equivalent to milk. Soy milk has attracted interest because it is a good source of protein and lower in fat than cow's milk (*see* Table 1).

Soy milk has also attracted interest not only as an alternative to cow's milk but also as a major source of isoflavones. Isoflavones are plant compounds found predominantly in legumes (peas, beans, and lentils, and so on). They form one class of a wider group of chemicals known as phytoestrogens *(2)*. Soybeans and soy products, such as soy milk, are perhaps the most common food source of isoflavones and contain large amounts of the isoflavones genistein and daidzein *(3)*, but other legumes, especially clovers, contain higher total levels and, in addition to genistein and daidzein, also contain formononetin and biochanin *(4)*. The amount of phytoestrogens found in each soy protein depends on the processing technique used and its relative abundance in the specific soy product. The secondary soy products (milk or flour) contain lower amounts of the isoflavones than the primary products. Different brands of soy milk vary in isoflavone content, ranging from 1.3–21.1 mg total isoflavones/100 g wet weight (*see* Table 2). The isoflavones are covalently bound to glucose and, when ingested by humans, are enzymatically cleaved in the gut to the active forms. Phytoestrogens' metabolism varies from person to person, and women metabolize them more efficiently than men *(6)*.

Research into the health benefits of phytoestrogens has used numerous food sources, including soy protein, soy milk, and extracted isoflavones. They are all included for discussion in later sections; concentrating only on studies using soy milk would ignore a large body of highly relevant evidence.

From: *Beverages in Nutrition and Health*
Edited by: T. Wilson and N. J. Temple © Humana Press Inc., Totowa, NJ

Table 1
Nutritional Content of Soy Milk in Comparison With Cow's Milk
(Whole, Semi-Skimmed, and Skimmed)*

	Soy (plain)	Whole (average)	Semi-skimmed (average)	Skimmed (average)
Protein (g)	2.9	3.2	3.3	3.3
Fat (g)	1.9	3.9	1.6	0.1
Carbohydrate (g)	0.8	4.8	5.0	5.0
Energy (kcal)	32	66	46	33
Calcium (mg)	13	115	120	120

*Data taken from McCance and Widdowson's The Composition of Foods (1).

2. LACTOSE INTOLERANCE

Lactose, a disaccharide of glucose and galactose, is a sugar particular to milk and milk products. Its universal presence in milk means that all newborn mammalian species have the appropriate enzyme, lactase, to breakdown this sugar. However, after weaning, lactase activity declines rapidly in all species, including humans. Without lactase, milk drinking may produce diarrhea and abdominal pain and distension. This is because unabsorbed lactose exerts an osmotic effect in the small bowel and results in large amounts of fluid and sugar entering the large bowel. In the large bowel, the sugar is rapidly fermented, producing gas, and, if enough lactose is present, osmotic diarrhea ensues (7). Lactose intolerance is common in adult populations worldwide, except for adults with a northern European background. Even among these people, it is estimated that 5–15% may be alactasic (8). For those who are lactose intolerant, soy milk provides an alternative to cow's milk.

Cow milk allergy (CMA) induces a large spectrum of clinical manifestations in infants and children. These manifestations mainly affect the gastrointestinal (GI) tract, skin, and, more rarely, the respiratory tract (9). The severity of the disease varies with a patient's age, atopic status, and clinical presentation (9). It is estimated that CMA occurs in ≤ 2% of all children in the first 3 yr of life (9). Soy protein formula is the preferred food for children with IgE-mediated CMA, because it has lower immunogenicity and allergenicity than cow-milk formula, and better palatability than hydrolyzed formulas (9).

3. CANCER

Soy milk and, more generally, isoflavone intake have primarily been associated with endocrine responsive cancers, including prostate cancer, but particularly breast cancer. Most of the research has examined soy products in general but also extracted isoflavones, and findings are relevant, whatever the food source.

Interest has focused on soy intake and breast cancer, due to the relatively low breast cancer mortality rates in Asian countries, where soy foods are commonly consumed. In Japan, for example, the breast cancer mortality rate is about one quarter of that in the United States (10). In addition, a lower proportion of breast biopsies from Asian women

Table 2
Isoflavone Content (mg/100 g Wet Weight) of Soy Milk*

Isoflavone	N (number of individual values)	Mean	SE	Minimum	Maximum
Daidzein	14	4.45	0.75	1.14	9.84
Genistein	16	6.06	0.84	1.12	11.28
Glycitein	5	0.56	0.09	0.36	0.86
Total isoflavones	14	9.65	1.76	1.26	21.13

*Data taken from the USDA-Iowa State University Database on the Isoflavone Content of Foods (5). SE, standard error.

contain hyperplasia, atypical hyperplasia, and apocrine metaplasia than breast biopsies from American women (11,12). The evidence linking isoflavone or soy intake with breast cancer risk comes from several sources.

In vitro studies have established that isoflavones are weakly estrogenic, because they have the ability to weakly bind to mammalian estrogen receptors. Genistein has the strongest affinity for mammalian estrogen receptors, approx 100 times fewer than 17β-estradiol, whereas daidzein and equol bind approx 1000 times fewer (13). Although these weak estrogens bind to the estrogen-receptor complex, they do not stimulate a full estrogenic response of estrogen-receptor replenishment and protein synthesis. They may, thus, act paradoxically as both estrogens and antiestrogens (14). There are hundreds of in vitro studies showing that genistein inhibits the growth of a range of both hormone-dependent and hormone-independent cancer cells, including breast cancer with an IC_{50} between 5 and 40 μmol/L (15). In vitro studies of genistein suggest that it also inhibits the metastatic activity of breast cancer cells independent of its effects on cell growth (16).

Apart from antiestrogenic action, the mechanism whereby isoflavones reduce cell growth, particularly in estrogen-receptor-negative cells, has yet to be fully elucidated. Although their antioxidant properties must contribute to the anticancer effects observed in vitro (17), it is likely that these effects are also due to their inhibitory actions on several enzymes involved in signal transduction, including tyrosine protein kinases (18), MAP kinase (19), and ribosomal S6 kinase (20). Genistein inhibits the DNA topoisomerase II activity (21), inhibits angiogenesis (22), and increases the in vitro concentrations of transforming growth factor β (23). However, many of these effects have been observed at far higher concentrations than would be found in vivo, so caution is warranted in the interpretation of some of this early work.

A majority of studies in animal models (both rat and mice) show that isoflavone supplementation may prevent mammary tumors induced by chemical carcinogens. Seven out of nine studies have shown lower numbers of tumors in rats whose diets were supplemented with soy isoflavones compared to those that were fed standard diets, and no study showed an increase in the number of tumors (2). These effects were not seen when feeding products that were treated to remove the isoflavones (24). The chemopreventive effects are generally attributed to isoflavones' antiestrogenic characteristics.

Although there is supportive evidence from in vitro and animal studies that isoflavone intake may influence the risk of breast cancer, there are few studies on this association in humans. Epidemiologic studies indicate that, in populations with a high isoflavone intake, the risk of breast cancer is reduced *(25–27)* and that, within ethnic groups whose diets are traditionally high in isoflavone intake, a move to a Western lifestyle (including diet) has led to an increase in breast cancer incidence *(28,29)*.

Since 1990, four case-control studies of breast cancer have evaluated the association between self-reported soy intake and breast cancer. These studies were conducted in the Chinese population of Singapore *(30,31)*, Shanghai and Tianjin in China *(32)*, Japanese in Nagoya, Japan *(33)*; and Asian Americans (Chinese, Japanese, and Filipino Americans) residing in San Francisco, CA, and Oahu, HI *(34)*. Study designs varied between the four studies, with those in China and in America population based, whereas those conducted in Japan and Singapore were hospital based. The sample size was largest in Japan, intermediate in China and the United States, and smallest in Singapore. The study in Asian Americans had a smaller age range than those conducted in Asia. In all four studies, adjustment was made for some relevant dietary factors and menstrual and reproductive factors in the analysis, but adjustment for total energy was made only in the Chinese study. In China, there was no association between soy intake and breast cancer risk. This lack of association was seen in both premenopausal and postmenopausal women *(32)*. In Singapore, high soy intake was associated with a reduced risk in premenopausal women but not in postmenopausal women *(30,31)*.

The findings from the studies were as follows. In premenopausal women, high consumers (≥ 55.0 g/d soy product) showed a 60% (95% CI 0.2, 0.9) reduced risk compared with low consumers (< 20.3 g/d) *(30,31)*. Similarly in Japan, a high bean curd intake was associated with a statistically nonsignificant reduced breast cancer risk in premenopausal women but not in postmenopausal women. However, in both groups of women, there was no association between miso soup intake, which was categorized in the food-frequency questionnaire as daily or occasional-to-never, and breast cancer risk *(33)*. Among Asian Americans, tofu intake was associated with a lower risk of breast cancer in both premenopausal and postmenopausal women. Similar results were obtained after adjustment for relevant menstrual and reproductive factors and selective dietary factors *(34)*. Asian American women in the highest intake group (> 120 times/yr) showed a 30% reduced risk (95% CI 0.4, 1.0) compared with women in the lowest intake group (< 12 times/yr). Analysis by migrant status showed a significant protective effect in non-US born American Asians but not in Western-born Asian Americans.

These four case-control studies show some suggestive evidence for a protective association between soy intake and breast cancer risk, but the results, overall, are inconclusive. There are no obvious reasons for the differences in findings between these studies, but the adjustment for dietary factors was not identical. Thus, there may be significant errors due to confounding, because soy intake may be a marker for other lifestyle aspects.

The studies discussed reviewed soy intake as a marker for isoflavone status. Only two studies have, to date, reviewed isoflavone levels or their metabolites in biological fluids. Ingram et al. *(26)* carried out a case-control study of 144 patients with breast cancer and an equal number of age-matched healthy controls in Australia. Examining excretion data in quartiles, when equol (a metabolite of daidzein) excretion increased, the relative risk of breast cancer was significantly reduced. The risk for the highest quartile of excretion of equol, after adjustment for confounding variables, was one quarter that of the lowest quartile. Daidzein showed a similar pattern, but the trend was not significant. The analyses for genistein were not reliable to report results. These results were surprising, because the total phytoestrogen intake of the study subjects, as estimated from the urinary phytoestrogen excretion, was low *(35)*. A similar, though preliminary, study, also conducted in Australia but this time in women who were postmenopausal, found that those with breast cancer had lower 24-h urinary daidzein excretion than controls ($p = 0.03$) and a trend toward lower genistein ($p = 0.08$) *(36)*.

3.1. Intervention Studies—Hormone Endpoints

Several studies have reviewed the effect of isoflavone supplementation on hormonal endpoints, which can then be theoretically related to breast cancer risk *(2)*. Cassidy et al. *(37,38)* showed that isoflavone-rich soy consumption extends the length of the follicular phase and, therefore, overall menstrual cycle and decreases serum concentrations of follicle-stimulating hormone (FSH) and luteinizing hormone (LH). More recently, a 1-mo crossover intervention study using soy milk (113–202 mg/d isoflavone content) or an isoflavone-free soy milk (< 4.5 mg/d isoflavones), with a 4-mo washout between phases, analyzed the effect on the metabolism of 17β-estradiol *(39)*. Higher levels of two putative carcinogenic metabolites of 17β-estradiol (4- and 16α-hydroxyestrogen) and lower amounts of anticarcinogenic metabolites (2-hydroxyestrogens) are associated with a greater risk of breast cancer. An isoflavone-rich diet increased the cycle mean daily urinary excretion of 2-hydroxyestrone, whereas the mean daily excretion of 16α-hydroxyestrone did not change. The ratio of 2-hydroxyestrone to 16α-hydroxy-estrone was higher during the isoflavone-rich diet (2.6 ± 0.34) than during the isoflavone-free diet (2.0 ± 0.32; $p = 0.01$). These results suggest that isoflavones increase the metabolism of endogenous estrogens to the protective 2-hydroxylated estrogens in women, and this may play a role in lowering 17β-estradiol levels and, therefore, reduce breast cancer risk *(39)*. The results of two human studies, however, suggest that soy consumption may exert estrogenic effects on breast tissue and highlight the fact that caution is necessary at this stage.

3.2. Intervention Studies—Breast Cancer-Related Endpoints

In a 6-mo study by Petrakis et al. *(40)*, feeding soy protein isolate (containing 37.4 mg genistein/d) caused an increase in both the secretion of breast fluid and the number of atypical cells in it; this was seen in both premenopausal and postmenopausal women. However, this was a pilot study, which did not include a control group.

In another study, this time in premenopausal women, by McMichael-Phillips et al. *(41)*, the DNA synthesis rate by breast cells taken from biopsies of normal breast tissue from women with benign or malignant disease was enhanced by 14 d of soy feeding (60 g/d, equivalent to 45 mg isoflavones) before surgery.

From these intervention studies, it is obvious that the link between isoflavones and breast cancer has yet to be fully established, whereas the mechanisms involved also must be further elucidated. The heterogeneity of response to isoflavone exposure, which depends on gut microflora activity, necessitates an increase in the numbers of subjects required for an adequately powered study *(2)*. In addition, the dilemma over whether isoflavones act as estrogens or antiestrogens in humans is further complicated by recent work identifying a novel second estrogen receptor, ERβ, to which isoflavones bind *(42)*. Finally, emerging animal study evidence suggests that short-term neonatal and prepubertal exposure to dietary isoflavones decreases carcinogen-induced breast cancer by increasing the proportion of differentiated cells in the mammary gland *(43)*. This supports the concept that the protective effect of the traditional Asian diet occurs early in life *(44)*, which may explain why epidemiologic studies focusing on adult intake have, to date, been unimpressive.

Therefore, in vitro and animal evidence suggests that dietary isoflavones, whether soy milk or other soy forms, may be protective against the development of breast cancer. Epidemiologic evidence remains inconclusive, and, although case-control studies have produced convincing evidence that increased dietary isoflavone intake correlates with reduction in breast cancer risk, early intervention studies have produced conflicting results. Furthermore, well-designed research should elucidate the role of these compounds/foods in breast cancer etiology.

4. OSTEOPOROSIS

Estrogen replacement therapy is highly effective at reducing the rate of bone loss and can also replace lost bone *(45)*. Epidemiologic data suggest that osteoporosis is approximately one third as common in Japanese women (who consume a diet rich in soy products) compared with those on a Western diet *(46)*. However, there are many confounding factors distinguishing Asian women from Western women (lifestyle, sociocultural, and morphologic factors), whereas the extent to which this difference is genetic is also unknown *(47)*.

Animal studies demonstrate a favorable effect of isoflavones on bone: an isoflavone-rich diet partially prevents bone loss induced by ovariectomy in female rats *(48)*.

Studies in women have concentrated on ipriflavone, a synthetic isoflavone, and have shown that this compound (of which approx 10% of the ingested dose is converted to the natural phytoestrogen daidzein), slightly prevents bone loss in women treated with a gonadotrophin-releasing hormone agonist *(49)*. In another placebo-controlled study, 98 women with an established diagnosis of osteoporosis were given ipriflavone, 200 mg/3 times d. After 2 yr of treatment, the placebo-treated group lost 3.5% of bone mass, but those treated with ipriflavone maintained or slightly increased their bone density *(50)*. A further placebo-controlled study with 453 participants and the same study design showed similar results after 2 yr *(51)*.

Numerous studies show that ipriflavone not only prevents bone loss but also increases bone mass *(52,53)*. However, ipriflavone is a synthetic derivative used at pharmacologic doses, and its effects cannot, therefore, be extrapolated to those of natural phytoestrogens or of soy milk *(47)*.

Potter et al. *(54)* reported that in women who were postmenopausal an isoflavone-rich diet for a 6-mo period slightly increased lumbar bone mineral density (2%), but this was a short-term study conducted on a small number of women. Another study examined the effects of soy isoflavones on bone turnover markers for > 3 mo and found small beneficial effects, although the authors concluded that they were unlikely to be of clinical significance *(55)*.

Another study examined the effect of three daily servings of whole soy foods (approx 60 mg/d) for 12 wk on osteoporosis markers of women who were postmenopausal *(56)*. A significant serum osteocalcin increase was observed, but no change in bone-specific alkaline phosphatase was noted, confirming that the situation is complicated.

Therefore, although isoflavones prevent bone loss under experimental conditions, their effect, and that of soy milk, must be confirmed by longer term larger studies, with a careful choice of suitable endpoints.

5. CORONARY HEART DISEASE

The protective role of a soy-rich diet on coronary heart disease (CHD) has been hypothesized based on the decreased incidence of CHD in Asian countries. However, Asian lifestyles are distinct from Western lifestyles in several ways, e.g., their diet is much lower in saturated fat and higher in fiber *(57)*.

One study examined the associations between dietary isoflavone intake and CHD risk factors in women who were postmenopausal. Isoflavone consumption did not vary by age, exercise, smoking, education, or years postmenopausal. In adjusted analyses, however, genistein, daidzein, and total isoflavone intake were positively associated with high-density lipoprotein (HDL) cholesterol and inversely associated with insulin levels after a glucose challenge *(58)*. These observations suggest that isoflavone exerts effects that will decrease the risk of CHD.

Isoflavones in the form of soy milk may affect CHD risk by numerous mechanisms. Isoflavones can act as antioxidants *(2)* and may inhibit LDL oxidation *(59)*. Kapiotis et al. *(60)* observed that LDL oxidation products, assayed as thiobarbituric acid-reactive substances, were strongly inhibited by genistein, somewhat inhibited by daidzein, but not affected by genistin (the glycosylated form of genistein) or control. Furthermore, both genistein and daidzein protected against cytotoxic effects of oxidized LDL, as assessed by cellular morphologic features, and lactate dehydrogenase release by cultured endothelial cells. Genistein also inhibits hydrogen peroxide production and increases the activity of antioxidant enzymes, such as catalase, superoxide dismutase, glutathione peroxidase, and glutathione reductase *(59)*. A protective/antioxidant effect has been shown by phytoestrogen supplementation on the susceptibility of LDL to oxidation in another study *(61)*. Six healthy volunteers received 19 mg/d isoflavones for 2 wk. Lag phases of LDL oxidation curves were reduced postsupplement compared with baseline values. Another study, however, failed to show an inhibition of lipid peroxidation after 8 wk of isoflavonoid supplementation in subjects with high-normal blood pressure *(62)*, measuring urinary F-2-isoprostanes. This study was randomized, double-blind, and placebo-controlled and included relatively large numbers of subjects ($n = 59$).

A meta-analysis of studies published in 1995 concluded that: "Soy protein rather than animal protein significantly decreased serum concentrations of total cholesterol, LDL cholesterol and triglycerides" *(63)*. Of the 38 studies reviewed, 89% reported a net decrease in plasma cholesterol that averaged approx 9% for an intake of approx 47 g soy protein daily. However, 77% of the studies included in the meta-analysis had 95% confidence intervals that included zero.

Since the meta-analysis, several well-controlled studies have been carried out, and the results of these have varied *(64)*. There are several potential explanations for this variability.

Merz-Demlow et al. *(65)* suggest that the effect of isoflavones on lipids may be related to menstrual cycle phase. The food matrix may also be important, and Lichtenstein *(64)* suggests that the effect of isoflavones is somewhat dependent on whether the isoflavones are ingested in isolation or as an enriched preparation of those endogenously present in soy.

A recent study observed a reduction in LDL cholesterol in 156 men and women by an average of 6%. This resulted from a mean reduction of 9% among those with a raised baseline LDL cholesterol (> 4.29 mmol/L) and was only observed in men and women who were postmenopausal *(66)*. It may be that no difference was observed in the largely premenopausal sample set because they had a low-normal lipid status initially. The original meta-analysis also found a greater lowering effect in those with initially raised total cholesterol levels *(63)*.

The mechanism by which isoflavones reduce lipids is not established. Some studies suggest that isoflavones cause an increase in the excretion of bile acids and, therefore, enhance removal of cholesterol *(67)*. Others suggest that isoflavones initiate a hyperthyroid state *(68)*, because an increase in free thyroxine levels is seen after feeding soy protein to animal models *(69,70)*. A third suggestion is that isoflavones alter hepatic metabolism with augmented LDL and very LDL (VLDL) removal by hepatocytes *(59)*. Isoflavone supplementation in animal models reduces cholesterol levels, increases LDL degradation, and increases binding of radiolabeled LDL to receptors *(71)*. An isoflavone-rich diet lowers lipids in normal mice but not in LDL-receptor deficient mice; isoflavones may, therefore, increase LDL receptor activity *(72)*.

The protective isoflavone effect on CHD risk may be independent of both antioxidant and lipid effects. Isoflavones can have direct effects on the arterial wall, reducing vascular smooth muscle cell proliferation *(73)*. In macaques with preexisting atherosclerosis, fed either a soy+ or soy– diet for 6 mo, the soy– diet was associated with constriction of coronary arteries, whereas the soy+ diet was associated with a vasodilatory response. Intravenous genistein also produced a vasodilatory response *(74)*.

Nestel et al. *(75)* found no effect of a 5- to 10-wk intervention with an isoflavone tablet (80 mg/d) on either LDL oxidation or lipid levels, but found a significant (26%, $p < 0.001$ compared with placebo) improvement in systemic arterial compliance in 21 women who were menopausal and perimenopausal. This improvement is similar to what is achieved with conventional hormone replacement therapy *(76)*.

Finally, soy/isoflavones may affect atherosclerotic plaque formation. Atherosclerosis is initiated by monocytes binding to the endothelium and migrating to the intimal layer to develop into foam cells. This process is dependent on the transcription of adhesion molecules. Genistein inhibits the expression of ICAM-1 on human endothelial cells that have been cocultured with monocytes *(77)*.

The effect of soy has been examined in an apo-E mouse model, where soy protein isolate (SPI) was compared with casein *(78)*. The lesion area of the thoracic aorta in the SPI group was lower than in the casein group; therefore, SPI may reduce atherosclerotic lesion development. In a similar study, male monkeys were fed a soy+ diet (soy with isoflavones), a soy– diet (alcohol-extracted soy protein low in isoflavones), or a control diet consisting of a casein and lactalbumin mixture. Soy+ monkeys had lower total and LDL cholesterol and higher HDL cholesterol. Lesion development differed by diet, with the soy+ group having the smallest lesion area, followed by the soy– group and the casein group *(78)*.

Further work is required on the effects of isoflavones/soy milk on CHD risk, because the current epidemiological data are weak. There are, however, several possible mechanisms by which soy could reduce CHD risk, and this is a promising area of research.

6. NUTRITIONAL EQUIVALENCE TO MILK?

Giving a general estimate of the nutritional values of soy milk is difficult, because it differs considerably from brand to brand. Those labeled as "extra" or "fortified" have more calcium, vitamins A and D, and other nutrients, whereas flavored soy milk usually means more calories and sugar. Nutritionists recommend that those substituting soy milk for dairy milk should follow the recommended 2–3 servings/d and should use milk that has at least 30% of the daily requirement of calcium per serving.

For infant milk formulas, the distribution of nutrients in soy protein formulas is similar to that found in cow milk formulas. Several clinical studies show that feeding soy protein formulas to full-term infants is associated with normal growth, protein nutritional status, and bone mineralization *(9)*.

7. CONCLUSIONS

As cow's milk continues to attract a bad press, and the reported incidence of lactose intolerance increases, alternative milk sources will gain popularity. Soy milk, and soy products in general, which are rich in isoflavones, have attracted interest as potential health-promoting foods. Cell, animal, and, in particular, human studies are at an early stage, but these isoflavone-rich foods may have a role to play in endocrine-responsive cancer, osteoporosis, and CHD prevention.

8. MAIN POINTS FOR PRIMARY AND CLINICAL REVIEW

1. Soy milk has become more popular because it is tolerated by lactose-intolerant individuals and its protein and isoflavone content.
2. Soy isoflavones have weak estrogenic qualities and may be recognized by some estrogen receptors in the body.
3. Several studies suggest that soy consumption may be protective against cancer, especially breast and prostate cancer.
4. Soy consumption may also be protective against cardiovascular disease through effects on lipid profile and antioxidant effects, although the data are inconclusive.
5. For persons who cannot drink cow's milk, nutritionists suggest substitution with three servings of calcium-fortified soy milk per day.

REFERENCES

1. Holland B, Welch AA, Unwin ID, Buss, DH, Paul AA, Southgate DAT. McCance and Widdowson's The Composition of Foods. Royal Society of Chemistry, Cambridge, UK, 1991.
2. Bingham SA, Atkinson C, Liggins J, Bluck L, Coward A. Phyto-oestrogens: where are we now? Br J Nutr 1998;79:393–406.
3. Coward L, Barnes NC, Setchell KDR, Barnes S. Genistein and daidzein, and their glycoside conjugates: anti-tumor isoflavones in soybean foods from American and Asian diets. J Agric Food Chem 1993;41: 1961–1967.
4. Francis CM, Millington AJ, Bailey ET. The distribution of oestrogenic isoflavones in the genus Trifolium. Austr Vet J 1967;18:47–54.

5. Food and Nutrition Information Center. Accessed April 25, 2002, from http://www.nal.usda.gov/fnic

6. Lu LJ, Anderson KE. Sex and long-term soy diets affect the metabolism and excretion of soy isoflavones in humans. Am J Clin Nutr 1998;68:1500S–1504S.

7. Garrow JS, James WPT. Human Nutrition and Dietetics. Churchill Livingstone, Philadelphia, PA, 1996.

8. Turner GK. Lactose intolerance and irritable bowel syndrome. Nutrition 2000;16:665–666.

9. Businco L, Bruno G, Giampietro PG. Soy protein for the prevention and treatment of children with cow-milk allergy. Am J Clin Nutr 1998;68:1447S–1452S.

10. American Cancer Society. Cancer Facts and Figures. American Cancer Society, Atlanta, GA, 1994.

11. Schuerch C, III, Rosen PP, Hirota T, et al. A pathologic study of benign breast diseases in Tokyo and New York. Cancer 1982;50:1899–1903.

12. Sasano N, Tamahashi N, Namiki T, Stemmermann GN. Consecutive radiography of breast slices for estimation of glandular volume and detection of small subclinical lesions. A comparison between Japan and Hawaii Japanese. Tohoku J Exp Med 1975;117:217–224.

13. Verdeal K, Ryan DS. Naturally-occurring estrogens in plant foodstuffs—a review. J Food Protection 1979;42:577–583.

14. Tang BY, Adams NR. Effect of equol on oestrogen receptors and on synthesis of DNA and protein in the immature rat uterus. J Endocrinol 1980;85:291–297.

15. Messina MJ. Legumes and soybeans: overview of their nutritional profiles and health effects. Am J Clin Nutr 1999;70:439S–450S.

16. Scholar EM, Toews ML. Inhibition of invasion of murine mammary carcinoma cells by the tyrosine kinase inhibitor genistein. Cancer Lett 1994;87:159–162.

17. Wei H, Wei L, Frenkel K, Bowen R, Barnes S. Inhibition of tumor promoter-induced hydrogen peroxide formation in vitro and in vivo by genistein. Nutr Cancer 1993;20:1–12.

18. Akiyama T, Ishida J, Nakagawa S, et al. Genistein, a specific inhibitor of tyrosine-specific protein kinases. J Biol Chem 1987;262:5592–5595.

19. Thorburn J, Thorburn A. The tyrosine kinase inhibitor, genistein, prevents alpha-adrenergic-induced cardiac muscle cell hypertrophy by inhibiting activation of the Ras-MAP kinase signaling pathway. Biochem Biophys Res Commun 1994;202:1586–1591.

20. Linassier C, Pierre M, Le Pecq JB, Pierre J. Mechanisms of action in NIH-3T3 cells of genistein, an inhibitor of EGF receptor tyrosine kinase activity. Biochem Pharmacol 1990;39:187–193.

21. Constantinou A, Kiguchi K, Huberman E. Induction of differentiation and DNA strand breakage in human HL-60 and K-562 leukemia cells by genistein. Cancer Res 1990;50:2618–2624.

22. Fotsis T, Pepper M, Adlercreutz H, Hase T, Montesano R, Schweigerer L. Genistein, a dietary ingested isoflavonoid, inhibits cell proliferation and in vitro angiogenesis. J Nutr 1995;125:790S–797S.

23. Kim H, Peterson TG, Barnes S. Mechanisms of action of the soy isoflavone genistein: emerging role for its effects via transforming growth factor beta signaling pathways. Am J Clin Nutr 1998;68:1418S–1425S.

24. Barnes S. Effect of genistein on in vitro and in vivo models of cancer. J Nutr 1995;125:777S–783S.

25. Adlercreutz H. Western diet and Western diseases: some hormonal and biochemical mechanisms and associations. Scand J Clin Lab Invest 1990;201:S3–S23.

26. Ingram D, Sander K, Kolybaba M, Lopez D. Case-control study of phyto-oestrogens and breast cancer. Lancet 1998;350:990–994.

27. Wu AH, Ziegler RG, Nomura AM, et al. Soy intake and risk of breast cancer in Asians and Asian Americans. Am J Clin Nutr 1998;68:1437S–1443S.

28. Buell P. Changing incidence of breast cancer in Japanese American women. J Natl Cancer Inst 1973;51:1479–1483.

29. Lee HP, Day NE, Shanmugaratnam K. Trends in cancer incidence in Singapore 1968-1982. IARC Scientific Publications 1988;91:1–161.

30. Lee HP, Gourley L, Duffy SW, Esteve J, Lee J, Day NE. Dietary effects on breast-cancer risk in Singapore. Lancet 1991;337:1197–1200.

31. Lee HP, Gourley L, Duffy SW, Esteve J, Lee J, Day NE. Risk factors for breast cancer by age and menopausal status: a case-control study in Singapore. Cancer Causes Control 1992;3:313–322.

32. Yuan JM, Wang QS, Ross RK, Henderson BE, Yu MC. Diet and breast cancer in Shanghai and Tianjin, China. Br J Cancer 1995;71:1353–1358.

33. Hirose K, Tajima K, Hamajima N, et al. A large-scale, hospital-based case-control study of risk factors of breast cancer according to menopausal status. Jpn J Cancer Res 1995;86:146–154.

34. Wu AH, Ziegler RG, Horn-Ross PL, et al. Tofu and risk of breast cancer in Asian-Americans. Cancer Epidemiol Biomarkers Prev 1996;5:901–906.

35. Messina M, Barnes S, Setchell KD. Phyto-oestrogens and breast cancer. Lancet 1997;350:971–972.

36. Murkies A, Dalais FS, Briganti EM, et al. Phytoestrogens and breast cancer in postmenopausal women: a case control study. Menopause 2000;7:289–296.

37. Cassidy A, Bingham S, Setchell KD. Biological effects of a diet of soy protein rich in isoflavones on the menstrual cycle of premenopausal women. Am J Clin Nutr 1994;60:333–340.

38. Cassidy A, Bingham S, Setchell K. Biological effects of isoflavones in young women: importance of the chemical composition of soybean products. Br J Nutr 1995;74:587–601.

39. Lu LJ, Cree M, Josyula S, Nagamani M, Grady JJ, Anderson KE. Increased urinary excretion of 2-hydroxyestrone but not 16-alpha-hydroxyestrone in premenopausal women during a soya diet containing isoflavones. Cancer Res 2000;60:1299–1305.

40. Petrakis NL, Barnes S, King EB, et al. Stimulatory influence of soy protein isolate on breast secretion in pre- and postmenopausal women. Cancer Epidemiol Biomarkers Prev 1996;5:785–794.

41. McMichael-Phillips DF, Harding C, Morton M, et al. Effects of soy-protein supplementation on epithelial proliferation in the histologically normal human breast. Am J Clin Nutr 1998;68:1431S–1435S.

42. Kuiper GG, Carlsson B, Grandien K, et al. Comparison of the ligand binding specificity and transcript tissue distribution of estrogen receptors alpha and beta. Endocrinology 1997;138:863–870.

43. Lamartiniere CA, Moore J, Holland M, Barnes S. Neonatal genistein chemoprevents mammary cancer. Proc Soc Exp Biol Med 1995;208:120–123.

44. Colditz GA, Frazier AL. Models of breast cancer show that risk is set by events of early life: prevention efforts must shift focus. Cancer Epidemiol Biomark Prev 1995;4:567–571.

45. Ettinger M, Genant HK, Cann CE. Long-term estrogen replacement therapy prevents bone loss and fractures. Ann Intern Med 1985;102:319–324.

46. Cooper C, Campion G, Melton LJ. Hip fractures in the elderly—a world-wide projection. Osteoporosis Int 1992;2:285–289.

47. Glazier MG, Bowman MA. A review of the evidence for the use of phytoestrogens as a replacement for traditional estrogen replacement therapy. Arch Intern Med 2001;161:1161–1172.

48. Arjmandi BH, Alekel L, Hollis BW, et al. Dietary soy bean protein prevents bone loss in an ovariectomised rat model of osteoporosis. J Nutr 1996;126:161–167.

49. Gambacciani M, Spinetti A, Piagesi L, et al. Ipriflavone prevents the bone mass reduction in premenopausal women treated with gonadotrophin-releasing hormone agonists. Bone Miner 1994;26:19–26.

50. Adami S, Bufalino L, Cervetti R, et al. Ipriflavone prevents radial bone loss in postmenopausal women with low bone mass over 2 years. Osteoporosis Int 1997;7:119–125.

51. Gennari C, Adami S, Agnusdei D, et al. Effect of chronic treatment with ipriflavone in postmenopausal women with low bone mass. Calcif Tissue Int 1997;61:S19–S22.

52. Kovacs AB. Efficacy of ipriflavone in the prevention and treatment of postmenopausal osteoporosis. Agents Actions 1994;41:86–87.

53. Passeri M, Biondi M, Costi D, et al. Effect of ipriflavone on bone mass in elderly osteoporotic women. Bone Miner 1992;19:S57–S62.

54. Potter S, Baum JA, Teng H, Stillman RJ, Shay NF, Erdman JR. Soy protein and isoflavones: their effects on blood lipids and bone density in postmenopausal women. Am J Clin Nutr 1998;68:S1375–S1378.

55. Wangen KE, Duncan AM, Merz-Demlow BE, et al. Effects of soy isoflavones on markers of bone turnover in premenopausal and postmenopausal women. J Clin Endocrinol Metab 2000;85:3043–3048.

56. Scheiber MD, Liu JH, Subbiah MTR, Rebar RW, Setchell KDR. Dietary inclusion of whole soy foods results in significant reductions in clinical risk factors for osteoporosis and cardiovascular disease in normal postmenopausal women. Menopause 2001;8:384–392.

57. Tham D, Gardner CD, Haskell W. Potential health benefits of dietary phytoestrogens: a review of the clinical epidemiological and mechanistic evidence. J Clin Endocrinol Metab 1998;83:2223–2235.

58. Goodman-Gruen D, Kritz-Silverstein D. Usual dietary isoflavone intake is associated with cardiovascular disease risk factors in postmenopausal women. J Nutr 2001;131:1202–1206.

59. Lissin LW, Cooke JP. Phytoestrogens and cardiovascular health. J Am Coll Cardiol 2000;35:1403–1410.
60. Kapiotis S, Hermann M, Held I, Seelos C, Ehringer H, Gmeiner BMK. Genistein, the dietary derived angiogenesis inhibitor, prevents LDL oxidation and protects endothelial cells from damage from atherogenic LDL. Arterioscler Thromb Vasc Biol 1997;17:2868–2874.
61. Tikkanen MJ, Wahala K, Ojala S, Vihma V, Adlercreutz H. Effect of soybean phytoestrogen intake on low density lipoprotein oxidation resistance. Proc Natl Acad Sci USA 1998;95:3106–3110.
62. Hodgson JM, Puddey IB, Croft KD, Mori TA, Rivera J, Beilin LJ. Isoflavonoids do not inhibit in vivo lipid peroxidation in subjects with high-normal blood pressure. Atherosclerosis 1999;145:167–172.
63. Anderson JW, Johnstone BM, Cook-Newell ME. Meta-analysis of the effects of soy protein intake on serum lipids. N Engl J Med 1995;332:276–282.
64. Lichtenstein AH. Got soy? Am J Clin Nutr 2001;73:667–668.
65. Merz-Demlow BE, Duncan AM, Wangen KE, et al. Soy isoflavones improve plasma lipids in normocholesterolemic, premenopausal women. Am J Clin Nutr 2000;71:1462–1469.
66. Crouse JR, Morgan T, Terry TG, Ellis J, Vitolins M, Burke GL. A randomised trial comparing the effect of casein with that of soy protein containing various amounts of isoflavones on plasma concentrations of lipids and lipoproteins. Arch Intern Med 1999;159:2070–2076.
67. Potter SM. Soy protein and serum lipids. Curr Opin Lipidol 1996;7:260–264.
68. Potter SM. Overview of the proposed mechanisms for the hypocholesterolaemic effects of soy. J Nutr 1995;125:606S–611S.
69. Forsythe WA. Soy protein, thyroid regulation and cholesterol metabolism. J Nutr 1995;125:619S–623S.
70. Lichtenstein AH. Soy protein, isoflavones and cardiovascular disease risk. J Nutr 1998;128:1589–1592.
71. Sirtori CR, Lovati MR, Manzoni C, et al. Soy and cholesterol reduction: clinical experience. J Nutr 1995;125:598S–605S.
72. Kirk EA, Sutherland P, Wang SA, Chait A, LeBoeuf RC. Dietary isoflavones reduce plasma cholesterol and atherosclerosis in C57BL/6 mice but not LDL receptor-deficient mice. J Nutr 1998;128:954–959.
73. Pan W, Ikeda K, Takebe M, Yamori Y. Genistein, daidzein and glycitein inhibit growth and DNA synthesis or aortic smooth muscle cells from stroke prone spontaneously hypertensive rats. J Nutr 2001; 131:1154–1158.
74. Honore EK, Williams JK, Anthiny MS, Clarkson TB. Soy isoflavones enhance coronary vascular reactivity in atherosclerotic female macaques. Fertil Steril 1997;67:148–154.
75. Nestel PJ, Yamashita T, Sasahara T, et al. Soy isoflavones improve systemic arterial compliance but not plasma lipids in menopausal and perimenopausal women. Arterioscler Thromb Vasc Biol 1997; 17:3392–3398.
76. Rajkumar C, Kingwell BA, Cameron JD, et al. Hormonal therapy increases arterial compliance in postmenopausal women. J Am Coll Cardiol 1997;30:350–356.
77. Takahashi M, Ikeda U, Masuyama JI, et al. Monocyte-endothelial cell interaction induces expression of adhesion molecules on human umbilical cord endothelial cells. Cardiovasc Res 1996;32:422–429.
78. Ni W, Tsuda Y, Sakono M, Imaizumi K. Dietary soy protein isolate, compared with casein, reduces atherosclerotic lesion area in apolipoprotein E-deficient mice. J Nutr 1998;128:1884–1889.

16 Human Milk and Infant Formula

Nutritional Content and Health Benefits

James K. Friel

1. WHAT IS THE BEST MILK FOR AN INFANT?

1.1. Recommendations from Authoritative Bodies

Current recommendations by the Canadian and the American Pediatric Societies are to breastfeed for the first year of life, with human milk being the primary source of milk *(1,2)*. Formula feeding is recommended for those who choose not to breastfeed. The consumption of whole or reduced-fat cow's milk is not recommended during the first year of life *(3)*. As of 2000, approx 68% of mothers in the United States initiate breastfeeding and 20% continue to 6 mo (Ross Mother's Survey). In Canada, 77% of children under the age of 3 yr were breastfed for some period of time (1996–1997 National Longitudinal Survey of Children and Youth [NLSCY]).

The first year of life is a time of more rapid growth, development, and maturation than any subsequent year. Body growth and development of the nervous system depend on an appropriate intake of calories and essential nutrients. The recent joint publication by the American and Canadian nutrition working groups, sponsored by the American Institute of Medicine, defines infancy as the period from birth to 12 mo of age, divided into two 6-mo periods *(4)*. The determination of the Adequate Intake (AI) during the first 6 mo of life for every nutrient is based on the average intake by full-term infants who are born to healthy well-nourished mothers and exclusively fed human milk. The mean intake of a nutrient was calculated based on the average concentration of the nutrient from 2 to 6 mo of lactation and assuming an average volume of milk intake of 780 mL/d. In the second 6 mo of infancy, AIs are based on nutrients available from 600 mL/d of human milk and that provided by the usual intake of complementary foods. Exclusive human milk feeding is the preferred method of feeding normal full-term infants for the first 4–6 mo of life, as recommended by most health professionals *(2,3)*. Although there are national regulations for upper and lower limits of nutrient content of infant formulas, specific Dietary Reference Intakes (DRIs) to meet the needs of formula-fed infants were not proposed. This was an error, because as a percentage of the total kinds of milk consumed during the first year of life *(5)*, formula is the milk food

From: *Beverages in Nutrition and Health*
Edited by: T. Wilson and N. J. Temple © Humana Press Inc., Totowa, NJ

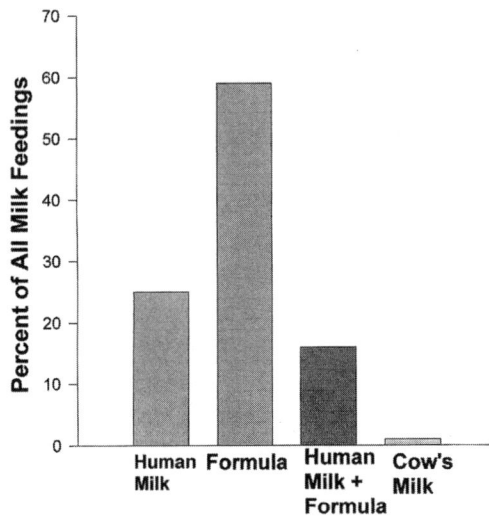

Fig. 1.

most consumed (Fig. 1). Not setting recommendations penalizes infants whose parents have chosen not to breastfeed or have switched to formula.

Breastfeeding is rarely contraindicated *(2)*. Infants who have galactosemia or whose mothers use illegal drugs, have untreated active tuberculosis, or have been infected with HIV should not breastfeed *(1)*. However, smoking, environmental contaminants, moderate alcohol consumption, or prescription and over-the-counter drugs use should not preclude breastfeeding.

With all the best intentions and technologic expertise, "humanized" infant formulas do not compare to mother's own milk. Therefore, it is logical and appropriate for health professionals to encourage human milk consumption whenever possible. However, once the information is presented, there is no justification for attempting to coerce women into making a feeding choice *(6)*.

Sometimes a formula-fed child and, rarely, a breastfed infant develop a sensitivity to cow's milk, either cow milk allergy (CMA) or lactose intolerance. The CMA incidence has been estimated to occur at 0.3–7.5% *(7)*. Secondary lactose deficiency occurs in infancy usually after a gastrointestinal (GI) disorder.

Although human milk is "uniquely superior" for infant feeding and is species specific, the most acceptable alternative is commercial formulas. Manufacturers do their utmost to mimic human milk. Presently, all substitute feedings differ markedly from human milk *(1)*. A "formula" is just that: an equation that is proprietary, consisting of a composite mix of nutrients, emulsifiers, and stabilizers that differs between manufacturers. Formulas in North America that are marketed for term infants are either (1) cow-milk based (casein or whey predominant), (2) soy-protein based, or (3) protein-hydrolysate based. The use of soy-based formulas, speciality formulas, or formulas for the feeding of the premature infant is beyond the scope of this review.

The success of formula manufacturers is due to: (1) aggressive marketing; (2) lack of support for breastfeeding from family, friends, and the medical profession; (3) cultural and public perception; (4) convenience; and (5) some government programs providing free infant formula. With the increase in working mothers, formula feeding has become a practical and an attractive alternative. Guidelines for formula composition have evolved over the years to provide not only what must be in a formula but also minimum and maximum levels. Standards may vary between countries.

1.2. Developing Countries

Historically, breastfeeding has been the preferred method of feeding in all countries. The introduction of formula feeding in developing countries has been extremely controversial. In 1981, the WHO/UNICEF "International Code of Marketing of Breast-milk Substitutes" *(8)* was endorsed by many countries. The code seeks to prevent formula promotion at the expense of breastfeeding. It does not ban infant formula but outlines inappropriate marketing practices. This is important because marketing techniques can be subtle. Organizations such as the Infant Feeding Action Coalition (INFACT) promote and protect breastfeeding. They believe that if the WHO code is properly implemented, breastfeeding rates will increase and infant health will improve. Unfortunately, these goals have been difficult to achieve. One reason for this is that the implementation of the WHO code may have a negative effect on the profits made by formula manufacturers.

2. NUTRIENT CONTENT OF BREAST MILK AND INFANT FORMULA

Specific nutrient requirements are expressed as the amount of nutrient needed per 100 kcal of total food intake. This reflects nutrient interaction and can be applied to foods of different caloric concentration. Human milk has a caloric density of 670 kcal/L. Most term formulas are designed to have the same caloric density.

The composition of a formula depends on many factors and differs between manufacturers. For example, cholesterol exists in human milk but is not added to formula because the public perceives cholesterol as "bad." Low-iron formulas are marketed, even though health professionals do not recommend their use as a standard feed. They remain on the market because the public and some health professionals perceive them as beneficial in dealing with problems such as colic and constipation. Companies will not remove their low-iron formula until "the other guy does" and as long as substantial consumer demand exists.

Human milk composition changes during feeding so that most of the fat in human milk occurs in the latter part of feeding, probably saturating the infant and providing a signal for terminating feeding. This does not occur in the formula-fed infant, because the formula composition is constant. The infant who is breastfed has more control over the amount consumed at a feeding than does the formula-fed infant *(6)*. Furthermore, frequent feedings with small amounts at each feeding, as seen in infants who are breastfed *ad libitum*, may lead to favorable metabolism changes *(9)*. These differences may affect feeding habits later in life.

2.1. Macronutrients: Protein, Lipids, and Carbohydrate

The protein content of human milk is high during early lactation (colostrum) and gradually declines to a low level of 0.8–1% in mature milk. The high protein concentration of colostrum results from high concentrations of secretory IgA and lactoferrin. These proteins provide protection against bacteria, giving benefits in early life beyond the role of building-blocks for tissue synthesis. Indeed, human milk is truly the first and foremost "functional food."

Milk proteins are separated into various classes, mainly caseins (10–50% of total) and whey (50–90% of total) proteins *(10)*. Milk fat globule membrane proteins and protein derived from cells present in milk comprise 1–3%. For a few years, manufacturers prepared their formulas with either a whey or a casein base. For the term infant, there is no nutritional advantage of whey-predominant over casein-predominant formulas. Interestingly, digested fragments of human casein, but not bovine casein, which is less well digested, may exert physiologic effects, such as enhancing calcium uptake by cells and playing a role in infant sleeping patterns *(10)*. Little is known about the role of hormones that are present in human milk and that may play a role in the developing infant.

Human milk contains significant amounts of linoleic acid (18:2, n-6: 10–12%), linolenic acid (18:3, n-3, 1–2%), and a small but significant amount of long-chain (n-6) and (n-3) fatty acids *(11)*. Although the total level of PUFA in human milk varies with the mother's intake, it is generally 13–20%. Long-chain fatty acids present in human milk and recently introduced in formula may confer some developmental advantage.

The primary carbohydrate source in human milk is lactose, with small amounts of other sugars. This is the principle carbohydrate of formulas as well. No minimum or maximum intake level of carbohydrate is set for North America. Corn syrup solids and/ or maltodextrin may be used as a carbohydrate source in certain formulas *(6)*.

2.2. Micronutrients: Minerals and Vitamins

2.2.1. MINERALS

Minerals can be divided broadly into macro (calcium, phosphorus, magnesium, sodium, potassium, chlorine, and sulphur) and micro (iron [Fe], zinc [Zn], copper [Cu], molybdenum [Mo], manganese [Mn], rubidium [Rb], cobalt [Co], iodine [I], and selenium [Se]) elements for physiologic purposes. Lead and aluminum *(12)* exist in human milk and may, ultimately, prove to be essential in trace amounts for humans, as shown in other species; however, in excess, they are problematic for human health.

In 19 women who gave birth to full-term infants, we found that mineral concentrations differed in human milk during the first 3 mo of lactation *(13)*. Zn, Cu, Rb, and Mo decreased with time. As for Zn and Cu, the decline in Mo suggests homeostatic regulation, implying possible essentiality for human infants. Cerium, cesium, lanthanum, and tin are not essential, and no consistent pattern in our data occurred that would indicate either maternal or dietary regulation. In general, the mineral content of human milk is not influenced by maternal diet, parity, maternal age, time of milk collection, or different breasts or socioeconomic status *(14)*.

The ultra-trace elements (< 1 µg/g dry diet/d) exist naturally in human milk but depend on protein sources in formulas where they occur as contaminants. Although many of these elements have no specified human requirement, we believe that recommendations for ultra-trace elements must be established. Our concern is that as preparation techniques for making more purified ingredients become available, less of these elements will occur in the normal diet of the formula-fed infant. A particular example is Mo, which is not usually added to infant formula but is essential *(15)*.

2.2.2. VITAMINS

Human milk has all the essential vitamins required by the infant, but it is low in essential vitamins D and K. Vitamin K is given to all infants at birth, and vitamin D (also considered a hormone) is usually recommended as a supplement for breastfed infants. Minimum and maximum levels of vitamins are regulated for formulas so that they are complete. Formula labels state the amount of all nutrients, including vitamins, that must be present when the shelf life expires. Because of this, "overage" is necessary because some vitamins will break down with time. Thus, as much as 60% over label claim might be present for different nutrients, primarily vitamins *(16)*.

2.2.3. SUPPLEMENTS

Supplement use for infants fed human milk is controversial. Some view supplements as undermining the integrity of human milk and implying that it is not adequate. Suggesting that human milk can be improved on is: " . . . like entering a minefield, one must tread carefully" *(17)*. Nonetheless, human milk is neither a perfect nor a complete food *(18)*. There are sufficient data to support vitamin K administration soon after birth to prevent hemorrhagic disease of the newborn and vitamin D supplements during early infancy to prevent rickets *(2,18)*.

A contentious nutrient is iron, because the amount of fortification required is not yet certain. Current practice is for iron supplements to be deferred until 4–6 mo of age, but formulas with a low content (< 4 mg/L) may lead to anemia. Some authorities *(18)* recommend iron supplements of 7 mg/d beginning in the first few weeks of life. Unpublished data from our laboratory support this recommendation, because we found a significant increase in iron status in infants receiving a modest iron supplement (7.5 mg/d). It was once believed that consuming iron-fortified formulas would result in intolerance and GI distress, but such theories have been discredited *(19)*. Fluoride supplements, once recommended for all infants, are no longer recommended during the first year of life *(18)*. Formulas that conform to specification of Canadian/American guidelines do not require supplementation with any minerals or vitamins, because they are complete. For a review of regulations for the nutrient content of infant formulas, *see* Fomon *(6)*.

2.3. Maternal Influences on Milk Content

In general, the content of protein, lipid, carbohydrate, energy, minerals, and most water-soluble vitamins in human milk is not affected by poor maternal nutrition *(20)*. Fat-soluble vitamins and fatty acids are affected by maternal diet *(21)*. There are mechanisms to ensure constant supply and quality of nutrients to the breastfed infant. The major difference between a breastfed and a formula-fed infant is that many of the components of human milk also facilitate the absorption of nutrients and have a function beyond nutrient requirements. Adding more of a nutrient to formula is not necessarily as good as having a bioactive component in human milk, even if present in small amounts (e.g., lactoferrin for both iron absorption and as a bactericide). There are many properties of human milk that attend to such detail for the benefit of the infant.

3. BIOACTIVITY OF HUMAN MILK AND FORMULAS

Human milk is "alive," that is, it has functional components that have a role beyond simply the provision of essential nutrients. According to *Dorland's Medical Dictio-*

nary, a tissue is "an aggregation of similarly specialized cells united in the performance of a single function." Human milk can be classified as a "tissue," which would alter the perspective on how human milk is viewed. There are active and functional ingredients in human milk whose role is evident and others for whom no clear role has been defined.

Bioactive compounds in human milk can be divided into several broad categories: (1) those compounds involved in milk syntheses, nutritional composition, and bioavailability, and (2) compounds that aid in protection and subsequent development of the infant. To date, many bioactive compounds have been identified in human milk, including cytokines immune factors, growth factors, hormones, antimicrobial agents, nucleotides, antioxidants, and enzymes (*see* ref. *22* for a review). Hormones, enzymes, cytokines for immunity, and cells present in milk have physiologically active roles in other tissues; therefore, it is reasonable to assume that they play a role in infant growth and development. Indeed, many bioactive compounds can survive the neonatal gut environment, thereby potentially exerting important physiologic functions *(22,23)*.

The composition of human milk varies. Nutrient content changes over time, so that the makeup of colostrum, transitional milk, and mature milk differ. Nutrient content also changes within the same feed, whereas formula content clearly does not. This is important to infant regulation of food intake.

Early postnatal exposure to flavor passed into human milk from the mother's own diet can predispose the young infant to respond to new foods. The transition from the breastfeeding period to the initiation of a varied solid food diet can be made easier if the infant has already experienced these flavors. Cues from breast milk can influence food choices and make safe new foods with flavors already experienced in breast milk *(24)*. Again, this does not happen with formula feeding.

Several cells exist in human milk. Macrophages, polymorphonuclear leucocytes, epithelial cells, and lymphocytes have been identified in human milk and have a dynamic role to play in the infant gut. These cells may offer systemic protection after transport across the "leaky gut," particularly in the first week of life *(25)*. Antiviral and antibacterial factors exist in human milk, with secretary IgA produced in the mammary gland being one of the major milk proteins *(10)*. There may even be a pathway from the infant back to the mother that tailors production of antibodies against microbes to which the infant has been exposed.

3.1. Enzymes in Human Milk

Enzymes serve to catalyze reactions and must be present only in small amounts to be effective. Hamosh *(22)* classifies enzymes in human milk into three categories: (1) those that function in the mammary gland, e.g., lipoprotein lipase, phosphoglucomutase, and antiproteases; (2) enzymes that might function in the infant, e.g., proteases, α-amylase (facilitates digestion of polysaccharides), and lysozyme (bactericidal); and (3) enzymes whose function is unclear, i.e., lactate dehydrogenase, DNase, and RNase. It is only recently that the physiologic significance of human milk enzymes has become appreciated. More than just protein, and not present in infant formulas, enzymes are another example of why human milk must be seen as alive. The enzymes in human milk have a more highly organized tertiary structure than enzymes from other tissues, which may be to protect function by resisting denaturation in the gut

(22). We believe that as well as serving an immediate function in the intestine, some enzymes may be transported across the gut or act in the body to offer protection to the infant.

Interestingly, amylase digests polysaccharides that are not present in human milk. Amylase is important after the initiation of such starch supplements as cereals *(22)*. It is as if the mammary gland is "thinking ahead" and assisting the infant gut in the transition to weaning. Milk-digestive lipase assists the newborn whose endogenous lipid digestive function is not well developed at birth.

Glutathione peroxidase (GHSPx) activity correlates with milk selenium concentration *(26)*. GHSPx may be related to fatty acid function or maintain milk integrity by neutralizing free radicals. We measured both GHSPx and superoxide dismutase for 3 mo in full-term milk and found high activity of both enzymes *(27)*. Because there are at least 44 enzymes whose substrates could be lipid peroxides or hydrogen peroxide *(22)*, these enzymes may protect the infant's gut.

3.2. Antioxidants

Recent interest has focused on the antioxidant properties of human milk. Several groups have reported the ability of colostrum *(28)* and mature milk *(29)* to resist oxidative stress, using several end points. This ability in human milk is heterogeneous rather than attributable to a specific compound. Infant formulas are less resistive to oxidative stress than is human milk. This is noteworthy, because formulas always have considerably more vitamins E and C, which are two of the more important antioxidants, than that found naturally in human milk *(30)*. Some researchers suggest that the attainment of adult levels of some antioxidants during infancy is dependent on human milk feeding *(23)*.

3.3. Should Infant Formulas Be Supplemented With Bioactive Ingredients?

We believe that infant formulas should be supplemented with bioactive ingredients *(29)*. Enzymes and long-chain polyunsaturated fatty acids are the more obvious additions. With recombinant technology, there are real possibilities of providing exciting alternatives to current infant formulations. This is the difference between seeing formula as a supply of nutrients or as a functional food. It is possible and realistic to modify manufacturing processes to preserve the biologic activity of certain molecules in the end product.

4. HEALTH BENEFITS OF HUMAN MILK

The health benefits of human milk are significant. Breastfeeding protects against numerous illnesses, particularly incidence and severity of diarrhea, otitis media, upper respiratory illnesses, botulism, and necrotizing enterocolitis *(21,23)*. Before advancements in hygiene, infants who were not breastfed did not fare well and mortality rates were as high as 90% *(5,21)*. Even with the use of current formulas, breastfed infants have lower incidences of many illnesses and are generally sicker for shorter times *(31)* than formula-fed infants. Breastfed infants have decreased incidence of diabetes, cancer, and cardiovascular disease (CVD) later in life *(32)*.

4.1. Growth

The most practical measure of the overall health and well-being of infants is growth. One would expect that with all the advantages of human milk, a breastfed baby would gain more weight (33). It is a puzzling phenomenon that growth of the exclusively breastfed infant is lower in weight-for-age than a formula-fed infant. The average difference at 12 mo will be 600 to 650 g, with no difference in height, so that a breastfed infant is leaner. There is probably more energy intake by a formula-fed infant. The relevance of increased growth in formula-fed infants is questionable, because no negative effects on functional outcomes have been observed in breastfed infants. We found that infants who had consumed home formulas made of evaporated milk grew more than either formula-fed or breastfed infants (34), yet they did not perform as well as infants fed human milk on tests of visual function (35).

4.2. Cognitive Development

There is controversy in this area, because it is difficult to conduct an ideal study. Breastfed infants have enhanced cognitive and neurologic outcomes in comparison to formula-fed infants (36–39). Small differences have been seen even into later childhood (37,39). Increased duration of breastfeeding and higher verbal IQ scores have been reported. Increasing the period of exclusive breastfeeding enhances infant motor development (40). We found enhanced visual acuity in full-term breastfed infants compared with formula-fed infants related to blood fatty acid levels (35). The explanation for these consistent observations is highly controversial. Possibly, there are components of human milk that enhance cognitive development. Other factors that may be responsible are the act of breastfeeding itself, maternal education, and social class.

Lucas reported improved neurologic development in infants fed human milk and sparked much debate concerning which factors truly explain the increased cognitive development in the human milk-fed infant (37). It is reasonable to assume that breast milk containing long-chain polyunsaturated fatty acids, enzymes, hormones, trophic factors, peptides, and nucleotides may enhance brain development and learning ability. Further, it is sensible to feed human milk whenever possible if any or all of the above differences are true. Whether an infant fed human milk has better development because of maternal factors or biologic factors does not lessen the value of enhanced development to the infant.

5. INTERNATIONAL ASPECTS OF BREASTFEEDING

The WHO attributes 7 of 10 childhood deaths in developing countries to just five main causes: pneumonia, diarrhea, measles, malaria, and malnutrition. All of them can be prevented, some specifically, by breastfeeding (41).

In nonindustrialized countries, the advantages of feeding human milk are easily seen and the use of a commercially available or home-prepared formula is not recommended (6). Home-prepared formulas are usually poorly designed and nutritionally inadequate. These problems are aggravated when there is an absence of a safe water supply, hygienic conditions, and adequate storage facilities.

Evidence from developing countries indicates that infants who are breastfed for fewer than 6 mo or not at all have a mortality rate 5 to 10 times higher in the second 6 mo of life than those breastfed for 6 mo or more *(8)*. Improper marketing of breast-milk substitutes still occurs and can lead to inappropriate feeding practices, resulting in malnutrition, illness, and death in developing countries *(42)*.

5.1. The Economics of Breastfeeding

It has been estimated that in the United States, $3.6 billion would be saved if the prevalence of exclusive breastfeeding rose only 11% *(43)*. Reduced health care costs, reduced employee absenteeism, and savings on formula purchase are all benefits of breastfeeding. The effect of savings on formula purchase would surely be more pronounced in Third-World countries. In fact, formula has become so expensive that it may not be an option in poorer countries. In countries "in transition," this may be more of an issue.

5.2. The Politics of Breastfeeding

Historically, most human infants have been breastfed. To enhance infant feeding practices, WHO and UNICEF launched the Baby-Friendly Hospital initiative in 1992. This policy encourages exclusive breastfeeding in the hospital soon after birth, with no other food or drink given unless medically indicated. This was done to encourage exclusive breastfeeding and discourage the introduction of supplementary formula feeding. Women who receive a "discharge pack" when leaving the hospital, which contains a breast pump rather than infant formula, will breastfeed for a longer period of time *(44)*.

"Exclusive" breastfeeding is defined as no other food or drink, not even water, except breast milk for at least 4 and, if possible, 6 mo of life. Using this criterion, rates for exclusive breastfeeding under 4 mo of age range from 4% to 23% in African countries. Rates are higher in European countries, with Sweden the highest at 61%. Where the advantages of breastfeeding have been widely publicized, breastfeeding rates are increasing, e.g., Australia, Canada, and the United States (http://www.who.int/nut/db_bfd.HTM).

In underdeveloped countries, breastfeeding is so ingrained into the many cultures and traditions of society that the pressure to breastfeed is intense. In fact, a woman can be ostracized from her community for formula feeding. This is why "free samples" are so insidious. If the milk supply dries up and a woman is forced to formula feed, she may become an outcast. HIV has altered perception on formula feeding as even UNICEF, who has been a supporter of breastfeeding, at one time considered providing formula to HIV-positive mothers to protect the infant. This idea has since been dropped. How this tragedy will be treated has not been decided.

If milk is not continually removed from the mother's breast, the ability to secrete milk is lost within 1 to 2 wk. It is common practice to offer an occasional bottle of formula. A better alternative would be for a mother to acquire a breast pump to have milk frozen for those times she is unable to feed.

6. SUMMARY

There is no doubt that human milk is the best food for the human full-term infant. The reasons are endless and convincing. Nonetheless, it is a challenge for the formula industry to make the best suitable alternative to human milk. There are, were, and always will be some women who are unable or choose not to follow recommendations to breastfeed for whatever reason (http://www.who.int/inf-pr-2001/en/note2001-07.html). We have a responsibility to those mothers and their infants to produce a formula that meets their needs. Future changes in infant formulas are likely to be designed to have a positive effect on physical, mental, and immunologic outcomes *(45)*. My hope is that formula will include bioactive ingredients that perform some of the same functions found in that exemplary fluid, human milk.

7. MAIN POINTS FOR PRIMARY AND CLINICAL REVIEW

1. Human breast milk provides the single best nutrition for full-term infants, and provides lactose as the primary carbohydrate, polyunsaturated fats, casein and whey proteins, minerals, vitamins, digestive enzymes, antibodies, components to improve nutrient absorption, and even immune cells.
2. Formula-fed infants tend to gain weight faster, are prone to become sick more frequently and for longer time periods, and possibly have slower cognitive development.
3. Breastfeeding is only contraindicated when the mother is HIV positive, although it may be temporarily precluded as a result of smoking, medication use, and alcohol consumption.
4. Infant formulas are designed to imitate breast milk, but lack cholesterol, the human profile of polyunsaturated fatty acids, and many of the biologically active components found in breast milk.
5. International policies for increased breast-feeding have had a positive impact on infant mortality, and, in the United States, it has been estimated that an 11% increase in breastfeeding would save $3.6 billion in health care costs.

REFERENCES

1. American Academy of Pediatrics. Breast feeding and the use of human milk. Pediatrics 1997;100: 1035–1039.
2. Canadian Paediatric Society, Dieticians of Canada, Health Canada. Nutrition for Healthy Term Infants. Minister of Public Works and Government Services, Ottawa, Canada, 1998.
3. American Academy of Pediatrics. The use of whole cow's milk in infancy. Pediatrics 1992;89:1105–1107.
4. Food and Nutrition Board. Institute of Medicine. Dietary Reference Intakes for Calcium, Phosphorus, Magnesium, Vitamin D and Fluoride. National Academy Press, Washington, DC, 1999, pp. 38–50.
5. Fomon SJ. Infant feeding in the 20th century: formula and breast. J Nutr 2001;131:409S–420S.
6. Fomon SJ. Recommendations for feeding normal infants. In: Nutrition of Normal Infants. Mosby, St. Louis, MO, 1993, pp. 455–458.
7. Bahna SL. Milk allergy in infancy. Ann Allergy 1978;41:1–13.
8. International Organization of Consumers Unions. In: Protecting Infant Health. Annelies A (ed.). Penang, Malaysia, 1986, pp. 36–39.
9. Jenkins DJA, Wolever TMS, Vinson U, et al. Nibbling vs gorging: metabolic advantages of increased meal frequency. N Engl J Med 1989;321:929–934.
10. Lonnerdal B, Atkinson S. Nitrogenous components of milk. A. Human milk proteins. In: Handbook of Milk Composition. Jensen UG (ed.). Academic Press, San Diego, CA, 1995, pp. 351–368.
11. Redenials WAN, Chen Z-Y. Trans, n-2, and n-6 fatty acids in Canadian human milk. Lipids 1996;31: 5279–5282.
12. Quarterman J. Lead. In: Trace Element in Human and Animal Nutrition. Mertz W (ed.). Academic Press, Orlando, FL, 1986, pp. 281–317.
13. Friel JK, Longerich H, Jackson S, Dawson B, Sutrahdar B. Ultra trace elements in human milk from premature and term infants. Biol Tr Elem Res 1999;67:225–247.

14. Lonnerdal B. Regulation of mineral and trace elements in human milk: exogenous and endogenous factors. Nutr Rev 2000;58:223–229.
15. Friel JK, Simmons B, MacDonald AC, Mercer CN, Aziz K, Andrews WL. Molybdenum requirements in low birth weight infants receiving parenteral and enteral nutrition. J Par Ent Nutr 1999;23:155–159.
16. Friel JK, Bessie JC, Belkhode SL, et al. Thiamine riboflavin, pyridoxine, and vitamin C status in premature infants receiving parenteral and enteral nutrition. J Ped Gastro Ent Nutr 2001;33:64–69.
17. Godel JC. Breast-feeding and anemia: let's be careful. Can Med Assoc J 2000;162:343–344.
18. Fomon SJ, Straus UG. Nutrient deficiencies in breast-fed infants. N Engl J Med 1978;299:355–357.
19. Nelson SE, Ziegler EE, Copeland AM, et al. Lack of adverse reaction to iron-fortified formula. Pediatrics 1988;81:360–364.
20. Lonnerdal B. Effects of maternal dietary intake on breast milk composition. J Nutr 1986;116:499–513.
21. Lonnerdal B. Breast milk: a truly functional food. Nutrition 2000;16:509–511.
22. Hamosh M. Enzymes in human milk. In: Handbook of Milk Composition. Jensen UG (ed.). Academic Press, San Diego, CA, 1995, pp. 388–427.
23. L'Abbe MR, Friel JK. Enzymes in human milk. In: Recent Advances in the Role of Lipids in Infant Nutrition. Huang V-S, Sinclair A (eds.). AOCS Press, Champaign, IL, 1998, pp. 133–147.
24. Mennella JA, Jagnow CP, Beauchamp GK. Prenatal and postnatal flavour learning by human infants. Pediatrics 2001;107:1–6.
25. Weaver LT, Lalver MF, Nelson R. Intestinal permeability in the newborn. Arch Dis Child 1984;59: 236–241.
26. Mannan S, Picciano MF. Influence of maternal selenium status on human milk selenium concentration and glutathione peroxidase activity. Am J Clin Nutr 1987;46:95–100.
27. L'Abbe M, Friel JK. Glutathione peroxidase and superoxide dismutase concentrations in milk from mothers of premature and full-term infants. J Ped Gastro Ent Nutr 2000;31:270–274.
28. Buescher ES, McIllherhan SM. Antioxidant properties of human colostrum. Pediatr Res 1988;24: 14–19.
29. Friel JK, Martin SM, Langdon M, Herzberg G, Buettner GR. Human milk provides better antioxidant protection than does infant formula. Pediatr Res 2002;51:612–618.
30. Ross Products Division. Ross Ready Reference. Abbott Laboratories, Columbus, OH, 1999.
31. Dewey KG, Heinig MJ, Nommsen-Rivers LA. Differences in morbidity between breast-fed and formula-fed infants. J Pediatr 1995;126:696–702.
32. Heinig, MJ, Dewey KG. Health advantage of breast feeding for infants: a critical review. Nutr Res Rev 1996;9:89–97.
33. Dewey KG, Heinig, MJ, Nommsen LA, Pearson JM, Lonnerdal B. Growth of breast-fed and formula-fed infants from 0 to 18 months: the DARLING study. Pediatrics 1992;89:1035–1041.
34. Friel JK, Andrews WL, Simmons BS, Mercer C, Macdonald A, McCloy U. An evaluation of full-term infants fed on evaporated milk formula. Acta Paediatr 1997;86:448–453.
35. Courage ML, McCloy U, Herzberg G, et al. Visual acuity development and fatty acid composition of erythrocytes. J Dev Behave Paediatr 1997;19:9–17.
36. Lancing CI, Patonga S, Weigelas-Capes N, Teven BCL, Boersma ER. Breastfeeding and neurological outcome at 42 months. Acta Paediatr 1998;87:1224–1229.
37. Lucas A, Morley R, Cole TJ, Lister G, Leeson-Payne C. Breast milk and subsequent intelligence quotient in children born preterm. Lancet 1992;339:261–264.
38. Friel JK. Cognitive development in breast-fed infants. J Hum Lact 1999;15:97–98.
39. Horwood LJ, Darlow BA, Mogridge N. Breast milk feeding and cognitive ability at 7–8 years. Arch Res Child Fetal Neonat Educ 2001;84:F23–F27.
40. Dewey KG, Cohen RJ, Brown KH, Rivera LL. Effects of exclusive breast feeding for four versus six months on maternal nutritional status and infant motor development. J Nutr 2001;131:262–267.
41. Wegman ME. Infant mortality in the 20th century, dramatic but uneven progress. J Nutr 2001;131: 4015–4085.
42. Wise J. Companies still breaking marketing code. Br Med J 1997;314:165.
43. Weimer JP. The economic benefits of breast-feeding. Economic Research Service. USDA. Report #13, 2001:1–14.

44. Dunghy CI, Christensen-Syalonski J, Losch M, Russel D. Effect of discharge samples on duration of breast-feeding. Pediatrics 1992;90:233–237.
45. Ryan AS, Benson JD, Flammang AM. Infants formulas and medical foods. In: Essentials of Functional Foods. Schmidt MK, Labuza TP (eds.). Aspen Publishers, Inc, Gaithersburg, MD, 2000, pp. 137–163.

17 Inclusion of Probiotics in Beverages

Can It Lead to Improved Health?

Knut J. Heller

1. INTRODUCTION

In 1965, the term "probiotic" was first used by Lilly and Stillwell *(1)* to describe "substances secreted by one microorganism which stimulate the growth of another." It was Parker *(2)* who, in 1974, used the term probiotic in the sense that it is used today. He defined probiotics as "organisms and substances which contribute to intestinal microbial balance." This definition implies beneficial association of certain microorganisms with the human host. Such an association was probably first suggested by Döderlein *(3)*, who proposed that lactic acid produced by vaginal bacteria prevented or inhibited growth of pathogenic bacteria. This idea was further advocated by Metchnikow *(4)*, who considered the longevity of the Caucasian population to be related to their frequent consumption of fermented dairy products. Although Metchnikow attributed the positive health effects to the dairy lactic acid bacteria present in the fermented products, other scientists soon suggested that lactic acid bacteria isolated from the intestines of healthy persons could be exploited for health purposes. One of these scientists was Henneberg *(5)* in Kiel, who proposed the use of an intestinal isolate of *Lactobacillus acidophilus* for production of "Acidophilus-Milch" or "Reform-Joghurt."

A valid definition of the term probiotic based on that by Havenaar and Huis in't Veld *(6)* is given by Schrezenmeir and de Vrese *(7)*: "A preparation of or a product containing viable, defined microorganisms in sufficient numbers, which alter the microflora in a compartment of the host and by that exert beneficial health effects in this host."

2. PROBIOTIC ORGANISMS

Probiotic bacteria of the genera *Lactobacillus* and *Bifidobacterium* are those most commonly used in foods and are described in Table 1. However, other lactic acid bacteria may also be probiotic. *Enterococcus faecium* (strains—Fargo 688 and PR88) has been described as being probiotic *(26,27)*, but is not considered a safe food organism in several countries. *Streptococcus thermophilus*, *Lactobacillus delbrueckii* subsp. *bulgaricus*, yogurt-, kumiss-, and kefir culture have all been proposed as being probiotic, because

From: *Beverages in Nutrition and Health*
Edited by: T. Wilson and N. J. Temple © Humana Press Inc., Totowa, NJ

Table 1
Bacterial Strains With Documented Probiotic Properties [a]

Species	Strains	Documented probiotic properties
Lactobacillus acidophilus	La5	Adherence to human intestinal mucus during rotavirus infection *(8)*
Lactobacillus casei	Shirota	Treatment and prevention of rotavirus diarrhea; lowering fecal enzyme activity; immune enhancer; reduction of recurrence of superficial bladder cancer *(9,10)*
Lactobacillus johnsonii	LA1	Immune enhancer—balancing intestinal microflora *(10–12)*
Lactobacillus paracasei	NFBC 338	Immunostimulation *(13)*
Lactobacillus plantarum	299V	Positive effects on irritable bowel syndrome *(14,15)*
Lactobacillus rhamnosus	GG	Prevention of antibiotic associated diarrhea; treatment and prevention of rotavirus diarrhea; treatment of relapsing *Clostridium difficile* diarrhea; prevention of acute diarrhea *(10,16–19)*
Lactobacillus reuteri	TM105	Antagonism against *Helicobacter pylori* *(20)*
Bifidobacterium animalis (lactis)	BB12	Prevention of travelers' diarrhea; treatment of antibiotic associated diarrhea; prevention of rotavirus diarrhea *(21–23)*
Bifidobacterium breve	Y8	Positive effect on irritable bowel syndrome *(24)*
Bifidobacterium infantis	Y1	Positive effect on irritable bowel syndrome *(24)*
Bifidobacterium longum	BB536	Treatment of antibiotic associated diarrhea *(25)*

[a] Only one strain per species is listed.

the corresponding products are beneficial for the digestive tract. However, there is no definite proof that the beneficial effects depend on the presence of viable microorganisms in these products. *Escherichia coli* strain Nissle is an enterobacterial Gram-negative bacterium that has been used as a pharmaceuticum but does not technically qualify as a probiotic or as a food additive *(28,29)*.

A whole species of bacteria cannot be considered probiotic, but only certain strains of that species. Table 1, which is by no means comprehensive, only lists one strain for each species. However, there may be several strains within a species for which probiotic properties have been documented. It should be emphasized that the use of the term "probiotic" in this communication is solely conceptual and is not related to proven health benefits.

3. PROBIOTICS AND HEALTH CLAIMS

There are several health effects attributed to the use of probiotics (Table 1; *see* ref. *10* for a review). Reduction of frequency and duration of diarrhea caused either by Rotavirus infection or by treatment with antibiotics are well documented, as are stimulation of cellular and humoral immunity and reduction of unfavorable metabolites or procarcinogenic enzymes in the colon (7). In addition, there is some evidence for health benefits induced by different probiotics, such as the reduction of *Helicobacter pylori* infection, reduction of allergic symptoms, relief from constipation, relief from irritable bowel syndrome, and cancer prevention. Not all of these effects can be brought about by a single probiotic strain. Research efforts, therefore, focus on the assignment of specific health effects to specific probiotic organisms.

4. BEVERAGES

To date, the majority of probiotic products are dairy based. Within this segment, yogurt-based products are the dominant product for the consumer. This may result from reasons of consumer perception related to the following. Fermented dairy products, such as yogurt, already have a reputation as a healthy food in folk medicine. Consumers are aware that fermented products contain viable microorganisms. The image of yogurt-like products as healthy food encourages daily consumption of probiotic products in rather large quantities. The use of dairy products as carriers for probiotics also has an important technological advantage, namely that many of these products have already been optimized for survival of the fermentation organisms. The existing technology can, therefore, be relatively easily adapted for survival of the probiotic bacteria in a product. For this reason, dairy-based products are the first choice when considering the production of probiotic beverages. It must, however, be noted that other fermented products (e.g., fermented vegetables) and beverages derived from such products may also serve as carriers for probiotic organisms.

5. GENERAL CONSIDERATIONS
FOR PROBIOTIC BEVERAGE MANUFACTURING

Numerous technological requirements must be met before particular organisms can be used in the production of probiotic beverages (30–33): they should survive in sufficient numbers in the product, their physical and genetic stability during storage of the product must be guaranteed, and all their properties essential for expressing their health benefits after consumption must be maintained during manufacture and storage of the product. In addition, they should not have adverse effects on taste, aroma, or product acidification.

To exploit the functional properties of probiotics, traditional dairy beverage processing methods may have to be modified to meet the probiotics' requirements. When this is not possible, other probiotic strains may be tested or new products developed. Attention must be paid to the parameters that are either necessary for or influence probiotic use in dairy beverages. Because fermented dairy products contain living bacteria, probiotic beverages must, therefore, be stored at a cool temperature to guarantee high survival rates of the probiotics and yield sufficient stability of the product (34,35). In addition, because the intestinal tract is considered the natural environment of probiotic bacteria, O_2 content and redox potential of the beverage are crucial factors for survival of the probiotic bacteria in the product (36).

Active microorganisms intensively interact with their environment by exchanging medium components for metabolic products. Therefore, attention must be paid to the chemical composition of the probiotic beverage, including the type and amount of carbohydrates available, the degree of hydrolysis of milk proteins (which determines the availability of essential amino acids), and the composition and degree of hydrolysis of milk lipids (which determines the availability of particular lipids, especially of short-chain fatty acids) *(37,38)*. On the other hand, the proteolytic *(39)* and lipolytic activities of the probiotics may alter the composition of the beverage through degradation of proteins and lipids. The latter two properties may considerably affect the product's taste and flavor *(37)*.

The quality of fermented probiotic products may be further affected by interactions between the different microorganisms present in the final product *(40)*. Synergistic interactions, such as those between the traditional yogurt bacteria *(41–44)*, may be beneficial for product manufacture and quality by accelerating fermentation or by enhancing the viabilities of the microorganisms present in the product. However, synergistic interactions are certainly less important than antagonistic interactions, which can be mostly attributed to bacteriocins. The latter are usually small peptides with antibacterial properties, produced by certain bacterial strains *(45,46)*. The ability to produce bacteriocins, and, thereby, attack pathogenic bacteria, has often been considered a desirable property of probiotics *(10)*. However, production of bacteriocins directed against starter bacteria may well be a limiting factor for combinations of starter and probiotic bacteria within a single product *(47)*. Other substances involved in potentially antagonistic effects are hydrogen peroxide, benzoic acid (produced from the minor milk constituent hippuric acid), biogenic amines (formed by decarboxylation of amino acids), and, certainly, lactic acid *(48–52)*.

For fermented dairy beverages, the timing of the addition of the probiotics to the product is critically important in determining the extent of the interaction of probiotics with the food matrix and starter organisms. Interactions may be minimized if the probiotics are added after fermentation and immediately before or even after cooling to below 8°C. Under these conditions, metabolic activities of starters and probiotics are drastically reduced. However, with extended storage, even small interactions may yield measurable effects.

Another important factor to consider is the physiologic state of the probiotics when they are added to the product. This state depends on the time of harvesting of the culture (whether in logarithmic or stationary phase), on the conditions causing growing cells to enter stationary phase (*see* following paragraph), on treatment of the probiotics during and after harvesting, and, finally, on the composition of the growth medium used to produce the probiotics in relation to the composition of the food to which they will be added. Similar considerations have already been made for the production of commercial starter cultures *(53)*.

Of special importance for the physiological state of probiotics added to a product are the conditions used to promote termination of growth of the probiotics and stability relative to shelf life. Bacteria from the logarithmic phase are usually much more susceptible to environmental stresses than those from the stationary phase *(54–56)*. This effect is caused by certain environmental factors signaling to the bacteria the transition from logarithmic to stationary phase *(57)*. For example, a starvation signal, triggered by depletion of carbon sources, is much more favorable for survival than a low pH in the presence of a high concentration of fermentable carbon sources.

If probiotic bacteria actively participate in fermentation, aspects of the chemical composition of the beverage and of interactions with the starter organisms become extremely important. However, because antagonisms between probiotics and starters result in retarded growth or complete inhibition of one of the bacterial components, such cases are relatively easy to identify. One important parameter in this respect is lactic acid production and concomitant pH reduction during fermentation and the resulting inhibition of the probiotic organisms.

6. SPECIFIC PROBIOTIC BEVERAGE PRODUCTS

6.1. Overview of Products

This section reviews beverages that are obtained by fermentation with probiotic organisms or from a basic beverage to which probiotics are added. Traditional fermented milk products (58) constitute the majority of probiotic beverages on the market, and their contribution to beverage choice is, therefore, emphasized. Some traditional products are considered probiotic, even without addition of or cofermentation with defined probiotic microorganisms. This is because the beneficial effects of these products on certain disorders of the intestinal tract have been well-known for a long time and are used in folk medicine. However, as stated, no definite proof is available that the beneficial effects of these products depend on the presence of viable microorganisms.

6.2. Traditional Fermented Milk Beverages

These beverages are produced from milk, whey, natural buttermilk, or mixtures of these. Their manufacture involves stirring the coagulum after fermentation to obtain drinkable properties. Often they are diluted with fruit juice, fruit syrup, or water or they are supplemented with fiber, cereals, or fruit extracts. Occasionally, polysaccharide-producing lactic acid bacterial strains are used for fermentation to enhance the viscosity of the products. In traditional manufacturing these products are made for consumption while fresh and contain large numbers of viable bacteria.

Airan is a traditional beverage of Central Asia, made from diluted yogurt. The microflora is often undefined and contains yogurt starter bacteria and yeasts. The latter are responsible for the observed alcohol content.

Buttermilk is an old traditional beverage first mentioned in India approx 2500 yr ago *(59)*. It is obtained during butter manufacture, as the serum that remains after the cream is churned into butter. Acid buttermilk, also called true buttermilk, is obtained from sour or cultured cream, using as starter culture *L. lactis* subsp. *lactis, L. lactis* subsp. *cremoris, L. lactis* subsp. *cremoris* biovar. *diacetylactis*, and/or *Leuconostoc mesenteroides* subsp. *cremoris*. Acid buttermilk may be fermented if acidity is below 0.45% titratable acidity.

Kefir is an old fermented milk, which originated in the northern Caucasus region. It has a complex microflora (*see* Table 2) organized in a specific macrostructure—the kefir grain—the matrix of which is formed by the polysaccharide kefiran. The presence of yeasts causes production of small amounts of alcohol (< 0.05%) and carbon dioxide, which makes kefir a refreshing dairy beverage. Before consumption, the kefir grains are removed using a sieve. Kefir can be an almost-ideal probiotic dairy product, because it contains several members of the flora described in Table 1. However, the market potential for this product is limited; its continued CO_2 production after being processed into retail

Table 2
The Kefir Microflora

Groups of microorganism	Species
Kefir grains: symbiotic, multistrain culture consisting of:	
Yeasts (10^7–10^8 cfu/g)	*Candida kefir, Saccharomyces cerevisiae, Kluyveromyces* etc.
Lactococci (10^7–10^8 cfu/g)	*Lactococcus lactis, Leuconostoc lactis, Leucon. mesenteroides*
Lactobacilli (10^8–10^9 cfu/g)	*Lb. kefir, Lb. fermentum, Lb. reuteri,*[a] *Lb. acidophilus,*[a] *Lb. casei,*[a] *Lb. brevis, Lb. buchneri*
Acetic acid bacteria (10^7–10^8 cfu/g)	*Acetobacter pasteurianus*

[a] Probiotic strains have been isolated from these species.

containers causes bulging of the lids of the containers, which implies spoilage to most consumers.

Kumiss probably originated in the central Asian steps and is named after ancient tribes of that region. Traditionally, it was prepared from raw mare's milk, but today, pasteurized mare's milk is used. The starter culture consists of *Lb. delbrueckii* subsp. *bulgaricus* and lactose-fermenting yeasts. The final product has an acidity of 0.9–1.25% titratable acidity and contains between 0.5 and 2.5% alcohol. Kumiss is regarded as a dietetic product and is used to treat GI disorders *(60)*. A therapeutic dose would be 1.5 L per day for adults, and about a third of that amount for children aged 8 to 15 yr.

Yogurt is traditionally produced with a thermophilic protosymbiotic culture of *S. thermophilus* and *Lb. delbrueckii* subsp. *bulgaricus*. Protosymbiotic in this respect means that both bacterial strains support one another's growth, resulting in accelerated fermentation. Because of the thermophilic nature of the starter culture, fermentation is carried out between 40° and 45°C. The time needed for fermentation may be as short as 2.5 h for the traditional protosymbiotic yogurt starter. A pH value lower than 4.8 is required to guarantee gel formation from coagulated milk protein *(61)*.

Compared with natural set and stirred yogurt, drinking yogurt has a lower content of nonfat solids (11–12%) *(62,63)*. Fermentation is performed with continuous stirring. Probiotics can easily be added during stirring of the product immediately before transferring to the final containers. Drinking yogurt is the fermented beverage that is, by far, the most often used as carrier for probiotics *(64)*. Goat milk is more suitable for yogurt beverage production than cow's milk. The curd is softer, more aqueous, and less firm. It is easily stirred, yielding a smooth and homogeneous product, which is believed to be easily digested because of the relatively small size of goat fat globules.

So-called "yogurt mild"—sold in several European countries—is produced with a thermophilic culture of *S. thermophilu* and *Lb. spec.*, the latter is usually *Lb. acidophilus*. For the manufacture of "yogurt mild," probiotic lactobacilli, together with *S. thermophilus*, may be used as starters, because they meet the legal requirements for this product (e.g., in Germany). However, production must be a compromise between the full expression of the potential health properties of the probiotic strain on the one hand, and the technologic suitability of the strain on the other. The latter must not only meet the criteria for good survival but also the criteria of fermentation properties and balanced interaction with the *S. thermophilus* starter strain used. This may mean that the strain used for manufacturing is not the one with the best health properties but the one with the best combination of functional and technologic properties.

6.3. Nontraditional Products

Nontraditional probiotic products, which are obtained by fermentation with a single probiotic strain and which do not use one of the standard dairy products as a carrier, have recently become increasingly popular. With such products, technologic restrictions are minimized as fermentation is directed toward maximum expression of the functional (health) properties of the probiotic strain. The only restriction that has to be considered is that the product must be acceptable for the consumer.

Acidophilus milk was first produced in the United States according to Rettger and Cheplin *(65)*. It is made from skim, partially skim, or whole milk. The starter culture consists of pure *Lb. acidophilus*, which should be a probiotic strain. *Lb. acidophilus* grows slowly in milk, which increases the likelihood of growth of contaminating microorganisms. To safeguard against this, sterilization or high-temperature pasteurization is recommended before fermentation. Acidophilus milk generally lacks a pleasant flavor and is often extremely sour. A general practice is, therefore, to add flavorings, sweeteners, and/or other lactic acid bacteria.

Yakult is a fermented skim-milk drink developed in Japan by Shirota in 1935 and first marketed there in 1955 *(66)*. The ingredients are water, reconstituted skim milk, glucose syrup, sugar, and flavoring. Each 65-mL bottle of Yakult contains 6.5 billion *Lb. casei* Shirota. Yakult does not contain preservatives and must be refrigerated until consumed. Several other fermented milk drinks—mostly differing in their microbial flora—are available in Japan from the Yakult company, whose latest development is Yakult light, a low-sugar version of the original Yakult drink.

6.4. Whey Beverages

In general, whey drinks are well suited for addition of or fermentation with probiotic lactic acid bacteria strains, because whey appeals to health-conscious consumers, is low in calories, is nutritious, is thirst quenching, and is less acidic than fruit juices. There are different methods for producing whey beverages. The cheapest method is to drain the whey from cheese vats, filter and pasteurize it, and then ferment it with a lactic acid bacterial starter culture. Sweet whey, obtained from rennet-coagulated curd, is more suitable than acid whey, because the latter is already fermented to a rather low pH by a culture that is optimized for cheese but not necessarily for whey beverage production. Whey drinks are often sweetened and flavored, with orange and lemon being the most compatible flavorings. The use of deproteinized whey has the advantages that the resultant beverages are clear, are not subject to sediment formation, and resemble soft drinks. The disadvantage is that the removal of the whey proteins lowers the protein content of the beverage.

6.5. Nondairy Beverages

Presently, nondairy probiotic beverages are just a theoretical alternative to the dairy-based probiotic products discussed in the previous sections. The first choice of such products could be fermented vegetable drinks for several reasons: production and storage conditions are already optimized for survival of the starter microorganisms, consumers know that these products contain viable microorganisms, and some of the bacteria with documented probiotic properties (e.g., *Lb. plantarum* 299v) *(14,15)* may also be used for fermentation.

Because they are recognized as a healthy food, fruit juices also have potential as carriers for probiotic microorganisms. However, the juices' low pH levels may be detrimental to the survival of the probiotic microorganisms during beverage storage. This certainly limits the development of fruit-based probiotic beverages.

7. HEALTH EFFECTS OF PROBIOTIC BEVERAGES

Documented health effects of some probiotic bacterial strains found in different kinds of foods are listed in Table 1, comprehensive overviews are presented in reviews by Saliminen, Isolari, and Salminene *(10)* and Rolfe *(66)*. A large body of literature on these health effects is available: a search at NCBI PubMed (http://www.ncbi.nlm.nih.gov/) using the search term "probiotic" yielded 900 hits in June 2002. This is an underestimate, because several dairy journals are not covered by PubMed. In contrast, the literature on the documented health effects of specific probiotic beverages is more limited. This is mostly because the probiotic properties of microbial strains have been tested in and documented for a particular food matrix (most often a yogurt-type fermented product). Subsequently, these strains have been applied in different food matrices, and the foods are then labeled as "probiotic." However, no further testing has been conducted to demonstrate that such foods are, indeed, probiotic. One exception is Yakult, the biological effects of which have been intensively studied since the latter half of the 1950s *(67)*.

8. CONCLUSIONS

Probiotic dairy products have been successful in recent years. In Germany, probiotic yogurt products have almost reached, and are expected to hold, a permanent share of approx 25% of the market for yogurt products. A similar development can be expected for dairy beverages, especially for yogurt type. However, for future success of such products in the market, it is important that health claims are supported by clinical studies. This has been the custom for many years for the nontraditional dairy beverages, which have been developed as new products for the promotion of a probiotic microbial strain. Health-conscious consumers have apparently accepted that concept and have made at least one of these products a big success.

Because probiotic products are consumed for their beneficial health effects, the matrices of the products, i.e., the products without probiotics, should already be widely accepted as healthy products by consumers. This is important to justify a high level of consumption. Besides dairy products, low-calorie beverages consumed for their thirst-quenching properties can also be ideal carriers for probiotics, because their regular consumption in rather large quantities is essential for health.

9. MAIN POINTS FOR PRIMARY AND CLINICAL REVIEW

1. Probiotic organisms in beverages alter the microflora of the host and thereby may exert beneficial health effects.
2. Consumption of probiotics is associated with a number of health claims that are largely related to prevention and/or treatment of digestive tract pathologies.
3. To produce a probiotic beverage, microorganisms must survive, be able to maintain physical and genetic stability during storage, and must not produce adverse effects on beverage taste or aroma.
4. Traditional probiotic beverages include fermented products, such as kefir, kumiss, and yoghurt; modern probiotic drinks include acidophilus milk in the United States, Yakult in Japan, and whey drinks.
5. Although fruit juices are well received by consumers, their acidic pH reduces the viability of probiotic bacteria.

REFERENCES

1. Lilly DM, Stillwell RH. Probiotics: growth promoting factors produced by microorganisms. Science 1965;147:747–748 (in German).
2. Parker RB. Probiotics, the other half of the antibiotics story. Anim Nutr Health 1974;29:4–8.
3. Döderlein A. The vaginal transsudate and its significance for childbed fever. Centralblatt für Bacteriologie 1892;11:699–700 (in German).
4. Metchnikoff E. The Prolongation of Life—Optimistic Studies. Heinemann, London, UK, 1908.
5. Henneberg W. About Bacillus acidophilus and Acidophilus-Milk (Reform-Yogurt). Molkerei-Zeitung 1926;40:2633–2635. (in German).
6. Havenaar R, Huis in't Veld JHJ. Probiotics: a general view. In: Lactic Acid Bacteria in Health and Disease, Vol. 1. Wood BJB (ed.). Elsevier Applied Science, London, UK, 1992, pp. 151–171.
7. Schrezenmeir J, de Vrese M. Probiotics, prebiotics, and synbiotics—approaching a definition. Am J Clin Nutr 2001;73(Suppl):361S–364S.
8. Juntunen M, Kirjavainen PV, Ouwehand AC, et al. Adherence of probiotic bacteria to human intestinal mucus in healthy infants and during rotavirus infection. Clin Diagn Lab Immunol 2001;8:293–296.
9. Aso Y, Akaza H, Kotake T, Tsukamoto T, Imai K, Naito S. Preventive effect of a *Lactobacillus casei* preparation on the recurrence of superficial bladder cancer in double-blind trial. Eur Urol 1995;27:104–109.
10. Salminen S, Isolauri E, Salminen E. Clinical uses of probiotics for stabilizing the gut mucosal barrier: successful strains and future challenges. Antonie van Leeuwenhoek 1996;70:347–358.
11. Link-Amster H, Rochat F, Saudan KY, Mignot O, Aeschlimann JM. Modulation of a specific humoral immune response and changes in intestinal flora mediated through fermented milk intake. FEMS Immunol Med Microbiol 1994;10:55–64.
12. Schiffrin EJ, Brassart D, Servin AL, Rochat F, Donnet-Hughes A. Immune modulation of blood leukocytes in humans by lactic acid bacteria, criteria for strain selection. Am J Clin Nutr 1997;66:515S–520S.
13. Collins JK, Thornton G, Sullivan GO. Selection of probiotic strains for human applications. Intern Dairy J 1998;8:487–490.
14. Molin G. Probiotics in foods not containing milk or milk constituents, with special reference to *Lactobacillus plantarum* 299v. Am J Clin Nutr 2001;73(Suppl):380S–385S.
15. Niedzielin K, Kordecki H, Birkenfeld B. A controlled, double-blind, randomized study on the efficacy of Lactobacillus plantarum 299V in patients with irritable bowel syndrome. Eur J Gastroenterol Hepatol 2001;13:1143–1147.
16. Gorbach SL, Chang TW, Goldin BR. Successful treatment of relapsing Clostridium difficile colitis with Lactobacillus GG. Lancet 1987;2:1519.
17. Guandalini S. Probiotics in the treatment of diarrhoeal diseases in children. Gastroenterol Intern 1998; 11:87–90.

18. Pelto L, Isolauri E, Lilius EM, Nuutila J, Salminen S. Probiotic bacteria down-regulate the milk-induced inflammatory response in milk-hypersensitive subjects but have an immunostimulatory effect in healthy subjects. Clin Exp Allergy 1998;28:1471–1479.

19. Kalliomäki M, Salminen S, Arvilommi H, Kero P, Koskinen P, Isolauri I. Probiotics in primary prevention of atopic disease: a randomised placebo-controlled trial. Lancet 2001;357:1076–1079.

20. Mukai T, Asasaka T, Sato E, Mori K, Matsumoto M, Ohori H. Inhibition of binding of Helicobacter pylori to the glycolipid receptors by probiotic Lactobacillus reuteri. FEMS Immunol Med Microbiol 2002;32:105–110.

21. Black FT, Andersen PL, Ørskov J, Ørskov F, Gaarslev K, Laulund S. Prophylactic efficiacy of lacto-bacilli on travellers diarrhea. Travel Med 1989;7:333–335.

22. Black FT, Einarsson K, Lidbeck A, Orrhage K, Nord CE. Effect of lactic acid producing bacteria on the human intestinal microflora during ampicillin treatment. Scand J Infect Dis 1991;23:247–254.

23. Saavedra JM, Baumann NA, Oung I, Perman JA, Yolken RH. Feeding of *Bifidobacterium bifidum* and *Streptococcus thermophilus* to infants in hospital for prevention of diarrhoea and shedding of rotavirus. Lancet 1994;344:1046–1049.

24. Brigidi P, Vitali B, Swennen E, Bazzocchi G, Matteuzzi D. Effects of probiotic administration upon the composition and enzymatic activity of human fecal microbiota in patients with irritable bowel syndrome or functional diarrhea. Res Microbiol 2001;152:735–741.

25. Orrhage K, Sjostedt S, Nord CE. Effect of supplements with lactic acid bacteria and oligofructose on the intestinal microflora during administration of cefpodoxime proxetil. J Antimicrob Chemother 2000;46:603–612.

26. Gardiner GE, Ross RP, Wallace JM, et al. Influence of a probiotic adjunct culture of Enterococcus faecium on the quality of cheddar cheese. J Agric Food Chem 1999;47:4907–4916.

27. Gardiner G, Stanton C, Lynch PB, Collins JK, Fitzgerald G, Ross RP. Evaluation of cheddar cheese as a food carrier for delivery of a probiotic strain to the gastrointestinal tract. J Dairy Sci 1999;82:1379–1387.

28. Lodinova-Zadnikova R, Sonnenborn U. Effect of preventive administration of a nonpathogenic *Escherichia coli* strain on the colonization of the intestine with microbial pathogens in newborn infants. Biol Neonate 1997;71:224–232.

29. Rembacken BJ, Snelling AM, Hawkey PM, Chalmers DM, Axon AT. Non-pathogenic *Escherichia coli* versus mesalazine for the treatment of ulcerative colitis: a randomised trial. Lancet 1999;354:635–639.

30. Gomes AMP, Malcata FX. Bifidobacterium spec. and Lactobacillus acidophilus: biological, bio-chemical, technological and therapeutical properties relevant for use as probiotics. Trends Food Sci Technol 1999;10:139–157.

31. Saarela M, Mogensen G, Fonden R, Matto J, Mattila-Sandholm T. Probiotic bacteria: safety, functional and technological properties. J Biotechnol 2000;84:197–215.

32. Heller KJ. Probiotic bacteria in fermented foods: product characteristics and starter organisms. Am J Clin Nutr 2001;73S:374S–379S.

33. Mattila-Sandholm T, Myllärinen P, Crittenden R, Mogensen G, Fondén R, Saarela M. Technological challenges for future probiotic foods. Int Dairy J 2002;12:173–182.

34. Shah NP, Lankaputhra WEV, Britz ML, Kyle WSA. Survival of *L. acidophilus* and *Bifidobacterium bifidum* in commercial yogurt during refrigerated storage. Int Dairy J 1995;5:515–521.

35. Roy D, Mainville I, Mondou F. Bifidobacteria and their role in yogurt-related products. Microecology Therapy 1997;26:167–180.

36. Dave RI, Shah NP. Effect of cysteine on the viability of yogurt and probiotic bacteria in yogurts made with commercial starter cultures. Int Dairy J 1997;7:537–545.

37. Fox PF, Law J, McSweeney PLH, Wallace J. Biochemistry of cheese ripening. In: Cheese: Chemistry, Physics and Microbiology, Vol. 1. Fox PF (ed.). Chapman and Hall, London, UK, 1993, pp. 389–438.

38. Fox PF, Wallace JM, Morgan S, Lynch CM, Niland EJ, Tobin J. Acceleration of cheese ripening. Antonie van Leeuwenhoek 1996;70:175–201.

39. Kunji ERS, Mierau I, Hagting A, Poolman B, Konings WN. The proteolytic systems of lactic acid bacteria. Antonie van Leeuwenhoek 1996;70:91–125.

40. Vinderola CG, Mocchiutti P, Reinheimer JA. Interactions among lactic acid starter and probiotic bacteria used for fermented dairy products. J Dairy Sci 2002;85:721–729.

41. Driessen FM, Kingma F, Stadhouders J. Evidence that *Lactobacillus bulgaricus* in yogurt is stimulated by carbon dioxide produced by *Streptococcus thermophilus*. Netherlands Milk Dairy J 1982; 36:135–144.

42. Radke-Mitchell LC, Sandine WE. Influence of temperature on associative growth of Streptococcus thermophilus and Lactobacillus bulgaricus. J Dairy Sci 1986;69:2558–2568.

43. Perez PF, De Antoni GL, Anon MC. Formiate production by Streptococcus thermophilus cultures. J Dairy Sci 1991;74:2850–2854.

44. Zourari A, Accolas JP, Desmazeaud MJ. Metabolism and biochemical characteristics of yogurt bacteria. A review. Lait 1992;72:1–34.

45. De Vuyst L, Vandamme EJ. Bacteriocins of lactic acid bacteria. Chapman and Hall, London, UK, 1994.

46. Dodd HM, Gasson MJ. Bacteriocins of lactic acid bacteria. In: Genetics and Biotechnology of Lactic Acid Bacteria. Gasson MJ, de Vos WM (eds.). Blackie Academic and Professional, London, UK, 1994, pp. 211–252.

47. Joseph PJ, Dave RI, Shah NP. Antagonism between yogurt bacteria and probiotic bacteria isolated from commercial starter cultures, commercial yogurts, and a probiotic capsule. Food Austr 1998; 50:20–23.

48. Desmazeaud M. Growth inhibitors of lactic acid bacteria. In: Dairy Starter Cultures. Cogan TM, Accolas J-P (eds.). VCH Publishers, New York, NY, 1996, pp. 131–155.

49. Sieber R, Butikofer U, Bosset JO. Benzoic acid as a natural compound in cultured dairy products and cheese. Int Dairy J 1995;5:227–246.

50. Weber H. Starter cultures in dairy industry. In: Mikrobiologie der Lebensmittel: Milch und Milchprodukte. Weber H (ed.). Behr's Verlag, Hamburg, 1996, pp. 105–152 (in German).

51. Lankaputhra WEV, Shah NP, Britz ML. Survival of bifidobacteria during refrigerated storage in the presence of acid and hydrogen peroxide. Milchwissenschaft 1996;51:65–70.

52. Leuschner RG, Heidel M, Hammes WP. Histamine and tyramine degradation by food fermenting microorganisms. Int J Food Microbiol 1998;39:1–10.

53. Sandine WE. Commercial production of starter cultures. In: Dairy Starter Cultures. Cogan TM, Accolas J-P (eds.). VCH Publishers, New York, NY, 1996, pp. 191–206.

54. Kolter R. The stationary phase of the bacterial life cycle. Annu Rev Biochem 1993;47:855–874.

55. Hartke A, Bouche S, Gansel X, Boutibonnes P, Auffray Y. Starvation-induced stress resistance in *Lactococcus lactis* subsp. *lactis* IL1403. Appl Envir Microbiol 1994;60:3474–3478.

56. Rallu F, Gruss A, Maguin E. *Lactococcus lactis* and stress. Antonie van Leeuwenhoek 1996;70: 243–251.

57. Wetzel K, Menzel M, Heller KJ. Stress response in Lactococcus lactis and Streptococcus thermophilus induced by carbon starvation. Kieler Milchwirtschaftl Forsch Ber 1999;51:319–332.

58. Kurmann JA, Rasic, Kroger M. Encyclopedia of fermented fresh milk products. Van Nostrand Reinhold, New York, NY, 1992.

59. Prakash OM. Food and drinks in Ancient India. Munshi Ram Manohar Lal, Oriental Booksellers and Publishers, Delhi-6, India, 1961.

60. Berlin PJ. Kumiss. Ann Bull IDF, International Dairy Federation, Brussels, Belgium, 1962, pp. 4–10.

61. Rasic JL, Kurmann JA. Yogurt. Technical Dairy Publishing House, Copenhagen, Denmark, 1978.

62. Teuber M, Geis A, Krusch U, Lembke J. Biotechnological procedures for production of food and feeding-stuffs. In: Handbuch der Biotechnologie. Präve P, Faust U, Sittig W, Sukatsch DA (eds.). R. Oldenbourg Verlag, München, 1994, pp. 479–540 (in German).

63. Robinson RK. A Colour Guide to Cheese and Fermented Milks. Chapman and Hall, London, UK, 1995.

64. Lourens-Hattingh A, Viljoen BC. Yogurt as probiotic carrier food. Int Dairy J 2001;11:1–17.

65. Rettger LF, Cheplin HA. Bacillus acidophilus and its therapeutic application. Arch Intern Med 1922; 29:357–367.

66. Rolfe RD. The role of probiotic cultures in the control of gastrointestinal health. J Nutr 2000;130: 396S–402S.

67. Yakult Central Institute for Microbiological Research. *Lactobacillus casei* Strain Shirota: Intestinal Flora and Human Health. Yakult Honsha Co., Tokyo, Japan, 1999.

VI NUTRITIONAL SUPPLEMENTATION AND WEIGHT CONTROL BEVERAGES

18 Beverages, Appetite, and Energy Balance

James Stubbs and Stephen Whybrow

1. BEVERAGES' CONTRIBUTIONS TO DIET AND OBESITY

1.1. Background: Recent Trends in Body Weight and Obesity

This chapter discusses the role of dietary beverages in appetite and energy balance (EB) control. The focus primarily relates to nonalcoholic beverages in the Western diet. Several other issues concerning tea, coffee, and alcoholic beverages are addressed in other chapters. To appreciate how beverages influence EB, we must examine the context in which beverages occur in our modern-day diet. Since World War II, the average composition of the Western diet has changed radically. This change has been paralleled by a change in the body size and composition of the average Western citizen.

Overweight and obesity prevalence have steadily increased in the last 50 yr in many countries. There has been a remarkable upturn in these trends in the last two decades. Currently, more than half the adult population of many Western countries are collectively overweight and obese. Childhood obesity has reached record levels in the United States and Europe. In the United States, there has been a virtual Tsunami of increase in obesity prevalence, which sweeps upward from West to East (1). In Europe, 15–20% of the population is obese. However, more than twice as many European adults are overweight and tracking toward obesity in the next 5 yr. Obesity prevalence is heavily associated with type 2 diabetes and other comorbidities. Obesity is notoriously difficult to treat. Even with the best of current dietary and drug treatments, sustained weight loss is ineffective, except for a minority (2).

What aspects of our modern environment are conducive to weight gain? It is generally accepted that, on average, Western populations are more sedentary than they used to be (3). Several cross-sectional studies strongly suggest that sedentariness is highly correlated with increased adiposity (4). There is also much evidence suggesting that the diet we eat (and drink) is heavily involved in the current pandemic of obesity (2). It has been argued that Western lifestyles are now so sedentary it is likely that energy intake (EI) still exceeds energy expenditure (EE) in a significant proportion of people. Indeed, recent longitudinal data from the NHANES datasets suggest that, on average, US adults gain 0.2–2.0 kg per year (5).

From: *Beverages in Nutrition and Health*
Edited by: T. Wilson and N. J. Temple © Humana Press Inc., Totowa, NJ

These observations must be considered as a backdrop to dietary intake data because a significant proportion of subjects in nutritional surveys underestimate the amount of food they are eating, because they are reporting intakes that are lower than EE without losing weight *(6)*. It is, therefore, often necessary to consider several sources of evidence in relation to each other. How is our diet likely to have changed in a way that is conducive to overconsumption, and how do beverages fit into this picture?

1.2. Recent Trends in Food and Fluid Intake

As human civilization has developed, the diet we consume has evolved to contain less fiber, more fat and readily assimilated carbohydrates (sugars and high glycemic index starches), and a higher energy density (ED) than was ingested in previous centuries *(2)*. The ED of the diet has increased, and the micronutrient density per unit of energy ingested has decreased because many modern foods are rich in refined fats and carbohydrates. Mela *(7)* has noted that, despite market access to a diet of virtually any composition, modern populations consume approx 38–42% fat by energy and a substantial proportion of EI from sugars or readily assimilated starches. Recent datasets suggest lower fat intakes of approx 33% EI from fat. Part of this effect will be a real reduction in fat intake, but part may also result from the phenomenon of misreporting. Approximately 60% of EI in the typical Western diet is derived from fats and sugars. It is well-established that the high fat content of modern diets is a major risk factor for weight gain *(see* the following section). Although this is true, there has been great disappointment that fat-reduction strategies induce only modest weight loss. This has led to further examinations of the role of types of carbohydrate in appetite and EB control and the importance of dietary ED as a factor that may undermine the beneficial effects of fat-reduction strategies *(8)*. There is growing evidence that sugars and high glycemic index starches can elevate EI, especially when their addition to foods increases ED. Sugars are also intensely sweet, and this property promotes active increases in food intake in some studies *(8)*. Beverages have significantly influenced the composition of the modern diet.

1.3. The Effect of Beverages on the Composition of Consumers' Diets

There has been a major shift in the consumption of beverage products in the last two decades. The dietary intake of fat from beverage sources in the form of milk has decreased dramatically, because the majority of the milk consumed is now skimmed and semiskimmed, as opposed to full-fat. This has led to a major decrease in the contribution of beverages to dietary fat intake in Western consumers *(9)*. Concomitant with the decrease in fat intake from milk is a dramatic growth in the market for carbohydrate-rich and low-energy (usually aspartame-sweetened) soft drinks. The increase in soft drinks rich in readily assimilated sweet carbohydrates has, indeed, been remarkable *(9)*. This growth is likely to have been stimulated, at least in part, by the low-fat food revolution and consumers' current preoccupations with avoiding fat in the diet through increased consumption of low-fat and lower fat foods and beverages *(10)*. To appreciate how these changes in the types of beverages are likely to affect body weight control, it is important to understand the relationship between diet composition, appetite, and EB.

1.4. The Relationship Between Diet Composition, Appetite, and Energy Balance

1.4.1. MACRONUTRIENTS AND APPETITE CONTROL

Numerous reviews have considered the means and mechanisms by which dietary macronutrients, macronutrient substitutes, and associated nutritional parameters, such as dietary ED, influence appetite and EB in humans *(2,8,10)*. The main points are summarized here. As they enter the diet, macronutrients have differing metabolizable energy coefficients. Average values for alcohol, protein, carbohydrate, and fat are 29, 17, 16, and 37 kJ/g. Fat and alcohol have a higher ED (energy/unit of wet weight of food eaten) than protein and carbohydrate *(2,8,10)*. Thus, high-fat foods are high in ED.

Importantly, the nutritional determinants of EI are multifactorial. Nutrients come in foods as mixtures; therefore, the satiating effect of a food is due to its combined effects of the nutrient content (and other attributes). To better understand how the nutritional properties of foods affect the EI and food intake of consumers living their normal lives in their natural environments, the relationships between diet composition, ED, EI, and food intake have been examined in a relatively large sample of men and women and the foods they eat. Consider the following five ideas in terms of this sometimes contradictory/multifactorial nature.

1. The different macronutrients do not all affect satiety to the same degree. There is a hierarchy in the satiating efficiency of protein, carbohydrate, and fat, such that per unit of energy ingested, protein suppresses appetite and subsequent EI to a greater extent than carbohydrate, which has a greater effect than fat *(2,8,10)*. This relationship has been demonstrated under several conditions and occurs as macronutrients come in the diet with differing EDs *(2,8,10)* (*see* Fig. 1). Caloric compensation can be defined as a unit decrease in EI for each unit of energy given as a particular nutrient. When given as solid food, protein produces supercaloric compensation (overcompensation), carbohydrate produces caloric compensation, and fat ingestion leads to subcaloric compensation (undercompensation).
2. When ingested at the same level of ED, protein is still the most satiating macronutrient *(2,8,10)*. Under these conditions, differences between carbohydrate and fat are less clear cut. Carbohydrate exerts a more acute effect on satiety than fat *(8,10)*.
3. Alcohol is exceptional in that its ingestion can stimulate food intake, and so induces counter-compensatory EI increases *(8,10)*. This may be related to alcohol being a drug with depressant effects on the central nervous system (CNS).
4. Dietary ED affects feeding behavior and EI *(8)*. A diet that has too low an ED will induce an energy deficit, determined by the rate at which low ED foods can be digested and absorbed. There is evidence that food intake increases in the longer term to offset this deficit. If a diet is higher in ED than that habitually consumed, overconsumption will occur, because the amount of food people eat is conditioned and there is relatively weak defence against excess EI *(2,8,10)*. There is a considerable body of evidence that both humans and animals prefer foods that are more ED to foods that are less ED *(8)*.
5. Certain types of protein, carbohydrate, and fats may exert different effects on appetite *(8,10)*. The effect of macronutrient subtypes on appetite control is a relatively novel area. Development of the properties of nutrients to manipulate appetite control is still in its infancy. Protein is the least well understood. The effects of different types of carbohydrate on appetite control are also unclear, and development of novel forms of carbohydrates to enhance satiety is in its infancy *(10)*. More is known about the effects of types

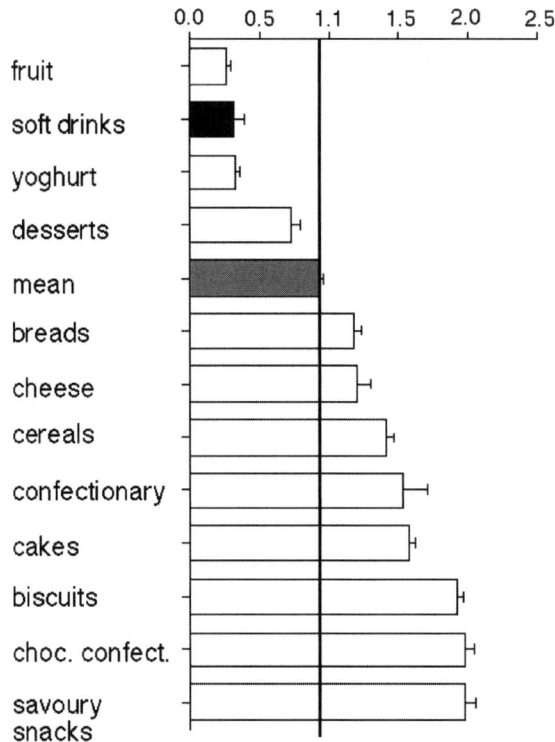

Fig. 1. The energy density (ED) of common snack foods. The ED of soft drinks is lower than the mean for solid snack foods.

of fat on appetite control, because the search for forms of fat do not predispose the general population to weight gain. Fat structure varies in terms of (1) chain length, (2) degree of saturation, (3) degree of esterification, and (4) by combining items 1 through 3 through the development of novel structured lipids. There is some evidence that fats with a shorter chain length and a higher degree of unsaturation exert a slightly protective effect against weight gain than longer chain or more saturated fats, respectively. There is little evidence that degree of fatty acid esterification influences appetite and EI (8). Currently, there is little information on the effects of structured lipids on appetite and EB. However, it can be envisaged that structured lipids can be developed to combine some of the individually modest effects of fat type on appetite and feeding behavior. Indeed, certain types of lipid have been added to yogurt to enhance satiety and limit EI (11). Evidence for the sustainability of the effect is lacking. In the future, specific nutrients can be tailored to exert quantitatively significant effects on appetite control, tissue deposition, and EB. In this context, certain isomers of conjugated linoleic acid (CLA) can be used to influence appetite and tissue deposition in animals and, perhaps, humans (12). The effects of CLA are not entirely understood but are near pharmacological in nature.

1.4.2. DETERMINANTS OF DIETARY ENERGY DENSITY

We conducted an analysis of the relationship between nutrients and water content and ED in 1032 ready-to-eat foods from the British food composition tables (13) and in the total diet of 73 free-living consumers self-recording their food intake for 7 d. The main factor decreasing dietary ED is water, and the main factor increasing ED is fat. Water is more important in ready-to-eat foods than the whole diet, but, in both cases, it has a greater effect on ED than fat (8,13). This suggests that increasing beverage consumption should decrease overall dietary ED, because the majority of soft drinks are considerably lower in ED than are most foods (see Fig. 1). The apparent contradictions of this suggestion with what is commonly observed in people is discussed in Subheading 2.1. of this chapter, and in Chapters 24 and 25.

1.4.3. DIETARY DETERMINANTS OF ENERGY INTAKE

Laboratory studies have revealed that the relationship between percent EI from each macronutrient and daily EI is hierarchical. Protein has a more negative slope than carbohydrate, and fat has a positive slope. A hierarchical order in the extent to which macronutrient ingestion correlates with a change in EI has been found elsewhere (2,8,10). In general, increases in the ED and percent fat in foods elevates EI. Percent energy from protein correlates negatively with EI, whereas percent energy from carbohydrate does not correlate with EI. Alcohol ingestion promotes increased EI. This is consistent with the work of de Castro and Mattes (14,15).

1.5. The Influence of Beverages on Diet Composition and Energy Intake

Beverages play a greater role than ever in the diet of Western consumers. They have helped to lower the fat intake and markedly elevate the intake of sugars and readily assimilated starches in the Western diet. Each of these effects has been equally impressive. For instance, Park and Yetley (16) examined the per-capita disappearance data for sweeteners and other sources of fructose in the United States during the past two decades. There was a considerable increase in the availability of free fructose (but not total fructose) in the food supply. For most gender/age groups, nonalcoholic beverages (e.g., soft drinks and fruit-flavored drinks) and grain products (e.g., sweet bakery products) were the major sources of fructose, nonalcoholic beverages were the major sources of added fructose, and fruits and fruit products were the major sources of naturally occurring fructose. Fructose intake alone averaged 8% of total daily EI. Prynne et al. (17) in the United Kingdom noted a rise in soft drink intake in 4-yr-old children from the 1950s to the 1990s.

In 2000, Troiano et al. (18) examined the contribution of beverages to energy and fat intakes of US children and adolescents. Remarkably, they found: "Beverages contributed 20–24% of energy across all ages and soft drinks provided 8% of energy in adolescents. Except for adolescent girls, beverage energy contributions were generally higher among overweight than nonoverweight youths; soft drink energy contribution was higher among overweight youths than among nonoverweight youths for all groups." In comparison to the data from the 1970s, these authors noted that although mean EI had changed little, there was a decrease in the percent EI from fat, in favor of carbohydrate. These data suggest that carbohydrate-rich soft drinks are playing a significant role in modifying the composition of the diet and, perhaps, also EI levels. Cavadini et al. (19) compared the food intakes of 12,498 US adolescents from 1965 to 1996. They found that both fat intake and total EI declined during this 31-yr period. Major shifts in beverage consumption included a change from full-fat to low-fat milks, although total milk consumption declined by

36%. This was accompanied by an increase in the consumption of soft drinks and noncitrus juices.

Ludwig et al. *(20)* conducted a prospective observational analysis of the relation between consumption of sugar-sweetened drinks and childhood obesity in 548 ethnically diverse schoolchildren who were studied for 19 mo. They found:

"For each additional serving of sugar-sweetened drink consumed, both body mass index (BMI) (mean 0.24 kg/m²; 95% CI 0.10–0.39; p = 0.03) and frequency of obesity (odds ratio 1.60; 95% CI 1.14–2.24; p = 0.02) increased after adjustment for anthropometric, demographic, dietary, and lifestyle variables. Baseline consumption of sugar-sweetened drinks was also independently associated with change in BMI (mean 0.18 kg/m² for each daily serving; 95% CI 0.09–0.27; p = 0.02)."

Dennison also points to the recent increase in fruit juice consumption in infants and children at the expense of milk intake. In a cross-sectional study of young children, Dennison et al. *(21)* found that consumption of ≥12 fl oz/d of fruit juice by young children was associated with short stature and with obesity.

Gibson *(22)* found: " ... an inverse association of nonmilk extrinsic sugars (NMES) with micronutrient intakes is of most significance for the 20% of children ... (aged 1.5–4.5 years) ... with diets highest in NMES." Gibson noted that lower intakes of milk, meat, bread, and vegetables and higher intakes of fruit juice largely explained the observed trends in micronutrient intake. Therefore, although a high level of soft drink consumption is associated with a lower percentage of EI from fat, high levels of soft drink intake can also displace micronutrients from the diet. The significance of this for body weight is discussed in the following section.

The effect beverages exert in increasing the percentage of energy from carbohydrates does not entirely result from an increase in sugar-rich soft drinks. Lee et al. *(23)* examined energy, macronutrient, and food intakes related to energy compensation in consumers who drink different types of milk, using the US Department of Agriculture's 1989–1991 nationwide food intake database. They found that total fat intake in drinkers of reduced-fat milk is significantly ($p \leq 0.05$) lower than that in drinkers of whole milk. Men, but not women, compensate for the reduced energy by increasing their carbohydrate intake. They also noted that through their reduction in total fat intake, several age groups of skim-milk drinkers have achieved the US dietary goal for fat intake (i.e., ≤30% of EI from fat).

The composition and sensory attributes of the diet have profound effects on appetite control. The current range of beverages available on the market has enormous potential to influence both the composition and sensory attributes of the diet. It, therefore, follows that they are likely to influence appetite and EB, and, hence, population levels of obesity. This leads to a discussion of the specific issues concerning beverages and appetite control.

2. SPECIFIC ISSUES CONCERNING BEVERAGES AND APPETITE CONTROL

2.1. Do Calories from Drinks Lead to a Higher EI Than Calories from Solid Foods?

Calories contained in drinks promote higher energy intakes than when the same number of calories is contained in solid foods. Because there are currently few high-fat beverages on the market, much of this discussion relates primarily to the effect of solutions rich in sugars or starch. Mattes *(14)* recently conducted a meta-analysis of feeding responses to either liquid or solid manipulations of the nutrient and energy content of the diet. The analysis suggests that the physical state of ingested carbohydrate intake may be important in influencing subsequent caloric compensation *(14)*. Wet carbohydrates induce hyperphagia in rodents *(24)*. DiMeglio and Mattes *(25)* have recently compared the effects of liquid vs solid carbohydrate on EI and body weight in humans. In a crossover design, 7 men and 8 women consumed dietary carbohydrate loads of 1.9 MJ/d as a liquid (soda) or solid (jelly beans) during two 4-wk periods separated by a 4-wk washout. Liquid carbohydrate promoted a positive EB, whereas a comparable solid carbohydrate elicited precise dietary compensation. They concluded that increased consumption of energy-yielding fluids could promote a positive EB.

This conclusion has been supported by the work of Raben et al. (personal communication), who investigated the effect of long-term (10 wk) supplementation with either sucrose or acaloric, intense sweeteners (primarily as drinks) on *ad libitum* food intake and body weight in overweight subjects. Two groups of overweight subjects (36 women, 6 men) consumed dietary supplements containing sucrose or artificial sweeteners in a parallel design. On average, the sucrose intervention supplemented 3.4 MJ/d and 152 g/d sucrose, whereas the sweetener intervention added 1.0 MJ/d and no sucrose. After 10 wk of 3.4 MJ/d sucrose supplementation, EI increased (2.6 MJ/d), as did dietary ED, the percentage of energy from sucrose (to 28%) and from carbohydrate. The percentage of energy from fat and protein decreased. On the sweetener-based diet, the only change was a small decrease in sucrose intake (by 4% of EI). Taken together, these studies suggest that excess EI can readily occur when subjects consume sweet monosaccharides, disaccharides, and maltodextrins in beverages.

2.2. Why Do Some Beverages Cause Overconsumption of Energy?

The evidence discussed suggests that energy contained in drinks (especially carbohydrates) does not induce compensatory reductions in food intake as efficiently as energy contained in solid foods. The following provides a possible explanation for this. It has been observed in rats and pigs consuming certain diets low in an essential nutrient (usually protein), that the animal can increase intake to satisfy requirements for that nutrient, at the expense of depositing extra energy as fat *(26,27)*. It is not clear to what extent foods or drinks low in protein and micronutrients lead to a greater intake of energy to attempt satisfaction of the requirements for certain essential nutrients. However, it has been noted in surveys that high levels of soft drink consumption can displace both protein and, to a greater extent, micronutrients from the diet and are associated with a high EI *(18–22)*. However, currently there is no clear evidence that the low intake of essential nutrients associated with high levels of soft drink intake actually drives an increase in EI. Although the arguments presented may help explain observations based on comparison of sugar drinks vs zero-energy drinks, these data do not explain higher EI from sugar drinks vs solid sugar-based foods.

Additional reasons why energy in drinks is less well compensated for than energy in solid foods may relate to the rate, timing, and density at which the energy is ingested. There may be a threshold in these parameters, below which energy is poorly detected. Another factor influencing the effect of carbohydrate-rich drinks on intrameal and intermeal satiety is the osmotic load that carbohydrates exert in the small intestine. When starches are digested, water is required to hydrolyze the glycosidic bonds. This slows digestion (and, hence, short-term food intake) and increases thirst. It is reasonable to hypothesize that these effects would enhance postingestive/preabsorptive satiety.

The process by which a food or drink enhances satiety involves several sequentially reinforcing steps or signals associated with the process of nutrient digestion, absorption, and metabolism. This has been termed the satiety cascade by Blundell *(2)*. Drinks are essentially solutions, which are likely to have minimal effect in limiting EI at the stage of digestion as they are already mechanically and chemically digested. Therefore, they are less likely to activate gastrointestinal satiety signals. Sweet carbohydrate-rich drinks with a water/carbohydrate ratio above 3/1 should exert maximal orosensory stimulation on intake and minimal osmotic EI reduction. The sensory properties associated with beverages, especially sweet beverages, exert a potent influence on the sensory stimulation to eat.

2.3. Beverages and the Sensory Stimulation to Eat: Sugar, Sweetness, and Artificial Sweeteners

2.3.1. Issues Relating to Sugar, Sweetness, and Artificial Sweeteners

The key issues in this controversy relate to what effect sweetness, with or without carbohydrate energy, has on appetite and EB *(28,29)*. There are three main hypotheses: (1) adding sweetness without calories to foods leads to lower EI levels than when sweetness with calories are added, (2) sweetness without calories leads to an increase in cephalic phase stimulation to eat, and (3) ingestion of sugars (sweetness with calories) lowers fat intake and, therefore, reduces the risk of overconsumption. There is little doubt that most animals display a preference for sweetness at an early age and that sweetness is a factor favoring the selection and subsequent ingestion of sweet foods. Conversely, different people exhibit markedly different preferences for sweetness intensities; therefore, simply adding sweetness to foods and beverages will not stimulate everyone to eat. Assuming that sweetness does, in general, stimulate the selection and consumption of these foods, the next question relates to whether sweetness with or without calories differently affects appetite and EI.

2.3.2. Does Sweetness Without Calories Lead to Lower Levels of Energy Intake and Body Weight Than Sweetness With Calories?

Despite the common assumption that replacing dietary sugars with intense sweeteners promotes a less positive (or even negative EB), there is a remarkable paucity of data to demonstrate this effect. The recent work by Raben (personal communication) lends support to this notion, at least when the substitution involves part of a day's mandatory intake. There is certainly little epidemiologic evidence to suggest that artificial-sweetener consumption correlates with lower body mass indexes (BMIs), or that increased artificial-sweetener consumption in the general population has contributed to any reduction in the prevalence of overweight or obesity. There are several possible reasons for this. Artificial sweeteners are probably popular among obese people, but this can be easily explained by reverse causation: obese people use artificial sweeteners because they are obese; it wasn't the artificial sweeteners that made them obese. Furthermore, Mela *(7)* has noted that artificial sweeteners are often used as food additives rather than sugar substitutes. Under these conditions, they are not likely to lower EI. A problem with the majority of laboratory studies that examine the effect of sweetness, sugars, and artificial sweeteners is that many are short-term and, therefore, do not address EB *(28)*.

2.3.3. DOES SWEETNESS WITHOUT CALORIES LEAD TO A CEPHALIC-PHASE STIMULATION TO EAT?

Most authors agree that the purely postingestive effects of aspartame do not stimulate intake *(28,29)*. Blundell and Rogers *(30)* initially reported that artificially sweetened drinks actually stimulate appetite. They suggest that sweetness without calories provides a sensory cue for carbohydrate calories, which leads to cephalic-phase physiologic changes that anticipate EI. They note that intense sweeteners only stimulate intake when a food has been sweetened with intense sweeteners or when a less sweet food has been compared with an isoenergetically equivalent food to which sweetness has been added (their "additive principle") and not when two foods of differing ED but the same level of sweetness are compared. They call this the "substitutive principle."

This area is bedeviled by methodologic controversies, such as the appropriate drink vehicle for the sweetener (water or a familiar soft drink), the time course of the experiment, and the participants. Blundell and Rogers *(30)* argue that the strongest experimental designs contain tests of both the additive and the substitutive principle. No long-term studies that address EB have yet achieved this dual testing. Black and Anderson *(31)* report that the use of aspartame-sweetened water leads to an acute short-term increase in subjective appetite in lean men, but that aspartame-sweetened carbonated soft drinks induce a transient suppression of appetite in similar subjects during a similar time frame. The issue is complicated because satiety can be transiently conditioned by starch-containing drinks that are paired with a given sensory cue, such as a specific flavor *(29)*. Once conditioned, similar levels of satiation can be transiently induced by the conditioning stimulus alone. Therefore, the effects of prior conditioning can influence the outcome of studies using vehicles that mimic the sensory properties of familiar foods.

In summary, there is little evidence that artificial sweeteners reliably decrease appetite or reduce EI but can, perhaps, prevent any excess EI that might otherwise occur when calories are provided as caloric sweetened drinks. There are instances when artificially sweetened drinks stimulate appetite and, less often, EI, usually when they are used as food additives rather than sugar substitutes or when ingested by subjects exhibiting dietary restraint *(32)*.

2.4. Sugar-Rich Drinks and the "Fat-Sugar Seesaw"

The epidemiologic data suggest that consumption of sugars (i.e., sweetness with calories) is associated with thinness. Yet, the same studies show that as sugar intake increases, so does EI *(33)*. This suggests that more physically active people select more sugars and, therefore, does not necessarily imply that increased sugar intake spontaneously promotes thinness. The "fat-sugar seesaw" means that fat and carbohydrates (especially sugar) reciprocally affect one another's intake *(33)*. Increasing sugar intake may, through the operation of the fat-sugar seesaw, displace fat energy from the diet *(33)* and decrease the excess EI risk. However, there are at least six limitations or inconsistencies in these simple arguments that fat is a risk for, and carbohydrates (especially sugar) a protector against, weight gains: (1) The major limitation of the epidemiologic studies is that they rely heavily on self-reported EI. Indeed, the fat-sugar seesaw disappears when misreporters are excluded from the data set *(34)*. (2) Ostensibly, the relationships mentioned are supported by data from laboratory studies *(10)*. However, as discussed, the evidence relating to the effects of sugar on EI is far more controversial. (3) There is a large bias in the literature when considering how adding specific nutrients to the diet affects appetite and EI. In the majority of studies, high-fat energy-dense foods have been compared to lower fat less energy-dense foods. Few studies have examined the effects of increasing the ED of the diet using readily hydrolyzed starches or sugars *(35)*. This is important, because the explosion of the low-fat food market has increased the availability of more energy-dense high-carbohydrate foods, especially drinks *(10)*. (4) Fats and sugars are generally not consumed in isolation, and both animals and humans show a strong preference for foods that are mixtures of fats and sugars *(36)*. The relationships derived from epidemiologic data separate and compare high-fat vs high-sugar (and low-fat) consumers. These studies do not consider the effects of fats and sugars in combination. (5) Although the epidemiologic data suggest a fat-sugar seesaw, high-sugar consumers are not low-energy consumers and may have more active lifestyles *(34)*. (6) Few, if any, studies have been specifically designed to detect changes in macronutrient selection.

Therefore, one must examine how incrementing both sugar and fat into the diet will affect feeding behavior and EI. Mazlan *(37)* has recently done this in a series of 7-d studies, using semisolid snacks. In these studies, the general effect of incrementing these mandatory snacks into the diet was to elevate total EI. Subjects did not compensate at all for the high-fat snacks into the diet and only compensated by 20–30% for the high-sugar snacks. The percentage of energy from fat and carbohydrate increased with fat and carbohydrate supplementation, respectively. However, when nutrient intakes were considered in absolute terms (grams), incrementing sugar into the diet did not displace fat and vice versa.

The general conclusion from these studies is that both fat-rich and carbohydrate-rich snacks of similar ED, sweetness, and palatability have similar effects in elevating EI. Recently, Whybrow *(38)* has shown similar effects, using commercially available snack foods in consumers living their normal lives in their home environments. These data can be considered in relation to the epidemiologic and intervention studies discussed in this chapter to conclude that the evidence that increasing intake of sugar-rich foods or drinks is not likely to lever fat out of the diet to the extent that it will prevent weight gain. On the contrary, the evidence suggests that supplementing the diet with carbohydrate-rich drinks is likely to elevate EI for the reasons discussed.

For the reasons mentioned, beverages are likely to be important in maintaining EB in those who are active. Indeed, there are a number of beverages that are formulated specifically as "sports drinks" (*see* Chapter 20). Several studies show that in active subjects, especially in conditions of high water turnover, carbohydrate-rich drinks enhance performance and well-being *(39)*. In addition, it has been suggested by Westerterp-Plantenga *(40)* that such stresses increase the preference for sweet drinks. High-energy beverages are also likely to be far more effective as clinical supplements than many solid foods. Indeed, there are numerous clinical supplements that are formulated as sip feeds.

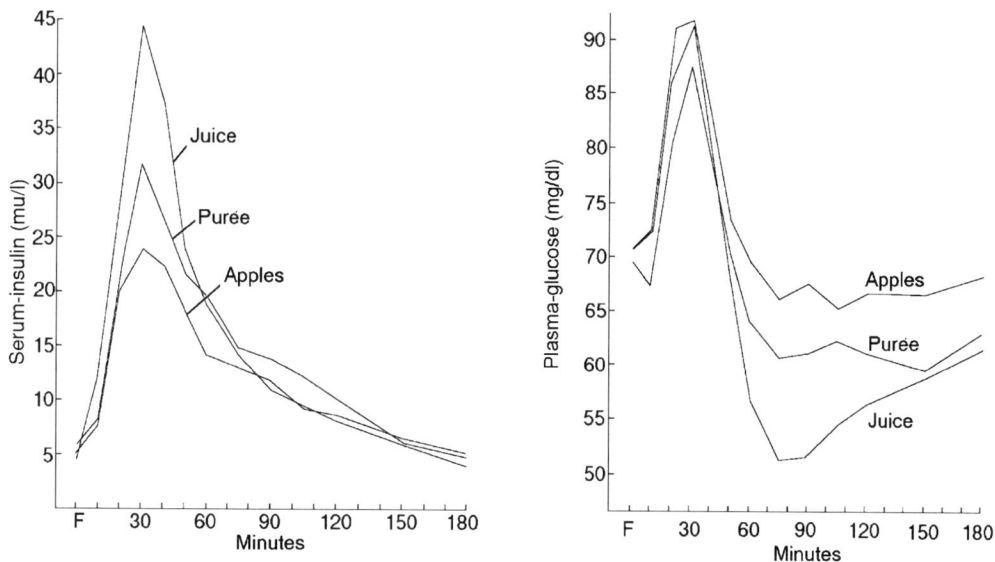

Fig. 2. The effects of disruption or removal of dietary fiber from apples on plasma glucose and insulin concentrations. Juice and purée were consumed in a time similar to that for the whole apples. To convert insulin values from mu/L to pmol/L, multiply by 7.175; to convert glucose values from mg/dL to nmol/L, multiply by 0.05551. From Haber et al. *(42)*.

3. BEVERAGES, GLYCEMIC INDEX, AND OBESITY

The low-fat food revolution has led to health messages promoting a greater intake of low-fat foods. Could it be that the increased consumption of energy-rich low-fat beverages is undermining the beneficial effects of fat reduction strategies? Most beverages are not only low in fat but are also high in readily assimilated carbohydrates with a high glycemic index. Roberts *(41)* recently reviewed this issue. Of six studies reviewed, four low-glycemic index treatments promoted satiation within a meal, whereas two did not. Between-meal satiety was less easy to predict, because three studies showed that low-glycemic index foods enhance postmeal satiety, although in two studies, high-glycemic index carbohydrates had the same effect. There was a similar lack of consensus relating to whether high- or low-glycemic index foods delay the return of hunger. The most consistent finding was that low-glycemic index foods reduce subsequent EI in short-term interventions.

Some reasons for the intake-restraining effect of less processed carbohydrates have been suggested by a most elegant study conducted by Haber et al. in 1977 *(42)*. They compared the same weight of whole apples ingested to apples that had been pureed (disrupting but not removing the structural fibers) or to apple juice, which contained the same energy but from which the fiber had been removed. Ten subjects ingested test meals based on the intact, pureed, or juiced apples, each containing 60 g available carbohydrate. Fiber-free juice could be consumed 11 times faster than intact apples and 4 times faster than fiber-disrupted puree. With the rate of ingestion equalized, juice was significantly less satiating than purée, and puree than apples (*see* Fig. 2). The authors noted that plasma glucose rose to similar levels after all three meals, but there was a striking rebound fall after juice and, to a lesser extent, after puree, which was not seen after apples.

Serum insulin rose to higher levels after juice and puree than after apples. These findings led the authors to suggest: "The removal of fiber from food, and also its physical disruption, can result in faster and easier ingestion, decreased satiety, and disturbed glucose homeostasis which is probably due to inappropriate insulin release. These effects favor over-nutrition and, if often repeated, might lead to diabetes mellitus" *(42)*. It is tempting to view this experiment as an allegory for the evolution of the Western diet, with reference to the role of carbohydrate-rich beverages in the low-fat food revolution.

Once carbohydrates are ingested and any primary interconvertions (e.g., fructose to glucose) are made, there is little reason to suppose that there is much difference between carbohydrates in their effects on satiety. The majority of differences likely result from sensory, preabsorptive, and absorptive phase events. The study by Haber et al. *(42)* illustrates how simple mechanical disruption or removal of structural carbohydrates by conversion of a food to a beverage can influence all three. This suggests that the effects of beverages on satiety operate primarily at the sensory, preabsorptive, and absorptive phases of ingestion. There is, however, little evidence to suggest that the glycemic index of beverages *per se* is important in relation to appetite and EB. One should remember that sugar has a lower glycemic index than many starches, and fructose is used as a caloric sweetener. To the best of our knowledge, there is currently little, if any, evidence to distinguish the effects of high- and low-glycemic index carbohydrates in beverages in relation to appetite and EB.

The evidence pertaining to beverages and body weight control suggests that modern calorific soft drinks are likely to be conducive to weight gain. The orosensory, nutritional, and physiologic effects of modern calorific soft drinks are more conducive to weight gain than weight control. However, these attributes of calorific beverages can be viewed as areas of potential to increase the function of beverages with reference to weight control.

4. THE FUNCTION OF BEVERAGES IN RELATION TO WEIGHT CONTROL

4.1. Tea and Catechins, Coffee, and Xanthines: Their Role in Thermogenesis

Caffeine is discussed more completely in Chapter 12, but with regard to energy issues, caffeine increases thermogenesis. Acute administration of 100 mg caffeine increased the resting metabolic rate of volunteers by 3–4% ($p < 0.02$) during 150 min *(43)*. Repeated doses (100 mg) at 2-h intervals during a 12-h period increased EE by 8–11% ($p < 0.01$) during the day but not the subsequent night *(44)*. This effect is similar in magnitude to that of numerous food ingredients deemed "neutraceutical" agents, because they have a small, but significant, effect on thermogenesis in acute studies *(44)*. These agents include green tea catechins (as more fully discussed in Chapter 10), capsaincin, medium-chain triglycerides, and betel nuts. Although significant, the effect of these ingredients in isolation is rather small. However, caffeine has greater effects on thermogenesis when combined with other agents that influence the sympathetic-adrenal axis, such as ephedrine. Likewise, Dulloo *(45)* argues that caffeine interacts with the green tea epigallocatechin gallate (EGCG) and stimulates thermogenesis through their interactions with sympathetically released norepinephrine. Relative to placebo, treatment with the green tea extract (50 mg caffeine and 90 mg EGCG) resulted in a significant increase in 24-h EE (4%; $p < 0.01$) and a significant decrease in 24-h respiratory quotient (RQ) (from

0.88 to 0.85; $p < 0.001$) without any change in urinary nitrogen excretion *(46)*. The same dose of caffeine alone had no effect on these parameters.

Therefore, it is possible that several of these agents can be combined in a beverage preparation, which has a significant effect on daily EE. The effect is still likely to be small, because, to date, any agents known to cause significant thermogenesis also have side effects. If such a preparation were formulated using neutraceutical ingredients, the question of sustainability of effects would arise.

4.2. Reduced-Fat Milks

When considering the success of various beverages in weight control, the role of population changes in milk consumption should not be forgotten. Although the topic of milk is also discussed in Chapter 14, the topic warrants some discussion here. The majority of milk consumed has changed in the last five decades from high-fat to low-fat versions. Johnson and Fary *(9)* report: " . . . in 1945 Americans drank > 4 times as much milk as soft drinks, whereas in 1997 they drank nearly 2.5 times more soft drinks than milk." Thus, consumers who have not replaced milk with soft drinks may have benefited from the increased consumption of low-fat milk products *(23)*. However, at least for the average US citizen, the problems for weight control associated with an increased consumption of carbohydrate-rich soft drinks literally outweigh the benefits of reducing the fat content of their milk.

4.3. The Use of Liquid Diets and Meal Replacers to Lose Weight

Given the discussion of the influence that beverages exert on EI and EB, it is remarkable that one of the most successful dietary approaches to weight management in the market involves the use of liquid meal replacers. This topic is also discussed in Chapter 19. There is a large body of literature demonstrating that meal-replacement therapy is, at least in the short- to medium-term, reasonably successful at getting the weight off *(47)*. The purpose of this discussion is not to document the literature regarding liquid meal replacers and low-calorie diets but to consider whether their role as beverages has any specific advantage over nonbeverage alternatives.

Wadden *(47)* summarized the effects of moderate and severe caloric restriction, largely using these products. He notes:

> *" . . . recent studies of the treatment of obesity by moderate and severe caloric restriction show that patients treated in randomized trials using a conventional 5 MJ/d reducing diet, combined with behavior modification, lose approx 8.5 kg in 20 wk. They maintain approximately two thirds of this weight loss 1 yr later. Patients treated under medical supervision using a low-calorie diet (1.7 to 3.4 MJ/d) lose approx 20 kg in 12 to 16 wk and maintain one half to two thirds of this loss in the following year. Both dietary interventions are associated with increasing weight regain over time."*

There is, however, no specific value in using beverages as the vehicle for the weight-reducing regimen. Liquid very low-calorie-diets (VLCDs) induce a faster weight loss than low-calorie diets in the first few months of treatment, because they prescribe a greater energy deficit. However, there is a point during weight loss beyond which the body attempts to prevent further loss of body tissue by changing one's physiology and behavior. Thus, the majority of people who lose weight regain it *(48)*. There is also evidence that those who lose weight faster regain it faster. This has, in some cases, been found with VLCDs *(47)*.

In the first few months of therapy, structured meal plans and behavior modification using liquid and semisolid products have certain advantages. These include the simplicity, convenience, and clear measure of EI and nutrient intake these products provide. There is little evidence to suggest that structured meal plans *per se* have any specific feature of their nutrient content that is conducive to weight control. One possible exception to this may be that many are fortified and are, therefore, nutritionally balanced. If a nutritional imbalance created by energy-rich fluids is implicated in weight gain (which for reasons explained earlier may be the case), then, by the same logic, beverages that are nutritionally balanced may be implicated in weight control. This hypothesis has yet to be tested. However, as with other methods of weight control, there is a high attrition rate in the longer term with these regimens. This points to an important need for the development of food and beverage products to maintain weight loss. This, of course, remains the Holy Grail of the weight-control industry.

Clearly, as weight loss proceeds, the ability to keep it off decreases *(47)*. This likely results from a greater physiologic drive to defend against tissue loss and also the difficulties people have in sustaining behavioral change. A considerable amount of work is required to define the mechanistic strengths and limitations of current dietary approaches to weight management (including beverages) before we can apply these findings to the control of body weight, through development of advanced products, tools, and advice tailored to meet the specific needs of individual consumers.

4.4. Aspartame-Based Low-Calorie Drinks

When intense sweeteners were first marketed, it was widely believed that their use as a sugar substitute would be a major dietary approach to weight management. There has since been an explosion in the market for sweetened beverages and foods containing these compounds. The effects of sugars, sweetness, and artificial sweeteners were discussed. There are, unfortunately, remarkably few long-term studies that have examined the efficacy of aspartame in dietary approaches to weight management. In 1997, Blackburn et al. *(49)* investigated whether the addition of the high-intensity sweetener aspartame to a multidisciplinary weight-control program would improve weight loss and long-term body weight control. They randomly assigned 163 women who were obese to consume or to abstain from aspartame-sweetened foods and beverages during 16 wk of a 19-wk weight-reduction program (active weight loss), a 1-yr maintenance program, and a 2-yr follow-up period. Women in both groups lost approx 10% of their initial body weight (10 kg) during active weight loss. Among women assigned to the aspartame group, aspartame intake was positively correlated with percentage of weight loss during active weight loss ($r = 0.32$, $p < 0.01$). During maintenance and follow-up, participants in the aspartame group experienced a 2.6% (2.6 kg) and 4.6% (4.6 kg) regain of initial body weight after 71 and 175 wk, respectively, whereas those in the no-aspartame group gained an average of 5.4% (5.4 kg) and 9.4% (9.4 kg), respectively. Weight loss was also correlated with exercise and eating control. This is in keeping with the observation that the more fat-reduction strategies people employ, the greater their chance of successful weight control *(50)*.

4.5. Drinks That Enhance Satiety

There has been a great deal of research examining how various nutritional and physiochemical attributes of beverages influence short-term satiety *(51)*. It is possible to enhance the satiating effects of drinks in several ways: (1) Using nutrients that have a higher satiety value. (2) Replacing carbohydrates with intense sweeteners. (3) Increasing the viscosity of drinks should enhance satiety *(52)*. Adding soluble fiber to beverages is one way that increased viscosity can be achieved. Soluble fiber delays the rate of glucose absorption from the gut and enhances short-term satiety. Psyllium (sold in the United States as Metamucil) is proven to both lower the blood cholesterol and help alleviate constipation. (4) Thermogenic neutraceutical ingredients may influence satiety, because, as a rule, agents that stimulate the sympathetic-adrenal axis suppress appetite. However, as seen from the evidence presented in this chapter, the development of the function of beverages in this respect is still in its infancy.

5. CONCLUSIONS

Obesity is rising dramatically in developed and developing countries despite the widespread adoption of fat-reduction strategies. This has led to research into how overconsumption is influenced by different types of carbohydrates and by foods vs beverages. Beverages have a large effect on the composition of the modern diet. There has been a shift in the last two decades away from whole-fat milk-based beverage in favor of lower-fat versions. This has also been accompanied by an increase in soft drink consumption per capita in the United States and numerous Western countries. In surveys of the general population, sugar-sweetened beverage intake is often, but not always, associated with higher levels of fatness. In addition, there is evidence that high soft drink intakes displace micronutrients from the diet. In children, there is also evidence of reduced stature and increased adiposity in children with high intakes of sugar-sweetened soft drinks. There is growing evidence that (mainly carbohydrate) energy from drinks promotes overconsumption, whereas solid carbohydrates promote caloric compensation. Part of this effect relates to the sensory properties of modern beverages being conducive to overconsumption. In addition, beverages activate fewer of the signals contributing to satiety than do solid foods. This is because many of these signals are associated with nutrient digestion and absorption. Because modern beverages are conducive to weight gain, there is considerable scope to develop the properties of beverages (viscosity, neutraceutical content, balance of nutrients, and soluble fiber) to enhance satiety and develop a range of products that assist in controlling body weight. This area is, however, in its infancy.

6. MAIN POINTS FOR PRIMARY AND CLINICAL REVIEW

1. Studies in children indicate that consumption of sugar-sweetened drink is associated with obesity.
2. Calories contained in drinks (especially carbohydrates) appear to promote higher energy intakes than when the same number of calories is contained in solid foods.
3. There is little evidence that artificial sweeteners reliably decrease appetite or reduce energy intake, but might possibly lower the energy intake that would occur when calories are provided as caloric, sweetened drinks.
4. Caffeine and green tea extracts tend to cause a small increase in energy expenditure.
5. There is little clear evidence that beverages are advantageous for weight reduction.

REFERENCES

1. Mokdad AH, Serdula MK, Dietz WH, Bowman BA, Marks JS, Koplan JP. The spread of the obesity epidemic in the United States, 1991-1998. JAMA 1999;282:1519–1522.
2. Blundell JE, Stubbs RJ. Diet and food intake in humans. In: International Handbook of Obesity. Bray GA, Bouchard C, James WPT (eds.). Dekker Inc., New York, NY, 1997, pp. 243–272.
3. The Allied Dunbar National Fitness. Survey commissioned by the Health Education Authority and Sports Council, Belmont Press, London, UK, 1992.
4. Martinez-Gonzalez MA, Martinez JA, Hu FB, Gibney MJ, Kearney J. Physical inactivity, sedentary lifestyle and obesity in the European Union. Int J Obes Relat Metab Disord 1999;23:1192–1201.
5. Kant AK, Graubard BI, Schatzkin A, Ballard-Barbash R. Proportion of energy intake from fat and subsequent weight change in the NHANES Epidemiological Follow-up Study. Am J Clin Nutr 1995; 61:11–17.
6. Goldberg GR, Black A, Jebb SA, et al. Critical evaluation of energy intake using fundamental principles of energy physiology. 1. Derivation of cut-off limits to identify under recording. Eur J Clin Nutr 1991;45:569–581.
7. Mela DJ. Understanding fat preference and consumption: applications of behavioural sciences to a nutritional problem. Proc Nutr Soc 1995;54:453–464.
8. Stubbs J, Ferres S, Horgan G. Energy density of foods: effects on energy intake. Crit Rev Food Sci Nutr 2000;40:481–515.
9. Johnson RK, Frary C. Choose beverages and foods to moderate your intake of sugars: the 2000 dietary guidelines for Americans-what's all the fuss about? J Nutr 2001;131:2766S–2771S.
10. Stubbs RJ, Mazlan N, Whybrow S. Carbohydrates, appetite and feeding behavior in humans. J Nutr 2001;131:2775S–2781S.
11. Burns AA, Livingstone MB, Welch RW, Dunne A, Rowland IR. Dose-response effects of a novel fat emulsion (Olibratrade mark) on energy and macronutrient intakes up to 36 h post-consumption. Eur J Clin Nutr 2002;56:368–377.
12. Atkinson RL, Gomez T, Clark RL, Pariza MW. Clinical Implications for CLA in the Treatment of Obesity. Program of the Annual Meeting, National Nutritional Foods Association, July 15–16, San Antonio, TX, 1998.
13. Stubbs RJ, Ferris S, Whybrow S. Dietary and phenotypic determinants of energy intake in 102 adults. Int J Obesity Relat Metab Disord 2001;25:S56.
14. de Castro JM, Orozco S. Moderate alcohol intake and spontaneous eating patterns of humans: evidence of unregulated supplementation. Am J Clin Nutr 1991;52:246–253.
15. Mattes RD. Dietary compensation by humans for supplemental energy provided as ethanol or carbohydrate in fluids. Physiol Behav 1996;59:179–187.
16. Park YK, Yetley EA. Intakes and food sources of fructose in the United States. Am J Clin Nutr 1993; 58(Suppl):737S–747S.
17. Prynne CJ, Paul AA, Price GM, Day KC, Hilder WS, Wadsworth ME. Food and nutrient intake of a national sample of 4-year-old children in 1950: comparison with the 1990s. Public Health Nutr 1999; 2:537–547.
18. Troiano RP, Briefel RR, Carroll MD, Bialostosky K. Energy and fat intakes of children and adolescents in the United States: data from the national health and nutrition examination surveys. Am J Clin Nutr 2000;72(Suppl):1343S–1353S.
19. Cavadini C, Siega-Riz AM, Popkin BM. US adolescent food intake trends from 1965 to 1996. West J Med 2000;173:378–383.
20. Ludwig DS, Peterson KE, Gortmaker SL. Relation between consumption of sugar-sweetened drinks and childhood obesity: a prospective, observational analysis. Lancet 2001;357:505–508.
21. Dennison BA, Rockwell HL, Baker SL. Excess fruit juice consumption by preschool-aged children is associated with short stature and obesity. Pediatrics 1997;99:15–22.
22. Gibson SA. Non-milk extrinsic sugars in the diets of pre-school children: association with intakes of micronutrients, energy, fat and NSP. Br J Nutr 1997;78:367–378.-
23. Lee HH, Gerrior SA, Smith JA. Energy, macronutrient, and food intakes in relation to energy compensation in consumers who drink different types of milk. Am J Clin Nutr 1998;67:616–623.

24. Ramirez I. Feeding a liquid diet increases energy intake, weight gain and body fat in rats. J Nutr 1987; 117:2127–2134.

25. DiMeglio DP, Mattes RD. Liquid versus solid carbohydrate: effects on food intake and body weight. Int J Obes Relat Metab Disord 2000;24:794–800.

26. Gurr MI, Mawson R, Rothwell NJ, Stock MJ. Effects of manipulating dietary protein and energy intake on energy balance and thermogenesis in the pig. J Nutr 1980;110:532–542.

27. Stirling JL, Stock MJ. Metabolic origins of thermogenesis induced by diet. Nature 1968;220: 801–802.

28. Anderson GH, Leiter LA. Effects of aspartame and phenylalanine on meal-time food intake of humans. Appetite 1988;11:48–53.

29. Booth D, Mather P, Fuller J. Starch content of ordinary foods associatively conditions human appetite and satiation, indexed by intake and eating pleasantness of starch-paired flavours. Appetite 1982; 3:163–184.

30. Blundell JE, Rogers PJ. Sweet carbohydrate substitutes (intense sweeteners) and the control of appetite: Scientific issues. In: Appetite and Body Weight Regulation: Sugar, Fat and Macronutrient Substitutes. Fernstrom JD, Miller GD (eds.). CRC Press, Boca Raton, FL, 1994, pp. 113–124.

31. Black RM, Anderson GH. Sweeteners, food intake and selection. In: Appetite and Body Weight Regulation: Sugar, Fat and Macronutrient Substitutes. Fernstrom JD, Miller GD (eds.). CRC Press, Boca Raton, FL, 1994, pp. 125–136.

32. Lavin, JH, French SJ, Read NW. The effect of sucrose- and aspartame-sweetened drinks on energy intake, hunger and food choice of female, moderately restrained eaters. Int J Obes Relat Metab Disord 1997;21:37–42.

33. Bolton-Smith C, Woodward M. Dietary composition and fat to sugar ratios in relation to obesity. Int J Obesity Relat Metab Disord 1994;18:820–828.

34. MacDiarmid JI, Vail A, Cade JE, Blundell JE. The sugar-fat relationship revisited: differences in con-sumption between men and women of varying BMI. Int J Obesity Relat Metab Disord 1998; 22:1053–1061.

35. Stubbs RJ, Johnstone AM, Harbron CG, Reid C. Covert manipulation of the energy density of high-carbohydrate diets: effect on *ad libitum* food intake in "pseudo free-living" humans. Int J Obesity Relat Metab Disord 1998;22:885–892.

36. Drewnowski A. Macronutrient substitutes and weight reduction practices of obese, dieting and eating disordered women. Ann NY Acad Sci 1997;819:132–141.

37. Mazlan N. Effects of Fat and Carbohydrate on Energy Intake and Macronutrient Selection in Humans [thesis]. Aberdeen University, Aberdeen, Scotland, 2001.

38. Whybrow S. Determinants of Food and Energy Intake and the Effects of Dietary Energy Density on Energy Intake in Humans. Queen Margaret University, Edinburgh, Scotland, 2002.

39. Stroud M. The nutritional demands of very prolonged exercise in man. Proc Nutr Soc 1998;57:55–61.

40. Westerterp-Plantenga MS, Verwegen CR, Ijedema MJ, Wijckmans NE, Saris WH. Acute effects of exercise or sauna on appetite in obese and non obese men. Physiol Behav 1997;62:1345–1354.

41. Roberts SB. High-glycemic index foods, hunger, and obesity: Is there a connection? Nutr Rev 2000; 58:163–169.

42. Haber GB, Heaton KW, Murphy D. Depletion and disruption of dietary fibre: effects on satiety, plasma-glucose, and serum-insulin. Lancet 1977;2:679–682.

43. Dulloo AG, Geissler CA, Horton T, Collins A, Miller DS. Normal caffeine consumption: influence on thermogenesis and daily energy expenditure in lean and postobese human volunteers. Am J Clin Nutr 1989;49:44–50.

44. Dulloo AG. Herbal simulation of ephedrine and caffeine in treatment of obesity. Int J Obes Relat Metab Disord 2002;26:590–592.

45. Dulloo AG, Seydoux J, Girardier L, Chantre P, Vandermander J. Green tea and thermogenesis: inter-actions between catechin-polyphenols, caffeine and sympathetic activity. Int J Obes Relat Metab Disord 2000;24:252–258.

46. Dulloo AG, Duret C, Rohrer D, Girardier L, Mensi N, Fathi M, et al. Efficacy of a green tea extract rich in catechin polyphenols and caffeine in increasing 24-h energy expenditure and fat oxidation in humans. Am J Clin Nutr 1999;70:1040–1045.

47. Wadden TA. Treatment of obesity by moderate and severe caloric restriction. Results of clinical research trials. Ann Intern Med 1993;119:688–693.
48. Garrow JS. Obesity and Related Diseases. Churchill Livingstone, London, UK, 1988, pp. 181–183.
49. Blackburn GL, Kanders BS, Lavin PT, Keller SD, Whatley J. The effect of aspartame as part of a multidisciplinary weight-control program on short- and long-term control of body weight. Am J Clin Nutr 1997;65:409–418.
50. Sigman-Grant M, Poma S, Hsieh, K. Update on the impact of specific fat reduction strategies on nutrient intakes of Americans. FASEB J 1998;12:A530.
51. Rolls BJ, Bell EA. Intake of fat and carbohydrate: role of energy density. Eur J Clin Nutr 1999;53 (Suppl):S166–S173.
52. Mattes RD, Rothacker D. Beverage viscocity is inversely related to postprandial hunger in humans. Physiol Behav 2001;74:551–557.

19 Nutritional Support Beverages in the Treatment of Malnutrition of the Elderly

Carrie Johnsen and Peter Glassman

1. MALNUTRITION IN THE ELDERLY

For the elderly, optimal nutrition goes hand in hand with optimal health, yet many elderly suffer from malnutrition or are at risk of poor nutrition. In the United States and Britain, researchers concluded that up to one third of ambulatory elderly and more than three fourths of homebound elderly are at moderate to high risk of malnutrition (1,2).

Although the prevalence of poor nutrition is surprisingly high, many clinicians do not readily recognize malnutrition or its underlying risks in day-to-day practice. For example, Mowe and Bohmer (3) reported that few malnourished patients in hospitals were recognized by their physicians as needing nutritional assessment. This problem also persists in ambulatory care. In a survey of primary-care physicians, Levine et al. (4) found that respondents were far more likely to address nutritional problems in patients who were overweight than to attempt to ascertain if their patients suffered from malnourishment.

Significant weight loss, gradual weight loss, or any type of unintentional weight loss is often the first indicator of malnutrition noted by the health care provider. Weight loss in the elderly, however, may result from several causes, not all of which are directly caused by inadequate intake. Physical changes associated with aging include a redistribution of body composition where muscle mass is largely replaced with fat mass (5). Older adults will then have a greater proportion of body fat and a lower proportion of muscle mass or lean weight compared with younger adults (6). This is significant, because lean weight or muscle mass is more dense than fat mass. Essentially, a lower weight may indicate a shift in body composition and a need to focus efforts on regaining lean mass for improved muscular function rather than on increasing caloric intake merely to gain weight. That is, the emphasis should be on getting stronger rather than fatter.

Underlying medical and environmental issues other than intake can also lead to malnutrition. Numerous medical and mental health conditions can interfere with the motivation or desire to obtain food, prepare food, and eat food. Even for those who have the desire or motivation, reduced social interaction and/or financial constraints may lead to

From: *Beverages in Nutrition and Health*
Edited by: T. Wilson and N. J. Temple © Humana Press Inc., Totowa, NJ

fewer and smaller meals *(5–7)*. Newly diagnosed dementia (of any type), depression, stroke, thyroid disease, diabetes mellitus, congestive heart failure, kidney disease, dysphagia, chronic pain syndromes, or cancer may all increase the risk for malnutrition; so, too, will dental problems that interfere with chewing and swallowing solid foods. Additionally, an underappreciated, yet not-infrequent, precursor, to malnutrition is alcohol abuse, especially in those who live alone. Elderly persons may be at risk for poor nutrition resulting from side effects from drug regimens containing many different types of drugs *(8)*. Many medications affect nutrition status by altering food intake, absorption, metabolism, and excretion of nutrients. They can decrease appetite, taste, and smell and cause gastronintestinal (GI) disturbances, such as nausea, diarrhea, and constipation. They can also affect cognition and mobility *(9–11)*. Such adverse effects may then be treated with new drugs or interventions, potentially worsening matters and further compromising nutrition and health.

2. MANAGEMENT RECOMMENDATIONS FOR MALNUTRITION

Resolving malnutrition and poor nutrition habits begins with correcting any underlying problems that interfere with obtaining, eating, or digesting food. For persons lacking in economic resources, there are several community resources, such as local senior centers and home delivery services (e.g., Meals on Wheels), that offer assistance. These services can provide at least one balanced meal per day, and senior centers have the advantage of increasing social contact. For patients with chewing problems or with poor dental hygiene, a referral to a dental health provider may be necessary. Physical limitations can be addressed with therapy, self-feeding skills training and devices, or feeding assistance. For selected patients, modifying drug regimens, as applicable, may improve appetite and desire to eat, as will the treatment of conditions that interfere with their motivation to eat (e.g., depression). A dietitian can assess poor eating habits and provide education about specialized diets and advice for improving intake to better meet needs.

It is the position of the American Dietetic Association (ADA) that "The best nutritional strategy for promoting optimal health and reducing the risk of chronic disease is to wisely choose a wide variety of foods" *(12)*. Thus, patients should be encouraged to eat a balanced diet that includes adequate protein, carbohydrate, and fat. They should adhere to a regular meal schedule of three small meals, with snacks in between. They must include variety at each meal with fruits, vegetables, breads and cereals, and a protein source. They should be advised to choose hearty, dense, whole-grain breads and cereals, and drink plenty of fluids from water, fruit or vegetable juices, milk, or soups *(13)*. Weight gain can be assisted relatively inexpensively by adding readily accessible easy-to-prepare high-calorie and high-protein snacks and/or beverages periodically throughout the day.

Additional vitamins and minerals from commercially manufactured supplements may help some people meet their nutritional needs *(12)* and may be needed in certain types of malnutrition, but it is not a sufficient answer to the problem. Epidemiological studies continue to indicate with certainty "the importance of diet and nutrition to optimize health and prevent disease" *(12)*. The potential benefit of supplementing diets with vitamins or minerals in generally healthy individuals is less clear. Studies demonstrate the positive health benefits of some supplements and uncertainty and even "ineffectiveness or adverse health effects" of others *(12)*. Therefore, it is beholden on health care professionals to look closely at claims made about such supplements. This is especially true with supplemental beverages, a source of nutritional supplements, because they are often heavily marketed to an unwary and often uneducated public, while, at the same time, oversight and regulation of supplements and their health claims by the Food and Drug Administration is limited in the United States (12).

Regarding increasing caloric intake by using manufactured nutritional support beverage products, there are little scientific data on the efficacy and effectiveness of these drinks when compared with other food sources, especially readily available foods. It is problematic, therefore, to know when such supplements are necessary or even appropriate. Much of contemporary advertising would have consumers believe that nutritional support beverages are part of a normal healthy lifestyle. In fact, the Federal Trade Commission has taken action to stop manufacturers from claiming that a nutritional supplement drink was "recommended" by doctors for healthy adults (12).

This brings us to several real considerations against the casual use of supplemental beverages to meet nutritional needs. First, some food components are clearly identified as having potential health benefits, such as dietary fiber, but are rarely found in supplemental beverages. Second, the composition of natural foods contains many yet-unidentified components that may have important health benefits. Third, even when beneficial constituents in foods and plants are identified, it is difficult to replicate the "complex matrix" of foods to achieve the same benefit and/or bioavailability in a supplement as that found in the original food or plant sources (12).

One thing that has become clearer as nutritional science has progressed is that we do not presently have the knowledge to formulate artificial solid or beverage diets that optimize health and prevent disease, as would be the case with eating numerous natural food sources and products (12). It is this message that is so often lost in the media blitz on consumers.

This might not be such a problem if physicians could supply consumers with needed information and act as a balance to media-based claims. However, physicians are part of the general population and are probably susceptible to many of the same biases instilled by advertising about nutritional supplement drinks. Ironically, many product labels state that the products should not be consumed without first discussing their use with a physician. Yet, physicians have little training in nutrition and poor knowledge of the subject (14) and, as discussed, do not often direct their nutritional assessments toward undernutrition (3,4). Moreover, as Steigh et al. (15) found in one health care center that physicians frequently prescribed nutritional support beverages to patients who either were not malnourished or, even more notably, should not have received a high-calorie mineral-rich commercial supplement beverage. These studies suggest that there is no guarantee that clinicians are able to correctly discern the benefits of nutritional support beverages and to target appropriate use. These few studies, taken together, emphasize the need to develop and implement criteria for appropriate use of nutritional support beverages.

3. ARE NUTRITIONAL SUPPORT BEVERAGES THE OPTIMAL THERAPY?

This brings us to the question of when nutritional support beverages should be considered as optimal or first-line therapy for malnutrition? Before trying to answer this question, it is important to recognize what is currently known about such beverages.

First, benefits of manufactured nutritional support beverages have been documented largely in institutionalized patients *(17)*. Extrapolating any positive outcomes achieved in institutionalized settings to community-dwelling populations may not be applicable. Second, even though one may be able to meet daily recommended needs for vitamins and minerals through the use of nutritional support beverages, the beverages often completely lack fiber and other important, yet often unknown, cofactors that allow proper use of vitamins, minerals, and energy. Third, patients may misuse the products as meal *replacements* instead of meal *supplements*, even when their use is accompanied by instructions from a registered dietician. Ensure®, Sustacal®, and Boost® are examples from the class of vaguely defined nutritional support beverages that have been marketed picturing healthy looking older adults enjoying active lives with product statements that encourage people to: "Use it as a snack, with a meal, or as an occasional meal on its own" *(16)*. In fact, it can take up to eight cans a day of a supplement to meet the minimum recommended energy needs of 1200 calories for a woman. When supplements are used as meal *replacements*, it can result in decreased energy and protein intake because the individual is relying only on the supplement for sustenance. Fourth, supplements are designed to be high in carbohydrate for energy but provide only moderate amounts of protein. Many easily prepared and readily accessible foods, including peanut butter, oatmeal, hearty soups, and cheese and crackers, offer superior sources of protein and calories than many manufactured supplements. In fact, many supplements are similar in content to candy bars. Table 1 lists comparative data on common food and supplement products.

Although supplements are clearly superior to candy bars in vitamin and mineral content, a balanced diet should be considered as the best source of bioavailable vitamins and minerals—and, ironically, some of the candy bars are better sources of fiber than commercial supplements. In any case, it is not clear which combination of nutrients, protein, energy, vitamins, trace elements, and particular types of fatty acids is responsible for optimal clinical benefit *(21)*. Supplements cannot mimic the potential of natural foods for providing that ideal combination of elements. The American Dietetic Association, in fact, says: "Much remains unknown about the biologically active components in food" and that all of the potentially beneficial components of foods have not been identified, let alone their appropriate amounts and combinations to achieve the benefits identified *(12)*.

Therefore, we strongly encourage using the patients' favorite foods and drinks, supplemented with nutritious, high-calorie, and high-protein snacks in a balanced diet, as a preferable method for improving calorie and protein intake. This approach is preferred to the use of manufactured supplement beverages.

A study by Unosson et al. *(21)* pointed out: "The goal of nutritional support in elderly patients is not only nutritional repletion, but also improved quality of life." We must remember that the eating process is both physiological and psychological. Real food stimulates smell and taste and provides fullness and satisfaction. Food choices can be tailored to individual likes and dislikes or accommodate dietary restrictions related to comorbidities. Commercial products cannot universally meet these needs, especially in the elderly. Sharing a meal, such as at a community senior center, helps meet the need of social interaction. These quality-of-life factors are certainly important and should not be discounted.

Table 1
Comparative Protein and Calorie Content
of Oral Supplements and Other Food Products *(8,18)*

Oral supplements/food products	Protein g	Calories
Nutritional support beverages		
Ensure® (8 fl oz)	8.8	250
Resource® Standard (8 fl oz)	9.0	250
Sustacal® (8 fl oz)	14.5	240
Enlive!® (8 fl oz)	10	300
NuBasics (8 fl oz)	8.75	250
Boost® (8 fl oz)	10	240
Candy bars		
Baby Ruth® (2.1 oz bar)	5.6	277
Snickers Bar® (2.16 oz bar)	5	280
Other snack foods		
Yogurt (low fat, flavored, 8 oz)	9	225
Instant breakfast (powder, 1.25 oz, whole milk, 8 oz)	15	280
Ice cream (1 scoop, vanilla)	12	250
Chocolate pudding (instant mix, 1 cup)	9	260
Bean soup (with ham, 1 cup)	12	231
Black bean soup (2 cups)	11	240
Baked beans (1 cup)	10	250
Peanut butter sandwich (2 tbsp peanut butter, 2 slices bread)	14	320
Cheese and crackers (cheddar, 2 oz, 5 saltine crackers)	15	288
Peanuts (dry roasted, 1.5 oz)	10	250
Granola (one-fourth cup, whole milk, 0.5 cup)	8	223
Cream of Wheat (made with whole milk)	10	325
Chili with beans (canned, 1 cup)	15	352
Oatmeal (cooked, 1 cup, whole milk, 0.5 cup)	10	221

4. EFFECTIVENESS AND COST-EFFECTIVENESS

Despite the strong recommendations for using real food sources whenever possible to meet nutritional needs, there is evidence that supports the effectiveness of nutritional supplement drinks in selected undernourished patient populations. As mentioned, several studies show that routine supplementation with nutrition support beverages results in increased body weight and muscle mass *(17,20,21)*. Only a few studies have directly compared the effect of using whole-food supplements and nutritional support beverages, although a limited comparison suggests that both methods of supplementation can improve nutritional status *(17,20)*.

Even without good scientific studies, it is reasonable to assume that nutritional support beverages have the same general effect when used as a short-term addition to balanced diets, as other high-calorie snacks. When used correctly, both will increase daily caloric intake and will, thus, help increase weight and energy stores in poorly nourished people, at least temporarily. The question is whether manufactured beverages are a cost-effective method for rectifying poor nutrition status among the community-dwelling population. From a payer's perspective, the cost of providing manufactured nutritional support beverages must be considered and, as a general rule of thumb, these supplements can only be called cost-effective if there are substantial health benefits above and beyond that seen with high-energy meals and snacks (20).

Such benefits might be seen if commercial supplements somehow provided more effective nutritional support or easier access to needed calories or protein or were somehow safer than natural food. However, this is unlikely to be and, although one might argue that supplemental beverages are easy to use, there are no good data to suggest that they are more tolerable or provide better access to calories and protein than nutritious whole-food snacks and beverages. On the contrary, as Baldwin (21) noted, many studies "highlight problems with use of and monitoring of patients taking nutritional supplements" and, more specifically, supplements are "frequently sweet-tasting drinks which may not be taken consistently due to monotony."

Notwithstanding logic or evidence of benefit, the demand for nutritional support beverages is booming. Baldwin (21) notes that the UK Department of Health expenditure on total nutrition support beverages was for $126 million in 1997 and is rising rapidly. This likely mirrors the expenditures on nutritional support beverages in other western countries. Increases in spending can result from the increased awareness of nutrition by the general public and by health care providers and/or marketing by manufacturers of nutritional supplements. Although none of these possibilities is necessarily bad, the issue is whether the benefits of consuming supplemental beverages (i.e., weight gain) in the short-term are sustainable to achieve the long-term beneficial health effects of decreased morbidity and mortality. As Baldwin states succinctly, "The data available suggest that nutritional supplements may enhance weight gain in the short term, but whether this can be sustained or whether survival and morbidity are also improved remains uncertain." Any use, especially long-term use of nutritional support beverages, may cost patients far in excess of usual food products. Thus, although supplemental beverages help to improve nutritional indices of physical health, we must also consider economic health, especially for those with fixed incomes, to form a complete picture.

One reason that use of commercial nutritional support beverages may be increasing is a shift in who is paying for it. By shifting the onus to pay for supplements onto health care systems, there is an underlying decrease in what patients are obligated to purchase. This causes a "medicalization" of poor nutritional status and allows patients and providers access to a beverage that can be used in lieu of purchasing and preparing food. Thus, patients and providers may be increasing demand by requesting supplements when food would do, especially when patients are relieved of the burden of paying for food products. This may provide short-term benefit but it is questionable whether health care systems are doing their patients, or themselves, any favors by freely providing nutritional support beverages rather than helping patients learn about nutritious foods that they could purchase on their own. In an ironic twist, health care systems that indiscriminately offer supplements may be not only promoting their use but also worsening the problem of poor dietary habits.

Any conclusive statement on the comparative benefit of food vs supplemental beverage must await properly conducted scientific studies. There is, as yet, little data suggesting that manufactured supplemental beverages are cost-effective, for most people, when compared to the most common form of nutritional support, namely food.

5. RECOMMENDATIONS ON APPROPRIATE USE OF NUTRITIONAL SUPPORT BEVERAGES

Given what we have written thus far, some may discount the use of manufactured nutritional support beverages altogether. However, we still would advocate using these products in particular circumstances. For example, a short-term trial use would be appropriate for patients who cannot ingest sufficient nutrients by eating solid food or cannot tolerate enough high-calorie snacks to resolve malnutrition. It would be prudent to use supplemental beverages for some defined period of time and then reassess the patient's weight and other nutritional indicators to see if the supplements are having the desired effect. Appropriate use might also include patients who are lactose intolerant, because many techniques for enhancing calorie and protein intake rely on dairy products. However, many nondairy high-calorie high-protein food sources are becoming available with the increase in popularity of soy milk and soy-based products.

Using manufactured products for patients requiring tube feeding may be appropriate with adequate monitoring by a dietitian to ensure that nutritional needs are being met. Again, the issue is to use the minimum amount of commercial supplement needed to sustain proper nutrition and rely as much as possible on natural or pureed-natural foods. For those people who cannot safely prepare meals, options include using community resources, such as Meals on Wheels, or local senior centers that can deliver or provide hot meals. If this is still not adequate, consideration can be given to using supplemental beverage products, but, because these are expensive and because cans are heavy to carry, simple store-bought nutritious snacks (e.g., granola bars) are a good first choice.

It is important to note that although manufactured supplemental beverage products are not particularly dangerous, they are contraindicated in patients who should avoid products high in carbohydrates, salt, and electrolytes (e.g., those with diabetes and chronic renal insufficiency). Therefore, these conditions should be ruled out before recommending manufactured supplements.

6. CONCLUSIONS

Available evidence suggests that early identification and treatment of malnutrition is beneficial for achieving and maintaining optimal health of the elderly. We believe that health care providers must routinely monitor their patients for the less obvious signs of early malnutrition. Patients with poor nutrition should have the underlying causes addressed in a prompt and efficient manner, and nutrition deficits should be reversed by using the most effective means while maintaining quality of life. Given the level of evidence, we do not feel that manufactured nutritional support beverages are preferred for the community-dwelling population. Rather, whenever possible, natural food sources in addition to education about healthy eating habits should be used as a primary method toward resolution. If these do not resolve, or do not begin to resolve, nutrition deficits, it is reasonable to use a nutritional support beverage in addition to other oral intake and close monitoring of supplement use.

7. MAIN POINTS FOR PRIMARY AND CLINICAL REVIEW

1. Malnutrition in the elderly is often underdiagnosed.
2. Dietary supplementation for at-risk elderly with vitamins and minerals is a common intervention, with beverages often being used as the vehicle.
3. Nutritional support beverages are heavily marketed.
4. These marketing efforts occur at the same time that oversight and regulation of supplements and their health claims by the Food and Drug Administration is limited.
5. The best nutritional strategy for promoting optimal health in the at-risk elderly is to encourage and educate them to eat a balanced diet, although certain conditions may exist where nutritional support beverages might be useful.

REFERENCES

1. Vailas LI, Nitzke SA. Screening for risk of malnutrition in Wisconsin's elderly. Wis Med J 1995;94: 495–499.
2. Bunidrick M. Nutritional screening of older South Carolinians: a pilot study. J SC Med Assoc 1995: 260–262.
3. Mowe M, Bohmer T. The prevalence of undiagnosed protein calorie undernutrition in a population of hospitalized elderly patients. J Am Geriatr Soc 1991;39:1089–1091.
4. Levine B, Wigren M, Chapman D, Kerner J, Bernman R, Rivlin R. A national survey of attitudes and practices of primary-care physicians relating to nutrition: strategies for enhancing the use of clinical nutrition in medical practice. Am J Clin Nutr 1993;57:115–119.
5. Bartlett S, Marian M, Taren D, Muramoto M. Geriatric Nutrition Handbook, Vol 5. Kluwer Academic Pub, New York, NY, 1997.
6. Niedert K, Dorner B, Gerwick C, Posthauer ME, Sichterman C (eds.). Nutrition Care of the Older Adult: A Handbook for Dietetics Professionals Working Throughout the Continuum of Care. The American Dietetic Association, Chicago, IL, 1998.
7. Sahyoun NR, Jacques PR, Dallal GE, Russell RM. Nutrition Screening Initiative checklist may be a better awareness/educational tool than a screening one. J Am Dietet Assoc 1997;97:760–764.
8. Johnsen C, East J, Glassman P. Management of malnutrition in the elderly and the appropriate use of commercially manufactured oral nutritional supplements. J Nutr Health Aging 2000;4:42–46.
9. Morrison G, Hark L. Medical Nutrition and Disease. Blackwell Science, Malden, MA, 1996, pp. 1–31.
10. Pronsky Z. Food-Medication Interactions, 11th Ed. Food-Medication Interactions, Birchrunville, PA, 2000, pp. 6–11.
11. Morley JE, Silver AJ. Nutritional issues in nursing home care. Ann Intern Med 1995;123:850–859.
12. Hunt J, Dwyer J. Position of the American Dietetic Association: food fortification and dietary supplements. J Am Diet Assoc 2001;101:115–125.
13. American Dietetic Association. Staying Healthy—A Guide for Older Adults. The American Dietetic Association, Chicago, 1998.
14. Temple NJ. Survey of nutrition knowledge of Canadian physicians. J Am Coll Nutr 1999;18:26–29.
15. Steigh C, Glassman P, Fajardo F. Physician and dietitian prescribing of a commercially available oral nutritional supplement. Am J Manage Care 1998,4:567–572.
16. Abbot Laboratories, Ross Products Division, Ensure® product information. Retrieved July 29, 2002, from http://www.ensure.com/OurProducts/Ensure.asp.
17. Potter J, Langhorne P, Roberts M. Routine protein energy supplementation in adults: systematic review. Br Med J 1998;317:495–501.
18. Bowes A. Bowes & Church's food values of portions commonly used (17th Ed. Rev. by Jean AT Pennington). Lipincott-Raven, Philadelphia, PA, 1998.
19. Unosson M, Larsson J, Ek AC, Bjurulf P. Effects of dietary supplement of functional condition and clinical outcome measured with a modified Norton scale. Clin Nutr 1992;11:134–139.
20. Allison SP. Cost-effectiveness of nutrition support in the elderly. Proc Nutr Soc 1995;54:693–699.
21. Baldwin C, Parsons T, Logan S. Dietary advice for illness-related malnutrition in adults. Cochrane Database Syst Rev 2001;2:CD002008.

VII BEVERAGES FOR PERFORMANCE ENHANCEMENT AND REHYDRATION

20

Sports Beverages for Optimizing Physical Performance

Ron J. Maughan

1. INTRODUCTION

Many different factors combine to produce a successful performance in sporting contests, with genetic endowment playing a large role. Other factors also intervene, but many of these also have a genetic basis, including the ability to adapt to a training program and the psychological factors that encompass motivation, competitiveness, and tactical awareness. Consistent intensive training is a major factor in the success of most elite performers, but there is a limit to the training load that can be sustained without illness or injury. Of those factors that can be altered by conscious effort, nutrition, which is perhaps only a small part of the overall picture, is important.

Nutritional support during training can enhance recovery between training sessions, allowing more consistent intensive training, with a reduced risk of illness, infection, and injury. Nutritional strategies can also be devised to maximize the adaptive changes occurring in muscle and other tissues in response to each training session *(1)*. Nutritional support may have its biggest effect in training rather than in competition, but the idea of an acute intervention that gives a competitive edge is intuitively attractive to athletes. In competition, there is scope for modification of the diet in the pre-event period, and, in some sports, for ingestion of food and/or fluids during the event itself. In events such as marathon running or cycling, this means taking drinks (and solid foods in cycling) without interrupting the exercise. In games such as tennis, there are regular breaks in play that provide opportunities for food and drink consumption. In most team games, there are no scheduled breaks, except for the half-time interval, but brief breaks in play do allow players to take drinks.

2. LIMITATIONS TO ENDURANCE PERFORMANCE

The major causes of fatigue in prolonged exercise are generally believed to be depletion of the body's limited carbohydrate store and the twin problem of dehydration and hyperthermia *(2)*. There is, however, no single clearly defined cause of fatigue in most exercise situations, and there are probably many different factors that contribute to the subjective sensation of fatigue and to the reduction in exercise capacity that occur in the

From: *Beverages in Nutrition and Health*
Edited by: T. Wilson and N. J. Temple © Humana Press Inc., Totowa, NJ

later stages of any intense exercise. The decision to slow down or to let the leaders go in a race situation is a conscious one, based on subjective assessment of the current physiologic status and the distance remaining. It would normally be possible to continue at the same speed, but not to sustain this to the end of the race. The brain, consciously or unconsciously, is, therefore, of paramount importance, and it may be that the cause of fatigue lies within the central nervous system (CNS) rather than in the periphery.

In most sports, especially team games, the outcome is determined by factors other than simple exercise capacity and there is a need to sustain skilled performance throughout the game. Most laboratory studies on the efficacy of fluid ingestion have used simple models of cycling or running at constant speed to the point of fatigue. The limitations of this approach have been recognized, and various other experimental models are now commonly used, including simulated time trial performance, multiple sprint shuttle running, and an assessment of the ability to maintain skill throughout exercise *(3,4)*.

3. AIMS OF FLUID INGESTION

Despite the definitive statement by the American College of Sports Medicine in its 1984 Position Stand on the prevention of thermal injuries in distance running that cool water is the optimum fluid for ingestion during endurance exercise *(5)*, there is a substantial body of evidence to support the suggestion that there are good reasons for consuming drinks containing added sugars, electrolytes, and flavoring ingredients. Commercially formulated sports drinks are intended to serve several purposes. These include:

    Supply of substrate
    Prevention of dehydration
    Electrolyte replacement
    Pre-exercise hydration
    Postexercise rehydration

To meet these various needs, the formulation of ingested beverages is likely to differ in some respects; in addition, because of the biological variability between individuals, no single formulation will meet the needs of all athletes in all situations. Taste preference further complicates the formulation of the ideal product. Although manipulation of the composition to suit the individual circumstances is not possible for the commercial manufacturers, understanding the issues involved will allow the consumer to make the best choice from the available options. The major components of the sports drink that can be manipulated to alter its functional properties are shown in Table 1. To some extent, these factors can be manipulated independently, although addition of increasing amounts of carbohydrate or electrolyte will generally be accompanied by an increase in osmolality, and alterations in the solute content will affect taste characteristics, mouth feel, and palatability.

4. CARBOHYDRATE CONTENT: CONCENTRATION AND TYPE

Carbohydrate ingested during exercise enters the blood glucose pool, if it is absorbed from the gastrointestinal (GI) tract. If performance is limited by the size of the body's limited endogenous liver or muscle glycogen stores, then exercise capacity should be improved when carbohydrate is consumed. Several studies show that glucose ingestion during prolonged intense exercise prevents the development of hypoglycemia by main-

Table 1
Characteristics of Carbohydrate-Electrolyte Sports Drinks

Carbohydrate type
Carbohydrate concentration
Osmolality
Electrolyte content—sodium and potassium
Anion content
pH and buffer capacity
Carbonation level
Flavoring ingredients
Vitamin content
Other ingredients (amino acids, herbal extracts, etc.)

taining or raising the circulating glucose concentration *(6–8)*. Beneficial effects of carbohydrate ingestion are seen during both cycling *(9)* and running *(10)*. As well as prolonging the time for which a fixed power output can be sustained, improvements are seen in time trial performance, in multiple sprint performance, and in the performance of skilled tasks, as well as in a reduced subjective perception of effort *(3,4)*. This ergogenic effect may be related to a sparing of the body's limited muscle glycogen stores by the oxidation of the ingested carbohydrate *(8,11)*, but other studies have failed to show a glycogen-sparing effect of carbohydrate ingested during prolonged exercise. The consensus view is probably that there is little or no sparing of muscle glycogen use, although glucose output from the liver is probably slowed as a result of the better maintenance of blood glucose concentration *(12,13)*. The primary benefit of ingested carbohydrate is probably its role in supplementing the endogenous stores in the later stages of exercise *(14)*. It is clear from tracer studies that a substantial part of the carbohydrate ingested during exercise is available for oxidation, but there is an upper limit of approx 1 g/min to the rate at which ingested carbohydrate can be oxidized, even when much larger amounts are ingested *(15)*. In hard exercise, the carbohydrate oxidation rate can reach 3–4 g/min, so the contribution from the exogenous supply is relatively small.

As well as providing an energy substrate for the working muscles, adding carbohydrate to ingested drinks promotes water absorption in the small intestine, provided the concentration is not too high. Because of the role of sugars and sodium in promoting water uptake in the small intestine, it is sometimes difficult to separate the effects of water replacement from those of substrate and electrolyte replacement when CHO-electrolyte solutions are ingested. Below et al. *(16)* have shown that ingestion of carbohydrate and water had separate and additive effects on performance capacity (Fig. 1) and concluded that dilute carbohydrate solution ingestion optimizes performance. Most reviews of the available literature have come to the same conclusion *(17–20)*.

In most of the early studies, the ingested carbohydrate was glucose, but the type of carbohydrate is not critical, and glucose, sucrose, and oligosaccharides are effective in maintaining the blood glucose concentration when ingested during prolonged exercise and in improving endurance capacity *(20)*. There are theoretical advantages in the use

- 6.5% improvement with large fluid volume
- 6.3% improvement with CHO
- Effects are additive

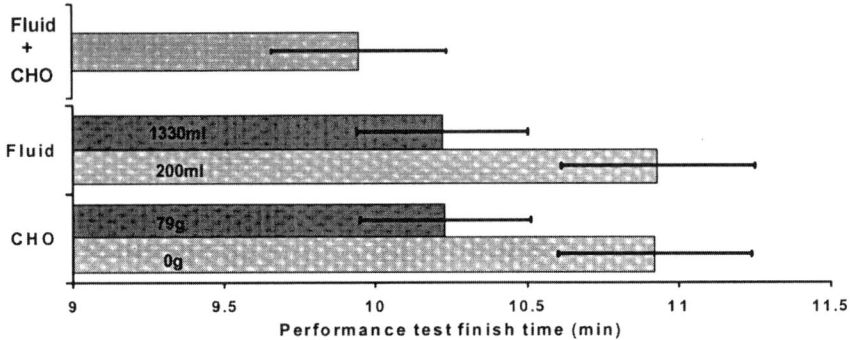

Fig. 1. Separate and additive effects of ingestion of water and carbohydrate on exercise performance. Note that a shorter time indicates a better performance. Redrawn from the data of Below et al. *(16)*.

of sugars other than glucose. Substitution of glucose polymers for glucose allow an increased carbohydrate content without an increased osmolality and may also have taste advantages, but the available evidence suggests that the use of glucose polymers or sucrose rather than free glucose does not alter the blood glucose response or the effect on exercise performance. Ingested fructose is generally less readily oxidized than glucose or glucose polymers, but mixtures of glucose and fructose in equal amounts may have some advantages. Fructose in high concentrations is generally best avoided because of the risk of GI upset. The argument advanced in favor of the ingestion of fructose during exercise, namely that it provides a readily available energy source but does not stimulate insulin release and consequent inhibition of fatty acid mobilization, is, in any case, not well founded: insulin secretion is suppressed during exercise. These studies have been reviewed by Maughan and Shirreffs *(20)*. There may be benefits in including several different carbohydrates, including free glucose, sucrose, and maltodextrin; this has taste implications that may influence the amount consumed and, by limiting the osmolality and providing numerous transportable solutes, may maximize the rate of sugar and water absorption in the small intestine *(21)*.

The optimum concentration of sugar to be added to drinks depends on individual circumstances. A high carbohydrate concentration delays gastric emptying, thus reducing the amount of fluid that is available for absorption, and also increases the rate of carbohydrate delivery. If the concentration is high enough to result in a markedly hypertonic solution, a transient net secretion of water into the intestine will result, and this will increase the danger of dehydration *(22)*. This may explain why high sugar concentrations (> 10%) can also result in GI disturbances *(23)*. Where the primary need is to supply an energy source during exercise, increasing the sugar content of drinks will increase the delivery of carbohydrate to the absorption site in the small intestine. Beyond a certain limit, however, simply increasing carbohydrate intake will not continue to increase the rate of oxidation of exogenous carbohydrate *(15)*. Dilute glucose-electro-lyte solutions may also be as effective, or even more effective, in improving perfor-mance as more concentrated solutions *(23)*, and adding as little as 90 mmol/L glucose may improve endurance performance *(24)*.

4.1. Osmolality

It has become common to refer to carbohydrate-electrolyte sports drinks as isotonic drinks, as though tonicity was their most important characteristic. The osmolality of ingested fluids is important, because this can influence the rates of both gastric emptying and intestinal water flux: both of these processes together determine the effectiveness of rehydration fluids at delivering water for rehydration. An increasing osmolality of the gastric contents delays emptying; increasing the carbohydrate or electrolyte content of sports drinks generally increases osmolality. The composition of the drinks and the nature of the solutes are, however, of greater importance than the osmolality itself *(20)*.

Although osmolality is identified as an important factor influencing the rate of gastric emptying of liquid meals, there is little effect of variations in the concentration of sodium or potassium on the emptying rate, even when this substantially changes the osmolality of the test meal *(25)*. The effect of increasing osmolality is most consistently observed when nutrient-containing solutions are examined, and the most significant factor influ-encing the rate of gastric emptying is the energy density *(26,27)*. There is some evidence that substituting glucose polymers for free glucose, which results in a decreased osmo-lality for the same carbohydrate content, may be effective in increasing the rate at which both fluid and substrate are delivered to the intestine. This has led to the inclusion of glucose polymers of varying chain length in the formulation of sports drinks. Vist and Maughan *(28)* have shown that there is an acceleration of emptying when glucose poly-mer solutions are substituted for free glucose solutions with the same energy density: at low (about 40 g/L) concentrations, this effect is small, but it becomes appreciable at higher (180 g/L) concentrations; where the osmolality is the same (as in the 40 g/L glucose solution and 180 g/L polymer solution), the energy density is of far greater significance in determining the rate of gastric emptying. This effect may, therefore, be important when large amounts of energy must be replaced after exercise but is unlikely to be a major factor during exercise when more dilute drinks are taken.

Water absorption occurs largely in the proximal segment of the small intestine, and, although water movement is itself a passive process driven by local osmotic gradients, it is closely linked to the active transport of solute. Osmolality plays a key role in the flux of water across the upper part of the small intestine. Net flux is determined largely by the osmotic gradient between the luminal contents and intracellular fluid of the cells lining the intestine. Absorption of glucose is an active energy-consuming process linked to the transport of sodium. The rate of glucose uptake is dependent on the luminal concentrations of glucose and sodium, and dilute glucose-electrolyte solutions with an osmolality that is slightly hypotonic with respect to plasma maximizes the rate of water uptake *(29)*. Solutions with a high glucose concentration do not necessarily promote an increased glucose uptake relative to more dilute solutions, but, because of their high osmolality, cause a net movement of fluid into the intestinal lumen *(30)*. This results in an effective loss of body water and exacerbates any preexisting dehydration *(22)*. Other sugars, such as sucrose or glucose polymers, can be substituted for glucose without impairing glucose or water uptake and may help by increasing the total transportable substrate without increasing osmolality. In contrast, isoenergetic solutions of fructose and glucose are isoosmotic, and the absorption of fructose is not an active process in man: it is absorbed less rapidly than glucose and promotes less water uptake *(31)*. The use of different sugars that are absorbed by different mechanisms and that might promote increased water uptake is supported by recent evidence from an intestinal perfusion study *(21)*.

Although most of the popular sports drinks are formulated to have an osmolality close to that of body fluids *(20)* and promoted as isotonic drinks, there is evidence that hypotonic solutions are more effective when rapid rehydration is desired *(29)*. It is argued that a higher osmolality is inevitable when adequate amounts of carbohydrate are to be included in sports drinks; however, the optimum amount of carbohydrate necessary to improve exercise performance has not been clearly established.

4.2. Electrolyte Composition and Concentration

The available evidence indicates that the only electrolyte that should be added to drinks consumed during exercise is sodium, which is usually added as sodium chloride *(20)*. Sodium stimulates sugar and water uptake in the small intestine and helps to maintain extracellular fluid volume. Most cola or lemonade soft drinks contain virtually no sodium (1–2 mmol/L); sports drinks commonly contain approx 10–30 mmol/L; oral rehydration solutions intended for use in the treatment of diarrhea-induced dehydration, which may be fatal, have higher sodium concentrations ranging from 30 to 90 mmol/L. Although a high sodium content may stimulate jejunal absorption of glucose and water, it makes drinks unpalatable; it is important that drinks intended for ingestion during or after exercise have a pleasant taste to stimulate consumption. Little thought is given to the choice of anion that accompanies sodium in functional beverages, but this has implications for osmolality, taste, pH levels, stability, and other factors.

When the exercise duration is likely to exceed 3–4 h, there may be advantages in adding sodium to drinks to avoid hyponatremia, which has occurred when excessively large volumes of low-sodium drinks are consumed. Physicians dealing with individuals in distress at the end of long-distance races are accustomed to dealing with hyperthermia and hypernatremia associated with dehydration, but it has become clear that a small number of individuals at the end of prolonged events may be suffering from hyponatremia in conjunction with either hyperhydration *(32,33)* or dehydration *(34)*. All reported cases have been associated with ultramarathon or prolonged triathlon events; most of the cases have occurred in events lasting more than 8 h, and there are few reports of cases when the exercise duration is fewer than 4 h. Noakes et al. *(32)* reported four cases of exercise-induced hyponatremia; race times were between 7 and 10 h, and postrace serum sodium concentrations were between 115 and 125 mmol/L. This is far below the normal range of approx 137–144 mmol/L (*see* Table 2). Estimated fluid intakes during the race were between 6 and 12 L and consisted of water or drinks containing low electrolyte levels; estimated total sodium chloride intake was 20–40 mmol. Frizell et al. *(35)* reported even more astonishing fluid intakes. Runners had an intake of 20–24 L of fluids (almost 2.5 L/h sustained for a period of many hours, which is in excess of the maximum gastric emptying rate that has been reported), with a mean sodium content of only 5–10 mmol/L in two runners who collapsed after an ultramarathon run and who were hyponatremic (serum sodium concentration: 118–123 mmol/L).

Table 2

Approximate Concentration, in mmol/L, of the Major Electrolytes
Present in Sweat, Plasma, and in Intracellular (Muscle) Water in Man[a]

	Plasma	Sweat	Intracellular
Sodium	137–144	40–80	10
Potassium	3.5–4.9	4–8	148
Calcium	4.4–5.2	3–4	0–2
Magnesium	1.5–2.1	1–4	30–40
Chloride	100–108	30–70	2

[a]The values are collated from several sources. *See* Maughan et al. *(45)* for further details.

These reports indicate that some supplementation with sodium salts may be required in extremely prolonged events where large sweat losses can be expected and where it is possible to consume large volumes of fluid. Most carbohydrate-electrolyte sports drinks intended for consumption during prolonged exercise contain a sodium concentration of approx 10–30 mmol/L, which is lower than the normal sweat sodium concentration (Table 2). Although the formulation of these drinks might represent a reasonable strategy for providing substrates and water (even though it can be argued that a higher sodium concentration would enhance water uptake and that a higher carbohydrate content would increase substrate provision), these recommendations may not be appropriate in all circumstances.

4.3. Flavoring Components

Taste is an important factor influencing the consumption of fluids. The thirst mechanism is insensitive and does not stimulate drinking behavior until some degree of dehydration has occurred *(36)*. This absence of a drive to drink is reflected in the small volumes of fluid that are typically consumed during exercise: in endurance running events, voluntary intake seldom exceeds 0.5 L/h *(37)*. Sweat losses normally exceed this, even in cool conditions, and a fluid deficit is, therefore, almost inevitable. Several factors influence palatability, and the addition of several flavors has been shown to increase fluid intake relative to that ingested when only plain water is available. Hubbard et al. *(38)* and Szlyk *(39)* found that the addition of flavorings resulted in an increased consumption (by approx 50%) of fluid during prolonged exercise. More recently, Bar-Or and Wilk *(40)* have shown that children's fluid intake during exercise presented with numerous flavored drinks is influenced by taste preference: under the conditions of this study, sufficient fluid to offset sweat losses was ingested only when a grape-flavored beverage was available. In many of these studies, added carbohydrates and/or electrolytes accompanied the flavoring agent, and the results must be interpreted with caution.

Given the need to add electrolytes to fluids intended to maximize the effectiveness of rehydration, there are clearly palatability issues that influence the formulation. Effective postexercise rehydration requires replacement of electrolyte losses as well as the ingestion of a volume of fluid in excess of the volume of sweat loss *(41)*. When sweat electrolyte losses are high, replacement with drinks with a high sodium content can result in an unpalatable product. This can be alleviated by substituting other anions for the chloride that is normally added. The addition of carbohydrate has a major effect on taste and mouth feel, and several different sugars with different taste characteristics can be added.

4.4. Other Active Ingredients

There is a trend for the formulation of sports drinks to be modified to include other components that might affect the functional characteristics of the drink. Many of the drinks aimed at the active individual include a range of vitamins and minerals, but it is agreed that these are not generally necessary. There is also little convincing evidence for beneficial effects of the addition of purported ergogenic compounds, such as taurine, ginseng, or aspartate *(42)*. There is more experimental evidence to support the use of caffeine *(43)*, and some evidence that glutamine supplementation may benefit athletes during intensive training periods *(44)*, but these compounds are not, at present, included in any of the commercially available products.

5. PROMOTING POSTEXERCISE RECOVERY

An effective strategy to promote recovery from exercise is vital for all athletes. The nature of the recovery process depends on the nature of the sport, the training and nutritional status of the athlete, the time in the training/competition cycle, and the time available before the next exercise bout. In some sports, where competition is infrequent and highly demanding, recovery relates to recovery between training sessions, which may be carried out two or even more times/day for prolonged periods. Good examples of such sports are marathon running and professional boxing. In other sports, such as professional basketball or baseball, or in professional road cycling, the greater part of the competition season, which lasts for several months, is occupied with almost daily competition, and recovery means preparing for the next day's competition.

Key issues in the recovery process for the athlete in training are:

Restorting fluid and electrolyte balance
Replenishing fuel stores
Stimulating the synthetic and catabolic pathways involved in the process of adaptation
Avoiding illness, infection, and injury
Psychological recovery

When recovery is discussed, the focus is normally on the first two of these processes, but the third and fourth are vital if performance capacity is to be enhanced in response to the training regimen and if overload and injury are to be avoided. Remodeling the tissues is a vital part of the adaptation to training. For the strength and power athlete, this means increasing the actin and myosin content of muscle to increase its force generating capacity. For the endurance athlete, the aim of training is to increase the muscle's content of mitochondrial enzymes, to promote the growth of new capillaries, and to activate other local changes that increase the capacity for aerobic metabolism. Overtraining, illness, and chronic fatigue have been identified as problems for some athletes, and there may be nutritional strategies to reduce the risks that inevitably accompany the sustained intensive training that is necessary to optimize performance. Psychological recovery in preparation for the next training session is also crucial if an intensive training program is to be sustained. Numerous other homeostatic mechanisms may also be involved, including restoration of acid-base status and restoration of thermal balance.

5.1. Restoring Fluid and Electrolyte Balance

In most sports, the physical effort involved leads to a rise in body temperature with a stimulation of sweating to maintain thermal balance. The extent of fluid and electrolyte losses during exercise depend on the volume of sweat lost and on the composition of the sweat. This, in turn, depends on the size and surface area of the individual, the intensity and duration of the exercise, the training and acclimation status of the individual, and the environmental conditions. Sweat losses also vary between individuals, making predictions of loss and, therefore, of the need for replacement difficult. Typical values for sweating rate range between 500 mL and 3 L/h, with the main electrolytes lost comprising sodium (20–80 mmol/L), chloride (20–60 mmol/L), and potassium (4–8 mmol/L). Formulating general guidelines for replacement strategies is, therefore, almost impossible, and individualization of rehydration strategies is essential *(20)*.

The important aspects of volume replenishment are the ingestion of an adequate quantity of fluid and replacement of electrolyte losses. The need for ingestion of fluid is obvious, and it is common to recommend that athletes drink 1 L of fluid for each kilogram of mass lost during training. It is now known, however, that the volume of fluid consumed must exceed that lost in sweat—perhaps by as much as 50%—if effective rehydration is to be achieved *(41)*. This stems from the need to allow for ongoing urine and other losses during the recovery period. Restoration of euhydration (a state of fluid balance) after exercise-induced sweat losses will not be achieved without replacement of the electrolytes lost in sweat *(45)*.

These electrolytes (especially sodium) prevent the drop in plasma sodium concentration and plasma osmolality that would occur with the ingestion of large volumes of plain water. If plasma osmolality and sodium concentration fall, a diuresis is initiated, leading to the prompt loss of a significant fraction of the ingested fluid *(46)*. The thirst mechanism is also inhibited by these changes, leading to the termination of drinking before a volume sufficient to meet the body's needs has been ingested *(47)*.

The addition of salt to drinks can prevent these changes in plasma composition, thereby reducing the urinary loss and maintaining the drive to drink. If food is eaten together with water, the electrolytes present in the food eaten may achieve this, but there are many situations, especially when the recovery time is short, when athletes may not be willing or able to tolerate solid food or when the amount and type of food eaten may not supply an adequate amount of sodium *(48)*. In this situation, the drinks consumed during the recovery period must provide sufficient electrolytes to replace the sweat losses. Because the electrolyte concentration of sweat varies so greatly between individuals, it is not possible to produce general recommendations that will meet the needs of all athletes in all situations. Nonetheless, the average sweat sodium concentration is approx 50 mmol/L, and this amount of sodium must be replaced to maintain volume homeostasis *(49)*. The ingestion of salt tablets is seldom necessary but may be contemplated when sweat losses are exceptionally high or if the food intake is limited.

5.2. Muscle Glycogen Resynthesis

Carbohydrate is the major fuel used by the muscles during high-intensity exercise, but the body's carbohydrate stores are small. The liver glycogen store amounts to only approx 80–100 g, and the total muscle glycogen content is only approx 300–500 g. This is sufficient to allow approx 1–3 h of continuous exercise at moderately high intensity exercise, but brief high-intensity sprints will cause rapid depletion of muscle glycogen. This must be replaced in the recovery period after training, and replenishment of the glycogen stores should be essentially complete between training sessions if an intensive training program is to be sustained *(50)*.

Several factors determine the extent and time of the replenishment of the glycogen stores after training. The body has a limited capacity for the conversion of noncarbohydrate substrates to glucose, the precursor of glycogen. The key factor in glycogen resynthesis is, therefore, the amount of carbohydrate supplied by the diet: other factors include the timing of carbohydrate intake, the type of carbohydrate ingested, and the type and amount of other macronutrients present in the food consumed. Of these, the amount of carbohydrate consumed is the most important single factor *(51)*.

For the athlete who is training at least once and perhaps 2 or 3 times/day and who also has to work or study, practical difficulties arise in meeting the demand for energy and carbohydrate. Most athletes find it difficult to train hard for some time after food intake, and the appetite is also suppressed for a time after hard exercise. In this situation, it is particularly important to focus on ensuring a rapid recovery of the glycogen stores between training sessions. This is best achieved when carbohydrate is consumed as soon as possible after training, because the rate of glycogen synthesis is most rapid at that time *(51)*. At least 50–100 g (1–2 g/kg body weight) should be consumed in the first hour, and a high carbohydrate intake continued thereafter. There is clearly a maximum rate at which muscle glycogen resynthesis can occur, and there is no benefit in increasing the carbohydrate intake to levels in excess of 100 g every 2 h *(50)*.

The type of carbohydrate is less crucial than the amount consumed, but there may be some benefit from ingesting foods with a high glycemic index at this time to ensure a rapid elevation of the blood glucose level. There is some limited evidence to suggest that foods with a high glycemic index (i.e., those that produce a substantial elevation of the blood glucose concentration) promote a more rapid synthesis of glycogen in the postexercise period. The addition of small amounts of protein to carbohydrate ingested at this time can also increase the rate of glycogen synthesis above that observed after ingestion of carbohydrate alone *(52)*. This effect has been attributed to an enhanced insulin secretion, but further experimental data are needed to confirm this.

5.3. Protein Synthesis and Tissue Remodeling

It is clear that a prolonged period of training causes substantial changes in the structural and functional characteristics of skeletal muscle and other tissues. Although major changes are not apparent in response to single exercise bouts, these changes must occur between training sessions. There is evidence of adaptive changes in muscle structure and function occurring in response to only a few exercise sessions *(53)*. These changes are different from those that are commonly observed after a single exercise bout, when the observed responses are largely catabolic in nature and manifest themselves as muscle damage and soreness *(54)*. Nonetheless, there must be adaptive changes involving synthesis of new proteins in response to each training stimulus. It is likely that the methods currently available are inadequate to measure these changes with any degree of reliability.

In the recovery period, muscle glycogen synthesis is a priority, but synthesis of new proteins should, perhaps, be viewed as being of equal or even greater importance. Because

ance time. Despite these rather unpromising findings, at least one sports drink containing BCAA is currently on sale.

8. PROMOTING HYPERHYDRATION

It has been suggested that if dehydration is one of the major factors contributing to fatigue in prolonged exercise, then increasing body water content before exercise should, by analogy with glycogen loading, improve performance. Drinking large volumes of plain water provokes a diuretic response, but some degree of temporary hyperhydration results when drinks with high (100 mmol/L) sodium concentrations are ingested. An alternative strategy that has been attempted with the aim of inducing an expansion of the blood volume before exercise is to add glycerol to ingested fluids. Glycerol exerts an osmotic action; although its distribution in the body water compartments is variable, glycerol expands the extracellular space and some of the water ingested with the glycerol is retained (75,76). The elevated osmolality of the extracellular space, however, results in some degree of intracellular dehydration, the implications of which are unknown. It might be expected, however, that the raised plasma osmolality will have negative consequences for thermoregulatory capacity. The evidence for improved thermoregulatory function and exercise performance after administration of glycerol and water before prolonged exercise is not entirely convincing at this stage (77,78).

9. FUTURE DEVELOPMENTS

It is unlikely that there will be major changes to the basic formulation of the mainstream sports drinks in the foreseeable future. These are based on a solid foundation of research that shows beneficial effects of ingestion of carbohydrates and water during exercise situations. There has been a move in the clinical oral rehydration field toward the use of hypotonic rather than isotonic drinks, but it is not clear that this will be adopted by the sports drink manufacturers, because they favor isotonic formulations. There are benefits of an increased sodium level for postexercise rehydration, but this may not have any benefit during exercise for most athletes. A separate postexercise drink may be attractive, and there may be scope for the addition of protein (or protein hydrolysates) to such a drink to promote protein synthesis after training. Many drinks currently contain a range of other ingredients, and it is easy to make claims for these that are attractive to the consumer. It is likely that the mainstream sports drinks, with a simple and well-proven sugar, salt, and water combination, will continue to dominate the sports drinks market.

10. MAIN POINTS FOR PRIMARY AND CLINICAL REVIEW

1. Water is the cheapest and most accessible beverage for optimizing physical performance.
2. Isotonic sports beverages containing electrolyte minerals, some carbohydrates, and flavoring may improve water reabsorption from the gut, energy supply, and the desire to drink during performance.
3. Sports beverages may help delay fatigue and prevent overtraining.
4. Sports beverages may also help with postexercise recovery of electrolytes and glycogen synthesis.
5. Although the tastes may change, the basic pattern of electrolytes and sugars present in current sports beverages is unlikely to change dramatically in the future.

REFERENCES

1. Pilegaard H, Keller C, Steensberg A, Helge JW, Pedersen BK, Saltin B, Neufer PD. Influence of pre-exercise muscle glycogen content on exercise-induced transcriptional regulation of metabolic genes. J Physiol 2002;541:261–271.
2. Maughan RJ, Leiper JB, Shirreffs SM. Fluids and electrolytes during exercise. In: Textbook of Sports Medicine. Garrett WE (ed.). Williams and Wilkins, Baltimore, MD, 2000, pp. 413–424.
3. Nicholas CW, Williams C, Lakomy HKA, Phillips G, Nowitz A. Influence of ingesting a carbohydrate-electrolyte solution on endurance capacity during intermittent high-intensity shuttle running. J Sports Sci 1995;13:283–290.
4. Welsh RS, Davis JM, Burke JR, Williams HG. Carbohydrates and physical/mental performance during intermittent exercise to fatigue. Med Sci Sports Exercise 2002;34:723–731.
5. American College of Sports Medicine. Position stand on prevention of thermal injuries during distance running. Med Sci Sports Exercise 1984;16:ix–xiv.
6. Costill DL, Bennett A, Branam G, Eddy D. Glucose ingestion at rest and during prolonged exercise. J Appl Physiol 1973;34:764–769.
7. Pirnay F, Crielaard JM, Pallikarakis N, et al. Fate of exogenous glucose during exercise of different intensities in humans. J Appl Physiol 1982;52:1620–1624.
8. Erickson MA, Schwartzkopf RJ, McKenzie RD. Effects of caffeine, fructose, and glucose ingestion on muscle glycogen utilisation during exercise. Med Sci Sports Exercise 1987;19:579–583.
9. Coggan AR, Coyle EF. Carbohydrate ingestion during prolonged exercise: effects on metabolism and performance. Exercise Sport Sci Rev 1991;19:1–40.
10. Tsintzsas OK, Liu R, Williams C, Campbell I, Gaitanos G. The effect of carbohydrate ingestion on performance during a 30-km race. Int J Sport Nutr 1993;3:127–139.
11. Hargreaves M, Costill DL, Coggan A, Fink WJ, Nishibata I. Effect of carbohydrate feedings on muscle glycogen utilisation and exercise performance. Med Sci Sports Exercise 1984;16:219–222.
12. Bosch AN, Dennis SC, Noakes TD. Influence of carbohydrate ingestion on fuel substrate turnover and oxidation during prolonged exercise. J Appl Physiol 1994;76:2364–2372
13. McConnell G, Fabris S, Proietto J, Hargreaves M. Effect of carbohydrate ingestion on glucose kinetics during exercise. J Appl Physiol 1994;77:1537–1541.
14. Coyle EF. Fuels for sport performance. In: Perspectives in Exercise Science and Sports Medicine. Vol. 10: Optimising Sport Performance. Lamb DR, Murray R (eds.). Benchmark Press, Carmel, IN, 1997, pp. 95–138.
15. Wagenmakers AJM, Brouns F, Saris WH, Halliday D. Oxidation rates of orally ingested carbohydrates during prolonged exercise in men. J Appl Physiol 1993;75:2774–2780.
16. Below P, Mora-Rodriguez R, Gonzalez-Alonso J, Coyle EF. Fluid and carbohydrate ingestion independently improve performance during 1 h of intense cycling. Med Sci Sports Exercise 1995;27:200–210.
17. Lamb DR, Brodowicz GR. Optimal use of fluids of varying formulations to minimize exercise-induced disturbances in homeostasis. Sports Med 1986;3:247–274.
18. Murray R. The effects of consuming carbohydrate-electrolyte beverages on gastric emptying and fluid absorption during and following exercise. Sports Med 1987;4:322–351.
19. Coyle EF, Hamilton M. Fluid replacement during exercise: effects on physiological homeostasis and performance. In: Perspectives in Exercise Science and Sports Medicine, Vol 3. Gisolfi, CV, Lamb DR (eds.). Benchmark Press, Carmel, IN, 1990, pp. 281–308.
20. Maughan RJ, Shirreffs SM. Fluid and electrolyte loss and replacement in exercise. In: Oxford Textbook of Sports Medicine (2nd ed.). Harries M, Williams C, Stanish WD, Micheli LL (eds.). Oxford University Press, New York, NY, 1998, pp. 97–113.
21. Shi X, Summers RW, Schedl HP. Effect of carbohydrate type and concentration and solution osmolality on water absorption. J Appl Physiol 1995;27:1607–1615.
22. Merson SJ, Shirreffs SM, Leiper JB, Maughan RJ. Changes in blood, plasma and red cell volume after ingestion of hypotonic and hypertonic solutions. Proc Nutr Soc, in press.
23. Davis JM, Burgess WA, Slentz CA, Bartoli WP, Pate RR. Effects of ingesting 6% and 12% glucose/electrolyte beverages during prolonged intermittent cycling in the heat. Eur J Appl Physiol 1988;57:563–569.

24. Maughan RJ, Bethell L, Leiper JB. Effects of ingested fluids on homeostasis and exercise performance in man. Exp Physiol 1996;81:847–859.
25. Rehrer NJ. Limits to Fluid Availability during Exercise. De Vriesebosch, Haarlem, Holland, 1990.
26. Brener W, Hendrix TR, McHugh PR. Regulation of the gastric emptying of glucose. Gastroenterology 1983;85:76–82.
27. Vist GE, Maughan RJ. The effect of increasing glucose concentration on the rate of gastric emptying in man. Med Sci Sports Exercise 1994;26:1269–1273.
28. Vist GE, Maughan RJ. The effect of osmolality and carbohydrate content on the rate of gastric emptying of liquids in man. J Physiol 1995;486:523–531.
29. Wapnir RA, Lifshitz F. Osmolality and solute concentration—their relationship with oral rehydration solution effectiveness: an experimental assessment. Pediatr Res 1985;19:894–898.
30. Gisolfi CV, Summers RW, Schedl HP. Intestinal absorption of fluids during rest and exercise. In: Perspectives in Exercise Science and Sports Medicine. Vol. 3: Fluid Homeostasis during Exercise. Gisolfi CV, Lamb DR (eds.). Benchmark Press, Carmel, IN, 1990, pp. 129–180.
31. Fordtran JS. Stimulation of active and passive sodium absorption by sugars in the human jejunum. J Clin Invest 1975;55:728–737.
32. Noakes TD, Goodwin N, Rayner BL, Branken T, Taylor RKN. Water intoxication: a possible complication during endurance exercise. Med Sci Sports Exercise 1985;17:370–375.
33. Noakes TD, Norman RJ, Buck RH, Godlonton J, Stevenson K, Pittaway D. The incidence of hyponatremia during prolonged ultraendurance exercise. Med Sci Sports Exercise 1990;22:165–170.
34. Hiller WDB. Dehydration and hyponatraemia during triathlons. Med Sci Sports Exercise 1989;21: S219–S221.
35. Frizell RT, Lang GH, Lowance DC, Lathan SR. Hyponatraemia and ultramarathon running. JAMA 1986;255:772–774.
36. Hubbard RW, Sandick BL, Matthew WT, et al. Influence of thirst and fluid palatability on fluid ingestion during exercise. In: Perspectives in Exercise Science and Sports Medicine. Vol. 3. Gisolfi CV, Lamb DR (eds.). Benchmark Press, Carmel, IN, 1990, pp. 39–95.
37. Noakes TD. Fluid replacement during exercise. Exercise Sports Sci Rev 1993;21:297–330.
38. Hubbard RW, Sandick BL, Matthew WT. Voluntary dehydration and alliesthesia for water. J Appl Physiol 1984;57:868–875.
39. Szlyk PC, Sils IV, Francesconi RP, Hubbard RW, Armstrong LE. Effects of water temperature and flavoring on voluntary dehydration in men. Physiol Behav 1989;45:639–647.
40. Bar-Or O, Wilk B. Water and electrolyte replenishment in the exercising child. Int J Sports Nutr 1996; 6:93–99.
41. Shirreffs SM, Taylor AJ, Leiper JB, Maughan RJ. Post-exercise rehydration in man: effects of volume consumed and sodium content of ingested fluids. Med Sci Sports Exercise 1996;28:1260–1271.
42. Williams MH. Nutritional Aspects of Human Physical and Athletic Performance. Charles C. Thomas, Springfield, IL, 1985.
43. Spriet LL. Ergogenic aids: recent advances and retreats. In: Perspectives in Exercise Science and Sports Medicine. Vol. 10: Optimising Sport Performance. Lamb DR, Murray R (eds.). Benchmark Press, Carmel, IN, 1997, pp. 185–238.
44. Newsholme EA, Castell LM. Can amino acids influence exercise performance in athletes? In: The Physiology and Pathophysiology of Exercise Tolerance. Steinacker JM, Ward SA (eds.). Plenum, New York, NY, 1996, pp. 269–274.
45. Maughan RJ, Owen JH, Shirreffs SM, Leiper JB. Post-exercise rehydration in man: effects of electrolyte addition to ingested fluids. Eur J Appl Physiol 1994;69:209–215.
46. Maughan RJ, Leiper JB. Effects of sodium content of ingested fluids on post-exercise rehydration in man. Eur J Appl Physiol 1995;71:311–319.
47. Nose H, Mack GW, Shi X, Nadel ER. Role of osmolality and plasma volume during rehydration in humans. J Appl Physiol 1988;65:325–331.
48. Maughan RJ, Leiper JB, Shirreffs SM. Restoration of fluid balance after exercise-induced dehydration: effects of food and fluid intake. Eur J Appl Physiol 1996;73:317–325.
49. Shirreffs SM, Maughan RJ. Volume repletion following exercise-induced volume depletion in man: replacement of water and sodium losses. Am J Physiol 1998;43:F868–F875.

50. Coyle EF. Timing and method of increased carbohydrate intake to cope with heavy training, competition and recovery. J Sports Sci 1991;9:29–52.

51. Ivy JL, Katz AL, Cutler CL, Coyle EF. Muscle glycogen synthesis after exercise: effects of time of carbohydrate ingestion. J Appl Physiol 1988;64:1480–1485.

52. Zawadzki KM, Yaspelkis BB, Ivy JL. Carbohydrate-protein complex increases the rate of muscle glycogen storage after exercise. J Appl Physiol 1992;72:1854–1859.

53. Green HJ, Jones S, Ball-Burnett ME, Smith D, Livesey J, Farrance BW. Early muscular and metabolic adaptations to prolonged exercise training in man. J Appl Physiol 1991;70:2032–2038.

54. Clarkson PM. Eccentric exercise and muscle damage. Int J Sports Med 1997;18: S314–S317.

55. Waldegger S, Lang F. Cell volume and gene expression. J Membr Biol 1997;162:95–100.

56. Lang F, Busch GL, Volkl K. The diversity of volume regulatory mechanisms. Cell Physiol Biochem 1998;8:1–45.

57. Low SY, Rennie MJ, Taylor PM. Modulation of glycogen synthesis in rate skeletal muscle by changes in cell volume. J Physiol 1996;495:299–303.

58. Low SY, Rennie MJ, Taylor PM. Signalling elements involved in amino acid transport responses to altered muscle cell volume. FASEB J 1997;11:1111–1117.

59. Rennie MJ, Low SY, Taylor PM, Khogali SE, Yao PC, Ahmed A. Amino acid transport during muscle contraction and its relevance to exercise. Adv Exp Med Biol 1998;441:299–305.

60. Nieman DC. Prolonged aerobic exercise, immune response, and risk of infection. In: Exercise and Immune Function. Hoffman-Goetz L (ed.). CRC Press, Boca Raton, FL, 1996, pp. 143–162.

61. Budgett R. Fatigue and underperformance in athletes: the overtraining syndrome. In: Benefits and Hazards of Exercise. MacAuley D (ed.) BMJ Books, London, UK, 1999, 172–183.

62. Walsh NP, Blannin AK, Robson PJ, Gleeson M. Glutamine, exercise and immune function. Sports Med 1998;26:177–191.

63. Pedersen BK, Bruunsgaard H, Jensen M, Toft AD, Hansen H, Ostrowski K. Exercise and the immune system—influence of nutrition and ageing. J Sci Med Sport 1999;2:234–252.

64. Nieman DC, Pedersen BK. Exercise and immune function. Sports Med 1999;27:73–80.

65. Packer L. Oxidants, antioxidant nutrients and the athlete. J Sports Sci 1997;15:353–363.

66. Levine SA, Gordon B, Derick CL. Some changes in the chemical constituents of the blood following a marathon race. JAMA 1924;82:1778–1779.

67. Newsholme EA, Castell LM. Amino acids, fatigue and immunodepression in exercise. In: Nutrition in Sport. Maughan RJ (ed.). Blackwell, Oxford, UK, 2000, pp. 153–170.

68. Davis JM. Nutritional influences on central mechanisms of fatigue involving serotonin. In: Biochemistry of Exercise IX. Maughan RJ, Shirreffs SM (eds.). Human Kinetics, Champaign, IL, 1996, pp. 445–455.

69. Wilson WM, Maughan RJ. A role for serotonin in the genesis of fatigue in man: administration of a 5-hydroxytryptamine reuptake inhibitor (Paroxetine) reduces the capacity to perform prolonged exercise. Exp Physiol 1992;77:921–924.

70. Blomstrand E, Hassmen P, Ekblom B, Newsholme EA. Administration of branched-chain amino acids during endurance exercise—effects on performance and on plasma concentration of some amino acids. Eur J Appl Physiol 1991;63:83–88.

71. van Hall G, Raaymakers JSH, Saris WHM, Wagenmakers AJM. Ingestion of branched-chain amino acids and tryptophan during sustained exercise—failure to affect performance. J Physiol 1995;486: 789–794.

72. Varnier M, Sarto P, Martines D, et al. Effect of infusing branched-chain amino acids during incremental exercise with reduced muscle glycogen content. Eur J Appl Physiol 1994;69:26–31.

73. Verger PH, Aymard P, Cynobert L, Anton G, Luigi R. Effects of administration of branched-chain amino acids vs. glucose during acute exercise in the rat. Physiol Behav 1994;55:523–526.

74. Mittleman KD, Ricci MR, Bailey SP. Branched-chain amino acids prolong exercise during heat stress in men and women. Med Sci Sports Exercise 1998;30:83–91.

75. Riedesel ML, Allen DL, Peake GT, Al-Qattan K. Hyperhydration with glycerol solutions. J Appl Physiol 1987;63:2262–2268.

76. Freund BJ, Montain SJ, Young AJ, et al. Glycerol hyperhydration: hormonal, renal and vascular fluid responses. J Appl Physiol 1995;79:2069–2077.

77. Montner P, Stark DM, Riedesel ML, et al. Pre-exercise glycerol hydration improves cycling endurance time. Int J Sports Med 1996;17:27–33.
78. Lyons T, Riedesel ML, Meuli LE, Chick RW. Effects of glycerol-induced hyperhydration prior to exercise in the heat on sweating and core temperature. Med Sci Sports Exercise 1990;22:477–483.

21 Improving the Effectiveness of Oral Rehydration Therapies

B. S. Ramakrishna

1. INTRODUCTION

Dehydration, or the loss of fluid and salt from the body, can be an uncomfortable and sometimes life-threatening disorder. In the healthy individual, dehydration may occur as a result of vigorous exercise, after exposure to extreme degrees of heat, or in industrial workers working in warm to hot ambient temperatures with protective clothing. The degree of dehydration determines the occurrence of symptoms and complications. Low levels of dehydration (2% loss of body weight or more) impair cardiovascular and thermoregulatory responses and reduce the capacity for further work or exercise *(1)*. Dehydration may also occur as a result of illness characterized by excessive loss of fluid from the body, such as in diarrhea or in diseases that lead to excessive vomiting or excessive loss of water in the urine. In these conditions, water loss may sometimes exceed 10% of body weight, and the disturbance of homeostasis may become life-threatening. Indeed, dehydration from diarrhea is a significant cause of morbidity and mortality in children in developing countries. Rehydration refers to the replacement of fluid and electrolytes to correct dehydration. In severe dehydration, particularly when there is ongoing fluid loss, as in diarrhea, rehydration must be achieved intravenously. In less severe dehydration (and in the absence of significant vomiting), the gastrointestinal (GI) tract has the capacity to absorb fluid rapidly and can be the route of rehydration. This chapter focuses exclusively on oral rehydration and briefly examines recent progress in the understanding of the mechanisms underlying intestinal absorption of fluid and electrolytes and how this understanding affects the design of beverages intended for oral rehydration. This chapter also distinguishes between oral rehydration solution (ORS), which was originally introduced for the treatment of dehydration in diarrhea, and other fluids (oral rehydration fluids, ORF) that do not meet the recommended formulation for ORS but can nevertheless be used to maintain hydration in selected situations. Such a distinction has been recommended by a Working Party of the World Congress of Gastroenterology 2002 *(2)*.

From: *Beverages in Nutrition and Health*
Edited by: T. Wilson and N. J. Temple © Humana Press Inc., Totowa, NJ

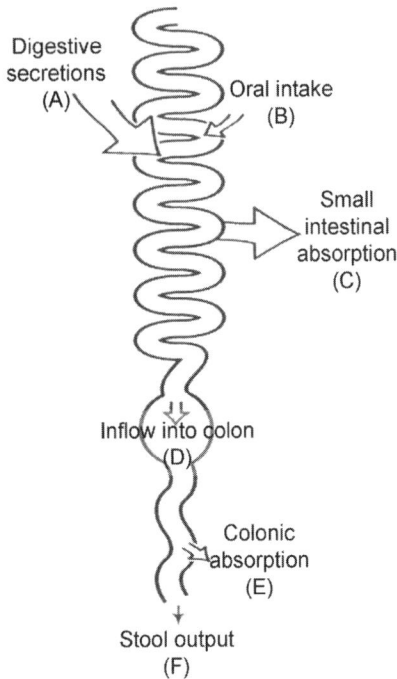

	Healthy adult	Maximal absorptive capacity	Severe cholera
A	7000		12000
B	2000		12000
C	7500	12000-22000	12000
D	1500		12000
E	1300	6000	1000
F	200		11000

Digestive secretions (A)

Oral intake (B)

Small intestinal absorption (C)

Inflow into colon (D)

Colonic absorption (E)

Stool output (F)

Fig. 1. Gastrointestinal handling of fluid handling in health and in diarrhea. Fluid fluxes (in mL) are representative figures calculated from various studies. In health, small intestinal loads derive from both ingested fluid and digestive secretions, whereas small intestinal and colonic absorption contribute to fluid salvage. The maximal absorptive capacity of the small intestine and of the colon is also shown. Severe cholera has been used as an extreme example of the remarkable derangements possible in some patients with diarrhea. Ingestion of large quantities of oral rehydration solution (ORS) is encouraged in the absence of vomiting to compensate for fluid secreted into the intestine. Although small intestinal absorption increases above basal levels, active (chloride and fluid) secretion continues alongside and large amounts of fluid enter the colon, where absorptive capacity is typically impaired. Increasing colonic absorptive capacity (using short-chain fatty acid precursors) can potentially increase colonic absorption and reduce fecal fluid loss in cholera.

2. PHYSIOLOGICAL BASIS FOR ABSORPTION OF ELECTROLYTES AND WATER FROM THE INTESTINE

Water absorption from the intestine and colon is entirely passive and linked to the active absorption of ions (e.g., sodium) or nutrients (e.g., glucose and amino acids). Active absorption implies the expenditure of energy for absorption and can occur against concentration or electrochemical gradients. Sodium is the major ion that is actively absorbed by the epithelial cells lining the intestine and colon, and its absorption is a significant driving force for water absorption. Chloride, another major ion in the diet, is either actively absorbed by epithelial cells coupled to sodium or absorbed passively through the paracellular pathway, depending on the segment of intestine that is under consideration.

Table 1
Pathways for Active Absorption in Different Levels of the Intestine

Segment of intestine	Absorptive pathway	Effect of aldosterone	Effect of cAMP and other secretagogues
Jejunum	Na-H exchange	Inhibited	Inhibited
	Glucose-Na cotransport	—	—
	Aminoacid-Na cotransport	—	—
Ileum	Coupled NaCl absorption	Inhibited	Inhibited
	Na channels	Enhanced absorption	—
	Glucose-Na cotransport	—	—
	Amino acid-Na cotransport	—	—
Proximal colon	Coupled NaCl absorption	Inhibited	Inhibited
	SCFA-linked NaCl absorption	—	—
Distal colon	Na channels	Enhanced absorption	—
	SCFA-linked NaCl absorption	—	—

Na-H exchange signifies sodium-hydrogen exchange; SCFA-linked NaCl absorption indicates elecroneutral sodium chloride absorption linked to short-chain fatty acids; — indicates that no effect on this process is known.

Different absorptive pathways predominate in different segments of the intestine, as shown in Table 1. The upper small intestine is responsible for absorption of glucose and other nutrients, after digestion within its lumen. Water absorption in the upper small intestine follows the absorption of nutrients, particularly glucose and amino acids. Perfusion studies of human jejunum have demonstrated that net sodium absorption ceased when luminal sodium concentration fell below 133 mmol/L *(3)*. The intercellular junctions between epithelial cells in the jejunum are permeable or "leaky" and allow the rapid movement of fluid either into or out of the intestinal lumen, depending on the balance between osmotic forces in the lumen of the intestine and the blood. Thus, if a meal or beverage with high sugar content (i.e., high osmotic load) is ingested, fluid quickly rushes into the lumen of the jejunum. On the other hand, rapid absorption of water occurs if the beverage is of lower osmolarity than plasma. In the ileum, different processes for sodium absorption predominate, and the junctions between the epithelial cells lining the intestine are less leaky, causing greater dependence of water absorption on sodium absorption. Sodium absorption is more avid and can occur even from a solution with a sodium concentration of 35 mmol/L *(3)*.

In the colon, the epithelial cells have a great capacity to absorb sodium. In addition, the intercellular junctions between epithelial cells in the colon are tight. These two attributes confer on the colon the ability to dehydrate the luminal contents. Perfusion studies have demonstrated sodium absorption from the colon, even when the concentration of sodium in the luminal solution is as low as 25 mmol/L *(4)*. Measurement of ileocecal flow in healthy adults, using slow marker perfusion, suggests that the normal colon absorbs approx 1500 mL water, 190 mmol sodium, and 95 mmol chloride daily *(5)*.

The colon's ability to absorb sodium and water is physiologically significant. Subjects who have had their entire colon removed are well adapted under normal circumstances but may become dehydrated when exposed to heat or a low-sodium diet or during diarrhea. In chronic dehydration, aldosterone secretion increases and the renin-angiotensin system is activated. The colon responds to both of these hormones by increasing sodium absorption via sodium channels *(6,7)* and coupled NaCl absorption *(8)*, respectively, allowing it to further conserve sodium and fluid in the adaptation of the body to dehydration.

One must recognize that the mechanisms responsible for sodium and water absorption in the healthy intestine may be altered in the presence of intestinal disease. In the healthy intestine, the normal sodium absorptive pathways remain intact and can be used for fluid absorption and for rehydration. On the other hand, sodium-hydrogen exchange and coupled NaCl absorption, which are the transport mechanisms responsible for the bulk of sodium absorption in health, are inhibited in diarrhea resulting from the cellular effects of the second messengers that mediate diarrhea (Table 1). Glucose-linked or amino acid-linked sodium absorption in the intestine is not inhibited in diarrhea, and this is the rationale for the use of oral rehydration solutions *(9)*. By administering sodium and other salts along with glucose, it is possible to stimulate sodium and water absorption from the intestine, even though fluid secretion (which is secondary to active chloride secretion) into the lumen of the intestine continues alongside. The composition of the rehydration fluid, therefore, depends, to a large extent, on the purpose for which it is intended, the specific absorptive pathway that is targeted, and the accompanying disturbances in homeostasis that it is designed to correct.

3. CONSIDERATIONS IN DESIGN OF REHYDRATION SOLUTIONS FOR USE WITH NORMAL INTESTINE

Dehydration may occur with excessive sweating and skin losses. Intense exercise can cause the loss of 1–3 L of fluid/h *(10)* and may be aggravated by warm climates. The fluid deficit typically ranges from 2–4% of body weight. At this level of dehydration, body fluid replacement can be achieved efficiently by oral rehydration, and intravenous (iv) rehydration is unnecessary. Ingested liquids are generally rapidly emptied from the stomach to reach the duodenum and jejunum, where maximum absorption is intended to take place. Studies in horses indicated that more than 90% of a single dose of 8 L fluid instilled into the stomach was emptied within 15 min *(11)*. However, in studies in exercising volunteers, ingestion of beverage of approx 23 mL/kg was accompanied by a gastric emptying rate of 13 mL/min, indicating that it would take nearly 2 h for the stomach to empty the ingested beverage *(12)*. The volume and nutrient content of the beverage ingested, but not its osmolarity, determine the rate of gastric emptying and must be considered in the design of oral rehydration beverages *(13)*. In the duodenum, water quickly moves into or out of the bloodstream, so that the osmolality within the lumen approaches 280–290 mOsm/kg by the time the contents enter the jejunum *(12,14)*. Bulk flow of water is, thus, a major consideration here, whereas the active sodium absorption mechanisms shown in Table 1 contribute to fluid absorption in the longer term. Although carbohydrate inclusion in the beverage provides substrate for oxidation and energy needs, the sugar concentration that is included is critical to ensuring efficient absorption. For instance, a 2% carbohydrate electrolyte drink was more efficient in replacing plasma volume and increasing physical performance than a 15% carbohydrate electrolyte drink *(15)*. Monosaccharides and disaccharides impose a high osmotic load, which likely interferes with fluid absorption from the duodenum and jejunum. Complex carbohydrates (e.g., glucose polymers) can, in theory, be advantageously used in this situation, because they are rapidly hydrolyzed in the jejunum to provide glucose for sodium and water absorption, without increasing luminal osmolarity *(16)*. The sweat and urinary losses during vigorous exercise have been calculated at approx 1800 mL water, 80 mmol sodium, and 33 mmol potassium per hour *(17)*. Some studies indicate that ingestion of water alone expands the plasma volume to the same extent as solutions containing electrolytes or carbohydrate and electrolytes but that the effect of water ingestion is comparatively ill sustained *(17)*. Animal studies suggest that isotonic plasma-like solution is more effective in restoring plasma volume than an equivalent amount of water *(18)*.

Debate regarding the composition of rehydration solutions designed for use during exercise relates to the carbohydrate and electrolyte composition. The current evidence regarding these parameters is summarized as follows. Sodium content and osmolarity of rehydration beverages does not significantly affect intestinal absorption of water or plasma volume changes during exercise *(12)*, but carbohydrate-containing solutions provided better hydration than plain water *(19)*. Sodium concentrations ranging from 25 to 50 mmol/L are adequate to provide hydration and restoration of cardiovascular function for rehydration after exercise *(20)*. Increasing the sodium content leads to more rapid restoration of plasma volume and removes the stimulus to drink further, whereas the complete absence of sodium rapidly removes the osmotic stimulus for absorption. Hence, sodium content at the lower end of the suggested range is optimal to strike a balance during rehydration *(21)*. All these observations relate to the ingestion of rehydration beverages during exercise, and there is evidence to indicate that rehydration carried out after exercise may require the use of fluids with higher sodium content *(22)*.

4. CONSIDERATIONS FOR THE DESIGN OF ORAL REHYDRATION SOLUTIONS FOR USE IN DIARRHEA

Diarrheal illness causes considerable morbidity and mortality in children in developing countries. Compiled health statistics indicate that mortality from diarrheal disease in children under the age of 5 yr has reduced to 1.8 million/yr compared to more than 3 million/yr a decade ago *(23)*. ORS was introduced in the 1960s after the recognition of glucose-linked sodium absorption as an important pathway of sodium and fluid absorption in the intestine and one that was intact in the secreting intestine in diarrhea *(9)*. ORS revolutionized diarrhea management, correcting dehydration and preventing unnecessary deaths, especially in children. The reduction in mortality resulting from the use of ORS made it one of the important medical advances of the 20th century, because of its simplicity and scope to save lives *(24)*. Nonetheless, global use of ORS has been considerably lower than expected.

Several reasons underlie this disappointing rate of ORS use in the community. Intravenous rehydration may be preferred because of its ease, particularly in developed countries *(25)*. The perception of ORS as a "nondrug" has also led to inadequate prescription and use *(26)*. The basis of ORS use is that the enterotoxins causing diarrhea do not impair sodium absorption linked to specific substrates (i.e., glucose and amino acids) *(9)*. Although it enhances fluid absorption from the secreting intestine, the glucose-based ORS that has, in the past, been recommended by the World Health Organization and UNICEF does not reduce intestinal secretion or diarrhea and may paradoxically increase diarrhea *(27)*. This was one factor responsible for poor use of ORS, especially by previous users *(28)*.

During the last 20 yr, numerous studies were conducted to develop an improved or "super" ORS that could, in addition to being effective therapy to treat and prevent dehydration, reduce the severity and duration of diarrhea. The inclusion of amino acid substrates (glycine, alanine, and glutamine) in ORS to replace or supplement the effect of glucose on sodium absorption did not prove advantageous compared with glucose ORS *(29)*. Glutamine, which is particularly interesting because of its role in providing energy to intestinal epithelial cells and its effects on immunity, was effective in reducing small intestinal secretion in experimental models of diarrhea. However, clinical trials in children with noncholera diarrhea did not show any advantage compared with glucose ORS *(30)*. Maltodextrins and cereal-based ORS were introduced to change the carbohydrate substrate in ORS, by providing glucose in the lumen at a reduced osmotic penalty compared with glucose ORS. Maltodextrin ORS did not show any advantage compared with glucose ORS *(29)*. The greatest promise came when several rice-based solutions were introduced to manage diarrhea. Meta-analysis of 15 evaluable clinical trials indicated that rice ORS was superior to glucose ORS in cholera (leading to reduced stool output) but not in noncholera diarrhea in children *(31)*. Early refeeding of patients, commencing within 4 h after initiation of rehydration, has now become the standard of care in treating diarrhea, contrary to the earlier practice of withholding feeds. This possibly achieves some of the same effects as rice ORS. The ability of rice ORS to shorten diarrhea in cholera has been attributed to the low osmolarity of the solution, as well as a kinetic advantage resulting from the hydrolysis of starch end-products close to the sodium glucose cotransporter *(32)*. However, other factors, including a possible antisecretory factor found in rice *(33)*, could contribute to its effect in cholera.

The single most widely accepted change in the formulation of ORS for diarrhea has been in reduced osmolarity solutions. The glucose ORS that was recommended by the World Health Organization has an osmolarity of 311–331 mOsm/kg (*see* Table 2). Physiological studies established that reducing the osmolarity increases absorption of sodium and water from the proximal small intestine in both normal and secreting animals *(38,39)*. Following several clinical trials of reduced osmolarity ORS, a multicenter evaluation of hypoosmolar ORS was conducted, and the reduced osmolarity solution decreased stool output by 39%, ORS intake by 18%, and duration of diarrhea by 22% compared with standard ORS in children with diarrhea *(40)*. A second multicenter trial failed to demonstrate any benefit from reduced osmolarity solution in stool volume or diarrhea duration *(41)*. However, the need for unscheduled iv fluids was reduced by a third in the reduced osmolarity group compared with glucose ORS. There is general consensus that hypoosmolar ORS is preferable to treat diarrhea in children (which is usually the result of rotavirus or bacterial causes other than cholera), and that early refeeding is equally important in diarrheal management *(42)*. The goal of oral rehydration is to achieve reduction in mortality using a single rehydration fluid, which would be applicable in all clinical situations. In areas where cholera is prevalent, there has been worry regarding the

Table 2
Recommendations of Health Organizations and Professional Bodies
Regarding Composition of Oral Rehydration Solution for Use in Diarrhea

Solution	Na (mmol/L)	K (mmol/L)	Cl (mmol/L)	Citrate (mmol/L)	Other (mmol/L)	Glucose (mmol/L)	Osmolarity (mOsm/L)
WHO[a] (Citrate) 1976 (34)	90	20	80	10		111	311
WHO (Bicarbonate) 1976 (36)	90	20	80		HCO_3 30	111	331
ESPGAN 1992 (35)	60	20	60	10		74–111	200–250
AAP 1996 (36)	45–75	20	35–65	7–10		110–140	220–310
WHO (Resomal)[b] 2000 (37)	45	40	70	7	Mg 3 Zn 0.3 Cu 0.045	75	240
WHO 2002	75	20	65	10		75	245

WHO, World Health Organization; ESPGAN, European Society for Paediatric Gastroenterology, Hepatology and Nutrition; AAP, American Academy of Pediatrics.

[a]2002 WHO recommendations are proposed and in process.

[b]Resomal is intended for use in diarrhea in severely malnourished children.

use of hypoosmolar ORS in the community because of the possibility of developing symptomatic hyponatremia in a minority of patients with cholera and high purging rates. A recent clinical trial of the reduced osmolarity solution in 300 adult patients with cholera concluded that the new solution was as effective as the glucose ORS regarding hydration and diarrhea (43). Although hyponatremia (serum sodium below 130 mmol/L) was twice as common in the reduced osmolarity ORS group, it did not lead to symptoms in any patients. Persistent diarrhea, or diarrhea that lasts longer than 14 d, is seen in a small proportion of children who develop acute diarrheal illness. A recent trial examined the efficacy of reduced osmolarity solution on stool volume, need for rehydration fluid, and resolution of illness in infants with persistent diarrhea. The reduced osmolarity solution reduced stool volume by 40% and ORS requirement by approx 25% and hastened resolution of illness (44). Based on these lines of evidence, the World Health Organization is now changing its recommended formulation to a new solution containing 75 mmol/L sodium and 75 mmol/L glucose, which has considerably lower osmolarity than the previous recommended solution.

All the interventions (glucose, amino acids, and hypoosmolar solutions) described were targeted at small intestinal fluid absorption. Although it is true that the small bowel has the capacity to absorb between 12 and 22 L of fluid per day when needed, this capacity to absorb is compromised in diarrheal disease. The colon absorbs approx 1.5 L of water per day in health *(5)*. However, when stressed, as in diarrhea, the colon can absorb up to 6 L of water per day *(45)*. The reserve capacity of the colon to absorb fluid is tremendously important in diarrheal disease, where it acts to minimize fecal fluid losses *(46)*. The absorptive capacity of the colon is impaired by the effect of enterotoxins such as cholera toxin and *Escherichia coli* heat stable toxin *(47)*. Indeed, perfusion of the colon in patients with cholera indicate that colonic absorption of sodium and water is absent in these patients *(48)*. Therefore, it is likely that interventions specifically targeted at enhancing colonic absorption may limit diarrhea.

Fermentation of unabsorbed dietary carbohydrate by anaerobic bacteria in the colon results in the production of short-chain fatty acids (SCFA), of which acetate, propionate, and butyrate are found most abundantly in the human colon. SCFA are the primary stool anion, with concentrations ranging from 100 to 130 mmol/L. SCFA significantly increase sodium and water absorption from the normal human colon, through a process of linked ion exchanges across the luminal membrane of colonic epithelial cells *(49)*. This pathway of sodium absorption, i.e., that linked to SCFA, is not inhibited by cyclic AMP *(50)*. In addition, there is evidence from animal studies that SCFA may inhibit active chloride and fluid secretion in the colon caused by cholera toxin and other bacterial enterotoxins *(47,50,51)*. Restricting normal dietary intake during diarrhea reduces the availability of unabsorbed carbohydrate to the colon and leads to reduced SCFA concentration in the feces in patients with diarrhea *(52,53)*. SCFA are rapidly absorbed from all levels of the intestine and cannot be included in ORS because they would not be expected to reach the colon, their site of action. Amylase-resistant starch, nonstarch polysaccharides (e.g., pectin), and fructooligosaccharides are all different classes of carbohydrate that escape digestion in the small intestine to reach the colon for SCFA fermentation *(54)*. Of these, starch has a favorable profile of fermentation because significant production of butyrate results from its fermentation *(55)*. Incubation of stool from patients with cholera with starch resulted in SCFA production, indicating that the colonic flora in cholera retained the capacity to ferment carbohydrate *(56)*. On the basis of these studies, amylase-resistant starch was given to patients with cholera, along with ORS, assuming that SCFA resulting from its fermentation would increase colonic fluid absorption *(57)*. Addition of the amylase-resistant starch to ORS resulted in significant reduction in diarrhea (approx 30% reduction in stool volume after 12 h) and in diarrhea duration (reduced by approx 37%) in the test group compared with glucose ORS. Resistant starch ORS was also significantly better than rice ORS, which was included as another group for comparison.

Studies with rice ORS suggest that the response of the patient with cholera may differ from that of patients with other forms of diarrhea. It is, therefore, interesting to examine the evidence for the inclusion of indigestible carbohydrate (for fermentation to SCFA in the colon) in diarrhea other than cholera. Rotavirus is a major causative agent of diarrhea in infants and children. Pigs infected with transmissible gastroenteritis virus provide a model of rotavirus infection, and studies in these animals showed that diarrhea developed only in young animals but not in older animals *(58)*. Investigation of their intestinal and colonic content showed that infected animals of all ages secreted fluid into the small intestine. However, in contrast to older animals, the young ones demonstrated fluid secretion into the colon in addition to the intestine, which was associated with inability to ferment carbohydrate to SCFA in the colon. Experiments in rats show that recovery from osmotic diarrhea is accelerated by substrates, such as gum arabic or modified tapioca starch, which are potential sources for colonic fermentation *(59)*. Some of these inclusions in ORS may have other effects. Gum arabic promotes absorption by acting on nitric oxide *(60)*, which is another potential ingredient to include in ORS for the treatment of diarrhea. Diarrhea is also common in patients who receive enteral polymeric feeds directly through a tube into the stomach or intestine. Fluid secretion into the colon has been noted in these patients and may be responsible for diarrhea *(61)* and can be reversed by the presence of SCFA in the luminal fluid *(62)*. The role of colonic carbohydrate substrate in ORS for noncholera diarrhea was addressed by a study in children with diarrhea. Partially hydrolyzed guar gum (a soluble fiber designed to increase SCFA levels in the colon) was added to ORS as a source of fermentable carbohydrate. Children who received this ORS showed an 18% reduction in diarrhea duration and a trend to reduced stool volumes compared to glucose ORS *(63)*. The use of SCFA to manage diarrhea has also been indirectly shown in persistent diarrhea. In children with persistent diarrhea, addition of mashed green banana (high content of resistant starch) or pectin (soluble fiber) to therapy resulted in rapid recovery and reduced need for further rehydration compared with children given standard therapy *(64)*.

Addition of other constituents to ORS may also help early recovery from illness or prevent complications, such as persistent diarrhea and malnutrition. Vitamin A and zinc are nutrients essential for intestinal epithelial function; they are lost during any diarrheal illness *(65,66)*, and their depletion continues with prolonged illness. Deficiency of these micronutrients may, in turn, contribute to impaired intestinal mucosal function and persistence of diarrhea. It may, therefore, be appropriate to add micronutrients to ORS meant for the treatment of diarrhea in children *(67)*. Efforts have also been made to provide high carbohydrate content in ORS without increasing osmolarity to increase the energy density of ORS and, thus, to improve the nutrition of children with diarrhea. Complex carbohydrates, such as starch, provide energy without increasing osmolarity but increase ORS viscosity. In practice, this may be overcome by using α-amylase to partially hydrolyze the starch before adding it to ORS *(68)*, resulting in an energy-dense solution with osmolarity within the prescribed limits for ORS. This approach is experimental but may become commercially feasible if trials indicate that it is acceptable to the caregivers in the community.

5. CONCLUSION

The physiologic principles underlying the design and use of beverages intended for rehydration are now more clearly understood. The present state of our knowledge suggests that rehydration fluid composition should vary according to the specific conditions demanding their use. Rehydration in the presence of normal intestinal function can be conducted with several fluids, without leading to harmful side effects. The composition of these is, therefore, largely dictated by the additional benefits to be obtained from such fluids. On the other hand, rehydration in patients with diarrhea necessitates the use of a formulation complying with a narrower range of specific requirements. Multiple factors continue to hinder the general acceptance of rehydration fluids and beverages in the community. Physiologic, clinical, and operational research has already helped to optimize the composition of rehydration fluids to a considerable extent, but further progress in this area is expected.

6. MAIN POINTS FOR PRIMARY AND CLINICAL REVIEW

1. Normal losses of fluid from sweating can generally be easily replaced by reabsorption from the intestine using a 25–50 mmol/L sodium or 2% carbohydrate solution or a mixture of both.

2. In the late 1980s, diarrheal disease killed over 3 million children yearly, largely as a result of dehydration. Oral rehydration therapy (ORT) and its glucose-linked sodium absorption have massively reduced this.

3. ORT is inadequately prescribed to affected children, in part because it paradoxically increases diarrhea formation while improving patient fluid rehydration status.

4. WHO currently suggests that ORT solutions should contain 75 mmol/L sodium and 75 mmol/L glucose, which consists of a lower osmolarity than original formulations.

5. A rice-based ORT solution apparently helps anaerobic bacteria produce short-chain fatty acids that may improve colonic sodium and water reabsorption, in addition to inhibiting active chloride and water secretion stimulated by choleratoxin.

REFERENCES

1. Barr SI. Effects of dehydration on exercise performance. Can J Appl Physiol 1999;24:164–172.
2. Manatsathit S, Sabra A, Ramakrishna BS, et al. Acute diarrhea in adults. J Gastroenterol Hepatol 2002; 17(Suppl):S54-71.
3. Fordtran JS, Rector FC, Carter NW. The mechanisms of sodium absorption in the human small intestine. J Clin Invest 1968;47:884–900.
4. Billich CO, Levitan R. Effects of sodium concentration and osmolarity on water and electrolyte absorption from the intact human colon. J Clin Invest 1969;48:1336–1347.
5. Phillips SF, Giller J. The contribution of the colon to electrolyte and water conservation in man. J Lab Clin Med 1973;81:733–746.
6. Halevy J, Budinger ME, Hayslett JP, Binder HJ. The role of aldosterone in regulation of sodium and chloride transport in the distal colon of sodium depleted animals. Gastroenterology 1986;91:1227–1233.
7. Renard S, Voilley N, Bassilana F, Lazdunski M, Barbry P. Localization and regulation by steroids of the alpha, beta and gamma subunits of the amiloride-sensitive Na^+ channel in colon, lung and kidney. Pflugers Arch 1995;430:299–307.
8. Levens N, Peach M, Carey R, Poat J, Munday K. Changes in an electroneutral transport process mediated by angiotensin II in the rat distal colon *in vivo*. Endocrinology 1981;108:1497–1504.
9. Carpenter CCJ. The treatment of cholera: clinical science at the bedside. J Infect Dis 1992;166:2–14.
10. Rehrer NJ. Fluid and electrolyte balance in ultra-endurance sport. Sports Med 2001;31:701–715.
11. Leon LAS, Hodgson DR, Rose RJ. Gastric emptying of oral rehydration solutions at rest and after exercise in horses. Res Vet Sci 1997;63:183–187.
12. Gisolfi CV, Lambert GP, Summers RW. Intestinal fluid absorption during exercise: role of sport drink osmolality and [Na^+]. Med Sci Sports Exerc 2001;33:907–915.
13. Brouns F, Senden J, Beckers EJ, Saris WHM. Osmolarity does not affect the gastric emptying rate of oral rehydration solutions. J Parenteral Enteral Nutr 1995;19:403–406.
14. Fordtran JS, Locklear TW. Ionic constituents and osmolality of gastric and intestinal fluids after eating. Am J Digest Dis 1966;11:503–521.
15. Galloway SD, Maughan RJ. The effects of substrate and fluid provision on thermoregulatory and metabolic responses to prolonged exercise in a hot environment. J Sports Sci 2000;18:339–351.
16. Borgstrom B, Dahlqvist A, Lundh G, Sjovall J. Studies of intestinal digestion and absorption in the human. J Clin Invest 1957;36:1521–1536.
17. Sanders B, Noakes TD, Dennis SC. Water and electrolyte shifts with partial fluid replacement during exercise. Eur J Appl Physiol Occup Physiol 1999;80:318–323.
18. Marlin DJ, Scott CM, Mills PC, Louwes H, Vaarten J. Rehydration following exercise: effects of administration of water versus an isotonic oral rehydration solution (ORS). Vet J 1998;156:41–49.

19. Clapp AJ, Bishop PA, Smith JF, Mansfield ER. Effects of carbohydrate-electrolyte content of beverages on voluntary hydration in a simulated industrial environment. AIHAJ 2000;61:692–699.
20. Mitchell JB, Phillips MD, Mercer SP, Baylies HL, Pizza FX. Postexercise rehydration: effect of Na(+) and volume on restoration of fluid spaces and cardiovascular function. J Appl Physiol 2000;89:1302–1309.
21. Wemple RD, Morocco TS, Mack GW. Influence of sodium replacement on fluid ingestion following exercise-induced dehydration. Int J Sport Nutr 1997;7:104–116.
22. Galloway SD. Dehydration, rehydration, and exercise in the heat: rehydration strategies for athletic competition. Can J Appl Physiol 1999;24:188–200.
23. World Health Organization. The World Health Report 1999. WHO, Geneva, Switzerland, 1999.
24. Anonymous. Water with sugar and salt [editorial]. Lancet 1978;2:300–301.
25. Reis EC, Goepp JG, Katz S, Santosham M. Barriers to use of oral rehydration therapy. Pediatrics 1994;93:708–711.
26. Desjeux JF, Briend A, Butzner JD. Oral rehydration solution in the year 2000: pathophysiology, efficacy and effectiveness. Bailliere Clin Gastroenterol 1997;11:509–527.
27. Pierce NF, Banwell JG, Mitra RC, et al. Effect of intragastric glucose-electrolyte infusion upon water and electrolyte balance in Asiatic cholera. Gastroenterology 1968;55:333–343.
28. Greenough WB III. A simple solution. J Diarrhoeal Dis Res 1993;11:1–5.
29. Bhan MK, Mahalanabis D, Fontaine O, Pierce NF. Clinical trials of improved oral rehydration salt formulations: a review. Bull World Health Org 1994;72:945–955.
30. Duggan C. Glutamine-based oral rehydration solutions: the magic bullet revisited? J Pediatr Gastroenterol Nutr 1998;26:533–535.
31. Fontaine O, Gore SM, Pierce NF. Rice-based oral rehydration solution for treating diarrhoea. Cochrane Database Syst Rev 2000;2:CD001264.
32. Thillainayagam AV, Hunt JB, Farthing MJG. Enhancing clinical efficacy of oral rehydration therapy: is low osmolality the key? Gastroenterology 1998;114:197–210.
33. MacCleod RJ, Bennett HPJ, Hamilton JR. Inhibition of intestinal secretion by rice. Lancet 1995; 346:90–92.
34. World Health Organization. A Manual for the Treatment of Acute Diarrhoea, 2nd Ed. World Health Organization, Geneva, Switzerland, 1984.
35. ESPGAN Working Group. Recommendations for composition of oral rehydration solutions for children of Europe. J Pediatr Gastroenterol Nutr 1992;14:113–115.
36. American Academy of Pediatrics Provisional Committee on Quality Improvement. Practice parameter: the management of acute gastroenteritis in young children. Pediatrics 1996;97:424–435.
37. WHO. Management of severe malnutrition. World Health Organization, Geneva, Switzerland, 2000.
38. Lifshitz F, Wapnir RA. Oral hydration solutions: experimental optimization of water and sodium absorption. J Pediatr 1985;106:383–389.
39. Rolston DDK, Borodo MM, Kelly MJ, Dawson AM, Farthing MJG. Efficacy of oral rehydration solutions in a rat model of secretory diarrhea. J Pediatr Gastroenterol Nutr 1987;6:624–630.
40. International Study Group on reduced osmolarity ORS solutions. Multicentre evaluation of reduced osmolarity oral rehydration salts solution. Lancet 1995;345:282–285.
41. CHOICE Study Group. Multicenter, randomized, double-blind clinical trial to evaluate the efficacy and safety of a reduced osmolarity oral rehydration salts solution in children with acute watery diarrhea. Pediatrics 2001;107:613–618.
42. Szajewska H, Hoekstra JH, Sandhu B, et al. Management of acute gastroenteritis in Europe and the impact of the new recommendations. J Pediatr Gastroenterol Nutr 2000;30:522–527.
43. Alam NH, Majumder RN, Fuchs GJ, and the CHOICE study group. Efficacy and safety of oral rehydration solution with reduced osmolarity in adults with cholera: a randomised double-blind clinical trial. Lancet 1999;354:296–299.
44 Sarker SA, Mahalanabis D, Alam NH, Sharmin S, Khan AM, Fuchs GJ. Reduced osmolarity oral rehydration solution for persistent diarrhea in infants: a randomized controlled clinical trial. J Pediatr 2001;138:532–538.
45. Debongnie JC, Phillips SF. Capacity of the human colon to absorb fluid. Gastroenterology 1978; 74:698–703.

46. Read NW. Diarrhoea: the failure of colonic salvage. Lancet 1982;2:481–483.

47. Ramakrishna BS, Nance SH, Roberts-Thomson IC, Roediger WEW. The effect of enterotoxins and short chain fatty acids on water and electrolyte fluxes in ileal and colonic loops in vivo in the rat. Digestion 1990;45:93–101.

48. Speelman P, Butler T, Kabir I, Ali A, Banwell J. Colonic dysfunction during cholera infection. Gastroenterology 1986;91:1164–1170.

49. Rajendran VM, Binder HJ. Apical membrane Cl-butyrate exchange: mechanisms of short chain fatty acid stimulation of active chloride absorption in rat distal colon. J Mem Biol 1994;141:51–58.

50. Vidyasagar S, Ramakrishna BS. Effects of butyrate on active sodium and chloride transport in rat and rabbit distal colon. J Physiol 2002;539:163–173.

51. Charney AN, Giannella RA, Egnor RW. Effect of short chain fatty acids on cyclic 3'5'-guanosine monophosphate-mediated colonic secretion. Comp Biochem Physiol 1999;124:169–178.

52. Ramakrishna BS, Mathan VI. Colonic dysfunction in acute diarrhoea: the role of short chain fatty acids. Gut 1993;34:1215–1218.

53. Tazume S, Ozawa A, Yamamoto T, et al. Ecological study on the intestinal bacterial flora of patients with diarrhea. Clin Infect Dis 1993;16(Suppl):S77–S82.

54. Topping DL, Clifton PM. Short-chain fatty acids and human colonic function: roles of resistant starch and nonstarch polysaccharides. Physiol Rev 2001;81:1031–1064.

55. Scheppach W, Fabian C, Sachs M, Kasper H. The effect of starch malabsorption on fecal short chain fatty acid excretion in man. Scand J Gastroenterol 1988;23:755–759.

56. Ramakrishna BS, Selvi K, Srinivasan P, Mathan VI, Binder HJ. Fermentation of starch *in vitro* in human cholera: implications for therapy [abstract]. Gastroenterology 1994:106:A264.

57. Ramakrishna BS, Venkataraman S, Srinivasan P, Dash P, Young GP, Binder HJ. Amylase-resistant starch plus oral rehydration solution for cholera. N Engl J Med 2000;342:308–313.

58. Argenzio RA, Moon HW, Kemeny LJ, Whipp SC. Colonic compensation in transmissible gastroenteritis of swine. Gastroenterology 1984;86:1501–1509.

59. Teichberg S, Wingertzahn MA, Moyse J, Wapnir RA. Effect of gum arabic in an oral rehydration solution on recovery from diarrhea in rats. J Pediatr Gastroenterol Nutr 1999;29:411–417.

60. Rehman K, Wingertzahn MA, Harper RG, Wapnir RA. Proabsorptive action of gum Arabic. Regulation of nitric oxide metabolism in the basolateral potassium channel of the small intestine. J Pediatr Gastroenterol Nutr 2001;32:529–533.

61. Bowling TE, Raimundo AH, Grimble GK, Silk DB. Colonic secretory effect in response to enteral feeding in humans. Gut 1994;35:1734–1741.

62. Bowling TE, Raimundo AH, Grimble GK, Silk DB. Reversal by short chain fatty acids of colonic fluid secretion induced by enteral feeding. Lancet 1993;342:1266–1268.

63. Alam NH, Meier R, Schneider H, et al. Partially hydrolyzed guar gum-supplemented oral rehydration solution in the treatment of acute diarrhea in children. J Pediatr Gastroenterol Nutr 2000;31:503–507.

64. Rabbani GH, Teka T, Zaman B, Majid N, Khatun M, Fuchs GJ. Clinical studies in persistent diarrhea: dietary management with green banana or pectin in Bangladeshi children. Gastroenterology 2001;121:554–560.

65. Alvarez JO, Salazar-Lindo E, Kohatsu J, Miranda P, Stephensen CB. Urinary excretion of retinol in children with acute diarrhea. Am J Clin Nutr 1995;616:1273–1276.

66. Anonymous. Zinc and copper wastage during acute diarrhea. Nutr Rev 1990;48:19–22.

67. Strand TA, Chandyo RK, Bahl R, et al. Effectiveness and efficacy of zinc for the treatment of acute diarrhea in young children. Pediatrics 2002;109:898–903.

68. Vettorazzi C, Solomons NW, Brown KH, Shoemaker C. Amylase-treated rice flour oral rehydration solution with enhanced energy density. I. In vitro studies of viscosity, osmolality, and stability. Food Nutr Bull 1996;17:98–103.

VIII MARKETING AND SAFETY ISSUES OF BOTTLED AND TAP WATERS

22 The Nutritional Value of Bottled Water

Shelina M. Jamal
and Mark J. Eisenberg

1. INTRODUCTION

The human body is primarily comprised of water, which constitutes approx 90% of blood plasma, 80% of muscle tissue, 60% of red blood cells, and more than 50% of most other tissues *(1)*. Water is an extremely important nutrient for the body. Its functions vary from regulating body temperature to transporting waste products. Today's health-conscious society, now more than ever, focuses on the importance of water. An increase in health awareness and nutrition has fueled the billion-dollar bottled-water industry.

1.1. Types of Bottled Water

Water, the most abundant and familiar liquid on Earth, has been processed and modified to create the various types of bottled water available for commercial sale. Distilled water has been purified by passing it through an evaporation-condensation cycle. This type of water contains small quantities of dissolved solids *(1)*. Deionized water is water from which all ions have been removed by an ion-exchange process *(1)*. It is usually considered to be of higher quality than distilled water and is more economical to produce. Water purified using reverse osmosis is similar to deionized water. The only difference between the two is the process by which the water is purified. Reverse osmosis is reduced to a nonmineral state by passing it through a plastic membrane under pressure, which separates the water from other elements *(1)*. Mineral water contains large quantities of minerals, naturally collected by passing through various layers of earth and rocks to the well or spring. Finally, spring water is obtained naturally from an underground spring, without the benefit of drills or pumps *(1)*.

2. MARKET FORCES

During the past decade, bottled waters have flooded consumer markets. Walk down a grocery aisle in any town in the United States, Canada, Europe, or Asia, and there is a virtual tidal wave of bottled-water brands. The popularity of bottled water has increased substantially in countries throughout the world. During the past 10 yr, in North America

From: *Beverages in Nutrition and Health*
Edited by: T. Wilson and N. J. Temple © Humana Press Inc., Totowa, NJ

alone, sales of bottled water have increased by 400%, and one in five households now uses bottled drinking water (2). This $35-billion industry worldwide continues to grow, as water quality concerns and fitness/health awareness increase. In the United States in 1999, bottled-water sales exceeded $5.2 billion (1), allowing it to assume a prominent place in the North American diet. Deionized water refills are widely available in supermarkets. Bottled water containing mineral water, however, can cost upward of $1.40/L, more than a liter of gasoline. Regardless of the expense, according to the International Bottled Water Association, the average American consumes approx 0.5 L of bottled water per day. This is more than the average daily consumption of juice, milk, sports drinks, coffee, sodas, tea, or alcoholic drinks. Bottled-water consumption is second only to the consumption of tap water (approx 1 L/d).

Previously, consumers were unaware of the content of bottled water; they assumed it was healthier than tap water. In addition to its convenience, bottled water has made its mark as a fashion must-have. Manufacturers' marketing techniques have used this concept to increase sales. For example, one manufacturer has convinced consumers in Alberta, Canada (with all its pristine glaciers), to purchase an extremely high-priced imported French bottled water. The bottled-water boom, however, has transcended the elements of fashion and recently become a basic staple in the American household. Only recently have companies begun to cater to this market, leading to the plethora of waters now commercially available. Although many companies market bottled water, few offer optimum mineral- or vitamin-enhanced waters (see Table 1). For example, Gatorade's Propel Fitness Water is a flavored vitamin-packed water. However, no minerals are included. Coca-Cola's Dasani is purified water enhanced with low mineral concentrations. Clearly Canadian, in conjunction with Reebok, has released the new Reebok Fitness Water. This enhanced water beverage contains essential vitamins, minerals, and electrolytes. The mineral profile includes calcium, magnesium, zinc, selenium, potassium, chromium, and no sodium.

3. VERIFICATION STANDARDS

Significant differences exist between European and North American regulations for the bottled-water industry (see Table 2). In Europe, water with any level of mineralization is considered "mineral water," and no further modifications are allowed. In fact, European bottled mineral water may not be treated in any way to alter its original chemical and microbiologic composition. To be labeled as "spring," however, water may undergo permitted treatments, but, like mineral water, it must meet certain microbiologic criteria (3).

In the United States, the Food and Drug Administration (FDA) requires that "mineral waters" contain between 500 and 1500 mg/L of total dissolved solids, a combination of the dissolved minerals (4). To make the claim that a product is "very high in," "rich in," or an "excellent source of" a particular mineral, the product must contain a minimum of 25% of the mineral's Dietary Reference Intakes (5).

Recent changes have been made concerning recommended dietary intakes that must be clarified. In the past 50 yr, nutritional experts have established Recommended Dietary Allowances (RDA) in the United States and Recommended Nutrient Intakes (RNI) in Canada for various minerals and nutrients (6). A cooperative effort between the United States and Canada revised previous recommendations and created Dietary Reference

Table 1
Mineral Content of Commercially Available North American Bottled Waters

	Mineral content (mg/L)		
	Magnesium	Sodium	Calcium
A Sante	1	160	4
Adobe Springs	96	5	3
Arrowhead	5	3	20
Black Mountain	1	8	25
Calistoga	2	164	8
Canadian Glacier	0	1	1
Canadian Spring	3	2	11
Carolina Mountain	0	5	6
Clairval	7	13	20
Crystal Geyser Alpine Spring	6	13	27
Crystal Geyser Sparkling Mineral	1	30	2
Deer Park	1	1	1
Great Bear	1	3	1
La Croix	22	4	37
Lithia Springs	7	680	120
Mendocino	120	260	240
Monclair	12	475	8
Mountain Valley Spring	7	1	160
Naya	20	6	38
Ozarka	1	5	18
Poland Spring	1	4	1
Pure Hawaiian	0	0	0
Sierra	0	0	0
Sparkletts	5	15	5
Talawanda Spring	0	3	0
Talking Rain	2	0	2
Vichy Springs	48	1095	157
Zephyrhills	7	4	52

Adapted from ref. 27.
Reprinted with permission from Excerpta Medica Inc.

Intakes (DRI). Compared to the old RDAs and RNIs, DRIs incorporate the concept of preventing nutrient deficiencies as well as risk reduction for chronic conditions, such as heart disease, diabetes, hypertension, and osteoporosis.

The DRIs, RDAs, and RNIs are the daily nutrient intakes suggested, not as minimum requirements, but as generous allowances established by federal health regulations in the United States and Canada to meet the needs of most people (7). Each person may have slightly different needs resulting from differences in absorption and losses and overall diet composition. An intake below the recommended levels is not necessarily inadequate, but there is a greater chance of inadequacy if daily intake consistently falls below these levels.

Table 2
Mineral Content of North American Tap Water, North American Bottled Waters, and European Bottled Waters (mg/L)

	Ca^{2+}	Mg^{2+}		Na^+
	Males and Females	Males	Females[a]	Males and Females
Dietary reference intake, mg/d				
1–3 yr	500	80	80	Maximum
4–8 yr	800	130	130	recommended
9–18 yr	1300	240–410	240–360	intake of
19–50 yr	1000	400–420	310–320	2400 to 3000 mg
> 50 yr	1200	420	320	per day
North American tap water				
Surface water sources (n = 36)				
Mean ± SD	34 ± 21	10 ± 8		35 ± 41
Median	36	8		18
Range	2–83	0–29		0–169
Ground water sources (n = 8)				
Mean ± SD	52 ± 24	20 ± 13		91 ± 67
Median	48	12		83
Range	26–85	2–48		8–195
North American bottled waters				
Spring waters (n = 28)				
Mean ± SD	18 ± 22	8 ± 18		4 ± 4
Median	6	3		4
Range	0–76	0–95		0–15

(continued)

Table 2 (Continued)

	Ca^{2+}	Mg^{2+}		Na^+
	Males and Females	Males	Females[a]	Males and Females
North American bottled waters				
Mineral Waters (n = 9)				
Mean ± SD	100 ± 125		24 ± 42	371 ± 335
Median	8		7	240
Range	3–310		1–130	36–1095
European bottled waters				
Low mineralization waters (n = 40)				
Mean ± SD	60 ± 40		16 ± 19	13 ± 13
Median	54		14	9
Range	4–145		1–110	1–56
Moderate mineralization waters (n = 26)				
Mean ± SD	262 ± 139		64 ± 37	157 ± 197
Median	217		56	49
Range	78–575		9–128	2–660
High mineralization waters (n = 7)				
Mean ± SD	60 ± 59		16 ± 20	1151 ± 153
Median	33		9	1133
Range	5–176		4–60	900–1419

[a]For pregnant women, add 40 mg of Mg^{2+} per day.
Adapted from ref. 6.
Reprinted with permission from Blackwell Science Ltd.

DRIs have been established for various major minerals but not for all. For a few trace elements, no recommended daily amounts have been established. Rather, the US government has created Estimated Safe and Adequate Daily Intakes and Estimated Minimum Requirements. These standards provide reference values for the safe or minimum intakes of the trace elements.

3.1. Mineral Content

A variation exists in the mineral content of bottled waters commercially available in North America and Europe. Three minerals often included in bottled water, resulting from their presence in the earth's crust, are magnesium, calcium, and sodium. Magnesium and calcium, as explained later in this chapter, are advantageous for an individual's health. Including sodium, however, is not beneficial.

In a survey of approx 30 North American bottled waters, magnesium content ranged from 0 to 126 mg/L, calcium from 0 to 546 mg/L, and sodium from 0 to 1200 mg/L. The median concentrations for bottled waters in North America were 2.5 mg/L for magnesium, 5 mg/L for sodium, and 8 mg/L for calcium. For the European bottled waters, the median concentration for magnesium was 23.5 mg/L, 115 mg/L for calcium, and 20 mg/L for sodium (4). It is apparent that waters bottled in North America generally have low mineral contents relative to European bottled waters.

4. IMPLICATIONS FOR HUMAN HEALTH

If North Americans prefer to drink commercially available bottled waters, they should be selective when deciding which water to drink. As mentioned, the three minerals that are most commonly found in various brands of bottled water are magnesium, calcium, and sodium. Therefore, the levels of these elements can be useful as a basis for comparison. Individuals should select bottled water with an optimal mineral profile, i.e., high levels of magnesium, calcium, and little or no sodium. Unfortunately, few bottled waters available on the North American market fit this profile. In fact, North Americans may actually be more likely to drink mineral-*deficient* bottled water, such as spring waters, rather than mineral-*rich* bottled water. This can be attributed to the taste associated with mineral-rich bottled water, which is unfavorable to North Americans but pleasant to Europeans (6).

The minerals contained in bottled water aid in improving certain medical conditions. Minerals, such as magnesium, calcium, fluoride, copper, and selenium, all play beneficial roles in ailments, including cardiovascular disease (CVD), stroke, cancer, osteoporosis, dental caries, and arthritis. However, it is important to note that due to their mineral content, some bottled waters are not recommended for people with certain health conditions, such as kidney disorders (6).

Dietary intake of magnesium and calcium can be supplemented by drinking mineral-rich water. Children and individuals with poor dietary habits can especially benefit from this. Specifically, magnesium deficiency has been linked with sudden death, calcium inadequacy with osteoporosis, and excess sodium with hypertension. Drinking water that is high in magnesium and calcium and low in sodium will help people to achieve the RDAs. Because variations exist in the mineral content of commercially available bottled waters, understanding the potential beneficial and harmful effects of these minerals provides valuable information on which water to choose (6).

4.1. Magnesium

Approximately 60% of the total magnesium in the body is found in the bones, 26% in the muscles, and the remainder in soft tissues and body fluids. The organs with the highest magnesium concentration are the brain, heart, liver, and kidney (8). Magnesium is responsible for several biologic processes that influence membrane and mitochondrial integrity, such as the proper functioning of adenosine triphosphate (ATP). It is also essential for the synthesis and stability of nuclear DNA and for bone mineralization (9,10).

Magnesium in solution has a 30% higher rate of absorption than does magnesium from food (10). It is estimated that the body requires 220 to 410 mg of magnesium daily (10). The average magnesium intake in the United States ranges from 240 to 365 mg/d (9,11), but magnesium intake in specific North American population groups is often inadequate to meet daily requirements (11,12). The body can absorb only approx 50% of the magnesium present in food.

In some geographic areas, the magnesium in drinking water may provide 20–40% of magnesium intake. For example, a liter of water with a magnesium content of 100 mg/L contains 29% of the daily magnesium requirement of 350 mg/d (8). However, a liter of water that is low in magnesium (<10 mg/L) provides less than 3% of the daily requirement.

CVD rates are inversely related to water hardness (10). That is, rates of cardiovascular mortality and sudden death are 10% to 30% greater in soft-water areas (low in magnesium or calcium) than in hard water areas (high in magnesium or calcium) (10). Magnesium intake may have a cardioprotective effect and has been correlated with a reduction in rates of sudden death (13).

Magnesium is a key mineral involved in the maintenance of the cardiovascular system. It aids in lowering blood pressure and reducing the risks of hypertension and many different types of cardiovascular disease, such as arrhythmias, cardiac ischemia, sudden death, and myocardial infarction (14). Few studies have also indicated that magnesium may play a beneficial role in diabetes, cancer, asthma, stroke, leg and menstrual cramps, premenstrual syndrome, migraine, osteoporosis, and arthritis (8).

Animal and clinical studies support an inverse relationship between magnesium intake and sudden death. Magnesium deficiency promotes cardiac irritability, perhaps by causing malfunction of sodium-potassium ATPase (15). Clinical reports also suggest that in certain cases, intravenous (iv) magnesium can reverse cardiac rhythm disturbances (10). Magnesium deficiency may potentially lead to the development of myocardial ischemia and sudden death. Several animal studies have provided evidence supporting this theory (14). Other studies have related magnesium deficiency with pathologic changes in the heart that have been linked to chronic myocardial ischemia (16,17).

Dietary magnesium intake has also shown a strong inverse association with the incidence of type 2 or noninsulin-dependent diabetes mellitus (NIDDM). As magnesium intake increases, the number of NIDDM cases decreases, resulting in a proportional reduction in relative risk (18). Yajnik et al. (19) reported results establishing an association between low plasma magnesium concentrations and insulin resistance. Magnesium supplementation aids in glucose handling and has a beneficial effect on insulin sensitivity in patients with type 2 diabetes (20,21). Other studies have reported a decreased risk of diabetes in patients with the high magnesium intake (18). Magnesium intake, therefore, is a vital component of a healthy lifestyle that can be achieved through the consumption of magnesium-rich water.

4.2. Calcium

More than half of all North Americans consume inadequate levels of calcium. On average, adult women consume only 60% of the recommended daily calcium intake for their age. Calcium intake can be supplemented by the appropriate selection of drinking water. Calcium (Ca^{2+}) is the most abundant mineral in the body: the average human body contains approximately 1150 g. Bones and teeth comprise approx 99% of the body's calcium (22,23).

Calcium is vital to life. First, it is an integral part of bone structure, providing a rigid frame that holds the body upright and serves as attachment points for muscles, making motion possible. Calcium is a major component of mineralized tissues and is required for normal growth and development of the skeleton and teeth (24). Adequate calcium intake is needed for the acquisition of an individual's genetically determined bone mass (25).

Second, calcium intake can serve as a storage source, offering a readily available source of the mineral to the body fluids (26). It also helps to regulate muscle contraction, transmit nerve impulses, and regulate ion exchange across cell membranes. As well, it helps in the secretion of hormones, digestive enzymes, and neurotransmitters, including serotonin, acetylcholine, and norepinephrine (22). Calcium serves as a cofactor in calmodulin, a protein that relays messages and helps convey signals received at the cell surface to the interior of the cell. This is a critical factor in maintenance of normal blood pressure (22).

Studies show that when animals are fed calcium-deficient diets, their bones become susceptible to fracture. A low-calcium diet results in a loss of trabecular bone in adult cats, a generalized thinning of bone in dogs, and a decreased bone mass in young growing rats. The bones of experimental animals become weak and soft and have reduced density when their diets lack calcium, phosphorus, and vitamin D (27).

In children, calcium deficiency can progress to rickets, which results in bone deformities and growth retardation (22). In adults, calcium deficiency is associated with vitamin D deficiency, which can lead to osteomalacia, characterized by softening of the bones. Low calcium intake has been implicated as a determinant of several chronic conditions, including osteoporosis, hypertension, and colon cancer (22,24). However, ingesting too much calcium may lead to the formation of kidney stones (27,28). People with a history of kidney stone formation, therefore, might benefit from avoiding bottled waters with a high calcium content.

Naturally bioavailable calcium is found mainly in milk and milk products. Because the intake of these products is often low, many foods are now fortified with calcium (e.g., orange juice and bottled water). Calcium can also be found in small amounts in several vegetables, many of which contain binders that impede its absorption. Among the few vegetables that contain bioavailable calcium are mustard greens, parsley, broccoli, and kale (22).

The bioavailability of calcium in water is believed to be at least as high as that of milk and milk products (25). Approximately 20 to 40% of ingested calcium is absorbed by the body (26). The average North American bottled water contains only 8 mg/L (6). Therefore, only 1.6–3.2 mg of calcium out of every liter of bottled water consumed is absorbed.

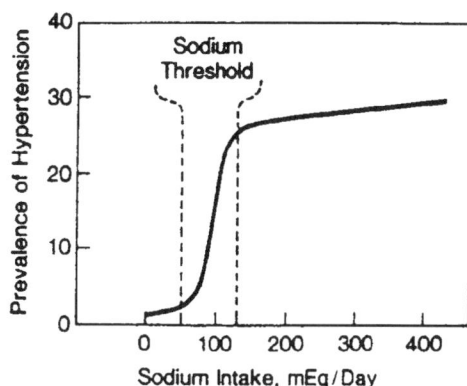

Fig. 1. Reproduced with permission, copyright 1984, American Medical Association. From ref. *42*.

However, selecting a bottled water with a high calcium content may help to achieve the daily recommended intake.

4.3. Sodium

Sodium is an essential mineral present in every cell and primarily found in the extra-cellular fluids, vascular fluids, and the intestinal fluids surrounding the cells *(29,30)*. Approximately 50% of the body's sodium is found in these fluids, and the remaining amount is in the bones. Normal sodium levels in the blood are maintained at 310–333 mg/100 mL *(22)*. Acid-base balance and the transmission of nerve impulses are important functions performed by sodium *(31)*.

Sodium is often added to food and beverages in the form of sodium chloride (salt) for two reasons, taste and the induction of thirst *(32)*. Salt intake and fluid consumption are directly related. A high-salt diet causes a rise in the blood's concentration of sodium and, in turn, causes an increase in thirst. Therefore, bottled waters that contain high sodium levels may lead to increased consumption of their product *(32)*. Excessive sodium intake, however, is associated with a common disease, high blood pressure.

In North America, one-fifth of the adult population is affected by hypertension *(33)*. High salt intake is believed to be an important contributor to its occurrence *(32–34)*. Sodium is believed to be the ion responsible for the hypertensive effects of a high salt intake. A highly significant relationship has been observed between average blood pressure and sodium intake in many populations around the world *(35)*.

Animal studies have also demonstrated that hypertension can be induced or made more severe by increasing sodium intake, and that hypertension can often be prevented by sodium restriction (*see* Fig. 1) *(36–38)*. For example, experimental animals have been made hypertensive by providing them with 1% and 2% saline solutions for drinking water. Cutler et al. *(39)* performed a meta-analysis of numerous studies that addressed the effects of salt restriction on blood pressure and concluded that a reduction of sodium intake to 1500 to 1700 mg/d (from an average of 2350 mg/d) would result in a decrease of 4 to 6 mmHg in systolic blood and of 2.3 mmHg in diastolic blood pressure.

Despite these health risks, several of sodium-rich foods are found in the North American diet. The addition of salt, primarily in foods, is appealing to taste but also increases thirst, therefore, increasing beverage consumption. The estimated minimum daily requirement of sodium for an adult (500 mg/d) *(22)* is easily achieved in any North American diets. Therefore, the FDA has not recommended a minimal sodium intake. However, the National Research Council has recommended limiting daily sodium intake to fewer than 2400 mg (6 g salt), and the American Heart Association recommends limiting sodium intake to 3000 mg/d *(22)*. Drinking 1 L of bottled water with a high sodium content (i.e., 1000 mg/L) may provide an individual with 45% of the maximum recommended daily sodium intake. By choosing a bottled water low in sodium, intake can be minimized.

4.4. Trace Elements

Bottled waters contain other minerals as well as trace elements that have important functions in the body. However, the concentration of these trace elements in most bottled waters is usually minimal in comparison with magnesium, calcium, and sodium. In addition, their daily requirements are usually met with a normal diet. Some examples include copper, iron, potassium, and zinc. Table 3 highlights the symptoms of deficiency/toxicity associated with elements often found in bottled waters other than the ones explained in this report.

One trace element of note is fluoride. Of the 90% of fluoride that is absorbed by the body, 50% is incorporated as an integral part of the tooth and bone structure. The average human body contains approx 2.6 g of fluoride *(22)*. A major function of fluoride is its role in protecting teeth. Fluoride attaches to hydroxyapatite, a crystal on the surface of teeth, making teeth strong and resistant to decay *(40)*. Fluoride deficiency, therefore, is related to a higher incidence of dental cavities, especially in children.

The leading source of dietary fluoride is drinking water. The ingestion of water containing high fluoride concentrations (> 2.0 mg/L), however, can cause pitting, mottling, and dulling of the teeth. Opponents of water fluoridation have claimed that fluoridating water increases the risk for various diseases. The safety and effectiveness of water fluoridation have been re-evaluated frequently, and no credible evidence supports an association between appropriate levels of fluoridation and toxic effects *(41)*.

Ingesting sufficient amounts of fluoride is especially important for children. A child who drinks nonfluoridated water will have a significant increase in the incidence of dental caries when compared with one who consumes fluoridated water. An optimal fluoride concentration should not exceed 1 mg/L. North American bottled waters often have low fluoride levels (i.e., < 0.3 mg/L), whereas European bottled waters exhibit the contrary, with levels exceeding the optimal level. Water fluoridation remains the most equitable and cost-effective method of delivering fluoride to all members of most communities, regardless of age, educational attainment, or income level *(5,41)*. If children are to consume bottled water, a water with adequate fluoride content should be used.

5. CONCLUSION

Water is essential to life. The mineral content of bottled water, if adjusted to optimal levels, can be of additional value to the consumer. Magnesium and calcium, two minerals

Table 3
Symptoms of Deficiency/Toxicity Associated With Elements Found in Bottled Waters

Element	Deficiency	Toxicity
Chromium	Decrease in metabolism	Rare except at extremely high doses; acts as gastric irritant Decreased control on blood sugar regulation
Copper	Atherosclerosis Anemia General weakness Impaired respiration	Rare except at extremely high doses; acts as gastric irritant
Fluoride	Higher incidence of cavities	Tooth/bone deformities Gastric irritant Pulmonary and cardiovascular (CV) disturbant
Iron	Anemia Fatigue, weakness, headaches, apathy	Can cause arterial vessel and other CV-related damage
Manganese	Rare; can cause poor growth Alter metabolism Osteoporosis	Can only occur through inhalation overdose Hallucinations, other psychiatric symptoms Nerve damage
Nitrate	Extremely rare	Methemoglobinemia (blue-baby syndrome) High doses can be carcinogenic
Phosphate	Rare; can cause muscle and bone weakness	Can occur in individuals with severe kidney dysfunction Bone weakness and fractures
Potassium	Extremely rare	Heart palpitations
Selenium	Rare; can cause tissue death and organ failure Premature aging CV disease	Rare; can cause hair and fingernail loss Gastric irritant
Zinc	Delayed growth and sexual maturity Prolonged wound-healing ability Can harm the fetus	Rare; can cause copper-deficiency anemia Impair immune function Gastric irritant

that are often not consumed in adequate amounts, can successfully be supplemented via the consumption of mineral water. Excessive sodium consumption leading to high blood pressure, however, can also result from some bottled waters. Therefore, it is imperative that the consumer is aware of the mineral content of the water he or she chooses to drink. A health-conscious consumer of bottled water should look for the following:

1. Calcium content as high as possible (levels up to 2500 mg/L have been proven safe in humans).
2. High magnesium level (at least 400 mg/L, excess magnesium is merely absorbed, broken down, and excreted in humans).
3. An absolute minimal level of sodium (preferably none).
4. Fluoride level close to 1.0 mg/L.

Mineral water is an excellent alternative beverage choice for today's active and health-conscious consumer. Not only does it provide a means of hydration, but it also serves as a means of ensuring nutritional mineral intake for all ages.

6. MAIN POINTS FOR PRIMARY AND CLINICAL REVIEW

1. Bottled water is produced in several different ways including distillation, reverse osmosis, and collection at a spring.
2. There has been heavy marketing of bottled water in recent years and as a result it is the second most popular beverage in the United States today (after tap water).
3. Bottled water is often perceived as healthier than tap water, though this is not always true.
4. In the United States, mineral water is bottled water required to contain between 500 and 1500 mg/L dissolved total minerals, and mineral water can be called "high in....", "rich in...", or "a good source of....." if the mineral is present at greater that 25% of the DRI for that mineral.
5. Mineral water can be beneficial by providing significant amounts of magnesium, calcium, and trace elements including fluoride, but may contain an excess of sodium.

REFERENCES

1. The Bottled Water Web. Retrieved July 30, 2001, from http://www.bottledwaterweb.com.
2. Bottled Water in the US. Beverage Marketing Corporation, New York, NY, 1995.
3. British soft drinks. Retrieved January 22, 2002, from http://www.britishsoftdrinks.com.
4. von Wisenberger A. The Pocket Guide to Bottled Water. Contemporary Books, Chicago, IL, 1991.
5. Canadian Food Inspection Agency. Section VI: Nutrient Content Claims. Section 6.2.6.4
6. Azoulay A, Garzon P, Eisenberg MJ. Comparison of the Mineral Content of Tap Water and Bottled Waters. J Gen Intern Med 2001;16:168–175.
7. Health & Welfare Canada. Nutrition Recommendations. The Report of the Scientific Review Committee. Supply & Services, Ottawa, Canada 1990.
8. Wester PO. Magnesium. Am J Clin Nutr 1987;45:1305–1312.
9. Cronin RE, Knochel JP. Magnesium deficiency. Adv Intern Med 1983;28:509–533.
10. Eisenberg, MJ. Magnesium deficiency and sudden death. Am Heart J 1992;124:544–549.
11. Jones JE, Manalo R, Flink EB. Magnesium requirements in adults. Am J Clin Nutr 1967;20:632–635.
12. Seeling MS. The requirement of magnesium by the normal adult: summary and analysis of published data. Am J Clin Nutr 1964;14:342–390.
13. Karppanen H. Epidemiological studies on the relationship between magnesium intake and cardiovascular disease. Artery 1981;9:190–199.
14. Elwood PC, Fehily AM, Sweetnam PM, et al. Dietary magnesium and prediction of heart disease. Lancet 1992;340:483.

15. Altura BM, Altura BT. Magnesium ions and contraction of vascular smooth muscles: relationship to some vascular dieseases. Fed Proc 1981;40:2672–2679.

16. Eisenberg MJ. Magnesium deficiency and cardiac arrhythmias. N Y State J Med 1986;86:133–136.

17. Altura BM. Sudden-death ischemic heart disease and dietary magnesium intake: is the target site coronary vascular smooth muscle? Med Hypotheses 1979;5:843–848.

18. Meyer KA, Kushi LH, Jacobs DR, et al. Carbohydrates, dietary fiber, and incident type 2 diabetes in older women. Am J Clin Nutr 2000;71:921–930.

19. Yajnik CS, Smith RF, Hockaday TDR, et al. Fasting plasma magnesium concentrations and glucose disposal in diabetes. Br Med J 1984;288:1032–1034.

20. Salmerón J, Manson JE, Stampfer MJ, et al. Dietary fiber, glycemic load, and risk of non-insulin-dependent diabetes mellitus in women. JAMA 1997;277:472–477.

21. Salmerón J, Ascherio A, Rimm EB, et al. Dietary fiber, glycemic load and risk of NIDDM in men. Diabetes Care 1997;20:545–550.

22. Macrominerals and Microminerals. In: Advanced Nutrition and Human Metabolism, 3rd Ed. Groff J, Gropper SS (eds.). Wadsworth, London, UK, 2000, pp. 371–417.

23. Matkovic V. Calcium metabolism and calcium requirements during skeletal modeling and consolidation of bone mass. Am J Clin Nutr 1991;54:245–260.

24. NIH Consensus Conference. Optimal calcium intake. JAMA 1994;272:1942–1950.

25. Couzy F, Kastenmayer P, Vigo M, Clough J, Munoz-Box R, Barclay DV. Calcium bioavailability from a calcium- and sulfate-rich mineral water, compared with milk, in young adult women. Am J Clin Nutr 1995;62:1239–1244.

26. Allen LH. Calcium bioavailability and absorption: a review. Am J Clin Nutr 1982;35:783–808.

27. Garzon P, Eisenberg MJ. Variation in the mineral content of commercially available bottled waters: implications for health and disease. Am J Med 1998;105:125–130.

28. Coe FL, Parks JH, Asplin JR. The pathogenesis and treatment of kidney stones. N Engl J Med 1992; 327:1141–1552.

29. Kinney JM, Jeejeebhoy DJ, Hill GL, et al. (eds.). Nutrition and Metabolism in Patient Care. WB Saunders, Philadelphia, 1988, pp. 61–88, 445–464, 701–726.

30. Somer E (ed.). The Essential Guide to Vitamins and Minerals. HarperCollins, New York, NY, 1995.

31. Tolonen M (ed.). Vitamins and Minerals in Health and Nutrition. Ellis Harwood, New York, NY, 1990, pp. 65–68, 148–175.

32. Roberts WC. From the editor: high salt intake, its origins, its economic impact, and its effect on blood pressure. Am J Cardiol 2001;88:1338–1346.

33. Kaplan NM. Clinical Hypertension (3rd ed.). Williams & Wilkins, Baltimore, MD, 1982, p. 6.

34. Prior IAM, Evans JG, Harvey HPB, et al. Sodium intake and blood pressure in two Polynesian populations. N Engl J Med 1968;279:515–520.

35. McCarron DA, Holly HJ, Morris CD. Human nutrition and blood pressure regulation: an integrated approach. Hypertension 1982;4(Suppl):2–13.

36. Haddy FJ, Pamnani MB. Role of dietary salt in hypertension. A review. J Am Coll Nutr 1995;14:428–438.

37. Stein PP, Black HR. The role of diet in the genesis and treatment of hypertension. A review. Med Clin North Am 1993;77:831–847.

38. Tobian L. Human essential hypertension: implications of animal studies. Ann Intern Med 1983;98: 729–734.

39. Cutler JA, Follmann D, Elliot P, et al. An overview of randomized trials of sodium reduction and blood pressure. Hypertension 1991;17(Suppl):27–33.

40. Position of the American Dietetic Association: The impact of fluoride on dental health. J Am Dietet Assoc 1994;94:1428–1431.

41. Fluoridation. A report by the American Council on Science and Health. June 1983.

42. Kaplan NM. Dietary salt intake and blood pressure [letter]. JAMA 1984;251:1429–1430.

43. Altruis Biomedical Network. Retrieved December 16, 2001, from http://www.daily-vitamins.com/rda.html.

23 Tap Water and the Risk of Microbial Infection

Christian Chauret

1. INTRODUCTION

Ever since Dr. John Snow demonstrated in the 1850s that cholera is a waterborne disease *(1)*, public health officials have been challenged by the need to provide the population with water free of infectious agents. The introduction of chlorine at the beginning of the 20th century has been a major factor in improving water quality, at least from a microbiological view. Although water quality in impoverished countries remains a major problem, in Western countries, mortality from consuming drinking water is low and good water quality is usually taken for granted. However, because of various issues, such as water shortages in some parts of the world, an increasing at-risk population due to aging and AIDS (individuals who are immunodeficient), as well as an aging infrastructure, water quality and distribution will likely be important problems in the 21st century. More specifically, one of the challenges facing the water industry today is to provide drinking water safe from disinfectant-resistant organisms (such as protozoan parasites), while at the same time minimizing the formation of harmful disinfection by-products (DBP) in drinking water.

2. WATERBORNE MICROBIAL PATHOGENS

Water can become contaminated with microbial pollutants from different sources, including human sewage and septic tanks, discharge of treated wastewater into source water, animal waste, and storm water. Wastewater can also serve as a source of contamination for municipal drinking water systems that are downstream from wastewater outfalls. These sources are reservoirs for various types of microbial agents, such as bacteria, viruses, and protozoa. In the United States, from data available from 1997–1998, the etiologic agent of waterborne disease outbreaks was a parasite or a bacterium in 35.3% and 23.5% of cases, respectively *(2)*. Of note, 29.4% of outbreaks had an unknown etiology. Both surface water and groundwater can be at risk. Therefore, there is a need for adequate water treatment to minimize the risk associated with the potential presence of microbial contaminants in water.

From: *Beverages in Nutrition and Health*
Edited by: T. Wilson and N. J. Temple © Humana Press Inc., Totowa, NJ

2.1. Protozoan Parasites

Waterborne protozoan parasites are characterized by the formation of (oo)cysts, which are the environmental stage in the life cycle of the parasite. Typically, these (oo)cysts are relatively resistant to environmental stresses and chemical disinfectants *(3)*. Therefore, encysted protozoan parasites may survive in source water. In addition, they may be difficult to inactivate using conventional water disinfectants. Because of their intrinsic resistance to various treatments, significant levels of protozoan parasites may survive during wastewater treatment and be released back into the environment in treated wastewater discharges *(4)*. In North America, protozoan parasites of concern include *Cryptosporidium parvum*, *Giardia lamblia*, *Toxoplasma gondii*, and emerging parasites, such as microsporidia.

2.1.1. CRYPTOSPORIDIUM PARVUM

Members of the genus *Cryptosporidium* are coccidian protozoan parasites that cause intestinal illnesses in humans and animals and spread through contaminated water, contaminated foods, and close contact. *C. parvum*, which has oocysts measuring 4–6 μm in diameter, is the predominant species responsible for cryptosporidiosis in humans *(5)*. This microorganism causes abundant watery diarrhea, sometimes associated with abdominal pain, nausea, vomiting, and fever *(5)*. *C. parvum* infects many different mammals, including cattle and humans *(6)*. Individuals who are immunocompromised or immunologically naïve are particularly prone to persistent infections, which are often fatal *(7)*. Oocysts of this organism are released into the environment through the feces of an infected host *(5)*. In the environment, the oocyts can survive for several months while remaining viable *(3)*. In addition, oocysts are extremely resistant to chemical disinfectants used for water treatment *(8,9)*.

2.1.2. GIARDIA LAMBLIA

Members of the genus *Giardia* are protozoan parasites (flagellates) that infect the upper portion of the small intestine in humans and in several different mammals, causing giardiasis with stomach cramps, diarrhea, nausea, and fatigue *(10)*. It is the most commonly detected parasite in stool specimens. The usual mode of transmission is fecal-oral. Children in day-care centers, schools, and nurseries, as well as people who are immunologically compromised are especially at risk *(10)*. These parasites are commonly passed between family members through the fecal-oral route. The cyst, which is the environmentally stable stage, is characteristically oval in shape, ranging from 8 to 14 μm. After the cyst stage, the second stage in the life cycle of *Giardia* is the parasitic trophozoite, which commonly inhabits the duodenum and initiates the infection process. *Giardia* cysts are considered common biologic contaminants of North American surface waters. Many waterborne outbreaks of giardiasis have been reported in the last few decades *(10)*. Most waterborne outbreaks are associated with filtration failures in water treatment plants or have occurred in small communities where water treatment was minimal *(11)*. *Giardia* cysts are generally more easily inactivated by chlorine (and other disinfectants) than *Cryptosporidium* oocysts. In addition, because they are larger than oocysts, *Giardia* cysts are more readily removed by coagulation and sand filtration.

2.1.3. TOXOPLASMA GONDII

T. gondii, like *Cryptosporidium*, is a coccidian protozoan parasite. It is endemic throughout the world and commonly found in birds, mice, and cats *(12)*. Its oocyst is slightly larger than the *Cryptosporidium* oocyst. The disease (toxoplasmosis) is typically transmitted to humans via contact with cat feces and ingestion of oocysts. In human adults, it causes a mild disease, which is often asymptomatic. In more severe cases, it causes retinitis and/or lymphadenopathy. In pregnant women, however, there is a chance of transferring the parasite to the fetus *(13)*. Congenital infections may produce stillbirth or may result in severe abnormalities (liver problems, hydrocephalus, or blindness, etc.). People with AIDS are susceptible to *Toxoplasma*, which often causes acute encephalitis *(14,15)*.

2.2. Bacterial Pathogens

Bacteria are abundant in feces, which contain up to 10^{12} bacteria per gram. As a result, fecal contamination of sources of potable water may introduce several bacterial pathogens into drinking water. Common and potential waterborne bacterial agents of disease include *Salmonella* sp, *Escherichia coli*, *Pseudomonas aeruginosa*, *Aeromonas hydrophila*, mycobacteria, *Helicobacter pylori*, and various opportunistic bacteria. A few of these are described in the following sections.

2.2.1. ESCHERICHIA COLI O157:H7

This Gram-negative bacterium is an enterohemorrhagic strain of *E. coli*, which was first isolated in 1982 *(16)*. It produces a shiga-like toxin and causes diarrhea characterized by bloody stools, especially in children and the elderly. If left untreated, the infection may lead (in 5–10% of patients) to hemolytic uremic syndrome, a form of kidney damage that is potentially fatal to children and other susceptible individuals *(17)*. This bacterium is ubiquitous in cattle farms, where it can persist for years *(18)*. The infection is often spread through contaminated foods, such as hamburger meat *(19)*. Waterborne transmission has also been documented, often in cases in which cow manure contamination of water occurred *(20,21)*. The organism can also survive for at least 6 mo in water, contributing to its ability to contaminate potable water *(18)*. In addition, human carriers can serve as a source for *E. coli* O157:H7 by shedding the bacteria in their feces, and the infection is then transmitted by the fecal-oral route. Of those individuals who experienced the clinical disease, young children reportedly shed the bacteria for longer periods after resolution of symptoms than do older children and adults *(22)*. The severity of illness affects the shedding duration.

Municipal wastewater may possibly act as a reservoir for *E. coli* O157:H7 in the environment because sewage contains high *E. coli* concentrations even after conventional treatment, and treated wastewater is often discharged into rivers that are used for recreational activities *(23)*. Few studies have examined the survival of *E. coli* O157:H7 in wastewater and its fate during wastewater treatment. This bacterium can survive, and even grow, in wastewater over a wide temperature range (10–29°C) *(24)*. Detectable levels of the cells survived for extended periods (ranging from 49 to 84 d) in river water at 25°C, and some of these cells can enter a nonculturable (i.e., undetectable) state in water *(25)*.

2.2.2. *AEROMONAS HYDROPHILA*

This Gram-negative bacterium is present in fish and an opportunistic human pathogen commonly occurring in surface waters supplying municipal drinking water systems *(26,27)*. It is increasingly recognized as an emerging waterborne pathogen, causing hemorrhagic septicemia or red sore disease in fish, and it was recently placed on the US Environmental Protection Agency (EPA) Contaminant Candidate List. As an opportunistic human pathogen, it causes water-associated wound infections and has often been isolated from patients with diarrhea in the absence of other enteric pathogens, which suggests that it has some involvement in human intestinal illnesses *(28,29)*. In drinking water, the main concern is that *A. hydrophila* may become part of the biofilm, thus, potentially leading to future waterborne outbreaks *(28,30)*. Studies conducted in Europe, Asia, and North America have reported widespread presence of *Aeromonas* in water distribution systems *(26,27,29,31–34)*.

2.2.3. MYCOBACTERIA

Atypical mycobacteria, such as *Mycobacterium avium/M. intracellulare* (MAC), are common soil and water bacteria that cause secondary infections in patients with AIDS and other individuals who are compromised. In patients who are immunocompromised, the infection is often disseminated throughout the body *(35)*. In other patients, such as the elderly and people with predisposing lung conditions, it causes pulmonary infections *(36)*. MAC was recently placed on the EPA Contaminant Candidate List. These bacteria are often present in drinking water, where they grow as part of the biofilm on pipe surfaces *(37)*.

2.3. Viral Pathogens

More than 140 different viral pathogens may contaminate water and wastewater, causing various types of infection, such as intestinal diseases (e.g., Norwalk agent, rotaviruses, echoviruses), respiratory diseases (e.g., adenoviruses, coxsackieviruses), skin rash (echoviruses), aseptic meningitis (e.g., coxsackieviruses, echoviruses), hepatitis (hepatitis A virus), and paralysis (e.g., polioviruses) *(38)*. One of the problems associated with viral contamination of water is the difficulty in isolating and detecting the viral agents from drinking water. Viruses are often present in small numbers and, in addition, most of them difficult to culture in vitro. Therefore, large sample volumes must be processed and analyzed for verification of their presence. However, with recent advances in molecular technology, detection has become easier.

3. DRINKING WATER TREATMENT AND DISTRIBUTION

3.1. Overview of Water Treatment

Most surface and groundwater sources used to supply potable water contain microbial and/or chemical contaminants. It is, therefore, essential to adequately treat water to minimize the health risk associated with its consumption. The treatment often includes source protection (or watershed management), which typically involves physical barriers to minimize animal and human activities, as well as regulations to restrict urban/industrial/agricultural wastewater discharges into source water. These regulations may also restrict recreational activities (swimming and boating, etc.) in source water.

In addition to source protection, water treatment plants are designed to inactivate and/ or remove most water pollutants. Most water treatment facilities use a conventional multibarrier treatment approach, commonly referred to as "conventional water treatment plants." In the United States, more than 100 million people receive their water from such plants *(38)*. Water treatment may vary from plant to plant but typically includes a preliminary treatment that consists of screening large particles. Often, chlorine (prechlorination) or an alternative disinfectant is also applied directly to raw water. Although prechlorination does achieve microbial removal, its main purpose is typically to minimize taste and odor problems *(39)*. Preliminary treatment is followed by coagulation and flocculation. Coagulation rapidly mixes water with a coagulant (aluminum sulfate, or ferric chloride). Flocculation is a slow mixing of water and the coagulant to form the floc, an agglomeration of small colloidal particles (which contain microorganisms as well as organic material) *(39)*. Sedimentation (or clarification) is the next step, in which settable solids (such as the floc) sediment by gravity in large sedimentation basins. Remaining suspended solids (including microorganisms) are removed by filtration. Typical filters used for water treatment consist of granular material, such as sand, anthracite, granulated activated carbon, and garnet sand *(40)*. Recently introduced is the new technology of membrane filtration, which shows great potential, especially for the removal of many microbial contaminants. The use of membranes is expected to increase in the future *(41)*. After filtration, the water then undergoes a final disinfection, often termed secondary disinfection, using chlorine (postchlorination) or an alternate disinfectant. This is further discussed below in the next section. At this stage, fluoride is also added to water to maintain the optimal levels needed for resistance to tooth decay *(42)*.

3.2. Disinfection

Disinfection is the inactivation of infectious microorganisms by adding a chemical disinfectant to water. The ideal water disinfectant should inactivate pathogenic microorganisms within a practical time period and over a range of water quality, be nontoxic to humans at the required doses, be palatable at required concentrations, persist in a water distribution system and maintain a residual concentration to prevent bacterial regrowth and contamination by infiltration, and be easy and inexpensive to measure and use.

In a water treatment plant, disinfection is typically the last barrier in water purification, and its main purpose is to achieve a reduction in pathogen numbers *(43)*. As mentioned, disinfectants are also often used where raw water enters the water purification plant (prechlorination). The use of chlorine in water treatment began early in the 20th century and remains the most widespread disinfectant in the water industry *(43)*. Other chemical disinfectants (or alternative disinfection strategies) include chloramination, ozonation, chlorine dioxide, and ultraviolet irradiation, this latter method being a physical means of achieving disinfection. Free chlorine remains the dominant choice for disinfection in North America, whereas monochloramine is the most common alternative to free chlorine. Each technology has some advantages under certain conditions. It is recognized, however, that with the exception of ozone, the use of chemical disinfectants alone may not be adequate to inactivate enough protozoan parasites in water to prevent waterborne outbreaks.

In the past decade, especially as *C. parvum* became recognized as a ubiquitous waterborne pathogen, research has focused on finding alternative disinfectants or disinfection methods that will provide more efficient inactivation of this protozoan parasite during water treatment, because oocysts can survive and remain infectious in chlorinated drinking water *(3)*. One of these alternative disinfectants is chlorine dioxide, which is a stronger oxidant than free chlorine. When using chlorine, the product disinfectant concentration and contact time (*Ct* values) must be at least 7000 mg · min/L to inactivate $2 \log_{10}$ (99%) of *C. parvum (44)*. Much lower *Ct* values are required when using chlorine dioxide to obtain similar levels of inactivation *(9)*. Among the other advantages attributed to chlorine dioxide is that it does not form many halogenated, and potentially carcinogenic, DBPs, which are typically associated with free chlorine. Chlorine dioxide does, however, react to form chlorite and chlorate *(45)*. The US EPA maximum contaminant level for chlorite is 1.0 mg/L.

Monochloramine (NH_2Cl) is produced when hypochlorous acid (HOCl) from chlorine reacts with ammonia (NH_3). Monochloramine is a less effective disinfectant than free chlorine; however, it is effective in controlling biofilms in distribution systems *(43)*. Its use is often recommended as a secondary disinfectant in systems having extensive biofilm problems *(46)*.

Ozone (O_3) was first used for water disinfection in Europe in 1906 *(47)*. Ozone forms free radicals in water, which inactivate microorganisms by affecting enzyme activity and DNA. Ozone is now more commonly used in North America as an alternative to chlorine for two reasons: (1) the recognition in the 1970s that chlorination leads to the formation of DBPs, and (2) the recent recognition of waterborne cryptosporidiosis as a major health problem, and the resistance of its causative agent to chlorine. Using ozone is one of the most efficient ways to inactivate parasites, such as *C. parvum*, during water treatment *(44,48)*. Its use, however, remains limited because of the cost of the technology.

In the past 5 yr, ultraviolet light (UV) has proved effective at inactivating significant levels of microorganisms in water, including protozoan parasites *(49)*. DNA molecules absorb light energy in the wavelength of 240–280 nm, and the resulting DNA damage is often in the form of dimerization of thymine molecules, which leads to lethal mutations. UV has many additional advantages, such as it is noncorrosive with no need for storage of toxic chemicals. UV irradiation also produces no known DBPs. Finally, it is relatively low maintenance, although fouling of the lamps can be a problem. Its use is expected to increase.

3.3. Water Distribution Systems

After treatment at the plant, drinking water is then distributed to consumers through a series of pipes and water reservoirs (e.g., water towers). This is known as the water distribution system, in which various problems may arise, leading to decreased water quality. The chemical disinfectant may react with various materials in the distribution system and be eliminated or reduced to a low level, thereby allowing microorganisms to survive. Bacterial regrowth may lead to deterioration of water quality, amplification of corrosion, generation of bad tastes and odors, and/or proliferation of macroinvertebrates *(50–55)*, and risk of gastroenteritis *(56)*. Biofilms that are present in distribution systems provide a range of environments for microorganisms, including aerobic and anaerobic sites. Biofilms are initially formed when encapsulated glycocalyx-producing bacteria become attached to the pipe wall or tubercle of a distribution system. These populations attract other microorganisms that can extract nutrients from by-products released by the metabolism of the biofilm members. Therefore, the site may become more diversified over time and develop mechanisms that resist disinfection. Biofilm control (typically an adequate disinfectant residual concentration in the distribution system) is now recognized as an important part of the operation of drinking water plants and distribution systems.

In addition to biofilm formation, distribution systems may be affected by microbial intrusion. Causes of such events can include uncovered reservoirs, improper water main repairs, cross connections, and transient negative pressures coupled with leaks. However, there is little information about the frequency of occurrence or the volume of contaminated water that can infiltrate distribution systems.

3.4. Disinfection By-Products and Cancer

The use of chemical disinfectants in water treatment also produces undesirable organic molecules known as DBPs. Some of these chemicals cause cancers in laboratory animals, and they are suspected carcinogens in humans as well *(57,58)*. Nevertheless, these chemical disinfectants are essential to provide good quality water and to minimize the biologic risk. "The risk of death from known pathogens in untreated water appears to be at least 100 to 1000 times greater than the risk of cancer from known DBPs in chlorinated drinking water," and the risk of illness from pathogens is at least 10,000 to 1 million times greater *(59)*. Trihalomethanes (THMs) and haloacetic acids (HAAs) are the most common DBPs detected when using chlorine for water disinfection *(60,61)*. THMs include chloroform, dibromochloromethane, bromodichloromethane, and bromoform, which are all considered potential human carcinogens at high doses or for long exposures *(60)*. HAAs include at least nine water-soluble chemicals. One of them, dichloroacetic acid, is also a probable human carcinogen, but tests in laboratory animals indicate that this would occur only in large doses.

An additional issue that is of great concern to certain water utilities is *N*-nitrosodimethylamine (NDMA) formation. The US EPA identifies NDMA as a probable human carcinogen. Its formation has been observed during treatment of drinking water *(62)* and, as such, has recently been considered to be a DBP. The mechanisms of NDMA formation and destruction are not yet understood. Once present in the aqueous environment, NDMA is relatively recalcitrant. Due to the likelihood of its carcinogenicity, regulatory limits are being set for NDMA concentrations in drinking water. For example, in California, a temporary action level of 0.02 µg/L was established in November 1999.

3.5. Regulations

In the United States, drinking water regulations are established by the EPA and were originally detailed in the Safe Drinking Water Act (SDWA) of 1974, which was amended in 1986 and 1996. The requirements for distribution system disinfectant residuals and microbial contaminants are regulated by the Surface Water Treatment Rule (SWTR), which was promulgated in June 1989. Because certain viruses and protozoa are more resistant to disinfection than bacteria, the SWTR increased disinfection requirements by incorporating strict inactivation criteria. Among others, the SWTR outlines distribution system disinfection requirements (secondary disinfection) to inactivate microbiologic pathogens for systems using surface water sources. For example, *Cryptosporidium* removal/inactivation must be at least 99%, whereas *G. lamblia* and enteric viruses must be removed/inactivated by 99.9% and 99.99%, respectively.

Under the SWTR, a measurable disinfectant residual must be maintained in the distribution system, or alternatively, heterotrophic bacterial counts must be less than 500 CFU/mL, in at least 95% of the samples from the distribution system each month, for any 2 consecutive mo. In Canada, similar criteria have recently been adopted by the Ontario Ministry of the Environment after a waterborne outbreak of *E. coli* O157:H7 in Walkerton. Ontario utilities using free chlorine must maintain at least 0.2 mg/L and, at most, 4 mg/L of free chlorine at all locations in the distribution system, whereas utilities applying chloramines must maintain at least 1 mg/L and, at most, 3 mg/L of chloramines at all locations *(63)*. In the United States, the Total Coliform Rule requires that a minimum disinfectant residual of 0.2 mg/L for free chlorine and 0.5 mg/L for chloramines be present throughout the distribution system. The 1996 amendments of the SDWA require the EPA to develop a series of rules to provide protection against microbial pathogens, while ensuring there are no health risks from DBPs. This led to the Disinfectants/Disinfection By-products (D/DBP) Rule, which established maximum residual disinfectant levels of 4.0 mg/L for chlorine or chloramine and 0.8 mg/L for chlorine dioxide.

3.6. Risk of Disease

Quantitative risk assessment for *Giardia* and enteric viruses are defined in the SWTR. The requirements are supposed to reduce *Giardia* cysts and enteric viruses to such low levels that the annual risk of giardiasis or enteric virus infection is < 1 in 10,000 (10^{-4}) per person *(64)*. This risk assessment analysis is based on: (1) the expected concentrations of *Giardia* cysts and viruses in surface sourcewater, (2) dose–response relationships (derived from human volunteer studies) for human infection from ingesting these microorganisms, and (3) required water treatment to reduce *Giardia* cysts and enteric viruses by 99.9% and 99.99%, respectively *(65)*.

The actual risk of enteric illness from drinking treated water from a surface water source was assessed in a series of epidemiologic studies now known as the "Payment studies" *(56,66)*. These studies were conducted in Laval (Canada), north of Montreal. The source of drinking water for the city is the "des Prairies" River, which is sewage contaminated. The water is treated using conventional treatment with ozonation. The studies compared intestinal illness rates in two sets of households (four sets in the second study; approx 300 households/set). One set used ordinary tap water, whereas the other set used reverse osmosis-filtered water in which pathogens were completely removed. In the second study (in 1997), a third set of households used distribution system tap water, whereas the fourth set used treated water bottled at water treatment plant and supplied to each household on a regular basis *(56)*. The results of these two studies revealed that intestinal illness rates were approx 25–35% (approx 15% in the second study) higher in tap water households. A dose-response relationship was seen, whereby increased intestinal illness was related to increased tap water consumption. These results were obtained, even though no pathogens were detected in tap water, which met all regular standards for quality, including coliform bacteria and turbidity *(56,66)*.

4. WATERBORNE OUTBREAKS OF INFECTIOUS DISEASES

As discussed, water treatment is an extensive process, which is highly regulated and monitored. Despite these facts, and for various reasons, water treatment is sometimes inadequate and waterborne outbreaks of disease occur. Waterborne outbreaks, especially the most severe ones, have sometimes served as a basis for the development of new technologies and/or new or improved regulations.

In the United States from 1971 to 1994, 740 waterborne outbreaks of disease were reported, affecting at least 571,000 individuals *(67)*. This total includes 403,000 cases from a single outbreak of cryptosporidiosis. The most recent data for the United States is for 1997–1998, in which 13 states reported 17 waterborne outbreaks of disease, causing an estimated 2038 persons to become ill *(2)*. Three recent examples of waterborne outbreaks of disease are discussed in the following sections. They illustrate various problems that may arise, depending on the nature of the treatment and the source of water used.

4.1. Walkerton (Canada)

In spring 2000, an outbreak of *E. coli* 0157:H7 occurred in Walkerton, Ontario; its source was the municipal drinking water *(21)*. This was the first such documented outbreak in Canada. The water supply was contaminated by agricultural wastes. Recent literature suggests that under certain water quality conditions, *E. coli* O157:H7 in the distribution system may be resistant to chlorination up to 0.5 mg/L *(68)*. However, another study indicated that *E. coli* O157:H7 isolates from cattle are sensitive to chlorination and are similar in resistance to that of wild-type *E. coli* isolates *(69)*.

Walkerton is a community of approx 5000 people. When the outbreak occurred, the town was obtaining its water from three groundwater wells with chlorination units. Two of these wells were in operation at that time *(70)*. Chlorination was the sole means of treatment of the groundwater. Overall, 1346 cases of gastroenteritis were reported, with an estimated number of cases to be more than 2300, and 65 patients requiring hospitalization *(70)*. The presence of *E. coli* O157:H7 was confirmed in 167 stool samples. Twenty-seven people developed hemolytic uremic syndrome, and six died *(70)*. Molecular analysis performed on water samples collected during the first few days of the outbreak confirmed the presence of *E. coli* O157:H7 in the water supply. In addition, historic data later indicated that one of the wells (well 5) was commonly subjected to contamination from surface water and high turbidity *(70)*. Apparently, heavy rains, due to an unusual storm in mid-May, washed infected cow manure into one of the municipal groundwater wells, triggering contamination of the whole distribution system and the onset of the epidemic. This was confirmed when the same type of *E. coli* O157:H7 was found in both human stools and cattle from a farm adjacent to well 5 *(70)*. Hydro-geologic data have since shown that rainwater drained from the cattle toward well 5. Because the water was simply chlorinated without additional treatment, the large amount of contamination could not be adequately treated in the distribution system.

This tragic incident is a warning signal that groundwater sources used for municipal water system must be better protected. Groundwater has always been considered a reasonably safe water source; that is why towns such as Walkerton simply use chlorination without additional treatment. In light of this outbreak, future regulation in Canada must address this issue.

4.2. Milwaukee, WI, United States

The most important waterborne outbreak of gastrointestinal (GI) disease ever documented occurred in Milwaukee, Wisconsin, in spring 1993. The outbreak eventually caused an estimated 403,000 cases, with approx 50 deaths, many of them individuals who were immunocompromised *(71)*. The disease was initially believed to be viral gastroenteritis. It was reported to the State Health Department on April 5, 1993, diagnosed on April 7, and followed by an advisory note that evening to the public to boil all drinking water. Records showed an increase in turbidity of the water produced by the southern water treatment plant from March 23 until April 9, when the southern plant was closed *(71)*. Stool analysis, as well as analysis of ice made from water in southern Milwaukee, revealed the presence of *C. parvum (71)*. An epidemiologic survey of nursing home residents showed that residents of the southern part of the city were 14 times more likely to have had diarrhea than residents of the northern part of the city, who received tap water from a different water treatment plant. The mean duration of illness was 12 d, and the average maximum number of watery diarrheal stools was 19 per day at the peak of illness. Watery diarrhea was the predominant symptom in most confirmed cases. However, other symptoms, such as abdominal pain, low-grade fever, weight loss, and vomiting, were also frequently observed *(71)*. The Milwaukee outbreak clearly demonstrated that waterborne cryptosporidiosis can result in a significant number of deaths, especially among individuals who are immunocompromised and immunonaive *(72)*.

An investigation showed that several factors may have contributed to water contamination, allowing the parasite to pass through the water treatment process. First, before the outbreak occurred, increased rainfall caused increased lake water turbidity and bacterial counts in Lake Michigan (the source water) *(73)*. Concurrently, the southern plant effluent (treated water) had a turbidity reading of 2.5 ntu, which is high *(73)*. Presumably, lake currents were responsible for contaminating the southern plant. In addition, the Milwaukee area has various environmental sources (dairy farms, wildlife, and human sewage) that could have contributed to the contamination of lake water. Finally, aluminum sulfate was the coagulant used until August 1992, when the plant started using polyaluminum chloride (PACl) *(73)*. Coagulant dosage was adjusted as needed based on laboratory results, but, because PACl had been used for less than a year, the historical records had not yet been developed *(73)*.

After the outbreak, Milwaukee implemented the use of ozonation at both plants. It also became obvious in Milwaukee, and elsewhere, that adequate particle (turbidity) monitoring must become part of water treatment. Nationwide, the Milwaukee outbreak was the trigger for an intensive research effort on *Cryptosporidium* and waterborne cryptosporidiosis and eventually led to the new regulations described.

4.3. Victoria (Canada)

The first documented waterborne outbreak of toxoplasmosis occurred in Victoria, British Columbia, Canada, in 1995. More than 220,000 residents receive treated water from the Humpback reservoir and distribution system *(74)*. In March 1995, several cases of acute toxoplasmosis were diagnosed in the greater Victoria area *(74)*. In total, 100 people, aged 6 to 83 yr, were diagnosed with the condition, and the estimated number of cases was between 2894 and 7718. In the 5 yr before this outbreak, no cases had been diagnosed in the area *(74)*. An epidemiologic study eliminated the most common sources of toxoplasmosis (unpasteurized milk, game meat, raw meat, sausage, and hamburger, etc.). A closer look at the data showed that the epidemic curve was bimodal, peaking in December 1994 and March 1995. In both cases, heavy rainfalls and increased reservoir water turbidity were noted before the outbreaks *(74)*. Domestic and wild cats, including cougars, are in the watershed and have access to the reservoir, which is not protected. Many of the captured animals were positive for *Toxoplasma*. Little is known about the environmental fate of *Toxoplasma* oocysts, as well as their resistance to disinfection. These oocysts are, however, similar to *Cryptosporidium* oocysts. It is, therefore, possible that they are also resistant to chlorine. Water treatment for Greater Victoria does not include filtration, and disinfection is accomplished with chloramines, a weaker chemical than chlorine. It is likely that contamination of the reservoir occurred during heavy rainfall and that the water treatment in Victoria was not adequate to remove or inactivate these protozoan parasites.

5. CONCLUSION

When a conventional water treatment plant is properly operated and maintained, the risk of disease to humans is minimized to an acceptable level (1 in 10^{-4} risk). Since the Safe Drinking Water Act was passed in the United States in 1974, regulations are now in place to promote and improve water treatment. Moreover, a lot of research is currently directed at balancing both biologic and chemical risks associated with the consumption of treated and disinfected water. However, as seen in the previous section, waterborne outbreaks of disease do occur but are often associated with either a failure in water treatment or an excessive pathogen load due to unexpected factors (unusually heavy rainfalls or domestic or wild animals in the watershed, etc.). A water treatment failure may be related to a problem during the operation of the plant (inadequate coagulation, faulty filters, improper disinfectant dosage) or a plant design issue (such as water treatment facilities that do not use filtration). Other issues that may affect water quality are aging infrastructure as well as increased urbanization, which puts additional stress on water resources (reservoirs and rivers, etc.).

An emerging issue for water treatment plant operators and managers is the risk of bioterrorism. Most experts agree that reservoirs are an unlikely target for bioterrorists and conventional water processes are considered effective against most biologic agents *(75)*. Chlorine, for example, would inactivate most, if not all, viral and bacterial agents. Additionally, the large quantity of water in most cities would significantly dilute a biologic agent, limiting its potential to cause harm. Potential danger may exist with the use of protozoan parasites, but these would have to be introduced in large amounts in systems that do not currently employ full conventional treatment.

6. MAIN POINTS FOR PRIMARY AND CLINICAL REVIEW

1. Tap water in both Third World and industrialized nations can become contaminated with protozoan, bacterial, and viral agents from various sources.
2. Water is disinfected by a variety of methods, including chlorine, ozone, and the use of UV light.
3. Some of these methods may have human health effects, although the health risk from untreated water is far greater.
4. Distribution systems represent a primary source by which microorganisms may be introduced into tap water after disinfection.
5. Recent large-scale water-borne infections in the United States and Canada include those mediated by *Escherichia coli*, *Cryptosporidium parvum*, and *Toxoplasma*.

REFERENCES

1. Snow J. On the Mode of Communication of Cholera, 2nd Ed. John Churchill, London, UK, 1855.
2. Barwick R, Levy D, Craun G, Calderon R. Surveillance for waterborne disease outbreaks—United States, 1997–1998. Morb Mortal Wkly Rep 2000;49(SS04):1–35.
3. Chauret C, Nolan K, Chen P, Springthorpe S, Sattar S. Aging of *Cryptosporidium parvum* in river water and their susceptibility to disinfection by chlorine and monochloramine. Can J Microbiol 1998;44: 1154–1160.
4. Chauret C, Springthorpe S, Sattar S. Fate of *Cryptosporidium* oocysts, *Giardia* cysts and microbial indicators during wastewater treatment and anaerobic sludge digestion. Can J Microbiol 1999; 45:257–262.
5. Fayer R. *Cryptosporidium* and *Cryptosporidiosis*. CRC Press, New York, 1999.
6. Bednarska M, Bajer A, Sinski, E. Calves as a potential reservoir of *Cryptosporidium parvum* and *Giardia* sp. Ann Agr Environ Microbiol 1998;5:135–138.
7. Casemore DP. Epidemiological aspects of human cryptosporidiosis. Epidemiol Infect 1990;104:1–28.
8. Finch GR, Black EK, Gyurek LG, Belosevic M. Ozone inactivation of *Cryptosporidium parvum* in demand-free phosphate buffer determined by in vitro excystation and animal infectivity. Appl Environ Microbiol 1993;59:4203–4210.
9. Chauret C, Radziminski C, LePuil M, Creason R, Andrews RC. Chlorine dioxide inactivation of *Cryptosporidium parvum* oocysts and bacterial spore indicators. Appl Environ Microbiol 2001;67: 2993–3001.
10. Hibler CP, Hancock CM. Waterborne giardiasis. In: Drinking Water Microbiology. McFeters GC (ed.). Springer-Verlag, New York, NY, 1990, pp. 271–293.
11. Fayer R, Ungar BLP. Cryptosporidium sp. and cryptosporidiosis. Microb Rev 1986;50:458–483.
12. Dubey JP, Speer CA, Fayer R. *Cryptosporidiosis* of man and animals. CRC Press, Boca Raton, FL, 1990.
13. Jones JL, Lopez A, Wilson M, Shulkin J, Gibbs R. Congenital toxoplasmosis: a review. Obstet Gynecol Surv 2001;56:296–305.
14. Leport C, Duval X. Toxoplasmosis, cerebral and AIDS-related opportunistic infections. Rev Prat 1999; 49:2271–2274.
15. Lanjewar DN, Surve KV, Maheshwari MB, Shenoy BP, Hira SK. Toxoplasmosis of the central nervous system in the acquired immunodeficiency syndrome. Int J Pathol Microbiol 1998;41:147–151.
16. Riley L, Remis R, Helgerson S, et al. Hemorrhagic colitis associated with a rare *Escherichia coli* serotype. N Engl J Med 1983;308:681–685.
17. Boyce TG, Swerdlow DL, Griffin PM. *Escherichia coli* O157:H7 and the hemolytic-uremic syndrome. N Engl J Med 1995;333:364–368.
18. Hancock D, Besser T, Lejeune J, Davis M, Rice D. The control of VTEC in the animal reservoir. Int J Food Microbiol 2001;66:71–78.
19. Willshaw GA, Thirlwell J, Jones AP, Parry S, Salmon RL, Hickey M. Vero cytotoxin-producing *Escherichia coli* O157 in beefburgers linked to an outbreak of diarrhoea, haemorrhagic colitis and haemolytic uraemic syndrome in Britain. Lett Appl Microbiol 1994;19:304–307.
20. Swerdlow DL, Woodruff BA, Brady RC, et al. A waterborne outbreak in Missouri of *Escherichia coli* O157:H7 associated with bloody diarrhea and death. Ann Intern Med 1992;117:812–819.
21. Waterborne outbreak of gastroenteritis associated with a contaminated municipal water supply, Walkerton, Ontario, Canada, May–June 2000. Can Comm Dis Rep 2000;26:170–173.
22. Belongia EA, Osterholm MT, Soler JT, Ammend DA, Braun JE, MacDonald KL. Transmission of *Escherichia coli* O157:H7 infection in Minnesota child day-care facilities. JAMA 1993;269:883–888.
23. Martin MT, Rivera IG, Clark DL, Olson BH. Detection of virulence factors in culturable *Escherichia coli* isolates from water samples by DNA probes and recovery of toxin-bearing strains in minimal o-nitrophenol-β-D-galactopyranoside-4-methylumbelliferyl-β-D-glucuronide media. Appl Environ Microbiol 1992;58:3095–3100.
24. Rajkowski KT, Rice EW. Recovery and survival of *Escherichia coli* O157:H7 in reconditioned pork-processing wastewater. J Food Prot 1999;62:731–734.
25. Wang G, Doyle MP. Survival of enterohemorrhagic *Escherichia coli* O157:H7 in water. J Food Protect 1998;61:662–667.

26. Kühn I, Allestam G, Huys G, et al. Diversity, persistence, and virulence of *Aeromonas* strains isolated from drinking water distribution systems in Sweden. Appl Environ Microbiol 1997;63:2708–2715.

27. Huys G, Kampfer P, Altweeg M, et al. *Aeromonas popoffii* sp. nov., a mesophilic bacterium isolated from drinking water production plants and reservoirs. Intern J System Bacteriol 1997;47:1165–1171.

28. Krovacek K, Faris A, Baloda S, Lindberg T, Peterz M, Månsson I. Isolation and virulence profiles of *Aeromonas* spp. from different municipal drinking water supplies in Sweden. Food Microbiol 1992;9: 215–222.

29. Hanninen ML, Salmi S, Mattila L, Taipalinen R, Siitonen A. Association of *Aeromonas* spp. with travellers' diarrhoea in Finland. J Med Microbiol 1995;42:26–31.

30. Burke V, Robinson J, Gracey M, Peterson M, Partridge K. Isolation of *Aeromonas hydrophila* from a metropolitan water supply: seasonal correlation with clinical isolates. Appl Environ Microbiol 1984;48: 361–368.

31. Havelaar AH, Versteegh JFM, During M. The presence of *Aeromonas* in drinking water supplies in the Netherlands. Zentralblatt Hygiene 1987;190:236–256.

32. Stelzer W, Jacob J, Feuerpfeil I, Schulze E. The occurrence of aeromonads in a drinking water. Zentralblatt Mikrobiol 1992;147:231-235.

33. Alavandi SV, Subashini MS, Ananthan S. Occurrence of haemolytic and cytotoxic *Aeromonas* species in domestic water supplies in Chenai. Indian J Med Res 1999;110:50-55.

34. Chauret C, Creason R, Jarosh J, Volk C, Robinson J, Warnes C. Detection of *Aeromonas hydrophila* in a drinking water distribution system: a field and pilot study. Can J Microbiol 2001;47:782–786.

35. Hoover DR, Graham NM, Bacellar H, et al. An epidemiologic analysis of *Mycobacterium avium* complex disease in homosexual men infected with human immunodeficiency virus type I. Clin Infect Dis 1994;20:1250–1258.

36. Contreras AM, Chung OT, Sanders DE, Goldstein RS. Pulmonary infection with nontuberculosis mycobacteria. Am Rev Respir Dis 1988;137:149–152.

37. Falkinham JO, Norton CD, LeChevallier MW. Factors influencing numbers of *Mycobacterium avium*, *Mycobacterium intracellulare*, and other mycobacteria in drinking water distribution systems. Appl Environ Microbiol 2001;67:1225–1231.

38. Bitton G. Wastewater Microbiology. Wiley-Liss, New York, NY, 1999.

39. American Water Works Association. Water Treatment, 2nd Ed. AWWA Press, Denver, CO, 1995.

40. Cleasby JL, Logsdon GS. Granular bed and precoat filtration. In: Water Quality and Treatment, 5th Ed. Letterman RD (ed.). McGraw-Hill, New York, NY, 1999, pp. 8.1–8.99.

41. Taylor JS. Membranes. In: Water Quality and Treatment, 5th Ed. Letterman RD, (ed.). McGraw-Hill, New York, NY, 1999, pp. 11.1–11.71.

42. Reeves TG. Water fluoridation. In: Water Quality and Treatment, 5th Ed. Letterman RD (ed.). McGraw-Hill, New York, NY, 1999, pp. 15.1–15.19.

43. Haas CN. Disinfection. In: Water Quality and Treatment, 5th Ed. Letterman RD (ed.). McGraw-Hill, New York, NY, 1999, pp.14.1–14.60.

44. Korich DG, Mead JR, Madore MS, Sinclair NA, Sterling CR. Effects of ozone, chlorine dioxide, chlorine and monochloramine on *Cryptosporidium parvum* oocyst viability. Appl Environ Microbiol 1990;56:1423–1428.

45. Lykins BW, Koffskey WE, Patterson KS. Alternative disinfectants for drinking water treatment. J Envir Eng 1994;120:745–758.

46. LeChevallier MW, Lowry CH, Lee RG. Disinfecting biofilm in a model distribution system. J Am Water Works Assoc 1990;82:85–99.

47. White GC. Handbook of Chlorination and Alternate Disinfectants, 2nd Ed. Van Nostrand Reinhold, New York, NY, 1992.

48. Finch GR, Black EK, Gyurek LG, Belosevic M. Ozone inactivation of *Cryptosporidium parvum* in demand-free phosphate buffer determined by in vitro excystation and animal infectivity. Appl Environ Microbiol 1993;59:4203–4210.

49. Bukhari Z, Hargy T, Clancy J. Medium-pressure UV for oocyst inactivation. J Am Water Works Assoc 1999;91:86–94.

50. O'Connor JT, Hash L, Edwards AB. Deterioration of water quality in distribution systems. J Am Water Works Assoc 1975;67:113–116.

51. Gerber NN. Volatile substances from actinomyces: their role in odor pollution of water. Crit Rev Microbiol 1979;7:191–214.
52. Mitcham RP, Shelley MW, Wheadon CM. Free chlorine versus ammonia-chlorine: disinfection, trihalomethane formation, and zooplankton removal. J Am Water Works Assoc 1983;75:196–198.
53. Volk C, Joret JC. Paramètres prédictifs de l'apparition des coliformes dans les réseaux de distribution d'eau d'alimentation. Sci Eau 1994;7:131–152.
54. LeChevallier MW, Welch NJ, Smith DB. Full-scale studies of factors related to coliform regrowth in drinking water. Appl Environ Microbiol 1996;62:2201–2211.
55. Geldreich EE. Microbial quality of water supply in distribution system. CRC Press, Boca Raton, FL, 1996.
56. Payment P, Siemiatycki J, Richardson L, Renaud G, Franco E, Prévost M. A prospective epidemiological study of gastrointestinal health effects due to the consumption of drinking water. Intern J Environ Health Res 1997;7:5–31.
57. Cantor KP, Lynch CF, Hildesheim ME, et al. Drinking water source and chlorination byproducts. I. Risk of bladder cancer. Epidemiology 1998;9:7–8.
58. Hildesheim ME, Cantor KP, Lynch CF, et al. Drinking water source and chlorination byproducts. II. Risk of colon and rectal cancers. Epidemiology 1998;9:29–35.
59. Regli S. Risk vs. risk: proposed decision tree for drinking water management. Health Envir Digest 1993; 7:3–6.
60. Cohn PD, Cox M, Berger PS. Health and aesthetic aspects of water quality. In: Water Quality and Treatment, 5th Ed. Letterman RD (ed.). McGraw-Hill, New York, NY, 1999, pp. 2.1–2.86.
61. Werderhoff KS, Singer PC. Chlorine dioxide effects on THMFP, TOXFP, and the formation of inorganic by-products. J Am Water Works Assoc 1987;79:107–113.
62. Najm I, Trussell RR. NMDA formation in water and wastewater. J Am Water Works Assoc 2001;93: 92–99.
63. Ontario Drinking Water Standard. Government of Ontario PIBS #4065e, 2001.
64. Regli S, Rose JB, Haas CN, Gerba CP. Modeling the risk from *Giardia* and viruses in drinking water. J Am Water Works Assoc 1991;83:76–84.
65. Rose JB, Haas CN, Regli S. Risk assessment and control of waterborne giardiasis. Am J Pub Health 1991;81:709–713.
66. Payment P, Franco E, Richardson L, Siemiatycki J. Gastrointestinal health effects associated with the consumption of drinking water produced by point-of-use domestic reverse-osmosis filtration units. Appl Environ Microbiol 1991;57:945–948.
67. Kramer MH, Herwaldt BL, Craun GF, Calderon RL, Juranek DD. Surveillance for waterborne-disease outbreaks: United States, 1993–1994. Mort Morb Wkly Rep 1996;45:1–33.
68. Lisle JT, Broadway SC, Prescott AM, Pyle BH, Fricker C, McFeters GA. Effects of starvation on physiological activity and chlorine disinfection resistance in *Escherichia coli* O157:H7. Appl Environ Microbiol 1998:64:4658–4662.
69. Rice EW, Clark RM, Johnson CH. Chlorine inactivation of *Escherichia coli* O157:H7. Emerg Infect Dis 1999;5:461–463.
70. The investigative report of the Walkerton outbreak of waterborne gastroenteritis. Bruce-Grey-Owen Sound Health Unit, Owen Sound, Ontario, Canada, 2000.
71. McKenzie WR, Hoxie, NJ, Neil J, et al. A massive outbreak in Milwaukee of cryptosporidium infection transmitted through the public water supply. N Engl J Med 1994;331:161–167.
72. Hoxie NJ, Davis JP, Vergeront JM, Nashold RD, Blair KA. Cryptosporidiosis-associated mortality following a massive waterborne outbreak in Milwaukee, Wisconsin. Am J Public Health 1997;12: 2032–2035.
73. Fox KM, Lytle DA. Milwaukee's *Cryptosporidium* outbreak: investigation and recommendations. J Am Water Works Assoc 1996;88:87–94.
74. Bowie WR, King AS, Werker DH, et al. Outbreak of toxoplasmosis associated with municipal drinking water. Lancet 1997;350:173–177.
75. Burrows WD, Renner SE. Biological warfare agents as threats to potable water. Environ Health Persp 1999;107:975–984.

IX MARKETING AND HEALTH ISSUES OF SOFT DRINKS

24 Liquid Candy

How Soft Drinks Harm the Health of Americans

Michael F. Jacobson

In 1942, production in the United States of carbonated soft drinks was approximately sixty 12-oz servings per person. The American Medical Association's (AMA's) Council on Foods and Nutrition *(1)* warned:

From the health point of view it is desirable especially to have restriction of such use of sugar as is represented by consumption of sweetened carbonated beverages and forms of candy which are of low nutritional value. The Council believes it would be in the interest of the public health for all practical means to be taken to limit consumption of sugar in any form in which it fails to be combined with significant proportions of other foods of high nutritive quality.

By 2000, soft-drink production had increased almost 10-fold and provided more than one third of all refined sugars in the diet, but the AMA and other medical organizations now are largely silent. This review discusses the nutritional effect and health consequences of massive consumption of soft drinks,[*] particularly for teenagers.

1. SOARING CONSUMPTION OF SOFT DRINKS

Carbonated soft-drink consumption in the United States has exploded during the past 40 yr (*see* Fig. 1). Those drinks now account for one out of four beverages consumed in America *(2)*. In 2001, Americans spent more than $61 billion *(3)* to buy 15 billion gallons of soft drinks *(4)*. That is equivalent to approx 55 gal, or 587 twelve-oz servings, per year, or 1.6 twelve-oz cans per day for every man, woman, and child. That is also more than twice the amount produced in 1974. Artificially sweetened diet sodas account for 24% of sales, up from 8.6% in 1970 *(5)*.

---

[*]This review does not cover sweetened noncarbonated beverages (bottled ice teas, fruit drinks and ades, etc.), which are nutritionally equivalent to carbonated beverages. Americans consume 15% as much fruit drinks, cocktails, and ades as soft drinks (US Department of Agriculture, Economic Research Service).

From: *Beverages in Nutrition and Health*
Edited by: T. Wilson and N. J. Temple © Humana Press Inc., Totowa, NJ

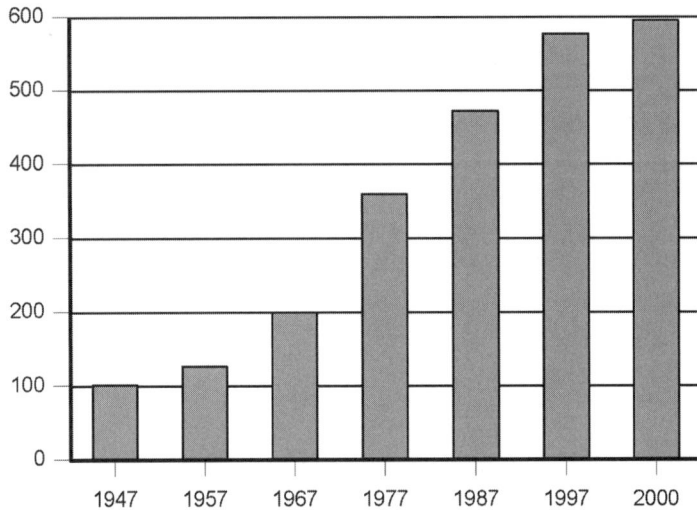

Fig. 1. Annual soft-drink production in the United States (12-oz cans/person).

Children begin drinking soda pop at a remarkably young age, and consumption increases through young adulthood. One fifth of 1- and 2-yr-old children consume soft drinks *(6)*. Those toddlers drink an average of 7 oz—nearly one cup—per day. Toddlers' consumption changed little between the late 1970s and mid-1990s.

Almost half of all children between 6 and 11 yr drink soda pop, with the average drinker consuming 15 oz per day, up slightly from 12 oz in 1977–1978. The most avid consumers are 12- to 29-yr-old males. Among teenagers aged 12–19 yr, boys who imbibe soda pop drink an average of 2.5 twelve-oz sodas (28.5 oz) per day *(see* Table 1). One fourth of 13–18-yr-old boy pop drinkers drink 2.5 or more cans per day, and 1 out of 20 drinks five cans or more *(6)* *(see* Table 2). Actual intakes are higher, because dietary surveys underestimate the quantities of foods people consume, and people may underestimate foods perceived as "bad."

Teenage girls also drink large amounts of soda pop. Girls who drink soft drinks consume approx 1.7 sodas/d. Women in their 20s average slightly more: two 12-oz sodas/d. One fourth of 13–18-yr-old female pop drinkers drink 2 or more cans per day, and 1 out of 20 drinks 3 cans or more *(6)*. By contrast, 20 yr ago, the typical (50th-percentile) 13–18-yr-old consumer of soft drinks (boys and girls together) drank 0.75 of a can/d, whereas the 95th-percentile teen drank 2.25 cans. That's slightly more than half of current consumption.

One reason, aside from the ubiquitous advertising, for increased consumption is that the industry has steadily increased container sizes. In the 1950s, Coca-Cola's 6.5-oz bottle was the standard serving. That grew into the 12-oz can, and now those are being supplanted by 20-oz bottles (and the 64-oz Double Gulp at 7-Eleven stores). The larger the container, the more beverage people are likely to drink, especially when they assume they are buying single-serving containers.

Also, pricing practices encourage people to drink large servings. For instance, at McDonald's restaurants, a 16-oz ("small") drink costs $1.04, whereas a drink 160%

Table 1

Consumption of Soft Drinks by 12–19-Yr-Olds (oz/d) and Percentage of Caloric Intakes

	Consumption[a]		Percent of caloric intakes[a]		Consumption[b]	
	Boys	Girls	Boys	Girls	Boys	Girls
1977–1978	7	6	3	4	16	15
1987–1988	12	7	6	5	23	18
1994–1996	19	12	9	8	28	21

[a] Nondiet soft drinks; includes nondrinkers.

[b] Regular and diet soft drinks; excludes nondrinkers.

Calculated from US Department of Agriculture Nationwide Food Consumption Survey, 1977–78; Continuing Survey of Food Intakes by Individuals (CSFII), 1987–88, 1994–96.

Table 2

Consumption of Regular and Diet Soft Drinks by 13–18-Yr-Olds
(oz/d; Excludes Nondrinkers)

	Percentiles					
	5	25	50	75	90	95
1994–1996 (boys)	6	12	20	30	44	57
1994–1996 (girls)	4	6	14	23	32	40
1977–1978 (boys and girls)	3	5	9	15	–	27

Percentile calculations by Environ, Inc.; data from USDA, CSFII, 1994–96. Figures for 1977–1978 calculated from Guenther (15).

larger (42-oz "super size") costs only 58% more ($1.64) (7). Similarly, at Cineplex Odeon theaters, a 20-oz ("small") drink costs $2.83, but one 120% larger (44-oz "large") costs only 24% more ($3.51) (8).

2. NUTRITIONAL EFFECT OF SOFT DRINKS

Regular soft drinks provide youths and young adults with hefty amounts of sugar and calories. Both regular *and* diet sodas affect Americans' intake of various minerals, vitamins, and additives.

2.1. Sugar Intake

Carbonated drinks are the single biggest source of refined sugars in the American diet (8). According to dietary surveys,[†] soda pop provides the average American with 7 tsp of sugars/d, out of a total of approx 20 tsp. Teenage boys get 44% of their 34 tsp of refined sugars a day from soft drinks. Teenage girls get 40% of their 24 tsp of sugar from soft drinks. Because some people drink little or no soda pop, the percentage of refined sugars provided by pop is higher among actual drinkers.

[†]Those dietary surveys find that consumers report consuming only 57% of all soft drinks produced. That suggests that the surveys greatly underestimate actual intake, even after allowing for the fact that some soft drinks are wasted or returned to manufacturers.

The US Department of Agriculture (USDA) recommends that people eating 1600 calories/d not eat more than 6 tsp a day of refined sugars, 12 tsp for those eating 2200 calories, and 18 tsp for those eating 2800 calories (9). To put those numbers into perspective, consider that the average 12–19-yr-old boy consumes approx 2750 calories and 1.5 cans of soda, with 15 tsp of sugars a day; the average girl consumes approx 1850 calories and 1 can with 10 tsp of sugars. Thus, teens almost reach their recommended refined-sugars limits from soft drinks alone. With candy, cookies, cake, ice cream, and other sugary foods, most teenagers largely exceed those recommendations. Considering only those who drink soda pop, soft drinks provide the average boy drinker, aged 13–18 yr old, with approx 30 tsp of refined sugars a day and the average girl with approx 20 tsp a day (6).

2.2. Calorie Intake

Lots of soda pop means lots of sugar, and that means lots of calories. Soft drinks are the fifth largest source of calories for adults (10). They provide 5.6% of all the calories that Americans consume and considerably more for adolescents (11,12). In 12–19-yr-olds, soft drinks provide 9% of boys' calories and 8% of girls' calories.[‡] Those percentages are triple (boys) or double (girls) what they were in 1977–1978 (Table 1). Note, too, that those figures include teens who consumed little or no soda pop. Boys and girls in the 75th percentile of soft-drink consumption obtained 12% of their calories from soft drinks, and those in the 90th percentile approx 18% of their calories (6).

2.3. Nutrient Intakes

Many nutritionists believe that soft drinks and other calorie-rich nutrient-poor foods can fit into a good diet. In theory, they are correct, but, regrettably, they ignore the fact that many people consume great quantities of soft drinks and meager quantities of healthful foods. One government study found that only 2% of 2–19-yr-olds met all five federal recommendations for a healthy diet (13). USDA's Healthy Eating Index found that on a scale of 0 to 100, teenagers had scores in the low 60s (as did most other age-gender groups). Scores between 51 and 80 indicate that a diet "needs improvement" (14).

Dietary surveys (6) of teenagers found that in 1994, only 39% of boys and 31% of girls consumed the number of servings of vegetables recommended by USDA's Food Pyramid. Even lower figures were seen for fruit (13% of boys and 15% of girls) and for dairy foods (29% of boys and 12% of girls). Moreover, most boys and girls did not meet the recommended amounts of grain and protein foods.

Those surveys (6) also found that few 12–19-yr-olds consumed recommended amounts of certain nutrients. For calcium, only 36% of boys and 14% of girls consumed 100% of the Recommended Dietary Allowance (RDA). Similarly low figures were also seen for vitamin A (36% of boys and 31% of girls) and for magnesium (34% of boys and 18% of girls). As teens doubled or tripled their soft drink consumption, they cut their milk consumption by more than 40%. In 1977–1978, boys consumed more than twice as much milk as soft drinks, and girls consumed 50% more milk than soft drinks. By 1994–1996, both boys and girls consumed twice as much soda pop as milk (and 20–29-yr-olds consumed three times as much). Teenage boys consumed approx 2-2/3 cups

---

[‡]Diet sodas, which provide no calories, constitute only 4% of soft-drink consumption by teenage boys and 11% by teenage girls, according to US Department of Agriculture surveys.

of carbonated soft drinks per day but only 1.25 cups of fluid milk. Girls consumed approx 1.5 cups per day of soft drinks, but less than 1 cup of milk. Compared to adolescents who did not drink soda pop, heavy drinkers of soda pop (26 oz/d or more) are almost four times more likely to drink less than 1 glass of milk a day (L. Harnack, personal communications, September 22, 1998).

In 1977–1978, teenage boys and girls who frequently drank soft drinks consumed approx 20% less calcium than nondrinkers. Heavy soft-drink consumption also correlated with low magnesium, riboflavin, and vitamins A and C intakes, as well as high intake of calories, fat, and carbohydrate (15). In 1994–1996, low calcium intake continued to be a special problem for girl soft-drink consumers (6).

Studies highlight the effect of soft drinks on calcium intake. A 1996 USDA study examined calcium consumption in a large sample of nonpregnant nonlactating women (16). The study correlated high intakes of soft drinks (added sugars were not analyzed) with low calcium intakes. The author stated: "Analysis of food consumption patterns indicated that women who failed to meet their calcium RDA consumed less milk and milk products than those who did meet their RDA.... They also consumed more regular soda." Women who met their calcium RDA consumed an average of 99 g (3 oz) of regular sodas per day, whereas those who did not meet their calcium RDA consumed 47% more regular soda, 146 g (5 oz) per day.

Another study found that carbonated-soda consumption was negatively associated with vitamin A intake in all age children, calcium in children younger than 12 yr, and magnesium in children aged 6 yr and older (17). The authors concluded: "A decrease of one glass of carbonated soda coupled with an increase of one glass of milk or juice could have a substantial effect on a child's daily nutrient intake."

A study by the USDA's Agricultural Research Service, analyzed 1994–1996 dietary intake data to understand the relationship between intake of added sugars (a substantial percentage of which is consumed in soft drinks) and other nutrients (18). That study provides strong evidence that foods and beverages high in added sugars are displacing more nutrient-rich foods in the American diet.

The researcher, Bowman, divided individuals into tertiles by intake of added sugars: light (< 10% of calories), medium (10% to 18% of calories), and heavy (> 18% of calories) consumers. She found that the medium and heavy consumers consumed 10% more calories than the light consumers. There was no difference in fat intake (grams) between light and heavy consumers of added sugars. However, heavy consumers, despite their higher caloric intake, consumed (in comparison with light consumers): 24% *less* dietary fiber; *less* of 15 different vitamins and minerals; and 15–20% *less* vitamins A, B_{12}, and C; folate; and magnesium.

The study concluded: "A remarkably lower percentage of [heavy consumers of added sugars] met their RDA for many micronutrients." It also found that disproportionately high percentages of lower income Americans (40%) and African Americans (44%) were heavy consumers of added sugars. Those figures compare to 33% of all individuals.

Bowman concluded:

Because of the increasing prevalence of obesity, consumers will be benefited by limiting intake of 'empty' calories, especially during childhood and adolescence.... It is important for consumers to recognize that they get large amounts of added sugars through processed foods and beverages.

Further, she cited the need for better food labeling:

Food labels contain information on total sugars per serving but do not distinguish between sugars naturally present in foods and added sugars. Better information on the food label is needed to help consumers make informed choices regarding added sugars. *(emphasis added)*

Another study reviewed adolescents' food consumption, based on USDA's national dietary surveys, between 1965 and 1996 *(19)*. The study found that decreases in raw fruits, nonpotato vegetables, and calcium-rich dairy foods coincided with "greatly increased" soft-drink consumption. Between 1965 and 1996, consumption of soft drinks (carbonated and fruit drinks) increased in adolescent boys from 19 to 50 oz/d and in adolescent girls from 16–35 oz/d. The study notes that those trends "are of most concern for females, who may be at greater risk of developing osteoporosis later in life."

Popkin, one of the authors of that study, said that the dietary changes during the past several decades may leave teenagers at higher risk of chronic ailments later in life, including heart disease, osteoporosis, and diabetes *(20)*. Popkin *(20)* said, "Sugar-loaded beverages are really just empty calories that block out healthy foods. I would tell parents to restrict their kids' soft drink and fruit-drink consumption." He said that people who indulge in too many soft drinks either get fewer nutrients than they should or they eat more food. A spokesperson for the American Dietetic Association *(21)* expressed concern that: "Soda is no longer considered a treat. Soda is now considered a given at a lot of peoples' tables. You're replacing nutritious calories with empty calories."

A study of children in grades 4–6 also found reason for concern *(22)*. Compared to children who did not drink soft drinks, children who consumed an average of 20 oz of soft drinks/d consumed substantially less fruit and more high-fat vegetables.

3. HEALTH IMPACT OF SOFT DRINKS

The soft-drink industry has consistently portrayed its products as being positively healthful, claiming that they are 90% water and contain sugars found in nature. A poster that the National Soft Drink Association *(23)* provided to teachers stated:

As refreshing sources of needed liquids and energy, soft drinks represent a positive addition to a well-balanced diet. . . . These same three sugars also occur naturally, for example, in fruits. . . . In your body it makes no difference whether the sugar is from a soft drink or a peach.

In 1998, Ivester *(24)*, then Coca-Cola's chairman and CEO, defended the marketing of soft drinks in Africa. He said: "Actually, our product is quite healthy. Fluid replenishment is a key to health. . . . Coca-Cola does a great service because it encourages people to take in more and more liquids."

In fact, soft drinks pose health risks because of both what they contain (for example, sugar and various additives) and what they replace in the diet (beverages and foods that provide vitamins, minerals, and other nutrients). The 2000 edition of the *Dietary Guidelines for Americans* recognizes the potential for adverse health effects from overconsumption of refined sugars. It states:

Intake of a lot of foods high in added sugars, like soft drinks, is of concern. Consuming excess calories from these foods may contribute to weight gain or lower consumption of more nutritious foods. . . . Limit your use of these beverages and foods (34).

Table 3
Prevalence of Overweight and Obesity Among American Children
(Percent)

Age (yr)	Year			
	1971–1974	1976–1980	1988–1994	1999–2000
6–11	4	7	11	15
12–19	6	5	11	16

Source: ref. 26.

Table 4
Prevalence of Overweight and Obesity
Among American Adults, 20–74 Yr (Percent)

	Year		
	1976–1980	1988–1994	1999–2000
Overweight	32	33	34
Obese	15	23	31
Overweight or obese	47	56	65

Source: ref. 36.

3.1. Obesity

Excess body weight increases the risk of diabetes and cardiovascular disease (CVD) and causes social and psychological problems in millions of Americans. Between 1971 and 1974 and 1999 and 2000, overweight rates in teenage boys soared from 6% to 15.5% and in teenage girls from 6% to 15.5% (*see* Table 3) *(26)*. Among adults, between 1976–1980 and 1999–2000, the rate of obesity more than doubled, from 15% to 31% (*see* Table 4) *(27)*. The overall rates of obesity plus overweight were 47% in 1976–1980 and 64.5% in 1999–2000.

Numerous factors—from lack of exercise to eating too many calories to genetics—contribute to obesity. Soda pop adds unnecessary nonnutritious calories to the diet. Nutritionists and weight-loss experts routinely advise overweight individuals to consume fewer calories—starting with empty-calorie foods, such as soft drinks. The National Institutes of Health recommends that people who are trying to lose or control their weight should drink water instead of soft drinks with sugar *(28)*.

Obesity rates have risen in tandem with soft-drink consumption, and heavy consumers of soda pop have high calorie intakes *(6)*. Although these observations do not prove that sugary soft drinks cause obesity (conceivably, heavy consumers may exercise more and need more calories), heavy consumption is likely to contribute to weight gain in many consumers.

One analysis found that soft drinks provide a larger percentage of calories to overweight youths than to other youths. The difference was most striking among teenage boys: soft drinks provide 10.3% of the calories consumed by overweight boys, but only 7.6% of the calories consumed by other boys. Calorie and fat intake did not differ between the two groups *(29)*.

A prospective study explored the relationship between soft-drink consumption and obesity *(30)*. The 19-mo study involved 548 children whose average age was just under 12 yr. Importantly, it found that the chances of becoming obese increased significantly with each additional daily serving of sugar-sweetened drink. It also found at the beginning of the study that consumption of sugar-sweetened drinks was associated with increased BMI (body mass index, a measure of overweight and obesity). Although the study was relatively small (37 children became obese during the 19 mo), it provides good evidence that soft drinks contribute to the obesity epidemic.

In another line of research, numerous studies indicate that calories consumed in liquids, rather than solids, are less likely to trigger satiety mechanisms and may play a significant role in obesity. This is further explored in Chapter 18. Those findings are of concern, because sweetened soft drinks are the largest source of added sugars in the average American's diet (sweetened fruit drinks are another significant major source).

In one study, researchers told subjects to add roughly 450 calories a day to their diets in the form of either a soft drink or jelly beans during two 4-wk periods separated by a 4-wk washout *(31)*. During the jelly-bean period, subjects compensated for the added calories by consuming roughly 450 fewer calories from other food. During the soft-drink period, the subjects failed to compensate, essentially adding 450 calories to their previous diet. The results of that recent study are consistent with earlier shorter studies, suggesting that liquid calories "add on," rather than displace, calories in solid foods *(32–34)*.

3.2. Bones and Osteoporosis

People who drink soft drinks instead of milk or other dairy products likely will have lower calcium intakes. Low calcium intake contributes to osteoporosis, a disease leading to fragile and broken bones. In 2002, the National Osteoporosis Foundation estimated that 10 million Americans had osteoporosis. Another 34 million had low bone mass and were at increased risk of osteoporosis *(35)*. Women are more frequently affected than men. Considering the low calcium intake of today's teenage girls, osteoporosis rates may well rise.

The risk of osteoporosis depends, in part, on how much bone mass is built early in life. Girls build 92% of their bone mass by age 18 yr *(36)*, but if they don't consume enough calcium in their teenage years, they cannot "catch up" later. That is why experts recommend higher calcium intakes for youths 9–18 yr than for adults 19–50 yr. Currently, teenage girls consume only 60% of the recommended amount, with soft-drink drinkers consuming almost one fifth less than nondrinkers *(6)*.

Although osteoporosis takes decades to develop, preliminary research suggests that drinking soda pop instead of milk can contribute to broken bones in children. One study found that children 3–15 yr old who had suffered broken bones had lower bone density, which can result from low calcium intake *(37)*.

A preliminary study by Grace Wyshak found strong associations between consumption of carbonated beverages and bone fractures in teenage girls *(38)*. Among active girls, the risk of bone fracture was almost five times greater in those who consumed colas compared with those who did not. Among all girls in this study, the risk of bone fracture was more than three times higher in those who consumed carbonated beverages of any kind than in nonconsumers. The author acknowledges limitations in the study (e.g., failure to ascertain amount of soft drinks and milk consumed), but stated:

In conclusion, nationally, there is great concern about the effects of carbonated-beverage consumption on obesity, tooth decay, osteoporosis, and other health problems. Concern about the health impact of carbonated-beverage consumption, in particular, the association with bone fractures in adolescent girls, is validated by our findings. Our findings have implications both for the health of teenagers and for the health of women at later ages.

In an editorial accompanying that article, a specialist in adolescent medicine stated that those "findings are alarming and warrant confirmation" *(39)*. He highlighted the sharp increase in soft-drink consumption and the sharp drop in milk consumption.

3.3. Dental Caries and Dental Erosion

Refined sugar is one of several important factors that promote dental caries. Soft drinks promote caries because they bathe the teeth of frequent consumers in sugar-water for long periods of time. An analysis of data from 1971 to 1974 found a strong correlation between the frequency of between-meal consumption of soda pop and caries *(40)*. Those researchers also considered other sugary foods in the diet and other variables. Soft drinks cause decay in certain surfaces of certain teeth more than in others *(41)*.

Tooth-decay rates in the United States have declined considerably in recent decades, thanks to such preventive factors as fluoride-containing toothpaste, fluoridated water, tooth sealants, and others. Nevertheless, caries remains a problem for some people. A large survey in California found that children (ages 6–8 and 15 yr) of less educated parents have 20% high rates of decayed and filled teeth *(42)*. A national study found that African American and Mexican American children (6 to 18 yr old) are twice as likely to have untreated caries as their white counterparts *(43)*. For people in high-risk groups, prevention is particularly important.

To prevent tooth decay, even the Canadian Soft Drink Association *(44)* recommends limiting between-meal snacking of sugary and starchy foods, avoiding prolonged sugar levels in the mouth, and eating sugary foods and beverages with meals. Unfortunately, many heavy drinkers of soft drinks violate each of those precepts.

The American Dental Association *(45)* has noted:

Though there is limited epidemiological evidence assessing the association between oral health and soft-drink consumption, it consistently indicates that soft drinks adversely affect dental caries and enamel erosion. Moreover, numerous in vitro and animal studies have consistently shown enamel erosion with the use of soft drinks. Given this evidence it would seem appropriate to encourage children and adolescents to limit their intake of soda.

3.4. Heart Disease

Heart disease is the nation's number one killer. Some of the most important causes are cigarette smoking, a sedentary lifestyle, and diets high in saturated fat, *trans* fat, and cholesterol. In addition, high-sugar diets may contribute to heart disease in people who are "insulin resistant." Those people, an estimated one fourth of adults, frequently have high levels of triglycerides and low levels of high-density lipoprotein (HDL) ("good") cholesterol in their blood. When they eat a diet high in carbohydrates, their triglyceride and insulin levels rise. Sugar has a greater effect than other carbohydrates *(46,47)*. The high triglyceride levels are associated with a high risk of heart disease *(48)*. Therefore, it is sensible for insulin-resistant people, in particular, to consume low levels of regular soft drinks and other sugary foods, although more researchers are urging that everyone reduce his or her intake of refined carbohydrates *(49)*. Research is needed on insulin resistance in adolescents.

3.5. Kidney Stones

Kidney (urinary) stones are one of the most painful disorders afflicting humans and one of the most common disorders of the urinary tract. According to the National Institute of Diabetes and Digestive and Kidney Diseases (NIDDK), a unit of the National Institutes of Health, more than 1 million cases of kidney stones were diagnosed in 1996 *(50)*. NIDDK estimates that 10% of all Americans will have a kidney stone during their lifetime. Several times more men, frequently between the ages of 20 and 40 yr, are affected than women. Young men are also the heaviest consumers of soft drinks.

After a study that suggested a link between soft drinks and kidney stones, researchers conducted an intervention trial *(51)*. That trial involved 1009 men who had suffered kidney stones and drank at least 5-1/3 oz of soda pop per day. Half the men were asked to refrain from drinking pop, whereas the others were not asked. During the next 3 yr, cola drinkers who reduced their consumption (to less than half their customary levels) were almost one third less likely to experience recurrence of stones. Among those who usually drank fruit-flavored soft drinks, which are acidified with citric acid rather than the phosphoric acid used in colas, drinking less had no effect. Although more research must be done to prove the cola-stone connection, the NIDDK includes cola beverages on a list of foods that doctors may advise patients to avoid.

3.6. Additives: Psychoactive Drug, Allergens, and More

Several additives in soft drinks raise health concerns. Caffeine, a mildly addictive stimulant, is present in most cola and "pepper" drinks, as well as some orange sodas and other products. The effects of this substance is reviewed in Chapter 12. Caffeine's addictiveness may be one reason why six of the seven most popular soft drinks contain caffeine *(52)*. Caffeine-free colas are available, but they account for only 5% of colas made by Coca-Cola *(53)*. On the other hand, Coca-Cola Co. and other companies have begun marketing soft drinks, such as Surge and Jolt, with 30–60% more caffeine than Coke and Pepsi.

Companies say they add caffeine as a flavoring. However, most regular cola soft-drink consumers cannot detect caffeine's flavor when the substance is consumed in soft drinks *(54)*. That suggests that companies add caffeine primarily for its physiological and psychological effects.

In 1994–1996, the average 13–18-yr-old boy who drank soft drinks consumed approx 1-1/3 cans/d. Those drinking Mountain Dew would have ingested 92 mg of caffeine from that source (55 mg caffeine/12 oz). That is equivalent to about one 6-oz cup of brewed coffee. Boys in the 90th percentile of soft-drink consumption consume as much caffeine as is in 2 cups of coffee; for girls, the figure is 1.5 cups of coffee.

One problem with caffeine is that it increases the excretion of calcium in urine *(55)*. Drinking 12 oz of caffeine-containing soft drink causes the loss of approx 20 mg of calcium, or 2% of the US RDA (or Daily Value). That loss, compounded by the relatively low calcium intake in girls who are heavy consumers of soda pop, may increase the risk of osteoporosis.

Caffeine can cause nervousness, irritability, sleeplessness, and rapid heart beat *(56)*. Caffeine causes children who normally do not consume much caffeine to be restless and fidgety, develop headaches, and have difficulty going to sleep *(57,58)*. Also, caffeine's addictiveness may keep people hooked on soft drinks (or other caffeine-containing beverages). One reflection of the drug's addictiveness is that when children aged 6–12 stop consuming caffeine, they suffer withdrawal symptoms that impair their attention span and performance *(59)*.

The amounts of caffeine in soft drinks can have distinct pharmacologic and behavioral effects. In one study, the caffeine equivalent of 2 to 3 cans of soft drink per day (100 mg/d) was sufficient to produce physical dependence, characterized by withdrawal symptoms of tiredness and headache if consumption were stopped. That study also found that 25 mg of caffeine is sufficient to suppress caffeine-withdrawal headache *(60)*. Another study shows that 40 mg of caffeine (roughly the amount in one can of soda) produces mood and performance effects *(61)*, whereas a third study shows that low doses of caffeine can have cognitive and performance effects, including cognitive effects at doses as low as 12.5 mg *(62)*.

The Australia New Zealand Food Authority has concluded that: (1) the amounts of caffeine in one or two cans of caffeinated soft drink can affect performance and mood, increase anxiety in children, and reduce the ability to sleep, though "the threshold dose for possible behavioral effects in children remains unclear…"; (2) typical doses of caffeine "may lead to withdrawal effects and some physical dependence in adults…. Further research will be required…in children"; and (3) there is little evidence for adverse cardiovascular effects *(63)*.

Several additives used in soft drinks cause occasional allergic reactions. Yellow 5 dye causes asthma, hives, and a runny nose *(64)*. A natural red coloring, cochineal (and its close relative carmine), causes life-threatening reactions *(65)*. Dyes can cause hyperactivity in sensitive children *(66)*.

In diet sodas, artificial sweeteners may raise concerns. Saccharin, which has been replaced by aspartame and other such sweeteners in all but a few brands, has been linked in human studies to urinary-bladder cancer *(67)* and in animal studies to cancers of the bladder and other organs *(68)*. The safety of acesulfame-K, which was approved in 1998 for use in soft drinks, has been questioned by several cancer experts *(69)*.

4. AGGRESSIVE MARKETING OF SOFT DRINKS

Soft-drink companies are among the most aggressive marketers in the world. They have used advertising and many other techniques to increase sales. For starters, companies ensure that their products are always readily accessible. Coca-Cola's *(70)* stated goal is to:

... make Coca-Cola the preferred drink for any occasion, whether it's a simple family supper or a formal state dinner. .... [T]o build pervasiveness of our products, we're putting ice-cold Coca-Cola classic and our other brands within reach, wherever you look: at the supermarket, the video store, the soccer field, the gas station—everywhere.

As one reflection of that marketing goal, Coca-Cola sells its soft drinks at 2 million stores, more than 450,000 restaurants, and 1.4 million vending machines and coolers *(71)*. Industry-wide, in 2000, 3 million soft-drink vending machines *(72)* dispensed tens of billions of drinks worth approx $16 billion *(73)*.

Soft-drink advertising budgets dwarf all advertising and public-service campaigns promoting the consumption of fruits, vegetables, healthful diets, and low-fat milk. In 2000, Coca-Cola Co., which accounts for 44% of the soft-drink market in the United States *(74)*, spent nearly $300 million on media advertising, and the entire industry spent more than $700 million *(75)*. Between 1986 and 1997, the top four companies spent $6.8 billion on advertising *(76)*.

In addition to media advertising, companies spend hundreds of millions of dollars a year on other forms of marketing, from coupons to sponsoring concerts. In 2000, Coca-Cola spent approx $400 million on promotional activities, on top of $293 million in television, magazine, and other media advertising for Coke, Diet Coke, and Sprite in the United States.

The major companies target children aggressively (though, to their credit, they have not gone after 4-yr-olds by advertising on Saturday morning television). Pepsi has advertised on Channel One, a daily news program shown in 12,000 junior high, middle, and high schools *(77)*. In addition, companies inculcate brand loyalties in children and boost consumption by paying school districts and others for exclusive marketing agreements. This marketing aspect is further examined in Chapter 25. For instance, Dr. Pepper paid the Grapevine Colleyville, Texas, School District $3.45 million for a 10-yr contract (it includes rooftop advertising to reach passengers in planes landing at the nearby Dallas/ Ft. Worth Airport) *(78)*. To reach youths after school, Coca-Cola is paying $60 million during 10 yr to the Boys & Girls Clubs of America for exclusive marketing rights in more than 2000 clubs *(79)*. Those exclusive marketing contracts typically result in heavier advertising and more vending machines.

Soft-drink (and fast-food) companies frequently link their brands to popular youth-oriented movies and music groups. Thus, in 2001, Coca-Cola was the exclusive global marketing partner for Time-Life-Warner's movie, *Harry Potter and the Sorcerer's Stone,* and reportedly spent $150 million on marketing related to that movie *(80)*. Coca-Cola and Pepsi-Cola have also paid pop-music stars Britney Spears, Christina Aguilera, and Jakob Dylan (Wallflowers band) to promote their products.

Soft-drink companies have been creating different products for different segments of the population. Low-calorie diet sodas have been aimed at women and caffeine-free products at parents. Some higher caffeine products are aimed at teenaged boys, whereas Pepsi Blue, Vanilla Coke, and Pepsi's Code Red are marketed to youths, minorities, or people who are tired of colas *(81)*.

In a particularly inappropriate marketing gambit, Pepsi, Dr. Pepper, and Seven-Up have encouraged feeding soft drinks to babies by licensing their logos to a major maker of baby bottles, Munchkin Bottling, Inc. Infants and toddlers are four times likelier to be fed soda pop out of those bottles than out of regular baby bottles *(82)*.

Table 5
Cost of Various Beverages[a]

Beverage	Cost ($)/container	Cost ($)/quart
Cola, supermarket brand	0.59/2 L	0.28
Coca-Cola	0.69/2 L	0.33
Pepsi-Cola	0.69/2 L	0.33
Bottled water (supermarket brand)	0.79/gall	0.20
Bottled spring water (supermarket brand)	0.89/gall	0.22
Seltzer water club soda (supermarket brand)	0.89/2 L	0.42
Milk	2.89/gall	0.70
	0.95/q	0.95
Orange juice, frozen concentrate (supermarket brand)	1.39/12-oz can	0.93 concentrate

[a]Prices at Washington-area stores, September 1998.

Although all those marketing efforts increase sales, perhaps the single most important factor fueling soft-drink sales is the relatively low cost of those products (*see* Table 5). Supermarket brands are particularly inexpensive, being as low as 28 cents/quart, but even Coca-Cola and Pepsi-Cola are available for 33 cents/quart when on sale. Milk costs two to three times as much, approx 70 to 95 cents/quart.

The soft-drink industry is aiming for continued expansion. Thus, the president of Coca-Cola has bemoaned the fact that his company accounts for only 1 billion of the 47 billion servings of all beverages consumed daily worldwide *(70)*.

5. RECOMMENDATIONS FOR ACTION

In part because of powerful advertising, ubiquitous availability, and low price, and, in part, because of disinterest on the part of health professionals, Americans consider soft drinks a routine snack and a standard appropriate component of meals instead of an occasional treat, as they were viewed several decades ago. Moreover, many of today's younger parents grew up with soft drinks, see their routine consumption as normal, and, so, make little effort to restrict their children's consumption of them.

It is a fact, though, that soft drinks provide enormous amounts of refined sugars and calories to a nation that does not meet national dietary goals and that is experiencing an obesity epidemic. The replacement of milk by soft drinks in teenage girls' diets portends higher rates of osteoporosis. Soft drinks may also contribute to dental problems, kidney stones, and heart disease. Additives may cause insomnia, behavioral problems, and allergic reactions and may slightly increase the risk of cancer.

The industry promises that it will do everything possible to persuade even more consumers to drink even more soda pop even more often. Parents and health officials must recognize soft drinks for what they are—liquid candy—and do everything possible to return those beverages to their former reasonable role as an occasional treat. Here are specific recommendations:

1. Individuals and families should consider how much soda pop they are drinking and reduce consumption accordingly. Parents should stock their homes with healthful foods and beverages that family members enjoy.

2. Physicians, nurses, and nutritionists routinely should ask their patients how much soda pop (and other low-nutrition foods) they are consuming and advise them, if appropriate, to decrease consumption.

3. Government regulatory agencies that control nutrition labeling should set a daily limit for refined sugars and require the amount of sugars and the percentage of the daily limit to be included on the label.

4. Organizations concerned about women's and children's health, dental and bone health, and heart disease should collaborate on campaigns to reduce soft-drink consumption.

5. Local, state, and federal governments should be as aggressive in providing water fountains in public buildings and spaces as the industry is in placing vending machines everywhere.

6. National and local governments should consider levying small taxes on soft drinks, as is already the case in California, New York, Arkansas, Chicago, and most Canadian provinces *(84)*. Arkansas raises $40 million/yr from that tax. If all states taxed soft drinks at Arkansas' rate (2 cents/12-oz can), they could raise $3 billion annually. Those revenues could fund mass-media campaigns to improve diets, build exercise facilities (bike paths and swimming pools, etc.), and support physical-education programs in schools. Unfortunately, current revenues simply go into the general treasury.

7. National or local governments could require chain restaurants to declare the calorie content of each item on menu boards or printed menus (where there is also room for listing saturated fat and sodium). Vending machines could also disclose the calorie content of each item.

8. School systems and other organizations catering to children should stop selling soft drinks, candy, and similar foods in hallways, shops, and cafeterias.

9. School systems and youth organizations should not enter into exclusive soft-drink marketing agreements. Those deals benefit the companies and schools at the expense of the students' health.

10. Independent scientific research should explore further the role of heavy consumption of soft drinks (and refined sugars) in nutritional status, obesity, caries, kidney stones, osteoporosis, and heart disease.

6. MAIN POINTS FOR PRIMARY AND CLINICAL REVIEW

1. Between 1942 and 2000, soft-drink production increased almost 10-fold, often at the expense of milk, and now provides more than one third of total dietary refined sugars, especially in children.

2. Soft-drink consumption increases calorie intake, but decreases overall nutrient intake.

3. The increase in soft-drink consumption is partly responsible for the increased incidence of obesity, osteoporosis, dental caries, and other diseases.

4. The $16 billion budget for marketing of soft drinks dwarf the small funds available for promoting the consumption of healthy beverages.

5. Consumers and health providers need to become more aware of the impact that soft drinks have on health and the cost of health care.

REFERENCES

1. American Medical Association, Council on Foods and Nutrition. Some nutritional aspects of sugar, candy and sweetened carbonated beverages. JAMA 1942;120:763–765.
2. National Soft Drink Assoc. Retrieved July 5, 2002, from http://www.nsda.com/SoftDrinks/index.html.
3. National Soft Drink Assoc. Retrieved July 5, 2002, from http://www.nsda.com/softdrinks/History/funfacts.html.
4. NSDA Web site. Retrieved July 5, 2002, from http://www.nsda.com/SoftDrinks/index.html and http://www.nsda.com/SoftDrinks/History/funfacts.html. http://eire.census.gov/popest/data/national/populartables/table01.php.
5. US Department of Agriculture (USDA), Economic Research Service. Beverages, per capita consumption, 1970–2000. Retrieved Aug. 7, 2002, from http://www.ers.usda.gov/Data/FoodConsumption/Spreadsheets/beverage.xls.
6. US Department of Agriculture Web site. Retrieved July 5, 2002, from http://www.barc.usda.gov/bhnrc/foodsurvey/home.htm.
7. National Alliance for Nutrition and Activity. From wallet to waistline: the hidden costs of super sizing. 2002.
8. Gibney M, Sigman-Grant M, Stanton Jr. JL, Keast DR. Consumption of sugars. Am J Clin Nutr 1995;62(Suppl):178S–194S.
9. US Department of Agriculture. The Food Guide Pyramid. Home Garden Bull 1996;252.
10. Subar AF, Krebs-Smith SM, Cook A, Kahle LL. Dietary sources of nutrients among US adults. J Am Dietet Assoc 1998;98:537–547.
11. Products from the CSFII/DHKS 1994–96, 1998, Washington, DC. US Department of Agriculture, Food Survey Research Group, 2002. Available at http://www.barc.usda.gov/bhnrc/foodsurvey/Products9496.html. Accessed September 25, 2002.
12. Troiano RP, Briefel RR, Carroll MD, Bialostosky K. Energy and fat intakes of children and adolescents in the United States: data from the National Health and Nutrition Examination Surveys. Am J Clin Nutr 2000;72(Suppl):1343S–1353S.
13. Munoz KA, Krebs-Smith SM, Ballard-Barbash R, Cleveland LE. Food intakes of U.S. children and adolescents compared with recommendations. Pediatrics 1997;100:323–329. Correction: Pediatrics 1998; 101:952–953.
14. USDA Center for the Healthy Nutrition Policy and Promotion, CNPP-5. Eating Index, 1994-96, July 1998. Retrieved July 10, 2002 from http://www.usda.gov/cnpp/insight9
15. Guenther PM. Beverages in the diets of American teenagers. J Am Dietet Assoc 1986;86:493–499.
16. Guthrie JF. Dietary patterns and personal characteristics of women consuming recommended amounts of calcium. Fam Econ Nutr Rev 1996;9:33–49.
17. Ballew C, Kuester S, Gillespie C. Beverage choices affect adequacy of children's nutrient intakes. Arch Pediatr Adolesc Med 2000;154:1148–1152.
18. Bowman S. Diets of individuals based on energy intakes from added sugars. Fam Econ Nutr Rev 1999;12:31–38.
19. Cavadini C, Siega-Riz AM, Popkin BM. US adolescent food intake trends from 1965 to 1996. Arch Dis Child 2000;83:18–24.
20. Vergano D, Sternberg S. Teens' thirst for sugar may mean bitter medicine later. USA Today July 24, 2000, p. 1D.
21. Warner J. Teens drinking too much soda, not enough milk. CBS HealthWatch. July 24, 2000. Retrieved August 21, 2000, from wysiwyg://15//http://cbshealthwatch . . ./HNews/HnewsPrint.asp?RecID=219641.
22. Cullen KW, Ash DM, Warneke C, de Moor C. Intake of soft drinks, fruit-flavored beverages, and fruits and vegetables by children in grades 4 through 6. Am J Pub Health 2002;92:1475–1478.
23. National Soft Drink Association. Soft Drinks and Nutrition. National Soft Drink Association, Washington, DC (undated).
24. Hays CL, McNeil, Jr, DG. Putting Africa on Coke's Map. New York Times, May 26, 1998, p. D1.
25. US Department of Agriculture, US Department of Health and Human Services. Nutrition and your health: dietary guidelines for Americans. Retrieved July 5, 2002, from http://www.health.gov/dietaryguidelines/dga2000/document/frontcover.htm.

26. Centers for Disease Control and Prevention, National Center for Health Statistics. Prevalence of over-weight and children and adolescents: United States, 1999–2000. Table 71. Retrieved October 14, 2002, from http://www.cdc.gov/nchs/products/pubs/pubd/hus/tables/2002/02hus071.pdf.

27. Centers for Disease Control and Prevention, National Center for Health Statistics. Prevalence of over-weight and obesity among adults: United States, 1999–2000. Table 70. Retrieved October 14, 2002, from http://www.cdc.gov/nchs/products/pubs/pubd/hus/tables/2002/02hus070.pdf.

28. NHLBI and Office of Research on Minority Health. Embrace Your Health! Lose Weight if You Are Overweight. US Department of Health and Human Services, NIH Publication No. 97-4061. 1997.

29. Troiano RP, Briefel RR, Carroll MD, Bialostosky K. Energy and fat intakes of children and adolescents in the United States: data from the national health and nutrition examination surveys. Am J Clin Nutr 2000;72(Suppl):1343S–1353S.

30. Ludwig DS, Peterson KE, Gortmaker SL. Relationship between consumption of sugar-sweetened drinks and childhood obesity: a prospective, observational analysis. Lancet 2001:357:505–508.

31. DiMeglio DP, Mattes RD. Liquid versus solid carbohydrate: effects on food intake and body weight. Int J Obes 2000;24:794–800.

32. DeCastro JM. The effects of spontaneous ingestion of particular food or beverages on the meal pattern and overall nutrient intake of humans. Physiol Behav 2993;53:1133–1144.

33. Mattes RD. Dietary compensation by humans for supplemental energy provided as ethanol or carbohy-drate in fluids. Physiol Behav 1996;59:179–187.

34. Rolls BJ, Kim S, Federoff IC. Effects of drinks sweetened with sucrose or aspartame on hunger, thirst and food intake in men. Physiol Behav 1990;48:19–26.

35. National Osteoporosis Foundation. Retrieved July 5, 2002, from http://www.nof.org/advocacy/preva-lence/index.htm.

36. Institute of Medicine. Dietary Reference Intakes: Calcium, Phosphorus, Magnesium, Vitamin D, and Fluoride. National Academy Press, Washington, DC, 1997, pp. 4–28.

37. Goulding A, Cannan R, Williams SM, Gold EJ, Taylor RW, Lewis-Barned NJ. Bone mineral density in girls with forearm fractures. J Bone Miner Res 1998;13:143–148.

38. Wyshak G. Teenaged girls, carbonated beverage consumption, and bone fractures. Arch Pediatr Adolesc Med 2000;154:610–613.

39. Golden NH. Osteoporosis prevention. A pediatric challenge. Arch Pediatr Adolesc Med 2000;154:542–543.

40. Ismail AI, Burt BA, Eklund SA. The cariogenicity of soft drinks in the United States. J Am Dent Assoc 1984;109:241–245.

41. Steinberg AD, Zimmerman SO, Bramer ML. The Lincoln dental caries study. II. The effect of acidulated carbonated beverages on the incidence of dental caries. J Am Dent Assoc 1972;85:81–89.

42. The Dental Health Foundation. A Neglected Epidemic: The Oral Health of California's Children. The Dental Health Foundation, Oakland, CA, 1997.

43. Vargas CM, Orall JJ, Schneider DA. Sociodemographic distribution of pediatric dental caries: NHANES III, 1988-1994. J Am Dent Assoc 1998;129:1229–1238.

44. Canadian Soft Drink Association. Retrieved November 28, 2001, from http://www.softdrink.ca.

45. Joint Report of the American Dental Association Council on Access, Prevention and Interprofessional Relations and Council on Scientific Affairs to the House of Delegates: Response to Resolution 73H-2000; Oct. 2001.

46. Hollenbeck CB. Dietary fructose effects on lipoprotein metabolism and risk for coronary artery disease. Am J Clin Nutr 1993;58:800S–809S.

47. Liu G, Coulston A, Hollenbeck C, Reaven G. The effect of sucrose content in high and low carbohydrate diets on plasma glucose, insulin, and lipid responses in hypertriglyceridemic humans. J Clin Endocrinol Metab 1984;59:636–642.

48. Stampfer MJ, Krauss RM, Ma J, et al. A prospective study of triglyceride level, low-density lipoprotein particle diameter, and risk of myocardial infarction. JAMA 1996;276:882–888.

49. Ludwig D. The glycemic index: physiological mechanisms relating to obesity, diabetes, and cardiovas-cular disease. JAMA 2002;287:2414–2423.

50. National Institute of Diabetes and Digestive and Kidney Diseases. Retrieved July 5, 2002, from http://www.niddk.nih.gov/health/kidney/pubs/stonadul/stonadul.htm.

51. Shuster J, Jenkins A, Logan C, et al. Soft drink consumption and urinary stone recurrence: a randomized prevention trial. J Clin Epidemiol 1992;45:911–916.

52. Beverage Digest. Retrieved September 9, 2002, from http://www.beverage-digest.com/editorial/ 020228s.php.

53. Beverage Digest. Retrieved September 9, 2002, from http://www.beverage-digest.com/editorial/ 990212s.html.

54. Griffiths RR, Vernotica EM. Is caffeine a flavoring agent in cola soft drinks? Arch Fam Med 2000;9: 727–734.

55. Barger-Lux MJ, Heaney RP. Caffeine and the calcium economy revisited. Osteoporos Intern 1995;5:97–102.

56. American Psychiatric Association. Diagnostic and Statistical Manual of Mental Disorders, 4th Ed. APA, Washington, DC, 1994.

57. Rapoport JL, Jensvold M, Elkins R, et al. Behavioral and cognitive effects of caffeine in boys and adult males. J Nerv Men Dis 1981;169:726–732.

58. Rapoport JL, Berg CJ, Ismond DR, Zahn TP, Neims A. Behavioral effects of caffeine in children. Arch Gen Psychiatr 1984;41:1073–1079.

59. Bernstein GA, Carroll ME, Dean NW, Crosby RD, Perwien AR, Benowitz NL. Caffeine withdrawal in normal school-age children. J Am Acad Child Adolesc Psychiatr 1998;37:858–865.

60. Evans SM, Griffiths RR. Caffeine withdrawal: parametric analysis of caffeine dosing conditions. J Pharmacol Exp Ther 1999;289:285–294.

61. Smith A, Sturgess W, Gallagher J. Effects of a low dose of caffeine given in different drinks on mood and performance. Hum Psychopharmacol Clin Exp 1999;14:473–482.

62. Smit HJ, Rogers PJ. Effects of low doses of caffeine on cognitive performance, mood and thirst in low and higher caffeine consumers. Psychopharmacology (Berl) 2000;152:167–173.

63. Australia New Zealand Food Authority. Report from the expert working group on the safety aspects of dietary caffeine. Retrieved July 6, 2000, from http://www.anzfa.gov.au/documents/pub04_00.asp.

64. US Food and Drug Administration. FD&C Yellow No. 5; labeling in food and drugs for human use. Fed Reg 1979;44:37,212–37,221.

65. Baldwin JL, Chou AH, Solomon WR. Popsicle-induced anaphylaxis due to carmine dye allergy. Ann Allergy Asthma Immunol 1997;79:415–419.

66. Weiss B, Williams JH, Margen S, et al. Behavioral responses to artificial food colors. Science 1980;207:1487–1488.

67. Hoover RN, Strasser PH. Artificial sweeteners and human bladder cancer: preliminary results. Lancet 1980;i:837–840.

68. Reuber MD. Carcinogenicity of saccharin. Env Health Perspect 1998;25:173–200.

69. Consumer group attacks artificial sweetener. Associated Press. August 1, 1996.

70. Coca-Cola Company. Annual Report. The Coca-Cola Company, Atlanta, GA, 1997.

71. Deogun N. A Coke and a perm? Soda giant is pushing into unusual locales. Wall Street Journal, May 8, 1997, p. 1.

72. Vending Times Census of the Industry 2001. Retrieved January 15, 2002, from http://vendingtimes.com/ census.htm.

73. Vending Times. 1998;38:15, 21, 22.

74. Beverage Digest. Retrieved November 28, 2001, from http://www.beveragedigest.com.

75. Chura H. Soft drinks: leading brands hold own, but flavored drinks gaining. Advertising Age, September 24, 2001, p. S8.

76. Beverage Digest. Retrieved September 9, 2002, from http://www.beverage-digest.com/editorial/ 980424.html.

77. Retrieved December 11, 2001, from http://www.channelone.com.

78. This school is brought to you by: Cola? Sneakers? USA Today March 27, 1998, p. 12A.

79. Gray S, Hall H. Cashing in on charity's good name. Chron Philanthropy July 30, 1998, p. 25.

80. Center for Science in the Public Interest (CSPI). Retrieved July 5, 2002, from http://www.saveharry.com.

81. Day S. Advertising: an old brand is back in America with ads for a young crowd. New York Times, July 5, 2002, p. C2.

82. Siener K, Rothman D, Farrar J. Soft drink logos on baby bottles: do they influence what is fed to children? ASDC J Dent Child 1997;64:55–60.

83. Jacobson MF, Brownell KD. Small taxes on soft drinks and snack foods to promote health. Am J Public Health 2000;90:854–857.

25 Marketing Soft Drinks to Children and Young Adults

Audrey Balay-Karperien, Norman J. Temple, and Marion Nestle

In an informal survey conducted by one of the authors (ABK), three Canadian and nine British mothers of children aged four to seven were asked if they would serve their children eight teaspoons of sugar in eight ounces of water. All of them said that they would never do it. Yet, all of them said that they would serve their children sugar-sweetened soda pop.

Children enjoy an occasional treat. However, evidence shows that young people throughout the world enjoy "liquid candy" (i.e., soft drinks) much more than occasionally. In fact, the amount of soft drinks young people consume has steadily increased during recent decades. Excessive soft-drink consumption is alarming, because it may pose significant risks to the health of young people. Consumption trends in the United States and health risks of soft drinks are reviewed in Chapter 24. That chapter also discusses the subject of marketing of soft drinks. Here, we further explore the subject, with a particular focus on the marketing of soft drinks to children and young adults. An especially alarming aspect of this story is that children and young adults consume soft drinks under pressure from sophisticated and aggressive marketers and with tacit approval from some ensnared elements of society.

1. ADVERTISING AND MARKETING OF SOFT DRINKS

An examination of the health effects of soft drinks reveals a paradox. The evidence of to the negative health effects of current levels of soft drink consumption is, on the whole, powerful to cause health advocates, including the World Health Organization, to caution countries, communities, schools, and individuals against the potential dangers of current trends. Yet, soft-drink consumption continues its steady climb. In 1995–1996, for example, soft drinks were the largest selling food category in Canadian grocery stores *(1)*. In 1999, Coca-Cola sold 160 brands of soft drinks in 200 countries, earning $2.4 billion in profit (which was actually less than in previous years) *(2)*.

Why are soft drinks so popular? Probably because carbonated soft drinks are supported by big business and advertised heavily to young people and the adults caring for them.

From: *Beverages in Nutrition and Health*
Edited by: T. Wilson and N. J. Temple © Humana Press Inc., Totowa, NJ

These companies do their utmost to promote their own positive image, yet their adver-tising never hints at the risks associated with soft-drink consumption. The information the soft-drink industry presents is sometimes potentially misleading. For example, the advertising industry touts soda pop as a desirable source of hydration and calories. To illustrate, in their online "Product FAQ" answering the question "Should I be concerned about the amount of sugar or calories in soft drinks?" Coca-Cola says:

> It may surprise you to know that the amount of sugar and calories in soft drinks is about the same as many fruit juices. An 8-ounce (240 mL) serving of Coca-Cola, for example, contains no more sugar and calories than 8 ounces (240 mL) of orange juice, and less sugar and fewer calories than 8 ounces (240 mL) of apple juice or grape juice. And, the body can't tell the difference between the natural sugar you get from fruit juice and that added to soft drinks.

Although this may be true, it ignores that numerous micronutrients and phytochemicals found in nutritious drinks are absent from soda pop. For example, a glass of milk (250 mL) provides 285 mg calcium, 33 mg magnesium, and 0.4 mg riboflavin, whereas a glass of orange juice (250 mL) provides 120 mg vitamin C, 27 mg magnesium, and 75 µg folate. In contrast, a can of soft drink provides none of these nutrients. That is why the consump-tion of soft drinks greatly increases the likelihood that the diet, as a whole, will have an inadequate content of various micronutrients, as documented in Chapter 24.

Some soft-drink promoters have challenged recommendations made by health agen-cies against sugar and soft-drink consumption by young people. To illustrate, although frequent consumption of soft drinks is considered to be a threat to oral health by virtually all dental associations (e.g., American, British, Canadian, Hong Kong), Coca-Cola states that: "The sugar in soft drinks has minimal effect on teeth because it's in a liquid form." Similarly, despite exhortations by public-health agencies to increase calcium intake in young people, a British report published by the soft-drink industry in 2001 applauds the finding that soft drinks have replaced milk in the diets of young people, stating that in the soft-drink industry "optimism was high because all consumer lifestyle trends point in favor of soft drinks and away from milk, hot drinks, or alcohol" (3).

Perhaps the most contentious aspect of soft-drink marketing to young people is "pour-ing rights" contracts (4). These are exclusive rights, usually bought with large lump-sum payments to school districts, followed by more payments during 5 to 10 yr in return for exclusive sales of one company's products in vending machines at schools. Approxi-mately 200 school districts in the United States were participating in such agreements by 2000 (5,6). The contracts may also include cash bonuses or incentives (e.g., a new car for a senior with perfect attendance and high grades) for exceeding sales targets (7). One contract, for instance, required all of a district's schools and preschool programs to use Coca-Cola products exclusively in all vending machines, athletic contests, booster club activities, and school-sponsored community events, where the company would pay addi-tional commissions on purchases exceeding minimum amounts, donate free Fruitopia drinks, provide drinks to fund-raising groups for resale, and include software, coupons, or other premiums for each vending machine placed (8).

The contracts involve considerable sales profits. A Pepsi official described such con-tracts as "a pretty high stakes business development," and a Coca-Cola official said that his company would "continue to be very aggressive and proactive in getting our share of the school business" (9).

For soft-drink companies, the benefits of these contracts go well beyond a stable base of sales in schools. Companies get constant advertising. Students get constant exposure to logos on vending machines, cups, sportswear, brochures, and school buildings. Even students too young or too difficult to reach by conventional advertising methods can get fully immersed in logos.

Selling pouring rights may give schools tangible rewards, too, but the contracts are laden with ethical and health concerns. In the United States, until sodas were permitted, milk was the only beverage provided to schoolchildren. However, from 1985 to 1997, as schools rapidly increased purchases of carbonated sodas, they decreased the amounts of milk they bought by nearly 30% *(10)*.

Because the payment that schools receive is contingent on soft-drink sales, there is an inevitable social cost. School administrators may find themselves pushing soft drinks to staff and students. The attractive returns could further compromise administrators by encouraging them to not comply with health recommendations and regulations. For example, administrators have, on occasions, defied regulations that restrict vending machines placement and when students can use them *(11)*. In response to this, legislation has been introduced to stop soft-drink companies from circumventing rules that discourage soft-drink sales during lunch periods *(12)*.

Students seeing school officials compromising nutritional principles and regulations for financial reasons may learn that the attitude that nutrition is ultimately unimportant. The negative consequences do not stop there. The contracts jeopardize not only individual nutrition habits but also the viability of nutrition programs needing adequate sales volume to survive *(13)*. School nutrition education is effective, especially when supported by meals served in school cafeterias; participants in school meal programs consume better diets than nonparticipants *(14,15)*. However, if school meals are replaced with foods of minimal nutritional value, diet quality can be expected to deteriorate. Indeed, evidence shows that when students have access to soft drinks, they are less likely to consume fruits, juice, and vegetables *(16)*. These threats to school nutrition education and meal programs may have damaging long-term consequences because a powerful tool for establishing healthy lifelong eating patterns has been thrown aside *(17,18)*.

2. OPPOSITION TO THE SOFT-DRINK GIANTS

The ongoing battle between food industry and health interests is certainly not a new development *(19)*. Regulators in the United States have been tinkering with regulations governing sales of soft drinks and other "foods of minimal nutritional value" in school lunch and breakfast programs for at least 50 yr. Some success has been achieved in regulating sales of unhealthy foods, including soft drinks, in public schools, but these moves have often been countered by deregulating legislation lobbied for by soft-drink companies, sometimes supported by education officials opposing restrictions on when or where soft drinks and other such foods may be sold.

One of the problems with numerous pseudo-juice products is the misleading labeling. Although the small print may follow the letter of the law, the big print may give a false impression. It is doubtful that most people appreciate that a "fruit beverage," a "fruit cocktail," a "fruit nectar," or a "fruit punch" has only a fraction of the fruit juice of a product labeled as "fruit juice." To make matters worse, all of them typically have images of fruit on their containers. Even though laws have attempted to regulate the content of labels (*see* Chapter 27), product names are much more difficult to control. Product name is probably more important to the consumer than what is actually listed on the ingredient listing. If the consumer reads the label small print, he or she finds out that US products with healthful names, such as, "Fruit Works," "Sunny Delight," "King Juice," "Fruitopia," and "Hi-C," contain a mere 5% actual juice by volume. Beverages such as these are typically fortified with vitamin C; however, their nutritional content is dubious, at best, based on actual juice content.

Health advocates lobby for guidelines and regulations to restrict sales of foods of minimal nutritional value and to expand the definition of such foods to include items such as dubious "juice" products. It may be that pricing, taxing, and other "environmental" strategies similar to those proposed to address current trends in obesity are important means for improving the diets of young people *(20,21)*.

In addition, health advocates are making their presence known in other arenas. When they perceive that regulations promote the commercial interests of the manufacturers of soft drink far more than they do children's health, advocates for health urge nations, communities, schools, and students to take effective action to counter this. Concerned advocates urge students to identify and resist school marketing, communities and states to require firm adherence to existing regulations, and school boards to disallow exclusivity agreements and pouring rights contracts altogether. Protests by those most affected are not always heeded, but, by the end of 2000, more than 30 American school districts had refused such deals after protests by parents, students, and school officials. This, too, may prove an effective counter strategy. The high potential to influence society through schools has certainly not escaped the soft-drink industry.

3. MAIN POINTS FOR PRIMARY AND CLINICAL REVIEW

1. The soft-drink industry often presents misleading information.
2. "Pouring rights" are contracts whereby money is paid to school districts in return for exclusive rights to place the company's products in vending machines at schools.
3. About 200 school districts in the United States were participating in such agreements by 2000.
4. There is growing opposition to this, and, by the end of 2000, more than 30 American school districts had refused such deals after protests by parents, students, and school officials.
5. Many pseudo-juice products (high in sugar but low in real fruit juice) have misleading labeling.

REFERENCES

1. Retrieved February 6, 2002, from http://www.softdrink.ca/prw96en.htm.
2. Endicott CR. 100 leading national advertisers, 43rd annual report. Advertising Age 1998;(Suppl): s3–s50.
3. The 2001 Sucralose Soft Drinks Report. Retrieved February 6, 2002, from http://www.officialsucralose site.com/report2001/SSDR_01_04-07.pdf.
4. Nestle M. Soft drink "pouring rights": marketing empty calories. Public Health Rep 2000;115:308–319.
5. General Accounting Office. Public Education: Commercial Activities in Schools (GAO/HERS-00-156). Washington, DC, 2000.

6. The Center for Commercial-Free Public Education. Retrieved from http://www.commercialfree.org. Accessed February 10, 2002.
7. Hays CL. Be true to your cola, rah! rah! Battle for soft-drink loyalties moves to public schools. New York Times, March 10, 1998, pp. D1, D4.
8. North Syracuse Central School District. Agreement with the Coco-Cola Bottling Company of New York, Inc., July 1, 1998.
9. Cherkassky I. Getting the exclusive. Beverage World 1998:97–101.
10. Daft L, Arcos A, Hallawell A, et al. School Food Purchase Study: Final Report. USDA, Washington, DC, 1998.
11. General Accounting Office. School lunch program: role and impacts of private food service companies (GAO/RCED-96-217). GAO, Washington, DC, August 1996.
12. Lawmakers are ready to enlist in the Cola wars. Nutr Wk May 14, 1999, p. 6.
13. USDA. Foods Sold in Competition with USDA School Meal Programs: A Report to Congress. January 12, 2001. Retrieved August 30, 2002, from http://www.fns.usda.gov.
14. Wildey MB, Pampalone SZ, Pelletier RL, Zive MM, Elder JP, Sallis JF. Fat and sugar levels are high in snacks purchased from student stores in middle schools. J Am Dietet Assoc 2000;100:319–322.
15. Contento I, Balch GI, Bronner YL, et al. The effectiveness of nutrition education and implications for nutrition education policy, programs, and research: a review of research. IV. Nutrition education for school-aged children. J Nutr Educ 1995;27:298–311.
16. Cullen KW, Eagan J, Baranowski T, Owens E, deMoor C. Effects of a la carte and snack bar foods at school on children's lunchtime intake of fruits and vegetables. J Am Dietet Assoc 2000;100:1482–1486.
17. WHO information series on school health. Document four. Nutrition: An Essential Element of a Health-Promoting School. World Health Organization, Geneva, 1998.
18. USDA. National school lunch program and school breakfast program: nutrition objectives for school meals; proposed rule. Fed Reg 1994;59:30218–30251.
19. Nestle M. Food Politics: How the Food Industry Influences Nutrition and Health. University of California Press, Berkeley, CA, 2002.
20. Nestle M, Jacobson MF. Halting the obesity epidemic: a public health policy approach. Pub Health Rep 2000;115:12–24.
21. Temple NJ, Nestle M. Population nutrition, health promotion, and government policy. In: Nutritional Health: Strategies for Disease Prevention. Wilson T, Temple NJ (eds.). Humana Press, Totowa, NJ, 2001, pp. 13–29.

X   LABELING ISSUES OF BEVERAGES

26 The Japanese Nutritional Health Beverage Market

Kohji Ohki, Yasunori Nakamura, and Toshiaki Takano

1. INTRODUCTION

The beverage market in postwar Japan started with carbonated and fruit-flavored drinks, following the trend of Western countries. More recently, several innovative beverage products have been developed, including fermented milk-flavored drinks, canned coffee, and teas. Today, Japan is recognized as leading the market in these categories. Nutritional/health beverages started with drinks that offered nourishment and tonic properties and/or nutrient supplements. In 1991, legislation was passed, Foods for Specified Health Uses (FOSHU), that approves labels that make health claims. As a result, many products have appeared and the market is continuing to develop rapidly and uniquely. The latest trends in the nutritional/health beverage market and the present situation of regulation on health claims are summarized in this chapter, with a focus on the Foods with Health Claims system, which started in 2001.

2. MARKET TRENDS

Because nutritional/health beverages include numerous products and it is difficult to give an exact definition for all the categories, there are several ways to classify the market. According to the leading Japanese analyst *(1)*, nutritional/health beverages may be categorized as follows:

1. *Nutritional drinks.* These provide nourishment and tonic properties and/or nutrient supplements (such as vitamins and minerals) and also some oriental drugs (such as ginseng). They are usually sold in small bottles, approx 100 mL. Some of these drinks are treated as quasidrugs under the control of the Pharmaceutical Affairs Law.
2. *Functional drinks.* These are represented by FOSHU products, with approved enhanced function claims.
3. *Nutritionally balanced drinks.* These are designed to supply nutrients in a balanced formulation for general use.

From: *Beverages in Nutrition and Health*
Edited by: T. Wilson and N. J. Temple © Humana Press Inc., Totowa, NJ

Table 1
Categories of Nutritional/Health Drinks and Market Size Changes

Category	Total sales in each year					
	1990	*1992*	*1994*	*1996*	*1998*	*2000*[a]
Nutritional drinks/ food category	155,900[b]	174,000	173,000	158,000	157,150	134,200
Nutritional drinks/ drug category						155,600
Functional drinks	87,000	65,800	64,950	58,600	58,400	50,500
Nutritional balanced drinks	2800	5500	7450	12,850	19,550	25,500
Sport drinks	190,500	176,800	208,500	205,500	219,700	245,850
Near water	2100	20,900	11,100	17,900	123,000	99,500
Soy milk	6920	7180	7600	7040	8700	12,300

[a] Estimate.

[b] Unit: 1 million yen.

4. *Sports drinks*. These provide athletes with water, in addition to carbohydrates and some minerals, vitamins, amino acids, etc., with adjusted osmotic pressure.
5. *Near water*. This is also formulated to supply water and essential minerals and vitamins.
6. *Soy milk*. This has a high protein content and has been consumed in Asia for many years. Recently, some ingredients, such as soy oligosaccharides, protein, and isoflavones, have been approved as FOSHU ingredients, and soy milk itself is often viewed as a health beverage.

The market data for these categories are shown in Table 1 *(1)*.

3. REGULATION COVERING NUTRITIONAL/HEALTH CLAIMS

Labeling of nutritional/health claims for these drinks is controlled mainly by three different laws. Food aspects are covered by the Health Promotion Law and the Food Sanitation Law. Medical aspects are covered by the Pharmaceutical Affairs Law. The laws for food category products include regulation of claims of the nutrient content, nutrient function, and any enhanced function. Presently, claims for "reduction of disease risk" have not been formalized and cannot be made.

Foods for special dietary use fall under the scope of the Health Promotion Law. This law covers special foods designed for people with specific dietary needs, such as infants, pregnant women, and patients with certain diseases, such as diabetes. In 1991, this law was revised to include FOSHU, which permits labeling of enhanced function claims. Such claims are based on individual evaluation and approval. In 1996, this law was again revised to systematize the rules for claims concerning nutrient content. Legislation on a nutrient function claim had not been made until recently, because health claims for vitamins and minerals were regulated as medical effects under the Pharmaceutical Affairs Law.

Recently, as a part of deregulation of the medical aspects of regulation, 15 types of medical claims, including the efficacy of vitamins and minerals and corresponding products sold only in drug stores, were changed to the quasidrug category. Quasidrugs consist

Table 2
Legal Category of Foods With Health Claims

Category	Possible claims
Drugs (including quasidrugs)	Medical
Foods with health claims	
Foods for specified health uses (individual approval system)	Enhanced function, nutrient content
Foods with nutrient function claims (standardized regulation system)	Nutrient function, nutrient content
Other foods (including so-called health foods)	Nutrient content

of products with mild effects, and involvement of a pharmacist is not required for their sale. As a result, restriction on places where these products may be sold have been removed.

Regarding the food aspects of regulations, in 2001, the system for Foods with Nutrient Function Claims was established. This allows health claims for 14 nutrients with proven functions. In this system, food products that meet a certain standard can be labeled with the claim by the manufacturer. The system for Foods with Nutrient Function Claims and the system for FOSHU, which was already established, were combined into the new Foods with Health Claims system. The differences in these regulatory criteria are shown in Table 2. Materials such as herbs, which are considered to have insufficient scientific evidence, are excluded from this standard and treated as "Other Foods." Inclusion of these items into the Foods with Nutrient Function Claims system has been left for later consideration. The regulation of categories of beverages is discussed in the following sections.

3.1. Quasidrugs (Nutritional Drinks/Drug Category)

This system treats supplemental beverage products as drug nutritional drinks and places them into four distinct classes:

1. *Vitamin agents drinks.* These supplement diets with beverages containing vitamins E and/or C needed by middle-aged and elderly people and those with physical fatigue.
2. *Health agents drinks containing vitamins.* These are beverages supplemented with nutrients and formulated as a nourishing tonic to fortify normal individuals of all ages who suffer from weak constitutions and/or physical fatigue.
3. *Calcium agent drinks.* This fortifies and supplements calcium required during particular periods of life, such as pregnancy and lactation and growth and development.
4. *Stomachic algefacient drinks.* This relieves and improves gastric distress.

Because most of the quasidrug beverages belong to the class of Health Agents Drinks containing Vitamins, the standards required for it are listed in Table 3.

Quasidrugs can be labeled with a modest medical claim, if it satisfies several requirements, including its effective components, quantity of the effective components, method and volume of ingestion, package portion, and good manufacturing practice for pharmaceuticals.

Table 3
Regulations Covering Health Agent Drinks Containing Vitamins

Aspects covered by the regulations	Regulations
Type of effective components	1. Vitamins B_1, B_2, and B_6 (must be contained in the final product) 2. Vitamins A, B_{12}, C, D, and E, nicotinamide, pantothenic acid, biotin, folic acid 3. Amino acids (including nitrogenous compounds such as taurine carnitine, dichloroacetic acid di-isopropyl amine, choline bitartrate, egg yolk lecithin) 4. Cholic acid, orotic acid, gamma orizanol, calcium, iron, magnesium, glucuronic acid, chondroitin sulfate, caffeine, inositol, glycyrrhizinate, gluconic acid, thioctic acid, rutin: these compounds are all regulated under their specific chemical names 5. Plant and animal ingredients (34 substances, including ginseng, royal jelly, garlic, etc.) The items in (2) to (5) can be optionally formulated with list (1) items that are compulsory.
Quantity of effective components	The quantity of effective components must be within the range between the lowest and highest limit, which are set for each effective component.
Method and volume of ingestion	One package portion must be designed to be ingested once daily as a single dose by a person aged 15 yr or over.
Efficacy claim	Efficacy of nourishment for the conditions, including asthenia, infirmity, physical fatigue, disease, and/or convalescence from debilitating diseases which weaken the patient physically, Astia (or gastrointestinal injury), abiotrophy (i.e., pus disorders), pyogenicity and anxiety conditions, pregnancy and lactation (i.e., before and after childbirth) can be labeled on the product.
Package portion	Unit of packaging is a mandatory 100 mL as the upper limit.

Foods with Nutrient Function Claims, described in the following section, can be labeled with nutrient functions. These are generic health claims that are validated and recognized widely in the scientific field. However, Foods with Nutrient Function Claims cannot be labeled with a medical claim, even though the medical claims for quasidrugs are modest. Foods with Nutrient Function Claims and quasidrinks, including nutritional drinks, are in separate classes.

3.2. Foods With Nutrient Function Claims

This system was first introduced in 2001, and the market for this genre is still in the early stages of development. As the regulations require only that the nutrient content be stated, all types of beverage may be included; products are not limited to specific characteristics, type of flavors, container size, etc. Currently, the permitted functional nutrients for labeling purposes are restricted to 12 vitamins and 2 minerals. The regulations

Table 4
The Standard Outline of Foods With Nutrient Function Claims

Name	Permitted labeling of nutrient function claims	Maximum/ minimum level
Vitamin A	Vitamin A is a nutrient that helps maintain vision in the dark. Vitamin A is a nutrient that helps keep skin and mucosa healthy.	600 µg (2000 IU)/ 180 µg (600IU)
Vitamin D	Vitamin D is a nutrient that promotes the absorption of calcium in the intestine and aids the development of bone.	50 µg (200 IU)/ 0.9 µg (35 IU)
Vitamin E	Vitamin E is a nutrient that helps protect fat in the body from being oxidized and maintains healthy cells.	150 mg/3 mg
Vitamin B_1	Vitamin B_1 is a nutrient that helps produce energy from carbohydrates and keeps skin and mucosa healthy.	25 mg/0.3 mg
Vitamin B_2	Vitamin B_2 is a nutrient that helps keep skin and mucosa healthy.	12 mg/0.4 mg
Niacin	Niacin is a nutrient that helps keep skin and mucosa healthy.	15 mg/5 mg
Vitamin B_6	Vitamin B_6 is a nutrient that helps produce energy from protein and keep skin and mucosa healthy.	10 mg/0.5 mg
Folic acid	Folic acid is a nutrient that aids in red blood cell formation. Folic acid is a nutrient that contributes to normal growth of the fetus.	200 µg/70 µg
Vitamin B_{12}	Vitamin B_{12} is a nutrient that aids red blood cell formation.	60 µg/0.8 µg
Biotin	Biotin is a nutrient that helps keep skin and mucosa healthy.	500 µg/10 µg
Pantothenic acid	Pantothenic acid is a nutrient that helps keep skin and mucosa healthy.	30 mg/2 mg
Vitamin C	Vitamin C is a nutrient that helps keep skin and mucosa healthy and has an antioxidizing effect.	1000 mg/35 mg
Calcium	Calcium is a nutrient necessary for the development of teeth and bones.	600 mg/250 mg
Iron	Iron is a nutrient necessary for red blood cell formation.	10 mg/4 mg

Note: β-carotene is the precursor of vitamin A and can, therefore, be labeled with the same nutrient function claims as vitamin A. The maximum/minimum level is 3600 µg and 1080 µg, respectively.

for an approved claim and upper and lower content limits for respective nutrients are listed in Table 4.

Once this new system is fully operational, it will extend its scope to cover additional nutrients not yet included, namely other vitamins and minerals, fatty acids, etc.

3.3. Foods for Specified Health Uses

FOSHU are foods that contain a functional ingredient for a specific physiologic purpose. Before health claims may be added to the label, the products must be evaluated individually with the submitted scientific evidence and approved by the Ministry of Health, Labor and Welfare. The main purpose of FOSHU is the prevention of lifestyle-related diseases which cause significant problems in Japan.

FOSHU, which started in1991, is the first approval system of health claims for foods by any national government in the world. FOSHU are defined as a part of Foods for Special Dietary Uses, according to the Health Promotion Law. In 1997 and 2001, the system was revised. Since the 2001 revision, efficacy and safety data are evaluated under the Health Promotion Law and the regulations of labeling are under the Food Sanitation Law.

Applicants must submit the following documents:

1. Sample of the entire package with labels and claims.
2. Explanation of how the product contributes to an improvement of diet and the maintenance/enhancement of health of the entire population, recommended daily intake, and considerations and precautions concerning intake.
3. Documentation providing clinical and nutritional proof of the product's function for maintenance of health and evidence of the quantity required.
4. Documentation concerning safety and stability.
5. Documentation of physical, chemical, and biological properties of the functional components of the product.
6. Results of nutrient analysis and energy calculation.
7. Results from quantitative and qualitative testing of components as nutrient constituents of the food and the testing methods.
8. Description of the production method and equipment of the factory, and a description of the quality control system.

The submitted documents are evaluated by experts from the Pharmaceutical Affairs and Food Sanitation Council. Actual analysis is then performed by the National Institute of Health and Nutrition. Finally, if the product has passed all these hurdles, the Ministry of Health, Labor and Welfare permits labeling of the claim on the product.

The outstanding feature of FOSHU products is the large amount of labeling information provided to the consumer. Functional components, health claims, reasons for approval, daily intake recommendations, and cautions are displayed on the label. When consumers wish to use FOSHU products, all the information required to make a personal selection, depending on individual needs, is available.

4. ACTUAL STATUS OF THE FOSHU PRODUCTS MARKET

As of December 19, 2001, 286 FOSHU products have been permitted. These consist of products targeting seven major functional categories: gastrointestinal (GI) conditions, blood cholesterol, blood lipids and body fat, blood pressure, blood glucose, mineral absorption, and teeth and bone. Table 5 lists the targets for benefit, ingredients, form of the product, and number of products.

The highest number of approved FOSHU items (58%) is for GI conditions. However, products approved for other health claims, such as blood cholesterol, blood lipids and body fat (16%), blood pressure (8.4%), and blood glucose (6.6%), are steadily increasing. This indicates a trend in the development and marketing of FOSHU products for lifestyle-related diseases.

Table 5

**Examples of Foods, Ingredients, and Health Claims
for Foods for Specified Health Uses (FOSHU) in Japan**[a]

Target for benefit	Foods[b]	Ingredients	Example of label statements
Gastrointestinal condition	Cultured milk (42), soft drink (20), lactic acid drink (18), powderd soft drink (15), carbonated beverage (6), others (68)	Oligosaccharide, dietary fiber, lactic acid bacteria	"~ increases intestinal bifidobactera and helps maintain a good intestinal environment"
Blood pressure	Soft drink (15), lactic acid drink (3), powderd soft drink (1), others (5)	Peptide, glycoside	"~ is suitable for people with high normal blood pressure"
Blood glucose	Soft drink (5), powdered soft drink (5), cultured milk (1), others (7)	Dietary fiber, polyphenol	"~ is helpful for those who are concerned about their blood glucose level and helps moderate absorption of sugars"
Blood cholesterol	Soft drink (14), powdered soft drink (4), soy milk (5), others (12)	Dietary fiber, protein, chitosan, diacylglycerol	"~ is helpful for people with a high blood cholesterol level to improve their diet pattern"
Blood lipids and body fat	Soft drink (1), others (9)	Protein hydrolysate, diacylglycerol	"~ helps reduce post-prandial blood trigly-cerides (triacylglycerol) levels"
Mineral absorption	Soft drink (9), others (5)	Peptide, mineral complex, oligosaccharide, heme iron	"~ is suitable for supple-menting calcium intake which tends to be insufficient in normal diets"
Others (teeth and bone)	Soft drink (1), soy drink (1), others (10)	Vitamin K_2, isofla-vone, sugar alcohol	

[a] *Source:* The Japan Health Food and Nutrition Food Association.
[b] Numbers in parentheses denote the numbers of products.

The market share of FOSHU products are: 32.5% soft drinks (including powdered drinks), 12.2% confectionery, 10.8% yogurt drinks, 8.7% lactic acid bacteria drinks, 7.4% table sugars, 6.3% noodles/cereals, 3.1% yogurt, and 18.9% others. Liquid foods, however, have achieved a much greater market share, namely 52.0%, indicating that this form of FOSHU product is more acceptable to Japanese consumers.

Before the revision of the regulations in 2001, products in tablet or capsule form were deemed to be medicines and no FOSHU products in these forms were approved. Since the deregulation on product shapes, much attention is now focused on whether the market share of products that have a tablet or capsule form will expand and occupy a major part of the FOSHU market.

Table 6
Market Size of Foods for Specified Health Uses

Target of benefit	Year (billion yen)		
	1997	1999	2001
Gastrointestinal condition			
Oligosaccharide	10.4	9.1	5.6
Dietary fiber	11.9	11.6	12.8
Lactic acid bacteria	97.9	186.3	317.1
Blood pressure	1.4	7.2	10.0
Blood cholesterol	0	0.4	2.8
Blood lipids and body fat	0	7.0	15.2
Mineral absorption	9.2	4.5	11.4
Blood glucose	0.7	0.5	18.4
Tooth decay	0	0.4	18.7
Total	131.5	226.9	412.1

Source: The Japan Health Food and Nutrition Food Association.

Total FOSHU sales in 2001 were 412 billion yen (approx $3.1 billion) (Table 6). The product category aimed at GI conditions (e.g., constipation relief) accounted for 81.4% of sales. The bulk of the sales were for lactic acid bacteria drinks, yogurt, and yogurt drinks (77%), which already had a big market as general items before FOSHU approval.

After 1997, several successful products appeared on the market that were developed as FOSHU and put on the market after FOSHU approval. These include "Ameal S" (Calpis), a lactic acid beverage with a claim for blood pressure moderation, and "Econa cooking oil" (Kao), with a claim for lowering of the postprandial blood triglyceride level. With the advantage of health claim labeling, these products have captured the major part of their respective functional food markets. In 2001, the market size of products for hypertension, including "Ameal S," was 10 billion yen, whereas that for blood cholesterol and lipids, including "Econa cooking oil," was 18 billion yen. In 2001, the tea drink "Bansourei Cha" (Yakult) expanded the market size of products in the blood glucose category (18 billion yen). The FOSHU products in beverage form for blood cholesterol and lipids have a small segment of the market, but this is expected to grow in the near future.

5. ILLUSTRATED DESCRIPTION OF EXAMPLES OF SUCCESSFUL FOSHU PRODUCTS

5.1. Lactic Acid Bacteria Beverage for Blood Pressure Moderation

Most of the FOSHU products designed to reduce high blood pressure are formulated using peptides, which inhibit the action of angiotensin I converting enzyme (ACE). "Ameal S" is the market leader.

"Ameal S" is prepared by fermenting milk with *Lactobacillus helveticus*, which is subsequently mixed with stabilizers, sweeteners, and flavors before being bottled and pasteurized. During the fermentation process, the *L. helveticus* proteases decompose milk casein proteins to produce the ACE inhibitory peptides valyl-prolyl-proline (VPP) and isoleucyl-prolyl-proline (IPP), collectively known as "Lactotripeptide" *(2)*. Labels on "Ameal S" claim that: "As this product contains "Lactotripeptide," it is suitable for those with high normal blood pressure level." The recommended intake is one bottle (160 g) per day, which provides 3.4 mg of the "Lactotripeptide." "Ameal S" is formulated to be low calorie (30 kcal/bottle), using fat-free skimmed milk, low-calorie sweeteners, aspartame, and sugar alcohol. Therefore, this product is also suitable for people concerned about diabetes, obesity, and hyperlipidemia.

In animal studies, VPP and IPP peptides showed an antihypertensive effect at a single oral administration in spontaneously hypertensive rats (SHR) *(3)*. To see if ACE inhibition occurs in the organs of SHR rats, sour milk containing VPP and IPP peptides was administered and ACE activity was measured in various organs *(4,5)*. ACE activity in the aorta of the sour milk group was significantly lower compared with that of a control group *(4)*. Also, high performance liquid chromatography (HPLC) analysis showed that VPP and IPP were present in the aorta of SHR after ingesting the sour milk *(5)*. These results suggest that VPP and IPP are absorbed from the intestine and delivered to the aorta, where they inhibit ACE activity and, consequently, exhibit antihypertensive activity.

In a clinical study, 30 hospital outpatients who were hypertensive and taking antihypertensive medication were randomly allocated to two groups *(6)*. Sour milk (100 g) or unfermented placebo milk drink was administered daily for 8 wk. In the sour milk group, 4 and 8 wk after ingestion, systolic blood pressure (SBP) decreased significantly by 9 and 14 mmHg, respectively. Diastolic blood pressure (DBP) showed the same trend. Thirty volunteers who were nonmedicated hypertensive (stage 1 and 2 according to the JNC VI classification) were recruited for a double-blind placebo-controlled study with a similar protocol *(7)*. In this study, "Ameal S" or placebo drinks were administered to subjects. The SBP of the test group decreased significantly by 8.6 mmHg after 2 wk and 12 mmHg after 6 wk of ingestion, compared with the initial SBP. This decrease was statistically significant when compared with that in the placebo group. In contrast, in a study with 26 volunteers who were normotensive subjected to the same protocol, no changes were seen in SBP, DBP, and all other blood parameters in both the sour milk and the placebo group *(8)*. In each clinical study, no adverse symptoms, such as coughing, were observed.

5.2. Tea Drinks Possessing Antihyperglycemic Action

The initial market for formulated tea-based drinks was successfully established using indigestible dextrins as an effective component. This market has now received a fresh impetus with the launch of a new tea drink called "Bansourei Cha," which is formulated with extract from leaves of guava, *Psidium guajava*. Guava is native to the tropical and subtropical zones.

The fruits, roots, and leaves have all been used in traditional medicine to treat diabetes. The leaf extract blocks α-amylase *(9)*, maltase, and sucrase activities. By inhibiting α-amylase activity in the intestine, it slows down the digestion and absorption of starches, thereby decreasing the demand for insulin and lowering blood sugar levels. The active substance in guava leaf extract that is responsible for the inhibition is believed to be ellagitannin, a polyphenol.

The product is packed in a 190-mL bottle formulated to contain a single dose, 70 mg, of polyphenols. The product label has been approved to claim that: "As guava polyphenol slows down the absorption of sugars, this product is suitable for those who are concerned about blood sugar levels." The recommended intake is one bottle at every meal, i.e., three bottles daily.

In a single-dose clinical study, 19 adult volunteers, with a body mass index more than 22, ingested 200 g of rice with 190 mL of guava leaf extract tea infusion or hot water as control. The tea drink group had significantly lower blood sugar levels than the control group at 30, 90, and 120 min after ingestion *(9)*. In another study, 16 adults with fasting blood sugar levels of more than 110 mg/dL (6.1 mmol/L) were given 190 mL of guava leaf tea extract three times a day (after each meal) for 12 wk. There was a significant reduction in blood sugar levels during the experiment. A decrease in blood insulin and C peptide was also observed, but this was not significant *(10)*.

5.3. Products for Modulation of Lipid Metabolism

There are several FOSHU-approved beverage products that are intended to help control blood cholesterol levels. These include drinks containing soy protein, low molecular sodium alginate, dietary fiber from psyllium husk, or phospolipid-binding soybean peptides. These ingredients bind with cholesterol and bile acids during their transit through the intestinal tract and inhibit their absorption, and, therefore, help to lower the blood cholesterol level *(11,12)*.

Another such product is a soft drink containing globin digest (i.e., acidic protease hydrolysate), which inhibits pancreatic lipase and enhances the activity of lipoprotein lipase and hepatic triglyceride lipase. The main effective component is reported as valyl-valyl-tyrosyl-proline peptides *(13)*. In a human study, a beverage with the globin digest inhibited the postprandial rise of triglyceride *(14)*. The recommended dosage is one bottle per meal, which is sold in 50 mL volume.

6. CONCLUSION

In Japan and oriental cultures, there is a traditional belief that medicine and food have the same origin. Scientific evidence has accumulated that food intake and ingestion of food components have a significant effect on the maintenance of health. Recently, legislation has been passed to support the appropriate food intake based on established scientific evidence.

Japan has a unique beverage culture, including the nutritional/health drinks. Many types of beverages have been developed and sold to meet consumer demand. The market for nutritional/health drinks is expected to expand further due to the aging of the population and the trend toward lifestyle changes.

7. MAIN POINTS FOR PRIMARY AND CLINICAL REVIEW

1. Food and beverage labeling claims in Japan are regulated by the Foods for Specified Health Uses (FOSHU) and the Foods with Nutrient Function claims.
2. FOSHU beverages contain a specific ingredient for a specific physiological purpose.
3. Under FOSHU, health claim approval for beverages is based on scientific evidence submitted to and approved by the Ministry of Health, Labor and Welfare.
4. Nutritional/health beverages are classified into the following types: nutritional drinks, functional drinks, nutritional balanced drinks, sports drinks, near water, and soy milk beverages.

5. Most FOSHU approvals are for gastrointestinal conditions, although approvals also exist for body fat and blood lipids, blood pressure, and glucose.

REFERENCES

1. 2001 Market Data of Japanese Processed Food No. 4. Fuji Keizai Co. Ltd.
2. Nakamura Y, Yamamoto N, Sakai K, Okubo A, Yamazaki S, Takano T. Purification and characterization of angiotensin I-converting enzyme inhibitors from sour milk. J Dairy Sci 1995;78:777–783.
3. Nakamura Y, Yamamoto N, Sakai K, Takano T. Antihypertensive effect of sour milk and peptides isolated from it that are inhibitors to angiotensin I-converting enzyme. J Dairy Sci 1995;78:1253–1257.
4. Nakamura Y, Masuda O, Takano T. Decrease of tissue angiotensin I-converting enzyme activity upon feeding sour milk in spontaneously hypertensive rats. Biosci Biotechnol Biochem 1996;60:488–489.
5. Masuda O, Nakamura Y, Takano T. Antihypertensive peptides are present in aorta after oral administration of sour milk containing these peptides to spontaneously hypertensive rats. J Nutr 1996;126:3063–3068.
6. Hata Y, Yamamoto M, Ohni M, Nakajima K, Nakamura Y, Takano T. A placebo-controlled study of the effect of sour milk on blood pressure in hypertensive subjects. Am J Clin Nutr 1996;64:767–771.
7. Kajimoto O, Nakamura Y, Yada H, Moriguchi S, Takahashi T. Hypotensive effects of sour milk in subjects with mild and moderate hypertension. J Jpn Soc Nutr Food Sci 2001;54:347–354 (in Japanese).
8. Itakura H, Ikemoto S, Terada S, Kondo K. The effect of sour milk on blood pressure in untreated hypertensive and normotensive subjects. J Jpn Soc Clin Nutr 2002;23:26–31 (in Japanese).
9. Deguchi Y, Osada K, Uchida K, et al. Effects of extract of guava leaves on the development of diabetes in the db/db mouse and on the postprandial blood glucose of human subjects. Nippon Nogeikagaku Kaishi 1998;72:923–931 (in Japanese).
10. Deguchi Y, Osada K, Chonan O, et al. Effectiveness of consecutive ingestion and excess intake of guava leaves tea in human volunteers. Nippon Shokuhin Shinsozai Kenkyuu Kaishi 2000;3:19–28 (in Japanese).
11. Imura T, Tanaka M, Watanabe T, Kanazawa T, Kudo S, Uchida T. Effect of soy protein on serum lipid in adult volunteers. Estimation of minimum daily intake of soy globulin. Ther Res 1996;17:2451–2456 (in Japanese).
12. Hori G, Wang MF, Chan YC, et al. Soy protein hydrolyzate with bound phospholipids reduces serum cholesterol levels in hypercholesterolemic adult male volunteers. Biosci Biotechnol Biochem 2001;65:72–78.
13. Kagawa K, Matsutaka H, Fukuhama C, Watanabe Y, Fujino H. Globin digest, acid protease hydrolysate, inhibits dietary hypertriglyceridemia and Val-Val-Tyr-Pro, one of its constituents, possesses most superior effect. Life Sci 1996;58:1745–1755.
14. Kagawa K, Matsutaka H, Fukuhama C, Fujino H, Okuda H. Suppressive effects of globin digest on postprandial hyperlipidemia in male volunteers. J Nutr 1998;128:56–60.

27 Labeling Requirements for Beverages in the United States

Leslie T. Krasny

Consumers have become increasingly interested in obtaining information about the health-related effects of food, and numerous products are promoted on that basis. It has been a challenge for regulatory agencies to implement a framework for labeling that permits the communication of truthful information, yet prevents the dissemination of false or misleading claims that could cause harm.

The labeling of nonalcoholic beverages in the United States is regulated by the Food and Drug Administration (FDA), pursuant to the Federal Food, Drug, and Cosmetic Act (FD&C Act) *(1)*. The labeling of alcoholic beverages is regulated by the Bureau of Alcohol, Tobacco and Firearms (ATF), pursuant to the Federal Alcohol Administration Act (FAA Act) *(2)*.

1. LABELING OF NONALCOHOLIC BEVERAGES

The term "label" means "a display of written, printed, or graphic matter upon the immediate container of any article...." *(3)*. "Labeling" is a broader term, encompassing "all labels and other written, printed or graphic matter upon any article or any of its containers or wrappers or accompanying such article" *(4)*. The word "accompanying" is interpreted broadly and does not require physical attachment. Thus, promotional materials available with a product at the point of sale are generally classified as labeling. Section 403(a) of the FD&C Act states that a food is misbranded "if its labeling is false or misleading in any particular."

Promotional materials other than labeling are considered advertising. The Federal Trade Commission (FTC) exercises primary jurisdiction over food advertising, pursuant to the Federal Trade Commission Act (FTC Act) *(5)*. A controversial issue is whether product information presented or available on a company's Internet website, including hyperlinks to third-party sites, is considered labeling or advertising. The distinction can be of great importance, because the FTC focuses on content in reviewing advertising, whereas the FDA examines both content and form in reviewing health-related labeling claims. Thus, a claim may be permissible under FTC standards but violate FDA standards. The FDA takes the position that information on a company website would most likely be considered labeling if the website is listed on a product label and the product is sold through the website *(6)*.

From: *Beverages in Nutrition and Health*
Edited by: T. Wilson and N. J. Temple © Humana Press Inc., Totowa, NJ

1.1. Required Label Information

The label of a nonalcoholic beverage must declare the product identity; net quantity of contents; ingredients; name and address of the manufacturer, packer, or distributor; and nutrition information. The required information must appear on the outer container or wrapper of the retail package or must be visible through a transparent wrapper *(7)*.

1.1.1. PRODUCT IDENTITY STATEMENT

The product identity statement, describing the nature of the product, is required to be displayed on the principal display panel (PDP) *(8)*. The product identity statement must be: (1) a name required by law (such as a standard of identity); (2) if there is no required name, the "common or usual" name of the food; or (3) in the absence of a required name or a common or usual name, an appropriately descriptive term or a fanciful name used by the public. For a dietary supplement, the product identity statement must include the term "supplement." A standard of identity mandates the use of specified ingredients, but a standardized food may be modified and still bear the standardized name, if a nutrient-content descriptor is used in conjunction with the product name *(9)*.

The product identity statement must indicate the presence, absence, or amount of any "characterizing" ingredient, if such information would have a material bearing on price or consumer acceptance, or if the labeling would be considered false or misleading without such information. An ingredient is characterizing if a product's label, by word, design, or vignette, makes a representation with respect to the ingredient. Detailed rules are applicable to the declaration of flavors in a product name, including whether the flavors are natural or artificial and whether the characterizing flavor is derived from the product whose flavor is simulated or from other substances that simulate, resemble, or reinforce the characterizing flavor *(10)*.

There is a separate regulation covering the common or usual name for beverages that contain fruit or vegetable juice *(11)*. The product name for a beverage containing less than 100% juice must include a qualifying term such as "beverage," "cocktail," or "drink." For multiple-juice beverages, whether diluted or single strength, any juices in the product name must be listed in descending order of predominance by weight, unless a characterizing juice is declared as a flavor (e.g., raspberry-flavored apple and grape juice drink). There is also a mandatory percentage juice declaration requirement, based on the soluble solids content of expressed juice (not from concentrate), or minimum Brix levels (for reconstituted juice) *(12)*. When a beverage is made from concentrate, the product name must indicate that fact.

1.1.2. INGREDIENT STATEMENT

The ingredient statement may appear on the PDP or on the information panel (IP) *(13)*. The statement must list all ingredients by common or usual name in descending order of predominance by weight *(14)*. "Incidental additives," substances that have no technical or functional effect in the product and are present at insignificant levels, are exempt from the ingredient listing requirement *(15)*. If a juice ingredient is so modified with respect to color, taste, or other organoleptic properties that it is no longer recognizable after processing or that its nutrient profile has been diminished to a level below the normal range, the nature of the modification must be included as part of the common or usual name in the ingredient statement. For dietary supplements, the source of a dietary ingredient must be declared, either in the ingredient statement or with the nutrition information.

In May 2001, the FDA issued a compliance policy guide (CPG) entitled *Statement of Policy for Labeling and Preventing Cross-Contact of Common Food Allergens*, which covers common allergens that cause 90% of allergic reactions: peanuts, milk, eggs, fish, crustacean shellfish, tree nuts, wheat, and soybeans *(16)*. The CPG clarifies that food allergens are not eligible for the incidental additive exemption to ingredient labeling because they are never present at "insignificant" levels. Moreover, the CPG urges manufacturers to implement production controls to prevent or reduce cross-contamination by allergens. In July 2001, the FDA asked for comments on additional steps that could be taken to identify products containing allergens and to reduce the risk of cross-contamination during production, including source or plain English labeling, labeling of substances currently exempt from ingredient declaration (incidental additives and allergenic components of flavorings, colors, and spices), and "may contain" advisory labeling *(17)*.

1.1.3. NET QUANTITY OF CONTENTS DECLARATION

The net quantity of contents must accurately reflect the contents in terms of weight, measure, or numeric count *(18)*. Metric labeling is required, in addition to traditional British units, pursuant to the American Technology Preeminance Act of 1991 *(19)*. The accuracy of the net quantity of contents declaration is determined by the FDA or individual states under compliance sampling criteria.

1.1.4. NUTRITION LABELING

The Nutrition and Labeling Education Act of 1990 (NLEA) amended the FD&C Act to require nutrition labeling for packaged foods *(20)*. Exemptions that may be applicable to beverages include small businesses, restaurant and other institution foods, ready-to-eat foods packaged on-site and not for immediate consumption, foods with no nutritional value, small packages, individual units in multiunit retail food packages, medical foods, and infant formulas. However, some exemptions are negated if there is a "nutrition claim or any other nutrition information on the label or in the labeling or advertising in any context, and in any form of expression, implicit, as well as explicit" *(21)*.

Before the NLEA, manufacturers were free to choose a serving size when reporting nutrition information. To facilitate nutritional comparisons between products, the FDA determined "reference amounts customarily consumed" (RACCs) for most food categories *(22)*. The appropriate RACC is converted to a serving size, expressed as a common household measure *(23)*. Unlike conventional foods, the reference amount for a dietary supplement is based on a manufacturer's recommended serving size for the product. However, if a supplement does not state a recommended serving size, the FDA assumes that a single unit (e.g., one can) is the serving size.

Nutrition labeling is mandatory for the following components/nutrients: calories, calories from fat, total fat, saturated fat, cholesterol, sodium, total carbohydrate, dietary fiber, sugars, protein, vitamin A, vitamin C, calcium, and iron. Nutrition labeling is voluntary for the following components/nutrients: calories from saturated fat, polyunsaturated fat, monounsaturated fat, potassium, soluble fiber, insoluble fiber, sugar alcohols, other carbohydrates, vitamin D, vitamin E, thiamin, riboflavin, niacin, vitamin B_6, folate, vitamin B_{12}, biotin, pantothenic acid, phosphorus, iodine, magnesium, zinc, and copper. However, the declaration of a "voluntary" nutrient becomes mandatory if the nutrient is the subject of a nutrient content claim or is added to a food as a nutrient supplement. A simplified format may be used when a product contains "insignificant" amounts of seven or more specified food components and nutrients *(24)*. In 1999, the FDA proposed a regulation to require that the amount of *trans* fat present in a product be declared in the nutritional facts box and issued a final rule in 2003.

The FDA has established Reference Daily Intakes (RDIs) for vitamins and minerals and Daily Reference Values (DRVs) for fat, saturated fat, cholesterol, total carbohydrates, fiber, sodium, potassium, and protein. The Percent Daily Value (%DV), a generic term covering DRVs and RDIs, must be provided for each declared nutrient other than sugars, except that declaration of the %DV for protein is not required unless the protein content of the product is of low quality.

The FDA's compliance policy for assuring the accuracy of nutrition information distinguishes between two classes of nutrients. Class I nutrients are added to foods, and Class II nutrients are naturally present. For Class I nutrients, the content must at least equal the declared value. For Class II nutrients, the content must at least equal 80% of the declared value. The different treatment of the two classes of nutrients is based on the fact that levels of ingredients added to formulated foods are more easily controllable than levels of naturally occurring nutrients.

1.2. Regulatory Categories

Section 201(f) of the FD&C Act defines "food" as (1) articles used for food or drink for man or other animals, (2) chewing gum, and (3) articles used for components of any such article. There are complex rules governing health-related labeling claims for food, which may vary by regulatory category. Thus, a product that meets the regulatory criteria for more than one category of food may bear different claims, depending upon the selection. The terms "functional food" and "nutraceutical" are not defined in the FD&C Act or regulations, although the General Accounting Office (GAO) defines functional foods as those that "claim to have health benefits beyond basic nutrition" *(25)*.

The Dietary Supplement Health and Education Act of 1994 (DSHEA) amended the FD&C Act to regulate dietary supplements as a category of food, with some separate requirements. A dietary supplement is a product that is intended to supplement the diet through ingestion, that contains one or more "dietary ingredients," that is not represented for use as a conventional food or sole item of a meal or the diet, and that is labeled as a dietary supplement *(26)*. Dietary ingredients include one or more of the following: a vitamin, a mineral, an herb or other botanical, an amino acid, or another substance intended to supplement the diet by increasing the total dietary intake of that substance, or a concentrate, metabolite, constituent part, extract, or combination of dietary ingredients. A "new" dietary ingredient is one that was not marketed in the United States before October 15, 1994. Dietary ingredients include substances that have been approved by the FDA as drugs but were available in the food supply or as dietary supplements before drug approval. Products intended for use to diagnose, cure, mitigate, treat, or prevent disease are classified as drugs.

Medical food is defined as a food specially formulated and processed to be consumed or to be administered enterally under the active and ongoing supervision of a physician and intended for the specific dietary management of a disease or condition for which distinctive nutritional requirements are established by medical evaluation *(27)*. Medical foods are exempted from nutrition labeling, nutrient content claim, and health claim requirements. The FDA is concerned that some products marketed as medical foods may not meet the statutory and regulatory criteria and has proposed reevaluating the regulations to ensure that these products are safe for their intended use; that claims are truthful, not misleading, and supported by sound science; and that the labeling adequately informs consumers about appropriate use *(28)*.

Foods for special dietary use supply particular dietary needs, which result from a physical, physiological, pathological, or other condition or from age (including infancy and childhood), or supplement the ordinary or usual diet with any vitamin, mineral, or other dietary property. The FDA has issued regulations requiring additional labeling information on certain foods marketed for special dietary use, such as weight loss/ maintenance, hypoallergenic, and infant foods *(29)*.

1.3. Allowable Ingredients

The definition of "food" encompasses all raw materials and any component of a food, including food additives. Under section 201(s) of the FD&C Act, a food additive is a substance, "the intended use of which results or may reasonably be expected to result, directly or indirectly, in its becoming a component or otherwise affecting the characteristics of any food." A food additive is deemed to be unsafe unless used in accordance with a food additive regulation *(30)*. However, substances generally recognized as safe (GRAS) for their intended use, "prior sanctioned" substances (permitted by the FDA before enactment of the Food Additives Amendment to the FD&C Act in 1958), and dietary ingredients used in a dietary supplement are excluded from the definition of food additive.

If there is no food additive regulation, manufacturers may rely on a self-determined GRAS position regarding the regulatory status of a beverage ingredient (at their risk) or may submit a GRAS notification to the FDA *(31)*. Information to be submitted as part of a GRAS notification includes the conditions of use (foods, levels, and purposes), the basis for the GRAS determination (scientific procedures or experience based on common use in food), and detailed information about the identity of the substance. Moreover, the notification must state the justification for concluding that there is a reasonable certainty the substance is not harmful under the intended conditions of use, based on consensus among qualified experts.

The FDA has sent numerous warning letters to conventional/functional beverage manufacturers who used ingredients such as lutein, ginkgo biloba, ginseng, echinacea, guarana, and bilberry extract in their formulations, questioning the manufacturers' basis for concluding that the ingredients are allowable. There are no food additive regulations authorizing the use of these substances, and, therefore, if the FDA does not agree that the substances are GRAS for their intended use, the beverages are considered adulterated.

DSHEA, which exempts dietary ingredients in dietary supplements from food additive requirements, shifts the burden of proof for product safety from the manufacturer to the FDA. Generally, the FDA must find that a dietary supplement "presents a significant or unreasonable risk of illness or injury" or an "imminent hazard to public health or safety" to take action against a marketed product. For a "new dietary ingredient," the manufacturer must notify the FDA 75 d before introducing the product, including substantiation that the new dietary ingredient can "reasonably be expected to be safe"

(32). Some companies that marketed beverages as dietary supplements under the less stringent DSHEA safety standard have had the FDA challenge the classification on the ground that the product was intended to be used as a conventional/functional food. In this regard, the FDA has concluded, in regulatory letters, that a claim such as "refreshing beverage" was evidence of positioning as a conventional/functional beverage rather than as a dietary supplement.

Another issue is the dietary supplement-drug distinction. A nicotine-laced water product was marketed as a dietary supplement alternative to smoking. The FDA concluded that the product is an unapproved drug under the FD&C Act, because the intended use is to treat or mitigate nicotine addiction (a disease). The FDA also found that the product does not meet the definition of a dietary supplement, because the active ingredient was approved for use as a drug before use in a dietary supplement.

1.4. Nutrient Content Claims

"Nutrient content claims" expressly or impliedly characterize the level of a nutrient in a food and must be authorized by regulation or by notification to the FDA based on a published authoritative statement by a scientific body of the United States *(33)*. The FDA permits nutrient content claims only if there is an established DRV or RDI for a nutrient and if claims are consistent with regulatory definitions. Undefined terms that are synonyms for defined terms may not be used, although there have been objections to this position. For example, the FDA considers the undefined term "with" to be an unauthorized nutrient content claim on the ground that it is a synonym for the defined terms "contains," "provides," and "good source" (10–19% of the DRV or RDI per serving).

If a beverage exceeds any of the following levels—13 g fat, 4 g saturated fat, 60 mg cholesterol, and 480 mg sodium per reference amount and per labeled serving size—no nutrient content claim may be made unless there is a "disclosure" statement adjacent to the largest claim on the panel: "See nutrition information for ___ content" *(34)*. However, a declaration of just the quantity of a nutrient per serving is not considered to be a nutrient content claim, because the level of the nutrient in the food is not characterized.

Nutrient content claims are either "absolute" or "relative." Absolute claims refer only to the nutrient content of the food bearing the claim. Relative claims compare the level of a nutrient in one food to the level of that nutrient in another food *(35)*. To ensure that comparisons are consistent and not misleading, the FDA has established two types of reference foods that may be used as a basis for comparison: similar foods and dissimilar foods within a product category. Less, fewer, and more claims may be based on either type. However, light, reduced, added, plus, fortified, and enriched claims may use only similar reference foods. For relative nutrient content claims, the label must bear a "related information statement" adjacent to the claim that discloses the identity of the reference food and the percentage or fraction by which the nutrient content has been reduced or increased. The label must also declare quantitative information comparing the level of the nutrient in the product (per serving) with the level of the nutrient in an appropriate reference food.

1.5. Health Claims

A health claim is "any claim made on the label or in labeling of a food, including a dietary supplement, that expressly or by implication, including 'third party' references, written statements (e.g., a brand name including a term such as 'heart'), symbols (e.g., a heart symbol), or vignettes, characterizes the relationship of any substance to a disease or health-related condition" *(36)*. For purposes of health claim requirements, a "substance" is defined as a specific food or component of food *(37)*. "Disease or health-related condition" means "damage to an organ, part, structure, or system of the body such that it does not function properly (e.g., cardiovascular disease), or a state of health leading to such disfunctioning (e.g., hypertension); except that diseases resulting from essential nutrient deficiencies (e.g., scurvy, pellagra) are not included in this definition" *(38)*.

In addition, if a health claim for a conventional/functional food is based on the presence of a substance at other than decreased levels, the substance must serve a traditional food purpose at levels necessary to justify the claim and must have been shown to be safe and lawful at the level at which it will be used in the food and the level at which it is expected to be consumed. The term "traditional food purpose" encompasses taste, aroma, nutritive value, or any other technical effect in food recognized by the FDA. "Nutritive value" is defined as having a "value in sustaining human existence by such processes as promoting growth, replacing loss of essential nutrients, or providing energy" *(39)*. The technical effects in food recognized by the FDA include: antimicrobial agents, antioxidants, colors, enzymes, flavors, formulation aids, nonnutritive sweeteners, nutrient supplements, nutritive sweeteners, oxidizing/reducing agents, pH control agents, and processing aids *(40)*.

Health claims require prior FDA approval or notification to FDA of authoritative status. To be approved by regulation, the FDA requires "significant scientific agreement" among qualified experts that the claim is supported by the "totality of publicly available scientific evidence" *(41)*. Dietary supplement manufacturers challenged the FDA's "significant scientific agreement" standard, urging that health claims be permitted with appropriate qualifications or disclaimers if the significant scientific agreement standard was not met. In *Pearson v. Shalala*, 164 F.3d 650 (D.C. Cir. 1999), the court ordered the FDA to consider the use of qualifications or disclaimers. The information to be submitted to the FDA in a petition to establish a health claim regulation must include a summary of the scientific data relied on and analytical data on the amount of the substance in foods likely to bear the claim.

In addition to approval of a health claim by regulation, the FDA may permit a health claim based on a published authoritative statement of a federal agency that has responsibility for the protection of the public health or research directly relating to human nutri-tion. Notification of the authoritative statement must be provided to the FDA at least 120 d before use on the label or in the labeling of the food. If the FDA does not take steps within the 120-d period to prohibit the proposed claim, the claim may be used on appropriate products.

Generally, a health claim may not be made for a conventional/functional food that exceeds specified levels of fat, saturated fat, cholesterol, and sodium. Under the so-called "Jelly Bean Rule," health claims approved by regulation are prohibited for most conventional/functional foods that do not contain, before fortification, at least 10% of the RDI or DRV of vitamin A, vitamin C, calcium, protein, or fiber per serving.

1.6. Structure/Function Claims

In contrast to health claims, structure/function claims may be made for conventional/functional foods and dietary supplements without previous authorization. DSHEA authorizes "statements of nutritional support" for the labeling of dietary supplements. The four types are: (1) statements that claim a benefit related to a classical nutrient deficiency disease, (2) statements that describe the role of a nutrient or dietary ingredient intended to affect the structure or function of the body, (3) statements that characterize the documented mechanism by which a nutrient or dietary ingredient acts to maintain structure or function, and (4) statements that describe general well-being from consumption of a nutrient or dietary ingredient. The manufacturer must have substantiation that the claim is truthful and not misleading.

DSHEA requires companies to notify the FDA within 30 d after the first use of structure/function claims in the labeling of a dietary supplement and to print the following disclaimer on the same label panel as the claim: "This statement has not been evaluated by the Food and Drug Administration. This product is not intended to diagnose, treat, cure or prevent any disease" *(42)*. Under the FDA's current interpretation of the FD&C Act, all structure/function claims made in the labeling of dietary supplements are subject to the notification and disclaimer requirements, although there is a strong argument, based on the statutory language, that only structure/function claims that fall within the definition of "health claims" are subject to the notification and disclaimer requirements.

Structure/function claims may also be made for conventional/functional foods, although the notification and disclaimer requirements are not applicable. The FDA takes the position that structure/function claims for conventional/functional foods must be based on the nutritive value of the food or nutrient, which is not a requirement for dietary supplements *(43)*. However, the FD&C Act and relevant case law do not compel that conclusion.

The FD&C Act and FDA regulations prohibit structure/function claims that refer to a disease ("drug" claims). The regulations specifically disallow claims that suggest that the product has an effect on a disease, refer to a characteristic sign or symptom of a disease, refer to a disease in the product name, or use pictures, symbols, or other means of suggesting a disease.

1.7. Healthy Claims

The term "healthy," and permitted synonyms, may be used to describe beverages that are low in fat and saturated fat, do not exceed established levels for sodium and cholesterol, and are a "good" source of at least one of six nutrients (vitamin A, vitamin C, calcium, iron, fiber, and protein) *(44)*.

1.8. Natural Claims

The FDA has not issued a regulation defining the term "natural" but has adopted a policy on the subject, which provides that "natural" means: "nothing artificial or synthetic has been included in, or has been added to, a food that would not normally be expected to be in the food" *(45)*. With respect to the classification of colors, any added color is considered to be artificial, even if the source of the color is natural *(46)*. An unresolved issue is the use of natural claims on products that contain synthetic forms of naturally occurring substances, such as ascorbic acid and citric acid, because the natural and synthetic forms are chemically identical.

1.9. Fresh Claims

The term "fresh," when used in labeling in a manner suggesting or implying that a beverage is unprocessed, means that the product is in its raw state and has not been frozen or subjected to any form of thermal processing or other form of preservation *(47)*. The FDA notes, as an example of a permissible use of the term, that pasteurized milk may be described as fresh because consumers commonly understand that milk is nearly always pasteurized. Use of the term as a sensory modifier, such as to describe taste, would be evaluated by the FDA on a case-by-case basis, taking into account the context of the claim and consumer perception regarding the processing of the product.

1.10. Directions for Use and Warnings

The manufacturer of a beverage must provide adequate directions for use or warnings, as appropriate. Usually, directions or warnings are found on dietary supplements and medical foods, although conventional foods may also have warnings, either as determined by the manufacturer or as required by regulation. For example, diet drinks that contain aspartame must state: phenylketonurics: contains phenylalanine *(48)*. Another example is that the label of any fresh (nonpasteurized) juice must bear a warning unless the processors can meet a specified pathogen reduction standard: "WARNING: This product has not been pasteurized and, therefore, may contain harmful bacteria that can cause serious illness in children, the elderly, and persons with weakened immune systems" *(49)*.

1.11. First Amendment Protection of Commercial Speech

On May 16, 2002, the FDA published a notice requesting public comment as to whether its regulations, guidances, policies, and practices comply with First Amendment case law, including its position that the Pearson ruling applied only to dietary supplements and that all health claims for conventional foods had to meet the "significant scientific agreement" standard *(50)*. In December 2002, the FDA announced the *Consumer Health Information for Better Nutrition* initiative, which is intended to provide consumers with greater information about the health benefits of foods. Importantly, the FDA decided to reverse its long-held position and to permit health claims that meet a "weight of the evidence" standard for both conventional foods and dietary supplements. The FDA also plans to use a "reasonable person" test to assess whether food labeling is misleading, consistent with the FTC standard for determining deceptive advertising. The new policy and procedures are described in an industry guidance document issued by the FDA, entitled *Qualified Health Claims in the Labeling of Conventional Foods and Dietary Supplements*.

1.12. Biotechnology Claims

Food biotechnology regulation is a highly controversial issue in the United States and internationally. Under the FDA's long-standing "substantial equivalence" policy, special labeling is required only when a bioengineered food contains potential allergens or otherwise differs from its traditional counterpart to the extent that the common or usual name is no longer adequate to describe the nature of the food.

The FDA released guidance to industry in January 2001, entitled "Voluntary Labeling Indicating Whether Foods Have Or Have Not Been Developed Using Bioengineering"

(51). The guidance sets forth the FDA's criteria for ensuring that voluntary claims concerning bioengineering are not false or misleading. The guidance notes that acronyms, such as GMO and GM, are not generally understood by consumers and should be avoided; that "genetically modified" applies to virtually all cultivated food crops; that NO GMOs is misleading, because most foods do not contain organisms; and that "free" should not be used unless there is a threshold established, in conjunction with readily available analytical methods. The FDA suggested statements that would be considered appropriate, if accurate, including: "We do not use ingredients that were produced using biotechnology."

1.13. Organic Claims

The Organic Foods Production Act of 1990 (OFPA) authorizes national standards for the marketing of raw and processed organic agricultural products in the United States for human and livestock consumption *(52)*. Regulations implementing the National Organic Program (NOP) were published in December 2000, with an effective date of October 21, 2002. The NOP applies to conventional organic beverages but does not cover dietary supplement beverages with organic claims. However, state organic programs (SOPs) may have broader coverage than the NOP.

There are four categories of products covered by NOP labeling regulations, based on organic content: 100%, 95% or more, 70–95%, and less than 70% (excluding water and salt). Beverages labeled as "100% organic" must be composed entirely of organically produced ingredients (including any processing aids). Beverages labeled as "organic" must contain at least 95% organically produced ingredients; the additional ingredients may be permitted nonorganic substances if not "commercially available" in organic form. Beverages labeled as "made with organic (specified ingredients or food groups)" must contain between 70% and 95% organically produced ingredients. Beverages containing less than 70% organic ingredients may use the term "organic" only on the information panel to identify organic ingredients. No organic ingredients, and no nonorganic ingredients in the first three categories, may be produced using biotechnology.

1.14. California Proposition 65 Warnings

The California Safe Drinking Water and Toxic Enforcement Act of 1986, Health and Safety Code §25249.5 *et seq.* (Proposition 65) requires California to maintain a list of chemicals known to the state to cause cancer or reproductive toxicity and provides that "no person in the course of doing business shall knowingly and intentionally expose any individual" to a listed chemical without first giving clear and reasonable warning. Proposition 65 permits private citizens to bring enforcement actions if officials do not file suit within 60 d after receiving notice of alleged violations.

The consumer aspect of the warning requirement does not apply to an exposure for which the responsible person can demonstrate that there is no significant risk, assuming lifetime exposure at the level in question (for carcinogens) or that there will be no observable effect, assuming exposure at 1000 times the level in question (for reproductive toxins). The required statement is "WARNING: This product contains a chemical known to the State of California to cause (cancer)/(birth defects and other reproductive harm)." There is an exemption for chemicals that are "naturally occurring" in food *(53)*.

2. LABELING OF ALCOHOLIC BEVERAGES

The ATF has jurisdiction over beverages in liquid form, intended for human consumption, that contain at least 0.5% alcohol by volume *(54)*. The ATF regulates the labeling of wine (exceeding 7% alcohol), beer, and spirits. The label of an alcoholic beverage must include the brand name, the class and type, the alcoholic content, and the net contents. The percentage of neutral spirits and the name of the commodity from which distilled must also be declared *(55)*. A Certificate of Label Approval (COLA) or exemption must be obtained from the ATF before marketing an alcoholic beverage.

The label of any alcoholic beverage container sold in the United States must contain a health warning statement separate from all other information: "GOVERNMENT WARNING: (1) According to the Surgeon General, women should not drink alcoholic beverages during pregnancy because of the risk of birth defects. (2) Consumption of alcoholic beverages impairs your ability to drive a car or operate machinery, and may cause health problems" *(56)*.

On March 3, 2003, the ATF issued a final rule on health claims and other health-related statements in the labeling and advertising of alcoholic beverages. As of June 2003, the regulations prohibit any health-related statement (including a specific health claim) in labeling or advertising that is untrue in any particular or tends to create a misleading impression. A specific health claim is considered misleading unless the claim is truthful and adequately substantiated by scientific evidence; properly detailed and qualified with respect to the categories of individuals to whom the claim applies; adequately discloses the health risks associated with both moderate and heavier levels of alcohol consumption; and outlines the categories of individuals for whom any levels of alcohol consumption may cause health risks. Furthermore, the ATF plans to consult with the FDA, as needed, on the use of specific health claims on labels of alcoholic beverages. If the FDA determines that a specific health claim is a drug claim under the FD&C Act, the ATF will not approve the label statement.

Health-related statements that are not specific health claims will be evaluated on a case-by-case basis to determine if they are misleading. Health-related directional statements (statements that refer consumers to a third party or other source for information regarding the effects of alcohol consumption on health) will be presumed misleading unless there is a disclaimer advising consumers that the statement should not encourage consumption of alcohol for health reasons, or a similar disclaimer *(57)*.

3. CONCLUSION

Labeling claims are an important source of health-related information and a driving force in the marketing of beverages. The usefulness and constitutionality of past labeling requirements were challenged by industry and consumers, and the regulatory positions were reevaluated. As a result, more flexible standards were adopted regarding health-related claims, focusing on the degree of substantiation and qualification. Consumers will now have greater access to truthful and nonmisleading labeling messages about the health benefits of foods.

4. MAIN POINTS FOR PRIMARY AND CLINICAL REVIEW

1. The labeling of nonalcoholic beverages in the United States is regulated by the Food and Drug Administration (FDA) (under the Federal Food, Drug, and Cosmetic Act,

FD&C Act), whereas the labeling of alcoholic beverages is regulated by the Bureau of Alcohol, Tobacco and Firearms (ATF) (under the Federal Alcohol Administration Act, FAA Act).

2. Nonalcoholic beverage labels must declare the product identity, net quantity of contents, ingredients, name and address of the manufacturer, packer or distributor, and nutrition information.
3. Nutrition labeling is mandatory for the following components/nutrients: calories, calories from fat, total fat, saturated fat, cholesterol, sodium, total carbohydrate, dietary fiber, sugars, protein, vitamin A, vitamin C, calcium, and iron.
4. Health claims require prior approval or authoritative status.
5. Structure/function claims may be made for conventional/functional foods and dietary supplements without prior authorization.

REFERENCES

1. 21 U.S.C. §§ 331 *et seq.*
2. 27 U.S.C. §§ 201 *et seq.*
3. 21 U.S.C. § 321(k) and 21 C.F.R. § 1.3(b).
4. 21 U.S.C. § 321(m) and 21 C.F.R. § 1.3(a).
5. 15 U.S.C. §§ 41 *et seq.*
6. FDA letter on labeling food products presented or available on the Internet. Retrieved November 1, 2001.
7. 21 C.F.R. § 1.20(a)-(e).
8. 21 C.F.R. § 101.3.
9. 21 C.F.R. § 130.10.
10. 21 C.F.R. § 101.22(i).
11. 21 C.F.R. § 102.33.
12. 21 C.F.R. § 101.30.
13. 21 C.F.R. § 101.3.
14. 21 C.F.R. § 101.4(a)(1).
15. 21 C.F.R. § 101.100(a)(3).
16. 66 *Fed. Reg.* 22240 (May 3, 2001).
17. 66 *Fed. Reg.* 38591 (July 25, 2001).
18. 21 C.F.R. § 101.105.
19. Pub. L. No. 102-245 (1991), codified at 15 U.S.C. § 278n.
20. 21 C.F.R. § 101.9.
21. 21 C.F.R. § 101.9(a).
22. 21 C.F.R. § 101.12(b).
23. 21 C.F.R. § 101.9(b).
24. 21 U.S.C. § 321(ff).
25. Food Safety Improvements Needed in Overseeing the Safety of Dietary Supplements and "Functional Foods," p. 3, GAO/RCED-00-156 (July 2000).
26. 21 C.F.R. § 101.9(f).
27. 21 C.F.R. § 101.9(j)(8).
28. 61 *Fed. Reg.* 6066 (November 29, 1996).
29. 21 C.F.R. Part 105.
30. 21 U.S.C. § 348.
31. 62 *Fed. Reg.* 18938 (April 17, 1997).
32. 21 C.F.R. § 190.6.
33. 21 C.F.R. § 101.13(b).
34. 21 C.F.R. § 101.13(g).
35. 21 C.F.R. § 101.13(j).
36. 21 C.F.R. § 101.14(a)(1).

37. 21 C.F.R. § 101.14(a)(2).
38. 21 C.F.R. § 101.14(a)(6).
39. 21 C.F.R. § 101.14(a)(3).
40. 21 C.F.R. § 101.70.
41. 21 C.F.R. § 101.14(c).
42. 21 U.S.C. § 343(r)(6).
43. 62 *Fed. Reg.* 49859, 49860 (September 23, 1997).
44. 21 C.F.R. § 101.65(d).
45. 58 *Fed. Reg.* 2407 (January 6, 1993).
46. 21 C.F.R. § 101.22(a)(4).
47. 21 C.F.R. § 101.95.
48. 21 C.F.R. § 172.804.
49. 21 C.F.R. § 101.17(g).
50. 67 *Fed. Reg.* 34942 (May 16, 2002).
51. 66 *Fed. Reg.* 4839 (January 18, 2001).
52. 7 U.S.C. § 6501 *et seq.*
53. 22 Cal. Code of Regulations, section 12507.
54. 27 U.S.C. § 214.
55. 27 C.F.R. § 5.39(a).
56. 27 C.F.R. § 16.21.
57. 68 *Fed. Reg.* 10076 (March 3, 2003).

XI CONCLUSIONS

28 Refining Beverage Nutrition to Provide Healthy Lives and Responsible Markets

David R. Jacobs, Jr., Norman J. Temple, and Ted Wilson

Beverages in Nutrition and Health is intended as a reference or classroom text source for health professionals, dietitians, physicians, university researchers, students, and beverage industry researchers and marketers. In a single book, it provides objective reviews on global health issues associated with beverages. The book, as a whole, is greater than the sum of its component chapters. Therefore, it is important to summarize the key messages contained in this book and the implication to our health; this is the first objective of this final chapter. The second objective is to describe how these health implications affect the beverage industry and how this industry affects its consumer base.

1. SUMMARY OF NUTRITION-RELATED OBSERVATIONS

One of the lessons that arises from this book is the rapid pace of diversification in the world of beverages in recent years. As a result, there is an impressive range of beverages now being marketed. This speaks volumes to human ingenuity, and reminds us of the importance of continued studies of how these beverages affect our health.

Clearly, international cross-fertilization of ideas has played a major role in this process. That, of course, has been a major goal of this book. It is our fervent hope, therefore, that this book will act as a catalyst for ongoing progress in the development of beverages that satisfy the needs and wants of the consumer, especially with regard to price and healthfulness.

The stage for understanding beverages and nutrition is set in the image presented by Grivetti and Wilson of prehistoric man searching for easily accessible water and the evolution of beverages. It is not a trivial observation that water, *per se* (that is, without consideration of minerals that might be dissolved in the water or microorganisms that might live in the water), is an essential nutrient. Water provides hydration; death ensues within days without water. An important question is, therefore, how do large human populations procure clean and healthful water? What other nutritionally important

From: *Beverages in Nutrition and Health*
Edited by: T. Wilson and N. J. Temple © Humana Press Inc., Totowa, NJ

substances come with that water? Chapters 22 and 23 discuss these issues, specifically for tap water and bottled water.

Chapter 23 reviews the issues related to the provision of safe tap water. In particular, an aspect of drinking water that we can never be complacent about is that of microbiologic contamination causing bacterial or parasitic infection. This problem has a habit of making a dramatic reappearance whenever it seems to have dropped off the radar screen. Chapter 23 provides a timely update on this important problem. Other issues discussed include using tap water as a vehicle to provide fluoride for the prevention of tooth decay and the risk of cancer that might be caused by water disinfection by-products (DBPs).

Chapter 22 documents that there are major differences among different bottled waters. As a result, some brands act as a vehicle for increasing our intake of minerals, such as calcium and magnesium, while also having a low content of sodium. Bottled water is an excellent alternative when tap water is not available or when it is not safe. However, for the large majority of consumers, bottled water typically has no nutritional advantage over tap water. Many bottled waters are not fluoridated. Therefore, as the market for bottled water expands, the dental advantage of fluoridation may be lost. The question of the relative microbiologic purity of tap water and of bottled water is an important topic that requires further investigation. Bottled water has become increasingly popular, and market forces encouraging the consumption of this product are powerful, yet rarely focused on health. As a result, there has been a recent dramatic increase in sales of bottled water in North America. Millions have been persuaded to consume copious amounts of a beverage that often costs considerably more than gasoline (measured as dollars/L) but is frequently inferior to tap water: a spectacular example of the triumph of commercialism over good sense.

Some questions about water remain. There is plenty of water on Earth; nevertheless, some regions are arid or parched, and water promises to become a major political issue in coming decades. The overarching question of how humankind will assure, or even achieve, equitable and necessary water rights is a formidable question that remains uncovered in this book and outside the scope of this book.

This book provides a comprehensive and informative epidemiologic review on the health associations of alcohol. There has been a recent explosion of epidemiologic and laboratory studies of alcohol. Given the findings of these studies, alcohol is increasingly becoming a fascinating drink in regard to nutrition. It is best known for its intoxicating, often pleasant, effect. Alcohol can also be a major source of antisocial behavior, family disruption, and motor vehicle deaths. For those who believe that alcohol should be prescribed more than proscribed, there is much to cheer in Chapter 2. Indeed, there has been a rapid accumulation of evidence in recent years documenting the beneficial health effects of moderate consumption of alcohol. That chapter restates the argument that it is alcohol—from any source—that is responsible for the prevention of coronary heart disease and that red wine has no particular additional benefit. The evidence cited is based almost entirely on epidemiology. Rimm and Temple suggest that: "Arguably, the most prudent policy is one that explains that alcohol in moderation will likely have several health benefits for people in middle age and above, while also stressing the hazards of abuse."

Coffee is a popular drink that has been suspected of causing harm and has been extensively studied. Fortunately, Tavani and La Vecchia (Chapter 9) provide reassurance that coffee is virtually free of suspicion as a cause of cancer, although it may induce a modest increase in risk of urinary bladder cancer. With coronary heart disease (CHD), however, we must be more cautious. Epidemiologic evidence indicates that three cups of coffee per day poses negligible risk, whereas five or more cups daily may increase risk by 40%. It must be stressed that epidemiology has its limitations. Particularly, the association between coffee and heart disease has been seen in case-controlled studies more so than in cohort studies. Case-controlled studies are more prone to error than are cohort studies. This controversy is clearly important and, hopefully, will be resolved by future cohort studies. An additional topic for consideration in future studies is the cholesterol-raising effect of cafestol, present in boiled coffee (1), a topic not directly reviewed in this book. However, overall, the consumption of three or fewer cups of coffee per day should not pose a threat to health.

Afaq and colleagues synthesize an impressive body of both epidemiologic and experimental evidence that tea, especially green tea, may provide significant protection against several chronic diseases, most notably cancer and cardiovascular disease (CVD). Green tea may also be helpful in diabetes, obesity, osteoporosis, and inflammatory disorders. Our best evidence is that the group of chemicals in green tea with the strongest claim to being the source of these remarkable benefits is the polyphenols, especially the catechins, of which (–)-epigallocatechin-3-gallate (EGCG) deserves special attention. Black tea has been much less studied experimentally than green tea, but the available epidemiologic evidence does suggest that black tea may also be healthful, especially regarding heart disease. In view of the countless millions around the world who drink tea, this whole area should be a priority for study. In particular, if we are ever to develop the ultimate supplement—one that is inexpensive, safe, and effective against a range of diseases—then tea may well be a source of some of its ingredients.

Chapter 11 by Schmitz, Kelm, and Hammerstone, indicates that cocoa has a chemical profile with similarities to that of tea. Furthermore, some experimental studies have indicated that it has physiologic effects that may be beneficial in preventing CVD, including antioxidant protection and effects on thrombosis. Unfortunately, there is a dearth of epidemiologic evidence. As with tea, no clinical trials have been conducted with clinical endpoints, such as incidence of heart disease. Although the recognition that the cocoa bean is a plant food that has great potential for health will be welcomed by chocolate-eaters generally, we may ask whether chocolate products, as typically prepared, are a vehicle for sugar and undesirable fat, or is it the reverse, a little exposure to sugar and fat opens the door to the widespread probable benefits of chocolate? Here we may ask how much of the cocoa bean makes it into a hot cocoa or a chocolate bar? According to Hershey Foods Corporation (2), which provides the US Food and Drug Administration (FDA) Standards of Identity for chocolate and cocoa products, semi-sweet chocolate is "a combination of chocolate liquor with added cocoa butter and sugar. To qualify, the product must contain at least 35% chocolate liquor. Though available in bars, this chocolate is most often found in baking chips." Dark and milk chocolate contain much less of the cocoa bean as a percent of weight.

The reader is properly warned by Craig that the effects on the body of phytochemicals may be a double-edged sword. Herbal teas are plant extracts that concentrate active principles. Some have beneficial health effects, others are popularly believed to have some, and some have been clearly demonstrated as toxic. Because color and scent are important in the lives of the herbal plants themselves, one may suspect that these phytochemicals have high biologic activity. Color and scent relate closely to taste and flavor in herbs. Craig provides a list of definitive sources in support of these concepts that many readers will find useful. Much more work is needed to properly evaluate the risks and benefits from the large range of herbal teas that are available and are consumed by millions.

Fruit and vegetable juices are extracts of whole foods. They might contain less nutritional value than the whole food, but they also might extract just what is nutritionally important. The popularity of orange juice is discussed in Chapter 5 by McGill, Wilson, and Papanikolaou and makes it an important nutritional vehicle, even though it lacks, among other things, the fiber found in the pulp and the limonene found in the peel. However, the nutritional value of juices also depends on processing and storage conditions. Chapter 6 reveals that processing and storage of orange juice may cause much greater losses of vitamin C and phytochemicals than has been previously assumed. More vitamin C is lost in orange juice stored in cardboard compared to plastic. By contrast, a lower loss is seen from frozen concentrate. Chapter 8 by Hadley, Schwartz, and Clinton, discusses the manifold real and potential benefits of tomatoes, but expresses concern about the large amount of sodium in commercially available tomato juices. Wilson comments on the possible benefits of cranberry juice for urinary tract and other aspects of health. He also discusses the variation in the amount of cranberry juice in cranberry drinks and how this reduces the possible health benefits that the consumer receives from cranberry drinks.

These chapters certainly underline the nutritional value of tomato and fruit juice, while simultaneously expressing some notes of caution. Two further notes of caution should also be made. First, Stubbs and Whybrow draw attention to the potential for excess fruit juice to contribute to obesity. Second, recent findings on grapefruit juice, as discussed by Kane, illustrate that a seemingly healthy drink can have unsuspected harmful effects, in this case, an interaction with certain drugs. Grapefruit juice should be consumed with caution by people taking drugs.

The chapters on wine, fruit and vegetable drinks, cocoa, tea, coffee, herbal teas, and soy milk are replete with references to the intense biologic activity of many phytochemicals, with special interest in, but not limited to, polyphenolic compounds such as flavonoids. These chapters highlight a recent trend in our fundamental understanding of nutrition. The traditional view is reductionist, with a strong focus on an individual constituent; independence between constituents is generally assumed but not investigated. For example, McLaren (3), in a 1981 book about deficiency diseases, was strongly focused on individual macronutrients and micronutrients and on maintaining intake of those substances above deficiency levels. He stated that food and nutrients are not synonymous, that many cultural, psychologic, and analeptic aspects to eating are not directly concerned with nutrients, but these aspects must be considered to encourage consumption of foods to ensure adequate nutrient intake. He remarked that food contains other substances besides nutrients that may be toxic or beneficial.

The more recent view incorporates the concept of food synergy, namely that the health influence of food (and drink) is the additive or synergistic effect of its constituents (4,5). Research guided by the principle of food synergy starts with the health effects of foods and compares findings to those for food parts, groups of constituents, or an individual constituent. The food synergy concept has evolved partly because there are so many compounds in plant foods, many are not even identified, and important epidemiologic associations have been seen for the food groups, namely whole grains, fruits, vegetables, legumes, and nuts. The traditional reductionist view that nutrition is about a few important nutrients was fostered by important discoveries concerning deficiency diseases such as protein-energy malnutrition, scurvy, pellagra, and rickets. As important as it was and is to understand deficiency diseases, the traditional view is unable to explain the association between various foods and the long-term risk of chronic disease among generally healthy people. The excitement about phytochemicals and food synergy is palpable in many of the chapters. These substances, sometimes called nonnutritive or nutritionally unclassified, could perhaps be brought into the nutritional fold by being recognized as micronutrients.

The apparent power of the many biologically active constituents of plant foods makes it plausible that plant-derived beverages, such as coffee, tea, and chocolate, have great potential for improving health and well-being.

Beverages that are animal products are described in chapters concerning human milk, cow's milk, and probiotics. Friel has reviewed the nutritional properties of breast milk and convincingly shown its superiority over formula. Although this is hardly a new story, its strength has grown considerably in recent years because we have learned more about breast milk. Friel describes human milk as "alive" and "a tissue," because it fulfills the *Dorland's Medical Dictionary* definition of a tissue: "an aggregation of similarly specialized cells united in the performance of a single function." For example, human milk is not the same drink a few days postpartum as it is after 3 mo and is different again after a year. Milk is responsive to the infant; nutrient content can change within a single feeding. Milk provides numerous enzymes that help the infant to respond to immune challenges. It even contains amylase, seemingly anticipating the child's future diet, given that the role of amylase is to digest cereal starches that are not found in human milk itself. This function of human milk has not been replicated in infant formula.

Cow's milk undoubtedly follows that same pattern of functionality but is optimized for calves, not for baby humans. The cow's milk available commercially is most likely mature, designed by nature for older calves. Nevertheless, cow's milk presents a diverse mixture of nutritive ingredients. McBean, Miller, and Heaney furnish evidence that cow's milk is protective against several diseases, including hypertension, osteoporosis, colorectal and breast cancers, kidney stones, and obesity. However, as they note, questions have arisen about the safety of full-fat milk, because the saturated fatty acids in milk fat have been shown in rigorous feeding studies to increase serum cholesterol, which is integrally related to atherosclerosis, the fundamental pathologic process in CHD (6). However, McBean et al. believe that the medical link of saturated fat intake to hypercholesterolemia and of hypercholesterolemia to heart disease "has always been tenuous . . . milk fat itself has never been directly linked to heart disease" (6).

The question of the health effects of milk fat is far from closed. For example, a recent feeding study found that at equal fat content, Jarlsberg cheese was less cholesterol increasing than butter (7). From the food synergy perspective, it is interesting to note that fat-soluble milk constituents are lost when milk fat is removed from milk. Whether these fat-soluble constituents are important is unknown. Of particular note, conjugated linoleic acid (CLA), which is present in milk fat, has anticarcinogenic properties (8,9).

Another ongoing debate in the world of beverages concerns the relative merits of cow's milk and soy "milk." Woodside and Morton review the health effects of soy-milk beverages. There is suggestive evidence that soy may help prevent breast cancer and CHD. Soy milk obviates the problem of lactose intolerance associated with cow's milk. The chapters on cow's milk and soy milk illustrate that nutrition is most certainly not rocket science: the choice of evidence to be cited and its interpretation can never be truly objective. What one person or team may believe is the best possible argument based on the available evidence, others may find contentious. Most likely, this debate will only be settled by a long-term controlled trial.

The consumer is being presented with a wide choice of modified forms of milk as a result of innovative developments. Chapter 17 by Heller and Chapter 26 by Ohki, Nakamura, and Takano describe the use of probiotics in milk products. Heller points out that milk-containing probiotics have positive health effects. We can confidently expect to see the appearance of new beverages that are both healthy and pleasant tasting.

An interesting question is whether the various constituents of beverages interfere in the effectiveness of beverages to bring about hydration? Weinberg and Bealer suggest that caffeine intake does not lead to significant diuresis; this view is in agreement with a recent review *(10)* but not all the literature *(11,12)*. The question of the relative abilities of different beverages to cause body hydration has not been adequately investigated and should be integral to understanding how beverages affect us. It would be helpful if we had more information on the relative hydrating action of, for example, water, tea, coffee, decaffeinated coffee, fruit juice, and caffeine-containing soft drinks.

Two chapters address beverages specifically intended for improved rehydration. Like so much else in nutrition, things are seldom as simple as they at first appear. Many physiologic principles underlying the design and use of beverages intended for rehydration have been learned in recent years, and special beverages for this purpose have been developed. Chapter 21 by Ramakrishna, on oral hydration therapies, and Chapter 20 by Maughan, with a focus on sports beverages, provide valuable information on how the composition of beverages can be best formulated to maximize the rate of water uptake from the intestine. Ramakrishna notes that the composition of rehydration fluids should vary according to the specific conditions demanding their use. According to Maughan, dehydrated extreme athletes need sodium in their rehydration fluids. However, the issue of sodium and its role, particularly in diarrhea, may be confusing in healthy thirsty (but not dehydrated) people outside the clinical context. Thus, sodium content should probably be relatively low in beverages designed for more casual athletes and those engaging in more routine activities. Maughan also discusses the ideal composition of sports drinks for improving performance in sports.

Beverages also exist for nutritional support of the elderly, although Johnsen and Glassman argue strongly that food is a better choice than specially formulated beverages. Such special formulations may replace food meals and, in doing so, from the food synergy perspective, worsen the overall nutritional status by causing the elderly person to have a reduced consumption of, for example, fiber and many phytochemicals. In addition, they are costly. Nutrition support beverages should be confined to select patients.

Three chapters in the book are critical of soft drinks. Jacobson calls soft drinks "liquid candy" and argues that the current epidemic of obesity is partly due to drinking large quantities of sugar in a liquid medium, lacking other food constituents that might provide counterbalance. Stubbs and Whybrow present evidence and theories in support of Jacobson's position. For example, it is believed that the liquid format allows for less time in the stomach than does a solid format with the same amount of sugar. For this or other reasons, the ingested energy may not be sensed by the body and positive energy balance may occur, leading to weight gain. If soft drinks are consumed frequently for a period of years, obesity may be expected. The potential harm caused by soft drinks go far beyond obesity, and this, too, is explored by Jacobson, with particular reference to children and teens. Every soft drink consumed is a missed opportunity to consume energy accompanied by a nutritious matrix of food constituents. Thus, the soft-drink consumer misses all the benefits discussed in the chapters on plant-derived beverages and milk.

2. NUTRITION OF BEVERAGES AND COMPETITIVE ADVANTAGE

Nutritional advantages of plant-based beverages and related foods are made clear in most of the chapters of this book. Most authors provide extensive evidence on the probable nutritional benefit of many phytochemicals, known and unknown, provided in a food matrix. The food matrix, providing a balance of biologically active constituents in a mix of low doses, is probably important; the potential danger of overreliance on single nutrients in supplement form was made clear by the failure of clinical trials of β-carotene and of other supplements to show benefit against cancer and heart disease *(13)*. Craig's discussion of herbal teas points to a clear distinction between food and pharmaceuticals: consumables with high doses of individual phytochemicals should probably be viewed as drugs, whereas those providing more moderate doses of individual phytochemicals in a natural plant matrix should be considered foods. Craig points out a tendency in the public and industry to use herbal drinks as medications, generally unregulated and with poor guidance in their use for the lay public. Caution is clearly warranted, because herbs may cause side effects, they may be contaminated with unlisted and possibly toxic ingredients, and the content of active ingredients may vary. Although not a plant-based beverage, the remarkable and responsive composition of human milk illustrates a similar point about variation in naturally occurring foods and the beverages that they often become.

In contrast to these naturally occurring foods, all existing infant formulas, meal replacement beverages, and, particularly, the extremely popular soft drinks are examples of foods on the market that serve limited nutritional purposes and may actually cause nutri- tional harm. Soft drinks are strongly suspected of contributing to obesity, and, because they supply energy but with little or no micronutrients, their consumption reduces the overall nutrient quality of the diet. Both infant formulas and meal replacement beverages, used to excess, may also worsen the overall nutrient profile.

Jacobson (Chapter 24), as well as Balay-Karperien, Temple, and Nestle (Chapter 25), are critical of the soft-drink industry. Many chapters in this book are political, because they espouse a view of how foods (beverages) should or should not be marketed. Articles from those affiliated with for-profit companies downplay potential adverse health effects, whereas those from unaffiliated health advocates revile the big business approach that opens the door to sales as the first priority. Both sides have points. Certainly, pouring rights (in which a soft-drink company contracts with a school district for the exclusive right to place its product in schools) can generate huge profits for the large soft-drink companies. The opportunity for marketing through large donations to school districts arises because local communities have often created funding shortfalls by cutting school budgets. Thus, although the soft-drink companies are providing a service with their multimillion-dollar contributions, the service and its consequences for the future health of the school children is provided as a sort of taxation without representation. The soft-drink company acts as the ultimate arbiter of which schools should get what. Although soft-drink companies generally provide only a minority of school districts funds, the funds are flexible. Hence, the school districts work to maximize that funding, while taking as a given status of state and local funding. This argument is ultimately political, because it concerns the basic system by which the community distributes goods and services to itself.

The final chapters of the book present information on laws and practice regarding labels and health claims. Like the chapters on soft drinks, these chapters are about politics and about marketing products. Compared with Japan, the United States is much more restrictive as to the permitted health claims. Krasny (Chapter 27) describes the American system for allowing health claims, whereas Ohki and colleagues (Chapter 26) describe the corresponding system in Japan. With a relatively restrictive system, Americans see comparatively few health claims on foods, whereas Ohki et al. describe a wide and proliferating variety of foods, more than half presented as beverages, that bear health claims. The various industrial groups supplying food operate in a competitive system and must strive to maximize profit. It is, therefore, clear that industry will take advantage of all marketing strategies available to it; a less restrictive health-claim system will result in more food industry interest in and statements about health benefits of foods.

A similar issue concerns how newly discovered scientific information is communicated and/or marketed to consumers. Journalists seemingly take all scientific statements as new truths, not conveying to the consumer that the latest scientific "discovery" may really be misleading (as it is one small part of a complex story) or may even be incorrect. Following their competitive mandate, companies also take advantage of the authority of scientists and the poor understanding of the average consumer. Thus, commercialism may be distorted when suggestive findings from epidemiologic and experimental studies are turned into supplements or added to foods, which then acquire the attractive label "functional." Although Wilson correctly points out that cranberry juice is a food with a specific function (prevention of formation of bacterial p-fimbriae) above and beyond, for example, the energy it provides, all foods are actually functional. The calcium now added to orange juice by many companies in one interpretation of our nutrition knowledge makes the orange juice functional, but in another interpretation merely adds a calcium supplement to a food that already has great functionality. The term "functional food" is in this sense a misnomer used for commercial advantage.

Green tea provides another example of possibly exaggerated commercial uses of scientific findings. Afaq and colleagues provide some evidence that green tea may assist with weight control. This justifies further investigation but can scarcely be described as a proven therapy. Yet, health food stores are already selling supplements containing green tea extracts as a quick fix for overweight. There are scores of other such examples. The purveyors of such supplements typically use evidence the way a person who is drunk uses a lamppost: more for support than illumination. Anecdotal evidence, the least reliable form of scientific research, is commonly used to "prove" how the supplement delivers "miracle" results.

Of course, in theory, consumers can be informed and individuals can make healthier choices. Certainly, there are individuals who do so. Why, then, are certain apparently less healthful foods so popular? Why don't academic or government nutritionists tell people unequivocally, for example, that soft drinks cause obesity, and why don't people take the advice and greatly reduce their consumption of these drinks? The answer to this question is not known. There are numerous elegant theories about what regulates human behavior and how to change it *(14,15)*. Nevertheless, interventions focused on either individuals or communities have had limited success *(16,17)*. In a strong sense, industry can only supply those foods that consumers will purchase. It is not hard to find examples of new products, e.g., breakfast cereals with lower salt, that have failed because the public did not accept them.

One wonders about what balance of regulation and cooperation, coupled with information from the research into the many aspects of the nutrition of beverages and solid foods presented in this book, might produce both a healthy economy and a healthy consumer base? The Model of Culture Bounded Change states that the four relevant societal sectors are linked to each other through their culture. Government, academia, industry, and consumers play different roles in the culture, but none can ever be too far out of step with the others. Consumers cannot eat food that is not available. Government cannot regulate so strongly that industry is not profitable. Industry cannot sell foods that people will not buy. If the information identified by academics about the nutrition of beverages is to be acted on for the benefit of the public health, government must play a role in regulation, akin to steering a ship, industry must play a role in supplying the healthy food. Consumers will vote with their pocketbooks for or against the actions taken. Although, as mentioned in connection with individually based interventions, consumers do not change quickly, they do change. In 1970, the typical American diet contained approx 40% of energy from fat; this figure now lies between 30% and 35%. What the Model of Culture Bounded Change suggests is that the various sectors must talk to each other and take planned actions, bearing in mind both profit and nutrition, to shift the culture to a more desirable nutritional status, especially with respect to their beverages choices.

3. CONCLUSION

The chapters in this book paint a picture of the remarkable diversity of the beverages now available. As with solid food, they run the spectrum from the nutritious, safe, and economic through to the unhealthy and overpriced. In the world of beverages, we see series of multifaceted clashes. We see a clash between good science telling us what is most healthy vs commercial hype telling us what we should drink for enjoyment. We see a clash because of different levels of credibility of the supporting scientific evidence used to form our opinions. There is also a clash between the accurate presentation of scientific information vs information that is distorted by journalists (usually resulting from a poor understanding of science) or by commercial interests (usually due to both scientific ignorance but, more importantly, due to greed for a quick dollar). Finally, there is a clash between government policies aimed at improving the public health and those focused only on improving economic issues. Anyone looking for simple answers to the relative health value of different beverages and how to achieve the ideal balance between health, personal freedom, and responsible economics will be disappointed.

One of our main aims in this book, and especially in this chapter, has been to identify areas that need further research. We have also discussed in this chapter the relative merits of different research strategies. Hopefully, this will encourage research into those questions that require investigation.

In conclusion, we can, perhaps, be forgiven for being pessimistically optimistic. The tremendous progress in research related to the health effects of beverages, combined with technological developments, leads one to expect that new beverages will steadily appear that combine the best of the present with new discoveries soon to be made.

REFERENCES

1. De Roos B, Van Tol A, Urgert R, et al. Consumption of French-press coffee raises cholesteryl ester transfer protein activity levels before LDL cholesterol in normolipidaemic subjects. J Intern Med 2000; 248:211–216.
2. Hershey Foods Corporation. Retrieved November 10, 2003, from http://www.hersheys.com/nutrition_consumer/identity_standards.shtml.
3. McLaren DS. A colour atlas of nutritional disorders. Wolfe Medical Publications, London, UK, 1981.
4. Messina M, Lampe JW, Birt DF, et al. Reductionism and the narrowing nutrition perspective: time for reevaluation and emphasis on food synergy. J Am Diet Assoc 2001;101:1416–1419.
5. Jacobs DR, Steffen LM. Nutrients, foods and dietary patterns as exposures in research: a framework for food synergy. Am J Clin Nutr, in press.
6. Steinmetz KA, Childs MT, Stimson C, et al. Effect of consumption of whole milk and skim milk on blood lipid profiles in healthy men. Am J Clin Nutr 1994;59:612–618.
7. Bong AS, Müller H, Lindbäck A, Pedersen JI. Effects of cheese and butter on serum lipid profile. Presented at the 26th International Dairy Federation World Dairy Congress, Paris, September 24–27, 2002.
8. Ha YL, Storkson J, Pariza MW. Inhibition of benzo(a)pyrene-induced mouse forestomach neoplasia by conjugated dienoic derivatives of linoleic acid. Cancer Res 1990;50:1097–2101.
9. Ip C, Scimeca JA, Thompson H. Effect of timing and duration of dietary conjugated linoleic acid on mammary cancer prevention. Nutr Cancer 1995;24:241–247.
10. Armstrong LE. Caffeine, body fluid-electrolyte balance, and exercise performance. Int J Sport Nutr Exerc Metab 2002;12:189–206.
11. Nussberger J, Mooser V, Maridor G, Juillerat L, Waeber B, Brunner HR. Caffeine-induced diuresis and atrial natriuretic peptides. J Cardiovasc Pharmacol 1990;15:685–691.
12. Neuhauser-Berthold, Beine S, Verwied SC, Luhrmann PM. Coffee consumption and total body water homeostasis as measured by fluid balance and bioelectrical impedance analysis. Ann Nutr Metab 1997; 41:29–36.
13. Omenn GS, Goodman GE, Thornquist MD, et al. Effects of a combination of beta carotene and vitamin A on lung cancer and cardiovascular disease. N Engl J Med 1996;334:1150–1155.
14. Lytle LA, Perry CL. Applying research and theory in program planning an example from a nutrition education intervention. Health Prom Pract 2001;2:68–80.
15. Bandura A. Social foundations of thought & action. A social cognitive theory. Prentice-Hall, Englewood Cliffs, NJ, 1986.
16. Luepker R, Perry CL, McKinlay SM, et al. Outcomes of a field trial to improve children's dietary patterns and physical activity. JAMA 1996;275:768–776.
17. Baranowski T, Lin LS, Wetter DW, Resnicow K, Hearn MD. Theory as mediating variables: why aren't community interventions working as desired? Ann Epidemiol 1997;7:S89–S95.

INDEX

About the Editors

Dr. Ted Wilson received his PhD from Iowa State University; he then worked for several years in the Departments of Biology and Cardiac Rehabilitation at the University of Wisconsin–La Crosse, and currently works in the Department of Biology at Winona State University in Winona, Minnesota. Dr. Wilson has taught courses in Nutrition, Physiology, and Cell Biology. His research examines the impact of dietary components on human nutrition and physiology, cancer, cardiovascular disease, and cardiac rehabilitation. Dr. Wilson has been interested in the validation of food health claims, with regard to the promotion of measurable physiological effects. He has also examined dietary influences on platelet aggregation, lipoprotein oxidation, arterial vasodilation, mechanisms for urinary tract infection, and plant phenolic analysis. Specific dietary components and supplements that he has studied include cranberry juice, apple juice, grape juice, wine, resveratrol, creatine phosphate, soy phytoestrogens, and tomatoes. Presently, Dr. Wilson conducts a USDA-sponsored study that investigates how cranberry juice consumption affects cardiovascular disease risk factors. *Beverages in Nutrition and Health* is the second book he has coedited with Norman Temple, the previous book is entitled *Nutritional Health: Strategies for Disease Prevention* (Humana Press, 2001).

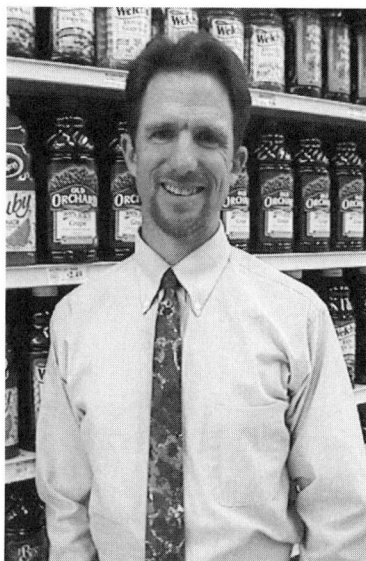

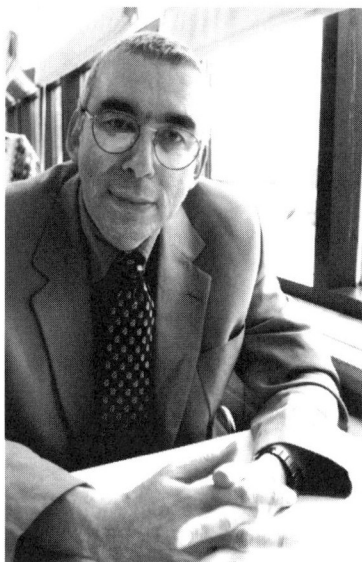

Dr. Norman J. Temple teaches nutrition at Athabasca University in Alberta, Canada, and develops distance education courses in nutrition and health. Dr. Temple's specialty is nutrition in relation to health, particularly the influence of dietary factors on heart disease and cancer. *Beverage Impacts on Health and Nutrition* is his sixth book on diet, health, and disease. He is coeditor with Denis Burkitt of *Western Diseases: Their Dietary Prevention and Reversibility* (Humana Press, 1994), which continued and extended Burkitt's pioneering work on the role of dietary fiber in Western diseases. He coedited with Dr. Ted Wilson the first edition of *Nutritional Health: Strategies for Disease Prevention* (Humana Press, 2001).

About the Series Editor

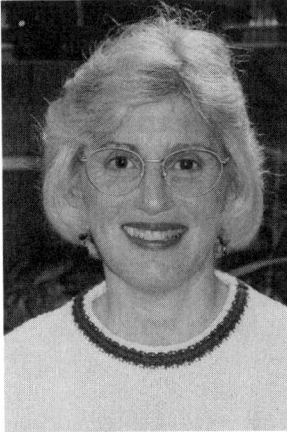

Dr. Adrianne Bendich is Clinical Director of Calcium Research at GlaxoSmithKline Consumer Healthcare, where she is responsible for leading the innovation and medical programs in support of TUMS and Os-Cal. Dr. Bendich has primary responsibility for the direction of GSK's support for the Women's Health Initiative intervention study. Prior to joining GlaxoSmithKline, Dr. Bendich was at Roche Vitamins Inc., and was involved with the groundbreaking clinical studies proving that folic acid-containing multivitamins significantly reduce major classes of birth defects. Dr. Bendich has co-authored more than 100 major clinical research studies in the area of preventive nutrition. Dr. Bendich is recognized as a leading authority on antioxidants, nutrition, immunity, and pregnancy outcomes, vitamin safety, and the cost-effectiveness of vitamin/mineral supplementation.

Dr. Bendich is the editor of nine books, including *Preventive Nutrition: The Comprehensive Guide for Health Professionals,* and is Series Editor of *Nutrition and Health* for Humana Press. She also serves as Associate Editor for *Nutrition: The International Journal of Applied and Basic Nutritional Sciences,* and Dr. Bendich is on the Editorial Board of the *Journal of Women's Health and Gender-Based Medicine,* as well as a member of the Board of Directors of the American College of Nutrition.

Dr. Bendich was the recipient of the Roche Research Award, a *Tribute to Women and Industry* Awardee, and a recipient of the Burroughs Wellcome Visiting Professorship in Basic Medical Sciences, 2000–2001. Dr. Bendich holds academic appointments as Adjunct Professor in the Department of Preventive Medicine and Community Health at UMDNJ, Institute of Nutrition, Columbia University P&S, and Adjunct Research Professor, Rutgers University, Newark Campus. She is listed in Who's Who in American Women.

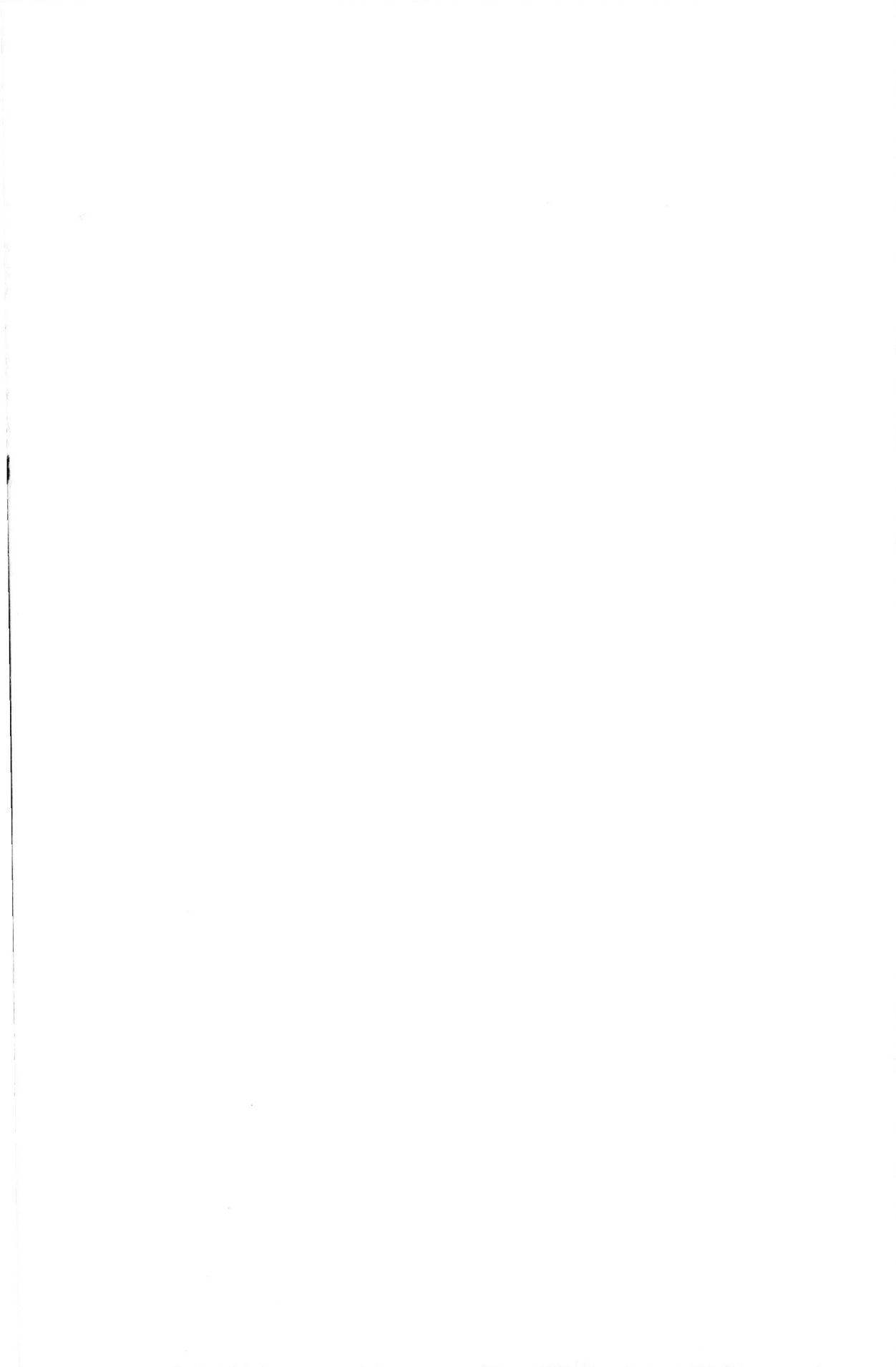

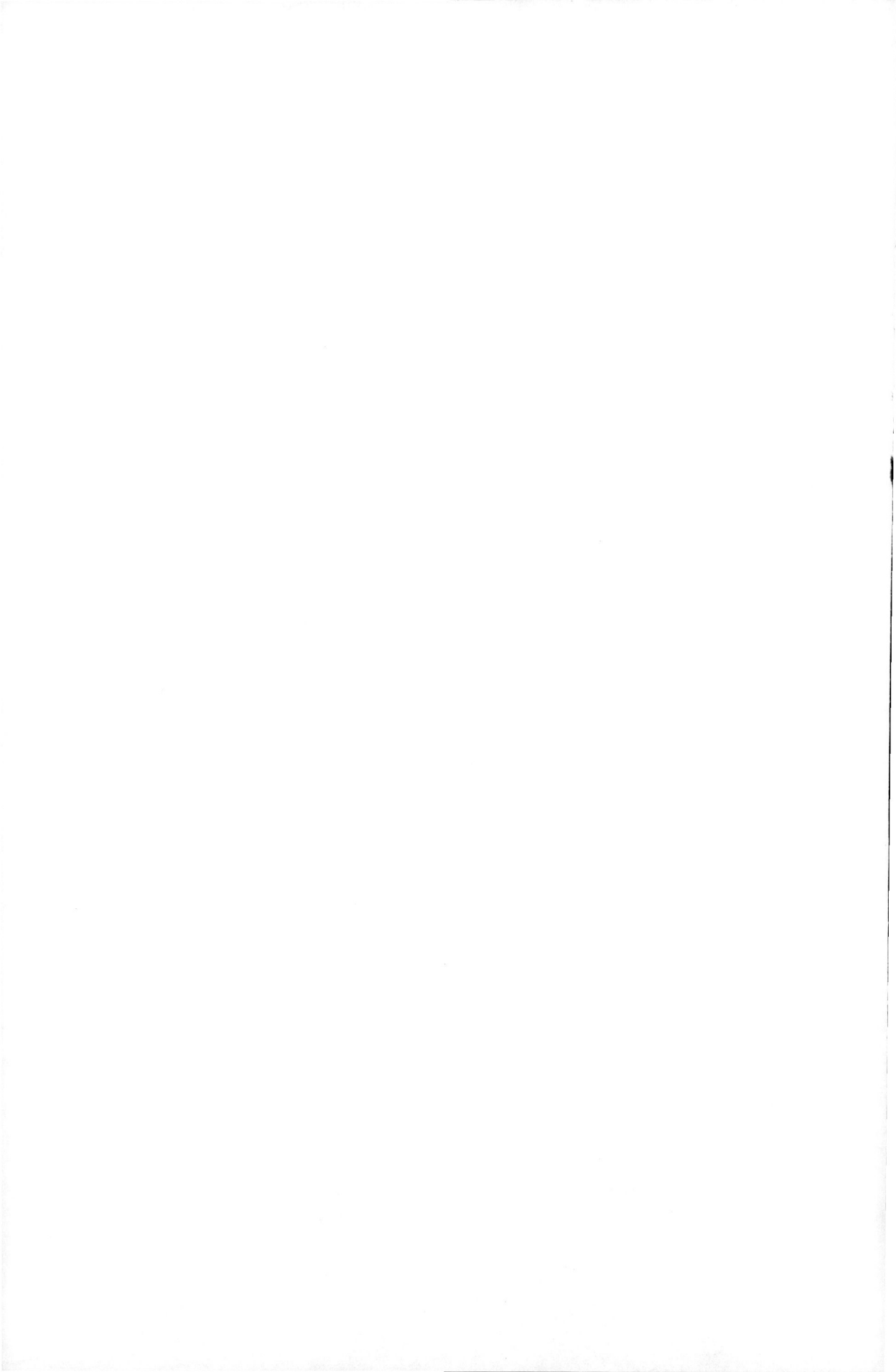

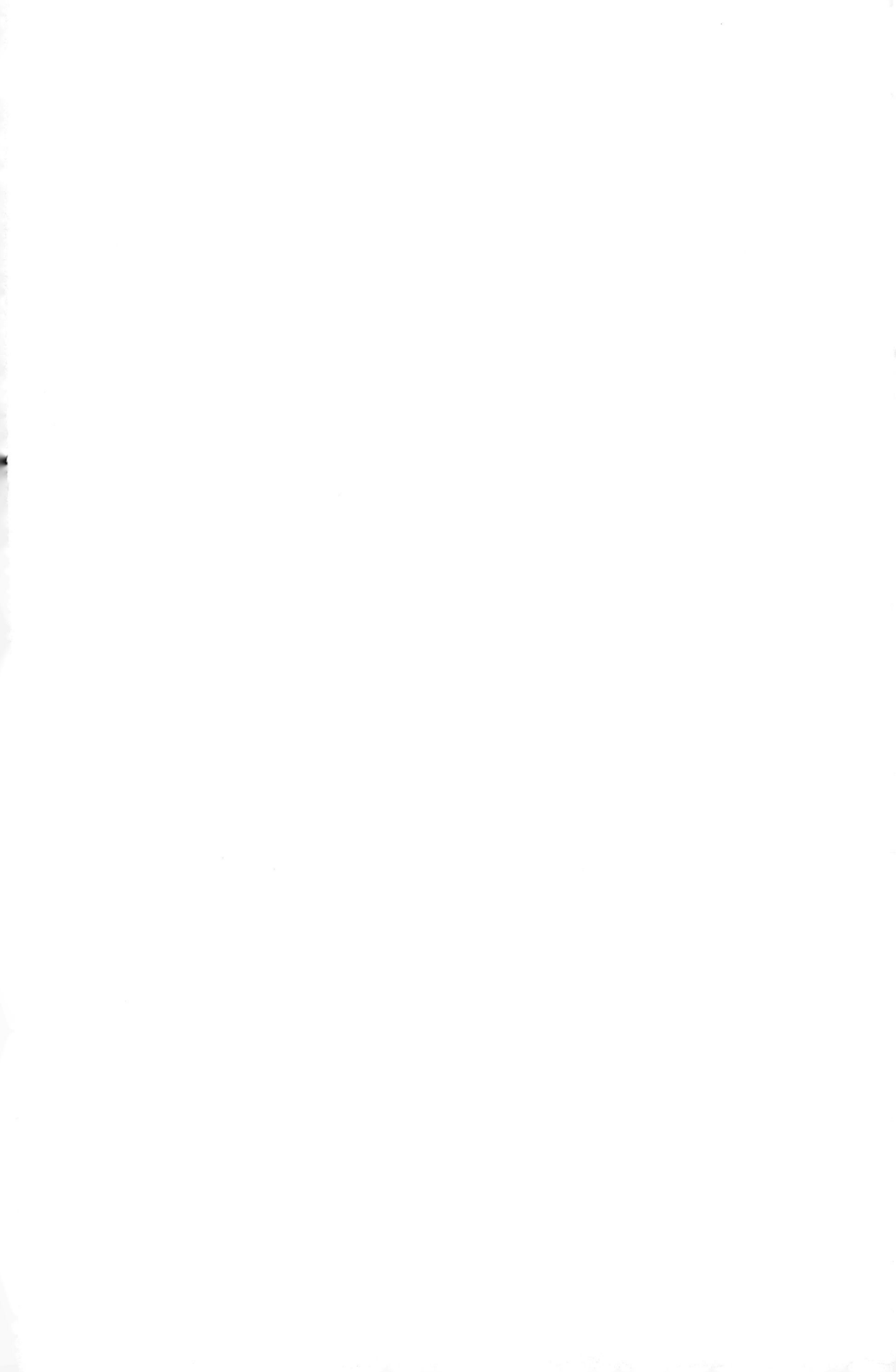

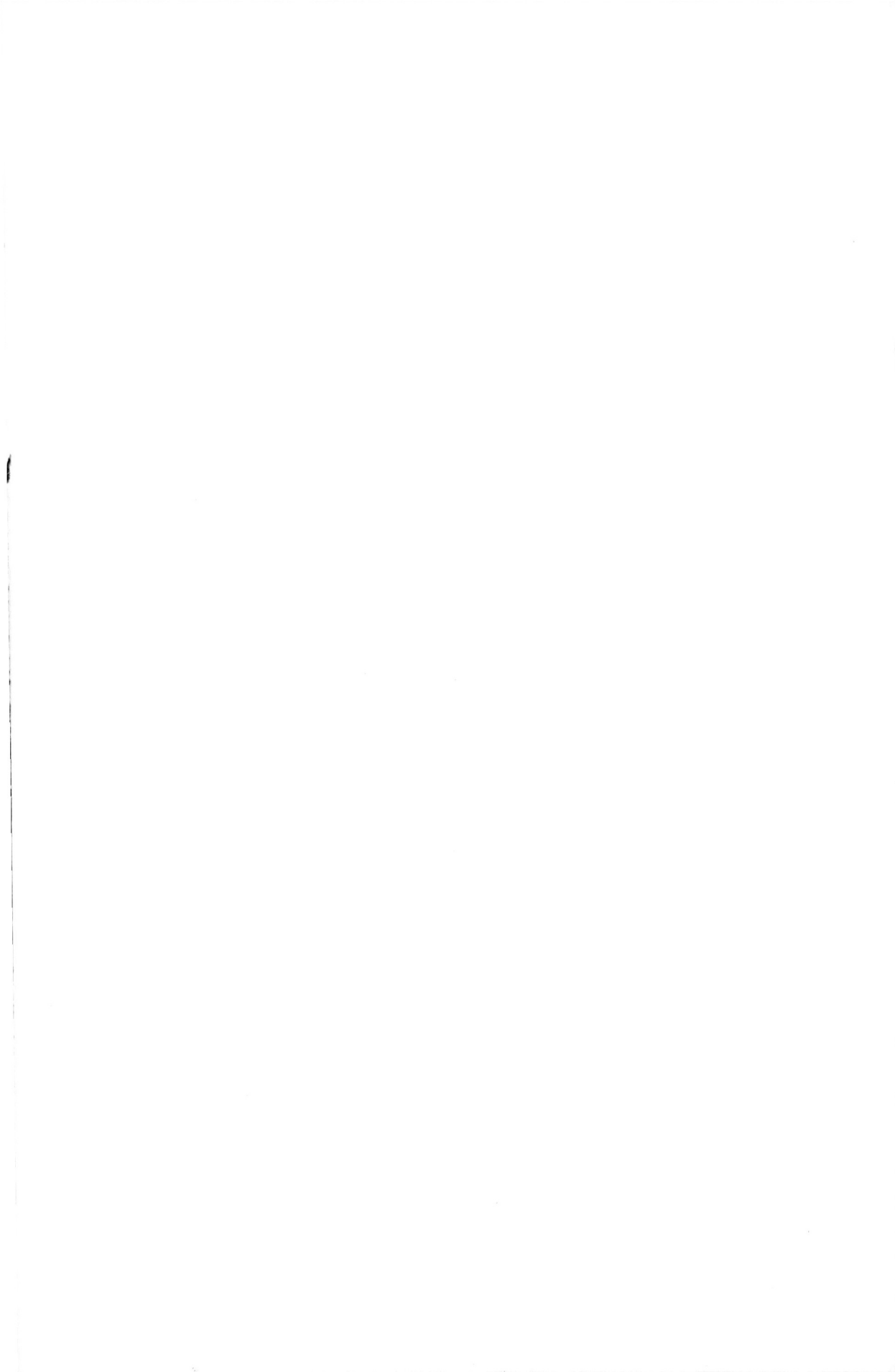